D1751852

Peripheral Nerve Lesions

Edited by M. Samii

With 225 Figures

Springer-Verlag
Berlin Heidelberg New York
London Paris Tokyo
Hong Kong Barcelona

Univ. Prof. Dr. med. M. Samii
Medical School Hanover
Director of Neurosurgical Clinic
City of Hanover
Nordstadt Hospital
Haltenhoffstraße 41
3000 Hannover 1, FRG

ISBN 3-540-52432-0 Springer-Verlag Berlin Heidelberg New York
ISBN 0-387-52432-0 Springer-Verlag New York Berlin Heidelberg

Peripheral nerve lesions / edited by M. Samii. p. cm. Includes index. ISBN 3-540-52432-0 (alk. paper). – ISBN 0-387-52432-0 (alk. paper) 1. Nerves, Peripheral – Wounds and injuries. 2. Nerves, Peripheral – Regeneration. I. Samii, Madjid. [DNLM: 1. Evoked Potentials, Somatosensory. 2. Nerve Regeneration – physiology. 3. Peripheral Nerve Diseases – diagnosis. 4. Peripheral Nerve Diseases – therapy. 5. Peripheral Nerves – injuries. WL 500 P44458] RD 595.P47 1990 617.4'83044 – dc20 DNLM/DLC for Library of Congress

This work is subject to copyright. All rights are reserved, whether the whole or part of the material is concerned, specifically the rights of translation, reprinting, reuse of illustrations, recitation, broadcasting, reproduction on microfilms or in other ways, and storage in data banks. Duplication of this publication or parts thereof is only permitted under the provisions of the German Copyright Law of September 9, 1965, in its current version, and a copyright fee must always be paid. Violations fall under the prosecution act of the German Copyright Law.

© Springer-Verlag Berlin Heidelberg 1990
Printed in Germany

The use of registered names, trademarks, etc. in this publication does not imply, even in the absence of specific statement, that such names are exempt from the relevant protective laws and regulations and therefore free for general use.

Product liability: The publishers can give no guarantee for information about drug dosage and application thereof contained in this book. In every individual case the respective user must check its accuracy by consulting other pharmaceutical literature.

Typesetting: Fotosatz-Service Köhler, D-8700 Würzburg
2114/3130-543210 – Printed on acid-free paper

Preface

The introduction of the operating microscope as a surgical tool revolutionized the treatment of peripheral nerve lesions. A new era thus began in the early 1960s, which led to a substantial improvement in the management of nerve lesions.

The results of nerve grafting techniques have demonstrated that, independent of the length of the defect, lesions can be successfully bridged. The free tissue transplants with microvascular anastomosis have also opened new, rewarding possibilities for peripheral nerve reconstruction procedures, facilitating the achievement not only of satisfactory anatomical but also of satisfactory functional results.

In order to evaluate the state of the art and reflect retrospectively on 25 years of microneurosurgical treatment of peripheral nerves, numerous outstanding scientists and clinicosurgical physicians were invited to Hanover in order to exchange their viewpoints and experiences. An active und fruitful discussion resulted which dealt with the many aspects of anatomy, pathology, clinical and neurophysiology, diagnosis, and with the surgery and physiotherapy which constitute modern-day peripheral nerve lesion treatment. The exciting ongoing experimental and clinical activities have led us to support the wish and idea to publish the scientific exchange which took place during the Hanover symposium.

I truly believe that the articles presented in this book cover so many interesting subjects concerned with peripheral nerve lesions that the book will serve the interested and dedicated physician involved with such cases as a reference work for the basics and also provide him with the therapeutic guidelines to assist him in his daily work.

My special gratitude and respect goes to the guest of honour, Sir Sydney Sunderland, a true pioneer, past and present. Also I am indebted to the authors and participants. The interdisciplinary exchange stimulates us to pursue this fascinating discipline further.

Zeiss, pioneers in the development of the operating microscope, supported our idea and sponsored our endeavours in every way. Without their assistance the symposium and this volume would not have been possible. Therefore I would like to thank the directors and their staff for all their work and commitment. Special mention must also go to Aesculap Werke AG and Contraves AG.

My gratitude is also due to Springer-Verlag and its staff for their excellent work and cooperation, as well as to Professor Löhr, Hamburg, for his work on the subject index. Among my staff, my grateful recognition goes to Dr. W. Bini for the organization of the symposium, as well as to Mrs. R. Nitsche and Dr. M. Ammirati for the revision of the manuscripts. Special acknowledgement is for Mrs. R. Nitsche for proof reading and skillfully bringing this volume to print, thereby coping with the immense amount of detailed work involved.

Hanover   Madjid Samii

Contents

Cellular Biology of the Experimental Peripheral Nerve Lesion.
G. W. Kreutzberg and M. B. Graeber (With 3 Figures) . . . 1

Muscle Response to Changes in Innervation. W. A. Nix 7

The Response of Sensory Ganglia and Spinal Cord to Injury.
H. Aldskogius. 11

Pathomorphology of Regenerating Peripheral Nerves.
J. M. Schröder (With 2 Figures) 22

Role of Neurotrophic Factors in Peripheral Nerve
Regeneration. D. Lindholm and H. Thoenen 29

Electrophysiological Changes Due to Motor Nerve Injury.
H. C. Hopf (With 6 Figures) 32

Somatosensory Regeneration Following Peripheral Nerve
Injury. A. Struppler and G. Ochs (With 3 Figures) 42

The Contribution of Both the Peripheral and Central Nervous
Systems to the Pain that Follows Peripheral Nerve Injury.
C. J. Woolf 51

Clinical Symptoms, Electrophysiological and Morphological
Findings in Traumatic Lesions of the Ischiadic Nerve in
Domestic Fowl. H.-E. Nau, M. Blank, M. A. Konerding,
P. Wenzel, and R. Werner (With 5 Figures) 58

Regeneration of Peripheral Nerves by Means of Muscle and
Nerve Transplants. M. Sparmann, G. Friedebold, and
T. Meyer (With 2 Figures) 66

Motor Recovery After Delayed Nerve Suture. H.-P. Richter . 70

Stimulation of Nerve Axon Outgrowth by Means of Fibrin
Adhesive with Added Melanotropic Neuropeptide.
O. Osgaard and N. H. Diemer 73

Nerve Regeneration in the Centrocentral Anastomosis.
J. M. González-Darder, J. Barberá, J. L. Gil-Salú,
and F. Garcia-Vázquez (With 3 Figures) 75

Biochemical Manipulation of the Microenvironment
in Experimental Nerve Regeneration Chambers.
H. Müller (With 2 Figures)........................ 81

Experimental Repair of Peripheral Nerve Injury Using Venous
Autograft. A. Leventis, A. Maillis, E. Singounas, P. Davaki,
and N. Karandreas (With 4 Figures) 88

Experimental Nerve Regeneration Under a Vein Graft in the
Rat. J. Godard, G. Coulon (†), G. Monnier, D. Rouillon,
G. Jacquet, and R. Steimle (With 6 Figures) 96

Rejection of Allogenic Nerve Grafts in a Genetic Model of the
Rat. E. Schaller, P. Mailänder, M. Becker, G. F. Walter,
and A. Berger (With 7 Figures) 104

Spinal Nerve Lesion and its Regeneration with and without
Nerve Suture: An Experimental Study in Rats. T. Wallenfang,
J. Bohl, J. P. Jantzen, and B. Wallesch (With 4 Figures)... 113

Limitation of Neuroma Formation by Fat Tissue. J. Weis
and J. M. Schröder (With 6 Figures) 124

The Blood-Nerve Barrier in Peripheral Nerve Injury,
Repair, and Regeneration. J. R. Bain, A. R. Hudson,
S. E. Mackinnon, F. Gentili, and D. Hunter (With 6 Figures) 130

Revascularization of Free Autologous Nerve Grafts.
G. Penkert and M. Samii (With 10 Figures) 143

Vascularization of the Peripheral Nerve After Epineural
Suture. M. Lehmann, M. A. Konerding, and M. Blank
(With 5 Figures) 149

Vascularization of the Peripheral Nerve in Laboratory Animals.
M. A. Konerding, M. Lehmann, and M. Blank
(With 9 Figures) 154

Primate Peripheral Nerve Anastomosis with CO_2 Laser.
J. E. Bailes, D. G. Kline, I. Ciric, A. R. Hudson, and
J. W. Cozzens 161

Laser-Assisted Sciatic Nerve Anastomoses and Transplants.
F. Ulrich, K. H. Reiners, and T. Sander (With 3 Figures) .. 165

Some Ultrastructural Aspects of Regeneration in 1.32 µm
Nd:YAG Laser-Assisted Peripheral Nerve Transplantation.
R. Schober, F. Ulrich, and T. Sander (With 6 Figures) ... 169

Experimental Peripheral Nerve Crush Lesion. I. Posttraumatic
Metabolic Responses of Spinal Motoneurons Over Time.
A. C. Nacimiento and C. Marx (With 5 Figures)....... 175

Experimental Peripheral Nerve Crush Lesion. II. Short-Term
Reinnervation Changes in Fast Muscle Fibers. G. Adler and
A. C. Nacimiento (With 6 Figures) 189

Structural Changes of the Peripheral Nerve After Pressure
Lesions in the Domestic Fowl. M. Blank, M. A. Konerding,
H.-E. Nau, and P. Wenzel (With 3 Figures) 197

Computed Tomography in Peripheral Nerve Pathology.
A. Alexandre, F. Di Paola, F. Di Toma, P. Cisotto,
D. Billeci, and A. Carteri 201

Initial Experiences with MRI in the Diagnosis of Peripheral
Nerve Lesions. W. E. Braunsdorf, H. D. Kuhlendahl,
F. Koschorek, and H.-P. Jensen (With 2 Figures) 204

Modern Imaging Procedures in Peripheral Nerve Lesions.
D. Stolke, U. Kunz, and V. Seifert (With 8 Figures) 206

Success of Sensory Evoked Potentials in Patients with Median
Compression Syndrome and Additional Neuropathy.
M. Conzen, R. Kramer, and F. Oppel (With 1 Figure) ... 212

Intraoperative Analysis of the Function of Peripheral Nerves
with Sensory Evoked Potentials. R. Stober 216

Functional Changes of Single Motor Units After Nerve Suture.
R. Dengler and R. B. Stein (With 4 Figures) 219

Outcome of Clinical Function in Relation to Motor, Sensory
Nerve Conduction, Somatosensory Evoked Potentials, and
EMG After Suture of Median and Ulnar Nerves.
W. Tackmann (With 2 Figures) 224

Intraoperative Somatosensory Evoked Potential Diagnoses in
Brachial Plexus Lesions. P. Mailänder, E. Schaller,
M. Möckel, A. Berger, and G. F. Walter (With 12 Figures) . 227

Postoperative Changes in Nerve Conduction Times After
Neurolysis of the Distal Median Nerve. S. A. Rath,
H. J. Klein, A. Kühn, and V. Wippermann (With 4 Figures) 233

Outcome of Traumatic Peripheral Neuromas After
Microsurgical Procedure. S. Bel and B. L. Bauer 239

Femoral Nerve Lesion in Surgery of the Hip. G. Bindl
(With 5 Figures) 243

Isolated Traumatic Nerve Lesions of the Extensor Pollicis
Longus and Brevis Muscles. C. Tizian and L. Döbler
(With 2 Figures) 248

Peripheral Nerve Involvement in Recklinghausen's Disease.
M. Tatagiba, A. Kleider, W. Bini, A. Sepehrnia,
J. Brennecke, G. Penkert, and M. Samii (With 4 Figures) . . 251

Clinical Aspects of Entrapment Neuropathies of Peripheral
Nerves. M. Mumenthaler. 258

Evaluation of the Various Routine Neurophysiological
Parameters in Diagnosis of Carpal Tunnel Syndrome.
L. Rabow and H. Holmgren 270

Relationships Between Preoperative Symptoms,
Electrophysiological and Intraoperative Findings,
and the Outcome in Patients with Carpal Tunnel
Syndrome. H.-E. Nau and B. Lange 273

Morphological and Pathogenetic Considerations in
Entrapment Syndromes. L. Gerhard, V. Reinhardt,
E. Koob, and H.-E. Nau (With 6 Figures) 278

Pitfalls in Surgery for Carpal Tunnel Syndrome.
H.-P. Richter and G. Antoniadis 288

Carpal Tunnel Syndrome: A New Surgical Approach.
P. Roccella, R. Ghadirpour, A. Migliore, and G. Trapella . 292

Anatomical Anomalies Causing Ulnar Neuropathy.
H. Kolenda, M. Schade, and E. Markakis (With 3 Figures) . 295

Neurolysis in Ulnar Nerve Entrapment Syndromes.
M. Samii (With 4 Figures) 298

Thoracic-Outlet Syndrome: Limitations of the
Neurophysiological Diagnosis. G. Krämer and A. Kleider . 302

Diagnosis and Surgical Management of the Thoracic-Outlet
Syndrome. A. Aghchi and J. Menzel (With 11 Figures) . . . 307

Retroperitoneal Hematoma with Femoral Neuralgia.
S. C. Tindall (With 1 Figure). 315

Timing Surgery in Nerve Lesions. G. Brunelli and
L. Monini (With 5 Figures) 317

Neurolysis. M. Samii 323

Free Vascularized Nerve Grafts. A. Berger, P. Mailänder,
and E. Schaller (With 9 Figures). 326

Caution in the Evaluation of Results of Peripheral Nerve
Surgery. D. G. Kline 335

Microsurgical Repair of Peripheral Nerve Lesions: A Study
of 150 Injuries of the Median and Ulnar Nerves.
J. Michon (†), P. Amend, and M. Merle (With 2 Figures) . . 343

Brachial Plexus Lesions

Operative Experience with Tumors of the Brachial Plexus.
    D. G. Kline, M. Lusk, and C. Garcia (With 4 Figures) . . . 359

Neurotization of the Avulsed Brachial Plexus. G. Brunelli,
    L. Monini, and F. Brunelli (With 3 Figures) 367

Special Considerations Regarding the Treatment of Brachial
    Plexus Lesions. M. Samii (With 9 Figures) 372

Schwannomas of the Brachial Plexus. A. Alexandre,
    P. Cisotto, D. Billeci, S. Cusumano, F. Di Paola, and
    A. Carteri (With 2 Figures) 386

Results of Brachial Plexus Surgery. G. Brunelli, L. Monini,
    and F. Brunelli 391

Selection of Brachial Plexus Cases for Operation –
    Based on Results. D. G. Kline (With 4 Figures) 396

Free Greater Omentum Transfer After Neurolysis for Actinic
    (X-Ray) Lesions of the Brachial Plexus. G. Brunelli,
    L. Monini, and F. Brunelli (With 4 Figures) 411

Dorsal Root Entry Zone Lesions for the Treatment of Post-
    Brachial Plexus Avulsion Injury Pain. A. H. Friedman,
    B. S. Nashold, and J. Carter (With 2 Figures) 416

Dorsal Root Entry Zone Coagulation for Control of
    Intractable Pain Due to Brachial Plexus Injury. M. Samii,
    E. Kohmura, H. Khalil, and C. Matthies (With 1 Figure) . . 422

Postoperative Treatment in Nerve Lesions. G. Brunelli and
    F. Brunelli (With 1 Figure). 427

Results of Brachial Plexus Surgery: Secondary Reconstruction.
    U. Laumann (With 4 Figures) 430

Subject Index 439

List of Contributors

Adler, G.: Neurosurgical Research Laboratory, Saarland University School of Medicine, 6650 Homburg/Saar, FRG
Aghchi, A.: Neurochirurgische Klinik, Städt. Krankenanstalten Merheim, Ostmerheimer Str. 200, 5000 Köln 91, FRG
Aldskogius, H.: Department of Anatomy, Karolinska Institute, Box 60400, 104 01 Stockholm, Sweden
Alexandre, A.: Department of Neurosurgery, Padova University School of Medicine, Treviso City Hospital, Treviso, Italy
Amend, P.: Centre Hospitalier Régional et Universitaire de Nancy, Hôpital Jeanne-D'Arc, Service de Chirurgie "D", Chirurgie Plastique et Reconstructive, B.P. 303, 54201 Toul Cedex, France
Antoniadis, G.: Division Neurosurgery, Fulda City Hospital, 6400 Fulda, FRG
Bailes, J. E.: Division of Neurosurgery, Evanston Hospital, Evanston JL, USA
Bain, J. R.: Division Plastic Surgery, Toronto General Hospital, 200 Elizabeth St., Toronto, Ont. M 5G 1L 7, Canada
Barberá, J.: Department of Neurosurgery, Faculty of Medicine, University of Cádiz, 11003-Cádiz, Spain
Bauer, B. L.: Clinic for Neurosurgery, Philipps-University Marburg, Baldingerstraße, 3550 Marburg, FRG
Becker, M.: Clinic of Plastic, Hand- and Reconstructive Surgery of the Medical School of Hanover, City of Hanover, Oststadt Hospital, Podbielskistr. 380, 3000 Hannover 51, FRG
Bel, S.: Clinic for Neurosurgery, Philipps-University Marburg, Baldingerstraße, 3550 Marburg, FRG
Berger, A.: Clinic of Plastic, Hand- and Reconstructive Surgery of the Medical School of Hanover, City of Hanover, Oststadt Hospital, Podbielskistr. 380, 3000 Hannover 51, FRG
Billeci, D.: Department of Neurosurgery, Padova University School of Medicine, Treviso City Hospital, Treviso, Italy
Bindl, G.: Abteilung für Unfall- und Wiederherstellungschirurgie, Katharinenhospital Stuttgart, Kriegsbergstr. 60, 7000 Stuttgart 1, FRG
Bini, W.: Neurochirurgische Klinik, Krankenhaus Nordstadt, Landeshauptstadt Hannover, Haltenhoffstr. 41, 3000 Hannover 1, FRG
Blank, M.: Institut für Anatomie, Universitätsklinikum Essen, Hufelandstr. 55, 4300 Essen 1, FRG
Bohl, J.: Department of Neuropathology, Joh. Gutenberg-University Mainz, Langenbeckstr. 1, 6500 Mainz, FRG
Braunsdorf, W. E.: Neurosurgical Clinic of Christian-Albrecht-University, 2300 Kiel, FRG
Brennecke, J.: Arzt für Pathologie, Kniggestr. 7, 3000 Hannover 1, FRG
Brunelli, F.: Clinica Ortopedica e Traumatologica dell' Universita di Brescia, Piazzale Ospedale Civile 2, 20124 Brescia, Italy

List of Contributors

Brunelli, G.: Clinica Ortopedica e Traumatologica dell' Universita di Brescia, Piazzale Ospedale Civile 2, 20124 Brescia, Italy
Carter, J.: Department of Neurosurgery, Duke University Durham Medical Center, Box 3807, Durham, North Carolina 27710, USA
Carteri, A.: Department of Neurosurgery, Padova University School of Medicine, Treviso City Hospital, Treviso, Italy
Ciric, I.: Division of Neurosurgery, Evanston Hospital, Evanston, IL, USA
Cisotto, P.: Department of Neurosurgery, Padova University School of Medicine, Treviso City Hospital, Treviso, Italy
Conzen, M.: Neurochirurgische Klinik, Krankenanstalten Gilead, Burgsteig 13, 4800 Bielefeld 13, FRG
Coulon, G. (†): Service d'Anatomie et de Cytologie Pathologique, Hôpital Jean Minjoz, 25000 Besançon, France
Cozzens, J.W.: Division in Neurosurgery, Evanston Hospital, Evanston, IL, USA
Cusumano, S.: Department of Neurology, Padova University School of Medicine, Treviso City Hospital, Treviso, Italy
Davaki, P.: Neurosurgical Department of Athens Polyclinic, Neurophysiological Department of Aeginition, University Hospital of Athens, Athens, Greece
Dengler, R.: Universitäts-Nervenklinik und Poliklinik, Neurologie, Sigmund-Freud-Str. 25, D-5300 Bonn 1
Diemer, N.H.: Institute of Neuropathology, University of Copenhagen, Frederik V Vej, 2100 Copenhagen Ø, Denmark
Di Paola, F.: Department of Neuroradiology, Padova University School of Medicine, Treviso City Hospital, Treviso, Italy
Di Toma, F.: Department of Radiology, City Hospital of Treviso, Padua University, Treviso, Italy
Döbler, L.: Clinic of Plastic, Hand- and Reconstructive Surgery, Clinic of the Main-Taunus-District, Lindenstr. 10, 6238 Hofheim/Taunus, FRG
Friedebold, G.: Oskar-Helene-Heim, Orthopädische Klinik und Poliklinik der Freien Universität Berlin, Clayallee 229, 1000 Berlin 33, FRG
Friedman, A.H.: Department of Neurosurgery, Duke University Durham Medical Center, Box 3807, Durham, North Carolina 27710, USA
Garcia, C.: Departments of Neurology and Neuropathology, Louisiana State University Medical Center, School of Medicine in New Orleans, 1542, Tulane Ave., New Orleans, LA-70112-2822, USA
Garcia-Vázquez, F.: Department of Neurosurgery, Faculty of Medicine, University of Cádiz, 11003-Cádiz, Spain
Gentili, F.: Department of Surgery, University of Toronto, 38 Shuter Street, Toronto, M5B 1A6, Canada
Gerhard, L.: Institut für Neuropathologie, Universitätsklinikum Essen, Hufelandstr. 55, 4300 Essen 1, FRG
Ghadirpour, R.: Department of Neurosurgery, S. Anna Hospital, Corso Giovecca 203, 44100 Ferrara, Italy
Gil-Salú, J.L.: Department of Neurosurgery, Faculty of Medicine, University of Cádiz, 11003-Cádiz, Spain
Godard, J.: Service de Neurochirurgie, Hôpital Jean Minjoz, 25000 Besançon, France
González-Darder, J.M.: Department of Neurosurgery, Faculty of Medicine, University of Cádiz, Dr. Marañon, 4, 11002-Cádiz, Spain
Graeber, M.B.: Department of Neuromorphology, Max-Planck-Institute for Psychiatry, Am Klopferspitz 18a, 8033 Martinsried, FRG
Holmgren, H.: Department of Clinical Neurophysiology, University of Linköping, Linköping, Sweden
Hopf, H.C.: Neurologische Klinik Joh. Gutenberg Universität Mainz, Langenbeckstr. 1, 6500 Mainz 1, FRG

Hudson, A. R.: Department of Surgery, University of Toronto, 38 Shuter
  Street, Toronto, M5B 1A6, Canada
Hunter, D.: Department of Surgery, University of Toronto, 38 Shuter Street,
  Toronto, M5B 1A6, Canada
Jacquet, G.: Service de Neurochirurgie, Hôpital Jean Minjoz, 25000 Besançon,
  France
Jantzen, J. P.: Department of Anaesthesiology, Joh. Gutenberg-University
  Mainz, Langenbeckstr. 1, 6500 Mainz, FRG
Jensen, H.-P.: Neurosurgical Clinic of Christian-Albrecht-University,
  2300 Kiel, FRG
Karandreas, N.: Neurosurgical Department of Athens Polyclinic,
  Neurophysiological Department of Aeginition, University Hospital of
  Athens, Athens, Greece
Khalil, H.: 17, Motanabii Str., Koubba Gardens, Cairo, Egypt
Kleider, A.: Psychiatrische Klinik Eichberg, Klosterstr. 4, 6228 Eltville, FRG
Klein, H. J.: Department of Neurosurgery, University of Ulm,
  Bezirkskrankenhaus, 8870 Günzburg, FRG
Kline, D. G.: Department of Neurosurgery, Louisiana State University Medical
  Center, School of Medicine in New Orleans, 1542 Tulane Ave.,
  New Orleans, LA 70112-2822, USA
Kohmura, E.: Dept. of Neurosurgery, Osaka University Medical School,
  1-1-50 Fukushima, Fukushima, Osaka 553, Japan
Kolenda, H.: Neurochirurgische Klinik der Georg-August-Universität,
  Robert-Koch-Str. 40, 3400 Göttingen, FRG
Konerding, M. A.: Institut für Anatomie, Universitätsklinikum Essen,
  Hufelandstr. 55, 4300 Essen 1, FRG
Koob, E.: Orthopädische Klinik, Abteilung für Handchirurgie,
  Universitätsklinikum Essen, Hufelandstr. 55, 4300 Essen 1, FRG
Koschorek, F.: Radiological Clinic of Christian-Albrecht-University,
  2300 Kiel, FRG
Krämer, G.: Department of Neurology, University Hospital, Langenbeckstr. 1,
  6500 Mainz, FRG
Kramer, R.: Neurochirurgische Klinik, Krankenanstalten Gilead, Burgsteig 13,
  4800 Bielefeld 13, FRG
Kreutzberg, G. W.: Department of Neuromorphology, Max-Planck-Institute
  for Psychiatry, Am Klopferspitz 18a, 8033 Martinsried, FRG
Kühn, A.: Department of Neurosurgery, University of Ulm,
  Bezirkskrankenhaus, 8870 Günzburg, FRG
Kuhlendahl, H. D.: Neurosurgical Clinic of Christian-Albrecht-University,
  2300 Kiel, FRG
Kunz, U.: Neurosurgical Clinic Hannover University Medical School,
  Konstanty-Gutschow-Str. 8, 3000 Hannover 61, FRG
Lange, B.: Neurochirurgische Klinik, Universitätsklinikum Essen, Hufelandstr.
  55, 4300 Essen 1, FRG
Laumann, U.: Orthopädische Abteilung, St. Marien-Hospital Borken,
  Am Boltenhof 7, 4280 Borken/Westf. 1, FRG
Lehmann, M.: Holsterhauser Str. 114, 4300 Essen 1, FRG
Leventis, A.: 9, Evzonon Street, Athens 11521, Greece
Lindholm, D.: Department of Neurochemistry, Max-Planck-Institute for
  Psychiatry, Am Klopferspitz 18a, 8033 Martinsried, FRG
Lusk, M.: Department of Neurosurgery, Louisiana State University Medical
  Center, School of Medicine in New Orleans, 1542 Tulane Ave.,
  New Orleans, LA 70112-2822, USA
Mackinnon, S. E.: Department of Surgery, University of Toronto,
  38 Shuter Street, Toronto, M5B 1A6, Canada

Mailänder, P.: Clinic of Plastic, Hand- and Reconstructive Surgery of the Medical School of Hanover, City of Hanover, Oststadt Hospital, Podbielskistr. 380, 3000 Hannover 51, FRG
Maillis, A.: Neurosurgical Department of Athens Polyclinic, Neurophysiological Department of Aeginition, University Hospital of Athens, Athens, Greece
Markakis, E.: Neurochirurgische Klinik der Georg-August-Universität, Robert-Koch-Str. 40, 3400 Göttingen, FRG
Marx, C.: Neurosurgical Research Laboratory, Saarland University School of Medicine, 6650 Homburg/Saar, FRG
Matthies, C.: Neurochirurgische Klinik, Krankenhaus Nordstadt, Landeshauptstadt Hannover, Haltenhoffstr. 41, 3000 Hannover 1, FRG
Menzel, J.: Neurochirurgische Klinik, Städt. Krankenanstalten Merheim, Ostmerheimer Str. 200, 5000 Köln 91, FRG
Merle, M.: Centre Hospitalier Régional et Universitaire de Nancy, Hôpital Jeanne-D'Arc, Service de Chirurgie "D", Chirurgie Plastique et Reconstructive, B.P. 303, 54201 Toul Cedex, France
Meyer, T.: Oskar-Helene-Heim, Orthopädische Klinik und Poliklinik der Freien Universität Berlin, Clayallee 229, 1000 Berlin 33, FRG
Michon, J. (†): Centre Hospitalier Régional et Universitaire de Nancy, Hôpital Jeanne-D'Arc, Service de Chirurgie "D", Chirurgie Plastique et Reconstructive, B.P. 303, 54201 Toul Cedex, France
Migliore, A.: Department of Neurosurgery, S. Anna Hospital, Corso Giovecca 203, 44100 Ferrara, Italy
Möckel, M.: Clinic of Plastic, Hand- and Reconstructive Surgery of the Medical School of Hanover, City of Hanover, Oststadt Hospital, Podbielskistr. 380, 3000 Hannover 51, FRG
Monini, L.: Clinica Ortopedica e Traumatologica dell'Universita di Brescia, Piazzale Ospedale Civile 2, 25100 Brescia, Italy
Monnier, G.: Laboratoire d'Explorations Fonctionnelles, Hôpital Jean Minjoz, 25000 Besançon, France
Müller, H.: Medizinische Universität Lübeck, Klinik für Neurochirurgie, Ratzeburger Allee 160, 2400 Lübeck, FRG
Mumenthaler, M.: Neurologische Klinik der Universität Bern, Inselspital, 3010 Bern, Switzerland
Nacimiento, A. C.: Neurosurgical Research Laboratory, Saarland University School of Medicine, 6650 Homburg/Saar, FRG
Nashold, B. S.: Department of Neurosurgery, Duke University Durham Medical Center, Box 3807, Durham, North Carolina 27710, USA
Nau, H.-E.: Neurochirurgische Klinik, Universitätsklinikum Essen, Hufelandstr. 55, 4300 Essen 1, FRG
Nix, W. A.: Department of Neurology, Joh. Gutenberg University Mainz, Langenbeckstr. 1, 6500 Mainz 1, FRG
Ochs, G.: Department of Neurology and Clinical Neurophysiology, Technical University Munich, Möhlstr. 28, 8000 München 80, FRG
Oppel, F.: Neurochirurgische Klinik, Krankenanstalten Gilead, Burgsteig 13, 4800 Bielefeld 13, FRG
Osgaard, O.: Copenhagen County Hospital, Department of Neurosurgery, 2600 Glostrup, Denmark
Penkert, G.: Neurochirurgische Klinik, Krankenhaus Nordstadt, Landeshauptstadt Hannover, Haltenhoffstr. 41, 3000 Hannover 1, FRG
Rabow, L.: Department of Neurosurgery, University Hospital Umeå, 90185 Umeå, Sweden
Rath, S. A.: Department of Neurosurgery, University of Ulm, Bezirkskrankenhaus, Ludwig-Heilmeyer-Str. 2, 8870 Günzburg, FRG

Reiners, K. H.: Department of Neurology, Düssseldorf University Medical
  School, Moorenstr. 5, 4000 Düsseldorf 1, FRG
Reinhardt, V.: Institut für Neuropathologie, Universitätsklinikum Essen,
  Hufelandstr. 55, 4300 Essen 1, FRG
Richter, H.-P.: Neurochirurgische Klinik der Universität Ulm im
  Bezirkskrankenhaus, 8870 Günzburg, FRG
Roccella, P.: Department of Neurosurgery, S. Anna Hospital,
  Corso Giovecca 203, 44100 Ferrara, Italy
Rouillon, D.: Service de Physiopathologie Respiratoire cérébrale et
  enzymatique, Hôpital Jean Minjoz, 25000 Besançon, France
Samii, M.: Neurochirurgische Klinik, Krankenhaus Nordstadt,
  Landeshauptstadt Hannover, Haltenhoffstr. 41, 3000 Hannover 1, FRG
Sander, T.: Department of Neurosurgery, Düsseldorf University Medical
  School, Moorenstr. 5, 4000 Düsseldorf 1, FRG
Schade, M.: Neurochirurgische Klinik der Georg-August-Universität,
  Robert-Koch-Str. 40, 3400 Göttingen, FRG
Schaller, E.: Clinic of Plastic, Hand- and Reconstructive Surgery of the
  Medical School of Hanover, City of Hanover, Oststadt Hospital,
  Podbielskistr. 380, 3000 Hannover 51, FRG
Schober, R.: Department of Neuropathology, Düsseldorf University Medical
  School, Moorenstr. 5, 4000 Düsseldorf 1, FRG
Schröder, J. M.: Institut für Neuropathologie, Klinikum der RWTH,
  Pauwelsstraße, 5100 Aachen, FRG
Seifert, V.: Neurosurgical Clinic, Hannover University Medical School,
  Konstanty-Gutschow-Str. 8, 3000 Hannover 61, FRG
Sepehrnia, A.: Neurochirurgische Klinik, Krankenhaus Nordstadt,
  Landeshauptstadt Hannover, Haltenhoffstr. 41, 3000 Hannover 1, FRG
Singounas, E.: Neurosurgical Department of Athens Polyclinic,
  Neurophysiological Department of Aeginition, University Hospital of
  Athens, Athens, Greece
Sparmann, M.: Oskar-Helene-Heim, Orthopädische Klinik und Poliklinik der
  Freien Universität Berlin, Clayallee 229, 1000 Berlin 33, FRG
Steimle, R.: Service de Neurochirurgie, Hôpital Jean Minjoz, 25000 Besançon,
  France
Stein, R. B.: Div. of Neuroscience, University of Alberta, 513 Heritage Medical
  Research Centre, Edmonton, Alberta T6G 2S2, Canada
Stober, R.: Klinik für Orthopäd. Chirurgie, Kantonsspital
  St. Gallen, 9007 St. Gallen, Switzerland
Stolke, D.: Neurosurgical Clinic, Hannover University Medical School,
  Konstanty-Gutschow-Str. 8, 3000 Hannover 61, FRG
Struppler, A.: Department of Neurology and Clinical Neurophysiology,
  Technical University Munich, Möhlstr. 28, 8000 München 80, FRG
Tackmann, W.: Neurologische Abteilung der Weserbergland-Klinik,
  3470 Höxter 1, FRG
Tatagiba, M.: Neurochirurgische Klinik, Krankenhaus Nordstadt,
  Landeshauptstadt Hannover, Haltenhoffstr. 41, 3000 Hannover 1, FRG
Thoenen, H.: Department of Neurochemistry, Max-Planck-Institute for
  Psychiatry, Am Klopferspitz 18a, 8033 Martinsried, FRG
Tindall, S. C.: The Emory Clinic, Section of Neurosurgery,
  1327 Clifton Road, NE, Atlanta, CA 30322, USA
Tizian, C.: Clinic of Plastic, Hand- and Reconstructive Surgery, Clinic of the
  Main-Taunus-District, Lindenstr. 10, 6238 Hofheim/Taunus, FRG
Trapella, G.: Department of Neurosurgery, S. Anna Hospital, Corso Giovecca
  203, 44100 Ferrara, Italy
Ulrich, F.: Department of Neurosurgery, Düsseldorf University Medical
  School, Moorenstr. 5, 4000 Düsseldorf 1, FRG

List of Contributors

Wallenfang, T.: Department of Neurosurgery, Joh. Gutenberg-University Mainz, Langenbeckstr. 1, 6500 Mainz, FRG
Wallesch, B.: Department of Neuropathology, Joh. Gutenberg-University, Langenbeckstr. 1, 6500 Mainz, FRG
Walter, G. F.: Institute of Neuropathology of the Medical School of Hanover, Konstanty-Gutschow-Str. 8, 3000 Hannover 61, FRG
Weis, J.: Institut für Neuropathologie, Klinikum der RWTH Aachen, Pauwelsstraße, 5100 Aachen, FRG
Wenzel, P.: Neurochirurgische Klinik, Universitätsklinikum Essen, Hufelandstr. 55, 4300 Essen 1, FRG
Werner, R.: Neurochirurgische Klinik, Universitätsklinikum Essen, Hufelandstr. 55, 4300 Essen 1, FRG
Wippermann, V.: Department of Neurosurgery, University of Ulm, Bezirkskrankenhaus, 8870 Günzburg, FRG
Woolf, C. J.: Cerebral Functions Research Group, Department of Anatomy and Developmental Biology, University College London, Gower Street, London WC1E 6BT, U.K.

Cellular Biology of the Experimental Peripheral Nerve Lesion

G. W. Kreutzberg and M. B. Graeber, Martinsried/FRG

The interruption of the continuity of axons, such as may occur with spinal or cranial nerve injury or as a result of compression or inflammation, leads to characteristic retrograde changes in the cell bodies of the affected neurons. These changes are part of a regenerative process which involves not only the lesioned neurons but also their microenvironment. Although regeneration may result in the anatomical restitution of a lesioned nerve, i.e., by neurite outgrowth and reinnervation of the musculature, functional recovery does not always take place.

The regenerative changes have been studied in our laboratory mainly in the facial nucleus. As a routine procedure the facial nerve is cut at the stylomastoid foramen. Rats, mice, and occasionally guinea pigs are used as experimental animals.

The Neuronal Metabolism During Regeneration

Since the classical experiments by Franz Nissl at the end of the last century, the morphological changes occurring after axotomy have been known as chromatolysis, retrograde reaction, or axonal reaction. The cell bodies of the affected neurons appear to be swollen, the Nissl substance becomes dispersed and more basophilic, the nuclei appear eccentric, and the cell surface is undulating (Fig. 1). Electron microscopy has shown an enormous increase in free ribosomes. These tend to accumulate within the cytoplasm and frequently form a "nuclear cap." The increased production of ribosomes is preceded by a synthesis of RNA which seems to be triggered by polyamines. This view is suggested by the rapid increase in activity of the neuronal key enzyme of polyamine synthesis, ornithine decarboxylase. Within 24 h after nerve transection the activity of this enzyme reaches about 300% of control values (Tetzlaff and Kreutzberg 1985). The elevated activity of the neuronal hexose monophosphate shunt which produces pentoses, i.e., ribose, may represent another prerequisite for the enhanced RNA synthesis (Tetzlaff and Kreutzberg 1984; Tetzlaff et al. 1986).

There is no doubt that the apparent increase in RNA and its associated organelles serves the de novo synthesis of additional and/or new neuronal proteins. However, these changes in protein synthesis are very selective. Several hundreds of proteins do not change at all, others are increased, and some

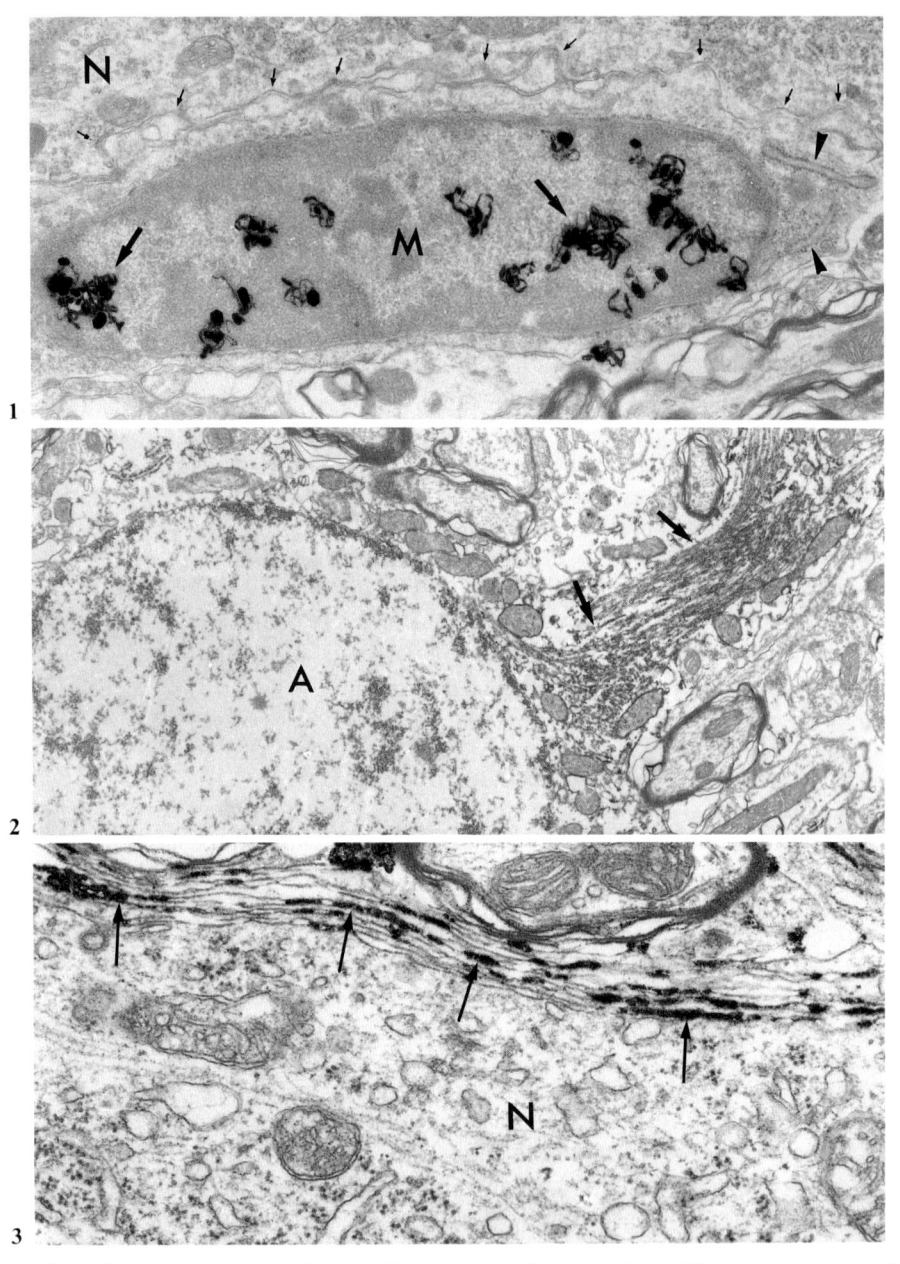

Fig. 1. Perineuronal microglial cell (*M*) 6 days after operation. Silver grains (*arrows*) overlying its nucleus indicate incorporation of radioactive [^{3}H]thymidine during premitotic DNA synthesis. Wide rough endoplasmic reticulum cisternae (*arrow-heads*) are typical of microglial cells. The neuronal (*N*) cell surface is undulating (*small arrows*). EM autoradiography. (×24000)

appear to be reduced (Bisby 1980). There seems to be a principle governing the changes in protein metabolism of the regenerating neuron. Proteins serving a more structural function, i.e., cytoskeletal proteins (beta-tubulin, calmodulin, actin) are preferentially synthesized; exceptionally, only the neurofilament proteins of 68 and 150 kDa are decreased (Tetzlaff et al. 1988a). In contrast to cytoskeletal components, proteins related to synaptic functions are diminished, e.g., enzymes concerned with transmitter metabolism and receptor proteins. The enzymatic changes have been studied in detail in the case of acetylcholinesterase (Kreutzberg et al. 1984). In the rat facial nucleus the activity of this enzyme is reduced by 30% 1 week after axotomy. However, in the guinea pig the same experimental conditions result in a selective reduction of the tetrameric isoenzymes. At the same time there is a dramatic increase (500%) in the 16s molecular form of acetylcholinesterase (Engel and Kreutzberg 1986). The function of this molecular form of acetylcholinesterase is probably unrelated to synaptic transmission. It is released from dendrites and undergoes anterograde axonal transport. Following secretion, it is found within the extracellular spaces of the facial nucleus and in basal membranes of local capillaries. Within the proximal nerve stump the intraaxonally transported enzyme is predominantly present in the plasma membrane of axonal sprouts. Here, the enzyme is also secreted and thereafter localized within the extracellular space (Engel et al. 1988). Unfortunately, the functional significance of these changes for neuronal regeneration is unclear. However, their possible relation to muscarinic-cholinergic mechanisms must be considered.

Glial Cells

Recently, interest has grown in the cellular reactions occurring in the neighborhood of regenerating motoneurons. As early as 1966 (see Kreutzberg 1981, 1982, 1986), the mitotic division of microglial cells was described in our laboratory. The number of microglial cells within the normal facial nucleus is low. However, as early as 2 days after the operation these normally quiescent cells become activated and begin to proliferate ("progressive microglia"). The proliferation reaches its peak about 4–6 days after the operation. This has been shown by light and electron microscopic [^{3}H]thymidine autoradiography

◄─────────────────────────────────

Fig. 2. Reactive astrocyte (*A*) of the regenerating facial nucleus 10 days following axotomy. Its glial filaments (*arrows*) are labeled by dark peroxidase/diaminobenzidine reaction product. EM immunocytochemistry. (× 15000)

Fig. 3. Stacks of lamellar astrocytic cell processes cover the surface of regenerating facial motoneurons (*N*) for several weeks following operation. Such an isolation has been observed even after reinnervation of the musculature. The plasma membrane of the astrocytic lamellae exhibits 5'-nucleotidase enzymatic activity (*arrows* point to enzymatic reaction product). (× 56000)

(Kreutzberg 1966, 1968; Graeber et al. 1988) together with the endogenous origin of these cells. The perineuronally proliferating microglial cells (Fig. 1) are in close contact with the regenerating motoneurons and appear to be involved in the displacement of axon terminals from the surface of neuronal somata and stem dendrites. This phenomenon, first described in the rat facial nucleus, has been confirmed in various systems and is now generally referred to as "synaptic stripping" (Blinzinger and Kreutzberg 1968). As a result, the axotomized neurons lose more than 80% of all afferent synaptic contacts from their somata.

In the course of studying the identity of the reactive microglial cells we found also that astrocytes participate in the retrograde changes following axotomy. Using light and electron microscopic immunocytochemistry (Graeber and Kreutzberg 1986) we have demonstrated that local astrocytes become stimulated by motoneuron axotomy and express the glial fibrillary acidic protein (GFAP; Fig. 2). Using two-dimensional SDS-PAGE the astrocytic increase in GFAP synthesis could be verified as early as 24 h after the operation (Tetzlaff et al. 1988b). GFAP is the major protein constituent of glial filaments (Eng 1985) and is considered to be a sensitive marker for astroglia responding to pathological tissue changes. The early increase in GFAP synthesis by reactive astrocytes is one of the earliest known glial responses to axotomy (Tetzlaff et al. 1988b). Electron microscopy demonstrated that the increase of GFAP immunoreactivity in the astrocytes of the regenerating facial nucleus is associated with an increased number of glial filaments and astrocytic processes (Graeber and Kreutzberg 1986). About 3 weeks after the operation the processes become ramified and form thin sheetlike or lamellar cell extensions. Subsequently, the lamellar processes become arranged in stacks covering virtually all neuronal surfaces (Fig. 3) except those of small dendrites and thus isolate them from their synaptic input (Graeber and Kreutzberg 1988). Such an insulation has been observed even after peripheral reinnervation of the musculature. However, there is no doubt that the early deafferentation of the axotomized neurons by microglial cells ("synaptic stripping") and the subsequent maintenance of this state by astrocytes has functional consequences. The delay in functional recovery of patients suffering from facial nerve trauma is a common clinical feature. Therefore, an underlying glial reaction should be taken into account if the peripheral reinnervation of the musculature appears to be normal, but functional deficits persist. The long-lasting deafferentation during motoneuron regeneration caused by glial cells may especially reduce the capability of performing fine movements as required, for instance, for mimic expression.

After the 2nd week following axotomy the reactive microglial cells leave the neurons and migrate into the neuropil. Since microglial cells are potentially cytotoxic macrophages (Rieske-Shows et al. 1987; Colton and Gilbert 1987; Streit and Kreutzberg 1988), it is possible that the separation of microglial cells from the regenerating motoneurons by lamellar astrocytic processes may have a neuroprotective function.

Dendrites

Today, it is generally accepted that synapse-bearing structures such as neuronal soma and dendrites undergo severe alterations during regeneration. The dendritic tree of the axotomized motoneurons shrinks as a whole (Sumner and Watson 1971). Whether this also leads to a loss of synaptic contacts is unknown but seems to be likely.

Recently, we have also observed that during regeneration neurons are able to develop somatic processes (Engel and Kreutzberg 1988). In particular, neurons in the dorsal vagal nucleus of the guinea pig seem to possess this capability. The processes grow out of the neuronal soma and partially cover the surface of the chromatolytic nerve cells. They are often arranged in stacks, and occasionally a growth cone or a single synaptic contact can also be seen. Therefore, the formations may be regarded as postsynaptic fibers, similar to dendrites. They are very common in vagal neurons. We also observed them arising from regenerating facial motoneurons, but these occurred rarely and were small in size.

Conclusions

Studies of the retrograde changes in motoneurons of cranial nerves have resulted in a complex picture of the fundamental changes in morphology, metabolism, and physiology of these cells. The changes in neuronal metabolism suggest an increased and modified production of macromolecules, especially proteins. They may reflect the efforts of the regenerating nerve cell to compensate for its lost axon. The accompanying glial reaction leads to a central deafferentation of the axotomized motoneurons. Up until 3 months after operation the overall number of axosomatic as well as axodendritic synaptic contacts appears to be reduced. Some neurons, i.e., of the guinea pig vagal nerve, may additionally develop new, pseudodendritic processes which surround the neuronal cell bodies. They are sometimes wrapped by astrocytic processes themselves.

We conclude from these observations that during regeneration cranial nerve nuclei exhibit profound changes in their synaptic organization. Obviously, this is of clinical relevance. Our findings may help to explain why patients suffering from a prolonged period of recovery after facial nerve trauma may be unable to regain full controll over fine movements although successful reinnervation of the musculature has taken place.

References

Bisby MA (1980) Changes in the composition of labeled protein transported in motor axons during their regeneration. J Neurobiol 11:435–445

Blinzinger K, Kreutzberg G (1968) Displacement of synaptic terminals from regenerating motoneurons by microglial cells. Z Zellforsch 85:145–157

Colton CA, Gilbert DL (1987) Production of superoxide anions by a CNS macrophage, the microglia. FEBS Lett 223:284–288
Eng LF (1985) Glial fibrillary acidic protein (GFAP): the major protein of glial intermediate filaments in differentiated astrocytes. J Neuroimmunol 8:203–214
Engel AK, Kreutzberg GW (1986) Changes of acetylcholinesterase molecular forms in regenerating motor neurons. Neuroscience 18:467–473
Engel AK, Kreutzberg GW (1988) Ultrastructural changes in the dorsal motor nucleus of vagus of the guinea pig during retrograde reaction. J Comp Neurol 275:181–200
Engel AK, Tetzlaff W, Kreutzberg GW (1988) Axonal transport of 16 s acetylcholinesterase is increased in regenerating peripheral nerve in guinea pig, but not in rat. Neuroscience 24:729–738
Graeber MB, Kreutzberg GW (1986) Astrocytes increase in glial fibrillary acidic protein during retrograde changes of facial motor neurons. J Neurocytol 15:363–373
Graeber MB, Kreutzberg GW (1988) Delayed astrocyte reaction following facial nerve axotomy. J Neurocytol 17:209–220
Graeber MB, Tetzlaff W, Streit WJ, Kreutzberg GW (1988) Microglial cells but not astrocytes undergo mitosis following rat facial nerve axotomy. Neurosci Lett 85:317–321
Kreutzberg GW (1966) Autoradiographische Untersuchung über die Beteiligung von Gliazellen an der axonalen Reaktion im Facialiskern der Ratte. Acta Neuropathol 7:149–161
Kreutzberg GW (1968) Über perineuronale Mikrogliazellen (Autoradiographische Untersuchungen). Acta Neuropathol, Suppl 4:141–145
Kreutzberg GW (1981) Neurobiologische Aspekte der Nervenregeneration. Arch Otorhinolaryngol 231:71–88 (Kongreßbericht)
Kreutzberg GW (1982) Acute neural reaction to injury. In: Nicholls JG (ed) Repair and regeneration of the nervous system, life sciences research report 24, Dahlem Konferenzen 1982. Springer, Berlin Heidelberg New York, pp 57–69
Kreutzberg GW (1986) Neurobiology of regeneration and degeneration. In: May M (ed) The facial nerve. Thieme, New York, pp 75–83
Kreutzberg GW, Tetzlaff W, Toth L (1984) Cytochemical changes of cholinesterases in motor neurons during regeneration. In: Brzin M, Barnard EA, Sket D (eds) Cholinesterases – fundamental and applied aspects. de Gruyter, Berlin, pp 273–288
Rieske-Shows E, Tetzlaff W, Czlonkowska A, Graeber M, Kreutzberg GW (1987) Microglia in culture. In: Althaus HH, Seifert W (eds) Glial-neuronal communication in development and regeneration. NATO ASI Series H, Vol. 2. Springer, Berlin Heidelberg New York Tokyo, pp 41–51
Streit WJ, Kreutzberg GW (1988) Response of endogenous glial cells to motor neuron degeneration induced by toxic ricin. J Comp Neurol 268:248–263
Sumner BEH, Watson WE (1971) Retraction and expansion of the dendritic tree of motor neurones of adult rats induced in vivo. Nature 233:273–275
Tetzlaff W, Kreutzberg GW (1984) Enzyme changes in the rat facial nucleus following a conditioning lesion. Exp Neurol 85:547–564
Tetzlaff W, Kreutzberg GW (1985) Ornithine decarboxylase in motoneurons during regeneration. Exp Neurol 89:679–688
Tetzlaff W, Graeber MB, Kreutzberg GW (1986) Reaction of motoneurons and their microenvironment to axotomy. In: Gilad GM, Gorio A, Kreutzberg GW (eds) Processes of recovery from neural trauma. Exp Brain Res, Suppl 13; 3–8
Tetzlaff W, Bisby MA, Kreutzberg GW (1988a) Changes in cytoskeletal proteins in the rat facial nucleus following axotomy. J Neurosci 8:3181–3189
Tetzlaff W, Graeber MB, Bisby MA, Kreutzberg GW (1988b) Increased glial fibrillary acidic protein synthesis in astrocytes during retrograde reaction of the rat facial nucleus. Glia 1: 90:95

Muscle Response to Changes in Innervation

W. A. Nix, Mainz/FRG

Motoneurons and the muscle they innervate are strongly dependent on each other for their normal development, physiological behavior, and maintenance. When nerve and muscle interact to produce movement, the motor unit is the smallest functional element within this system. The unit is composed of a single motoneuron and the muscle fibers that this neuron supplies. Within the unit, there is a mutual interaction of the constituents, so that disturbances of one component do not leave the other unaffected. This complex interdependence relies on a wide range of "trophic" interactions, which are made via synaptic contact, impulse, and trophic substance transmission.

Loss of Innervation and Muscle Atrophy

Disturbance of nerve-muscle interaction is most apparent in the sequelae of peripheral nerve damage when trophic interaction of nerve and muscle is interrupted. Without its neural supply the muscle quickly loses its tone, lacks the possibility for voluntary activation, and shows atrophy. The latter events involve primarily the contractile constituents of the muscle but also its 10%–25% of connective tissue [41]. Changes in this last component play a major role when newly reinnervated muscle must fulfill functional tasks. If loss of nerve continuity is the reason for muscle denervation, restoration of continuity is a therapeutic goal, but it will be pursued only if muscle tissue can be revived to a functional status. It is very difficult to establish how long this is possible after peripheral nerve injury. There are many observations which show that functional restitution of muscle is less after denervation periods of longer than 18–24 months than after earlier reinnervation [38].

After short-term denervation the reinnervated muscle fibers quickly regain their predenervation status [12]. However, after periods of 1 year or more this process can be hindered by degenerative changes within the muscle, which become more pronounced the longer the denervation exists. These alterations are usually dynamic since denervation may be followed by reinnervation, or the muscle fibers undergo a number of changes. There are animal studies which show that atrophy develops very quickly, so the about 30% of muscle is lost within the first 4 weeks after denervation and 60% after about 60 days [13, 39]. Thereafter, atrophy develops at a far slower rate. Because of atrophy and degradation of contractile protein, there is a relative increase in connective tissue, but parallel to this process connective tissue proliferates, which then leads to its absolute increase.

Findings differ regarding how far muscle fibers degenerate after denervation. Some investigators found a decrease in the number of muscle fibers after 16 months of denervation in rabbit [1, 39]. Others, for example, Bowden and Gutmann [5], could not confirm this finding in human muscle denervated up to 69 days [18]. It was shown that perimysial tissue increases in denervated muscle, but the increase in endomysial connective tissue takes place only when the total number of fibers in a fascicle is reduced [3].

The situation in human muscle has not been studied very well, as denervated muscle is no indication for a biopsy. In those human muscles that could be biopsied after many months or years of denervation a variety of changes could be seen. Appreciable increase in connective tissue could be recorded only from 4 months onwards, irrespective of the amount of muscle atrophy [4]. Those muscles which, in addition to denervation from direct mechanical trauma, suffered compartment syndromes or ischemia because of arterial or venous circulation disturbances or infection had severe fibrosis [4]. The small number of atrophic muscle fibers that remained were buried in a fibrous coffin which excluded their useful contribution to muscle contraction in case of reinnervation. These changes result in formation of contractures within the muscle and reduce mobility. That denervated muscle fibers can survive for many years is known from clinical cases in which fibrillation activity was recorded as long as 18–20 years after onset of paralysis due to poliomyelitis [40].

Loss of Innervation and Changes in Muscle Membrane Properties

An early sign of denervation is a drop in resting membrane potential of the muscle fiber, at first close to the endplate region and afterwards spreading over the whole membrane, of about 20 mV within 1–2 weeks. Furthermore, there is a large increase in specific muscle membrane resistance and a decrease in specific membrane capacitance together with a slowing of the action potential conduction rate [2, 6]. In normally innervated muscle acetylcholine receptors (AChR) are confined to the subsynaptic membrane. About 2 days after nerve section AChRs are exposed in the extrajunctional parts of the membrane [14]. At this time individual muscle fibers in animals start to contract spontaneously and asynchronously. This fibrillation can be seen in human muscle about 18 days after denervation [34]. All these changes allow a regenerating nerve to form new synapses at the membrane. Normally an innervated muscle fiber is refractory to innervation by a foreign nerve. The formation of AChRs suggests that membrane AChRs are necessary for synapse formation in the muscle membrane [11].

Effect of Nerve Stump Length

The time span between denervation and the above mentioned changes in muscle vary with the nerve stump length attached to the muscle. The longer the nerve stump, the later there evolves a drop in resting membrane potential [6], fibrillation activity [34], and denervation hypersensitivity of the membrane and electrical membrane changes [9, 10]. A delay also occurs in the degeneration process of the nerve branch terminals [8]. Two hypotheses explain this nerve stump effect. One proposes that changes in muscle are induced by breakdown products of the nerve end terminals. The other presumes trophic substances within the nerve stump that are transported with the fast axonal flow fraction to the endplate and released into muscle. It is known that axonal transport continues within a nerve distal to a cut.

Denervation changes the contractile properties of muscle so that denervated fast-twitch muscle slows down, and denervated slow-twitch muscle speeds up. Interestingly, these properties are not affected by nerve stump length, so that they must be controlled by a different mechanism.

Effect of Activity on Innervated Muscle

As mentioned above, the motor unit is the smallest functional element within a muscle, and all muscle fibers within a unit are biochemically homogeneous [24]. In general, two unit types can be distinguished. Type I units have slowly contracting muscle fibers that appear light when stained for myofibrillar ATPase at pH 9.4, and type II fibers are dark and rapidly contracting. Depending on the relative percentages of the two unit types within a muscle, the whole muscle contracts slowly or rapidly. Until recently it was unknown which influence governs the phenotypic expression of a muscle fiber. A major contribution to solving this question were the cross-reinnervation experiments by Buller and Eccles [7], who found that neural influence can change muscle properties. After denervation of the fast-twitch EDL the muscle was reinnervated with the nerve that normally supplies the slow-twitch soleus muscle; conversely, the denervated soleus muscle was reinnervated by the peroneal nerve. As a result of this cross-reinnervation the formerly fast-twitch EDL now contracted slowly, and the slow-twitch soleus muscle contracted more rapidly.

The neural influence that brought about these profound changes was at first thought to be a chemical trophic substance. However, Salmons and Vrbova [35] demonstrated that the influence which governs muscle phenotypic expression is the activity pattern that the nerve imposes on muscle. They superimposed onto the peroneal nerve innervating the EDL a slow, 10-Hz continuous activity pattern, which resembles the activity to which the slowly contracting soleus muscle is normally exposed. Thereby the fast-twitch EDL was transformed into a slowly contracting muscle. This change in activity pattern has a profound influence on muscle. The first step in transformation from fast- to slow-twitch activity is an increase in capillary density of the muscle that is followed by a change in contraction time [16]. Before the myofibrillar apparatus is changed, alterations take place in the sarcoplasmatic reticulum. The reduced capacity to bind Ca^{2+} and the diminished activity of Ca^{2+} ATPase slow muscle contraction and relaxation. The last step is a transformation of myosin into the form typical for a slowly contracting muscle. Under stimulation, there is an increase in mRNA activity which induces synthesis of enzymes typical for aerobic metabolism. Enzymes of the glycolytic and glycogenolytic pathways are degraded and resynthesized to a lesser degree than before, so that the enzyme composition of the muscle, which at first was anaerobic, resembles after about 3 weeks the composition of a muscle with aerobic metabolism. All these changes brought about by slow stimulation are reversible when the intermittent fast-activity pattern of the muscle's own nerve takes over again.

Effect of Activity on Denervated Muscle

One objection to this type of experiments is that in innervated muscle stimulation of the nerve might change the synthesis of trophic substances in the neuron, which then influences the muscle via axoplasmic transport. Therefore, it was necessary to stimulate denervated muscle to determine whether an activity pattern can substitute for the lost neural influence. Denervated soleus muscle of rats was stimulated with either an intermittent fast- or a continuous slow-impulse pattern, which left the muscle contracting slowly or induced fast-twitch characteristics, respectively [20, 21]. In denervated fast-twitch EDL muscle of rabbit a continuous 8-Hz stimulation induced the physiologic and biochemical characteristics of a slow-twitch muscle [27, 30, 33]. This indicates that muscle activity itself influences the metabolic properties without the need of a trophic factor. Even after 1 month of denervation electrical stimulation can influence denervated muscle [26]. However, in contrast to the experiments on rat muscle, stimulation of rabbit muscle did not retard atrophy. This shows either that a species-specific difference is involved, or that certain properties still need a trophic factor.

Special forms of electrical stimulation of denervated muscle can counteract denervation-induced changes of the muscle membrane. Membrane capacitance and muscle resting membrane potential [42] can be kept at its normal level and ACh hypersensitivity of the muscle membrane prevented [19].

Short-term electrical stimulation to prevent muscle atrophy acts in a different way than the above mentioned methods [27, 28]. To prevent muscle atrophy after peripheral nerve injuries electrical stimulation of denervated muscle is often used. To date there is no evidence that this therapeutic regime is effective. In animals denervation atrophy can be retarded, as was shown in a thorough study by Gutmann and Guttmann [12]. But an effect of stimulation was achieved only when muscle was stimulated under isometric conditions for at least 20 min each day. As denervation atrophy develops quickly, stimulation is only of use when started as early as possible after denervation. This sort of short-term isometric stimulation of muscle is effective because of the stretch that is applied to the fiber. This induces protein synthesis and counteracts denervation-induced protein degradation. This preserves even fast-contraction properties and fatigue resistance, as opposed to untreated denervated muscle [28]. Increased stretch tensions do not potentiate the effect of stimulation; rather, they induce connective tissue proliferation and form contractures which terminate any functional rehabilitation of the muscle after eventual reinnervation [28].

Electrical stimulation of muscle influences the genom [31, 32] and the muscle fiber and can induce different metabolic and physiologic changes. Therefore, studies are now under way to implement these possibilities in normal [36, 23] and diseased muscle [37].

Electrical Stimulation and Nerve Regeneration

In partially denervated muscle electrical long-term stimulation prevents terminal in favor of collateral sprouting [17]. This shows that muscle activity has an influence on nerve regeneration. From denervated muscle it is known that it emanates a factor that induces nerve growth in tissue culture [15]. It is not yet known whether long-term stimulation of denervated muscle interferes with this process and retards nerve growth. Short-term isometric stimulation does not retard or stimulate nerve regeneration [12]. Long-term stimulation of regeneration nerve enhances its regeneration [25, 29].

Retrograde stimulation of severed motoneurons enhances protein production and shows higher protein levels in the fast fraction of axoplasmic flow that is transported to the site of regeneration [22].

References

1. Adams RD, Denny-Brown D, Pearson CM (1962) Disease of muscle. Kimpton, London
2. Albuquerque EX, McIsaac RJ (1970) Fast and slow mammalian muscle after denervation. Exp Neurol 26:183
3. Banker BQ, Engel AG (1986) Basic reaction of muscle. In Engel AG, Banker BQ (eds) Myology, Vol I. McGraw-Hill, New York
4. Bowden RE (1954) Factors influencing functional recovery. In: Seddon HJ (ed) Peripheral nerve injuries. Medical Research Council, Special Report Series No. 282, London, pp 298–353
5. Bowden RE, Gutmann E (1944) Denervation and re-innervation of human voluntary muscle. Brain 67:273
6. Bray JJ, Hawken MJ, Hubbard JI, Pockett S, Wilson L (1976) The membrane potential of rat diaphragm muscle fibers and the effect of denervation. J Physiol 255:651
7. Buller AJ, Eccles JC, Eccles RM (1960) Interaction between motoneurons and muscles in respect of the characteristic speed of their responses. J Physiol 150:417
8. Card DJ (1977) Denervation: sequence of neuromuscular degenerative changes in rats and the effect of stimulation. Exp Neurol 54:251
9. Davey B, Younkin SG (1978) Effect of nerve stump length on cholinesterase in denervated rat diaphragm. Exp Neurol 59:168

10. Fernandez HL, Duell MJ, Festoff BW (1979) Neurotrophic control of 16S acetylcholinesterase at the vertebrate neuromuscular junction. J Neurobiol 10:441
11. Fex S, Sonesson B, Thesleff S, Zelena J (1966) Nerve implants in botulinum poisoned mammalian muscle. J Physiol 184:872
12. Gutmann E, Guttmann L (1944) The effect of galvanic exercise on denervated and reinnervated muscles in rabbit. J Neurol Neurosurg Psychiatry 7:7–17
13. Gutmann E, Zelena J (1962) Morphological changes in the denervated muscle. In Gutmann E (ed) The denervated muscle. Publishing House of the Czechoslovak Academy of Science, Prague, pp 57–102
14. Hartzell HC, Fambrough DM (1972) Acetylcholine receptors. Distribution and extrajunctional density in rat diaphram after denervation correlated with acetylcholine sensitivity. J Gen Physiol 60:248
15. Henderson CE (1986) Factors influencing motor nerve growth. In: Nix WA, Vrbova G (eds) Electrical stimulation and neuromuscular disorders. Springer, Berlin Heidelberg New York Tokyo, pp 46–49
16. Hudlicka O, Cotter MA, Cooper J (1986) The effect of long-term electrical stimulation on capillary supply and metabolism in fast skeletal muscle. In: Nix WA, Vrbova G (eds) Electrical stimulation and neuromuscular disorders. Springer, Berlin Heidelberg New York Tokyo, pp 22–32
17. Ironton R, Brown MC, Holland R (1978) Stimuli to intramuscular nerve growth. Brain Res 156:351
18. Karpati G, Engel WK (1968) Histochemical investigation of fiber type ratios with the myofibrillar ATPase reaction in normal and denervated skeletal muscle of guinea pig. Am J Anat 122:145
19. Lomo T, Westgaard RH (1975) Control of ACh sensitivity in rat muscle fibres. Cold Spring Habor Symp Quant Biol 40:263
20. Lomo T, Westgaard RH, Dahl HA (1974) Contractile properties of muscle: control by pattern of muscle activity in the rat. Proc R Soc Lond (Biol) 187:99
21. Lomo T, Westgaard RH, Engebretsen L (1980) Different stimulation patterns affect contractile properties of denervated rat soleus muscle. In: Pette D (ed) Plasticity of muscle. de Gruyter, Berlin, pp 297–309
22. Lux H, Schubert P, Kreuzberg G, Globus A (1970) Excitation and axonal flow: autoradiographic study on motoneurons intracellulary injected with a H3-amino acid. Ex Brain Res 10:197
23. Mannion JD, Hammond R, Stephenson LW (1986) Hydraulic pouches of canine latissimus dorsi muscle. Circulation Res 58:298
24. Nemeth PM, Pette D, Vrbova G (1981) Comparison of enzyme activities among single muscle fibres within defined motor units. J Physiol 311:489
25. Nix WA (1982) The effect of low frequency electrical stimulation on the denervated extensor digitorum longus of the rabbit. Acta Neurol Scand 66:521
26. Nix WA (1986) Maintenance of muscle integrity following denervation. In: Dimitrijevic MR, Kakulas BA, Vrbova G (eds) Recent achievements in restorative neurology 2: Progressive neuromuscular diseases. Karger, Basel, pp 332–340
27. Nix WA (1986) Effect of electrical stimulation on denervated muscle. In: Nix WA, Vrbova G (eds) Electrical stimulation and neuromuscular disorders. Springer, Berlin Heidelberg New York Tokyo, pp 114–124
28. Nix WA, Dahm M (1987) The effect of isometric short-term electrical stimulation on denervated muscle. Muscle & Nerve 10:136
29. Nix WA, Hopf HC (1983) Electrical stimulation of regenerating nerve and its effect on motor recovery. Brain Res 272:21
30. Nix WA, Reichmann H, Schröder JM (1985) Influence of direct low frequency stimulation on contractile properties of denervated fast-twitch rabbit muscle. Pflügers Arch 405:141
31. Pette D (1986) Regulation of phenotype expression in skeletal muscle fibers by increased contractile activity. In: Saltin B (ed) Biochemistry of exercise VI. International Series on Sport Sciences. Human Kinetics Publishers Champaign, Illinois 16:3

32. Pluskal MG, Sreter FA (1983) Correlation between protein phenotype and gene expression in adult rabbit fast-twitch muscles undergoing a fast to slow fiber transformation in response to electrical stimulation in vivo. Biochem Biophys Res Commun 113:325
33. Reichmann H, Nix WA (1985) Changes of energy metabolism, myosin light chain composition, lactate dehydrogenase isozyme pattern and fiber type distribution of denervated fast-twitch muscle from rabbit after low frequency stimulation. Pflügers Arch 405:244
34. Salafsky B, Bell J, Prewitt M (1968) Development of fibrillation potentials in denervated fast and slow skeletal muscle. J Physiol 215:637
35. Salmons S, Vrbova G (1969) The influence of activity on some characteristic of mammalian fast and slow muscle. J Physiol 201:535
36. Schmitt O (1986) Treatment of idiopathic scoliosis with daily short-term electrostimulation. In: Nix WA, Vrbova G (eds) Electrical stimulation and neuromuscular disorders. Springer, Berlin Heidelberg New York Tokyo, pp 132–143
37. Scott OM, Vrbova G, Hyde SA, Dubowitz V (1986) Effects of electrical stimulation on normal and diseased human muscle. In: Nix WA, Vrbova G (eds) Electrical stimulation and neuromuscular disorders. Springer, Berlin Heidelberg New York Tokyo, pp 125–131
38. Sunderland S (1978) Nerves and Nerve Injuries. Churchill Livingston, Edinburgh, p 508
39. Sunderland S, Ray LJ (1950) Denervation changes in mammalian striated muscle. J Neurol Neurosurg Psychiat 13:159
40. Weddell G, Feinstein B, Pattel RE (1944) The electrical activity of voluntary muscle in man under normal and pathological conditions. Brain 67:178
41. Weiss P, Edds M (1946) Spontaneous recovery of muscle following partial denervation. Am J Physiol 145:587
42. Westgaard R (1975) Influence of activity on the passive electrical properties of denervated soleus muscle fibres in rat. J Physiol 251:683

The Response of Sensory Ganglia and Spinal Cord to Injury*

H. ALDSKOGIUS, Stockholm/Sweden

Introduction

To achieve successful recovery of sensory functions after peripheral nerve injury, the affected population of sensory ganglion cells must (a) survive the axon injury, (b) produce axonal sprouts, (c) maintain and support the elongation of the sprouting axons, (d) participate in neuron-nonneuronal cell and neuron-target interactions, and (e) reintegrate properly in the functional system. Abundant clinical experience demonstrates that this series of events is frequently seriously disturbed. Over the last 10–15 years an increasing amount of information has accumulated which demonstrates that axotomized sensory ganglion cells undergo degenerative changes. The present report focuses on our present knowledge about the nature of these changes, the possible pathogenetic mechanisms for their development, and their possible significance for the deficient restitution of sensory functions after peripheral nerve injury.

In this context it may be useful to deal with sensory ganglion cell responses in two steps, a short-term and a long-term one. Most important, too, the neuronal response must be discussed in relation to the type of axonal injury. By far most of the experimental data obtained to date have been derived from studies in which the injured nerve has been either actively prevented from regenerating into the distal stump, or the conditions for such regeneration have been poor, such as when resection of several millimeters or more has been made. These two types of experiments are discussed initially, followed by a discussion of the changes after nerve crush. The experiments on which this presentation is based have been made mainly on rats, but to some extent also on cats, guinea pigs, and monkeys.

Short-Term Changes in Sensory Ganglion Cells

The response of sensory ganglion cells and their immediate environment in a short-term perspective includes (a) reorganization of the perikaryal metabolism, (b) morphological changes in the central projection territory, and (c) changes in the central synaptic transmission.

---

* This research was supported by the Swedish Medical Research Council (Project 5420) and by grants from the Karolinska Institute and the Åke Wibergs Foundation.

The main priorities of an axotomized neuron is to survive and to support and promote the outgrowth of a new axon. In line with these objectives, significant changes have been described in the synthesis of RNA and the enzymes involved in RNA metabolism (Austin and Langford 1980; Sjöberg and Kanje 1987). Fast axonal transport of proteins includes a number of new components in a molecular weight range (Redshaw and Bisby, 1985) that suggests a relationship to the so-called growth-associated proteins (Skene and Willard 1981). The rate of slow axonal transport is elevated and the amounts of actin and tubulin increased, while neurofilament protein levels are decreased (for review see McQuarrie 1983). This seems to be an adequate alteration since the newly formed sprouts and elongating axons have a high content of actin-containing microfilaments and microtubules.

While these growth-promoting changes are initiated, the production of substances involved in, or thought to be involved in, neural conduction and transmission are reduced. Thus, substance P is markedly reduced in sensory ganglia after axotomy and almost completely depleted in the superficial portion of the dorsal horn where the substance P containing primary afferent fibers terminate (Jessell et al. 1979). Interestingly, a similar observation has been made in a human autopsy case in which a limb amputation had been made (Hunt et al. 1982). Two enzymes which are present in different populations of sensory ganglion cells are fluoride-resistant acid phosphatase (FRAP) and carbonic anhydrase. These enzymes are normally synthesized in ganglion cell perikarya, transported into their processes, and presumed to play a role in the process of impulse conduction and/or synaptic transmission. Following peripheral nerve injury this is manifested as a reduced staining for FRAP in sensory ganglia as well as a depletion of FRAP in the substantia gelatinosa (Knyihar-Csillik and Csillik 1981). Similarly, staining for carbonic anhydrase is reduced in sensory ganglia and in the dorsal column where the central processes of many carbonic anhydrase positive ganglion cells are ascending (Peyronnard et al. 1986).

Another change which might be regarded as a result of a diminished emphasis on synaptic transmission is the reduction in opiate binding in the spinal cord dorsal horn (Fields et al. 1980), presumably reflecting a reduced synthesis of opiate receptors. Since the current notion is that these receptors are localized to terminals of C and A fibers, this reduction appears to be an event in the primary sensory neuron.

The changes may be a consequence not only of a reordering of metabolic priorities in the injured neurons but also of degenerative changes which have been shown to occur in the central termination area of the axotomized neurons (for review see Aldskogius et al. 1985). These degenerative changes have been shown with two independent techniques, the so-called suppressive silver stains and electron microscopy. Axons and axon terminals undergoing certain degenerative changes display a marked affinity for silver ions following oxidative treatment of the tissue sections. The result appears as black or dark brown granules, globules, and irregular fiberlike segments. Using this method, degeneration argyrophilia has been demonstrated in the deeper laminae of the spinal cord dorsal horn and in the dorsal column nuclei (Arvidsson et al. 1986), i.e., in areas where A fibers constitute the main (spinal cord) or only (dorsal column nuclei) primary afferent input. Ultrastructural changes have been described in the dorsal column nuclei and substantia gelatinosa. In the former, axons and axon terminals display marked swellings, which contain large amounts of tubular and vesicular profiles as well as dense bodies, which frequently appear as whorl-like structures (Persson et al. 1987). In the substantia gelatinosa two different types of changes have been reported – a gradual darkening of the axoplasm with retention of synaptic vesicle profiles (Csillik and Knyihar-Csillik 1981) and a depletion of synaptic vesicles leading to the appearance of "empty-looking" terminals. Some of these terminals seem to disappear eventually (Castro-Lopes et al. 1987).

In addition to these neuronal changes it is now also clear that changes in glial cells are in early and significant component of the reaction of primary sensory neurons to peripheral axotomy. Microglial cell numbers increase in superficial as well as deep layers of the spinal cord (Cova et al., in preparation), and astrocytes show signs of hypertrophy, as evidenced by increased immunocytochemical staining for glial fibrillary acidic protein (Gilmore and Leiting 1984). The implications of these alterations are unknown, but the participation in phagocytosis of degenerating neuronal profiles is one possible function (see Arvidsson 1986). Ultrastructural studies have described the appearance of concentric multilayered glial cell (probably astrocytic) processes surrounding what might be axonal elements, which do not seem to be in a state of irreversible degeneration (Knyihar-Csillik and Csillik 1981). This finding suggests the possibility that glial cells are actively involved in a disconnection of pre- and postsynaptic elements in some areas of the spinal cord after peripheral nerve injury.

Long-Term Changes in Sensory Ganglion Cells

One of the most significant consequences of sensory nerve injury is the occurrence of a substantial amount of nerve cell death in sensory ganglia, being in the range of 15%–30% of the total population of neurons in the affected ganglia (for review see Aldskogius et al. 1985; see also Arvidsson et al. 1986; Rich et al. 1987). In most cases the counts made include a population of cells not affected by the injury; for example, counts of L4–L5 ganglion cells in the rat after sciatic neurotomy also include cells with uninjured axons in lumbar dorsal rami and the saphenous nerve. Therefore, the figures just mentioned are likely to be underestimations of the "true" relative cell loss among the actually lesioned ganglion cell population.

This loss of ganglion neurons is obviously important to consider in relation to the central changes, which were described above. The central processes of dying ganglion cells will inevitably disintegrate. However, to what extent the degenerative or regressive changes in central axons and terminals are features of surviving neurons is unknown. A relevant piece of information in this context would be the time course of the cell death. Unfortunately, available data are somewhat inconsistent on these two points. Cell death was reported maximal at 3 weeks after sciatic neurotomy in one study (Rich et al. 1987) but to continue for at least 2 months in another, similar study (Arvidsson et al. 1986). At the thoracic level cell loss was found to begin 20 days after intercostal nerve transection and to continue for an additional period of about 1 month (Ygge and Aldskogius 1984). Thus, it would appear that the short-term central changes, including the central depletion of neuropeptides, FRAP and carbonic anhydrase as well as the non-neuronal changes, are manifest prior to the stage when cell death is established. In the light of these findings, one might interpret the initial central changes as being independent of nerve cell death, and the long-term ones as caused by cell death and a prolongation of the initial changes consequential upon lack of successful peripheral reinnervation.

Another aspect of importance in this context is whether the cell loss selectively affects certain neuronal type(s). The principal approach to resolve this issue has been to determine the distribution of ganglion perikaryal sizes in control and experimental ganglia and to analyze the fiber population in control and experimental dorsal roots. These analyses show that no selective loss in terms of ganglion cell size or dorsal root axon type appears to occur (Aldskogius et al. 1985). In the future, the possibility of using chemical ganglion cell markers might provide additional insights into this issue. Although the data available today indicate that cell death occurs evenly throughout the different ganglion cell populations, we must bear in mind that a differential response could exist within a set of ganglion cells which have so far been grouped together only on the basis of size.

Transsynaptic Changes

Peripheral axonal injury is accompanied by marked changes in central synaptic transmission. These include a decrease in so-called primary afferent depolarization (Horch and Lisney 1981), an expansion of receptive fields related to surrounding, uninjured nerves (Devor 1983; Markus et al. 1984), and a reduction in the A fiber mediated central inhibition (Woolf and Wall 1982). These changes are discussed in the chapter by Woolf in this volume. While these physiological changes are likely to have a presynaptic component, as judged by the extensive alterations described in previous sections, there is clearly also at least functional postsynaptic aspects. So far, however, clear evidence for morphological changes in second-order neurons are lacking.

Role of the Distal Stump and Trophic Factors

When comparing the effects after peripheral nerve transection, with or without deliberate prevention of peripheral reinnervation, with peripheral nerve crush, where regeneration and reinnervation is effective, important differences emerge. Thus, following crush, depletion of substance P in the dorsal horn is minimal (McGregor et al. 1984), and the marked physiological changes described above are absent (Wall and Devor 1981). FRAP in substantia gelatinosa does disappear, however, and reports of ultrastructural changes rather similar to those after nerve transection have been described in this area as well. A significant feature of the crush lesion is, however, that the enzyme in question returns after peripheral reinnervation has occurred, and the ultrastructure of the substantia gelatinosa is reported to become normal (Knyihar-Csillik and Csillik 1981). These findings clearly suggest a potential for the sensory ganglion cells to revert to normal, provided peripheral regeneration is functionally effective. However, there are other aspects to the reaction of sensory ganglion cells to crush regarding which we have no information at the present time. Therefore, it is not possible to state whether the entire system is normalized after this type of lesion.

The described differences between transection and crush become clear within a few days or weeks after the injury. Therefore, it is obvious that it is not reinnervation of the peripheral target which forms the basis for this difference but either the lesion itself or the distal stump, which is reached by the sprouting axons very rapidly after a crush. Recent data on changes in the expression of mRNA for nerve growth factor (NGF) and content of NGF in axotomized nerves, as well as experiments with the administration of exogenous NGF to axotomized sensory ganglion cells, provide evidence for the importance of the distal stump. Soon after axonal injury non-neuronal cells in the distal stump and in the most distal part of the proximal stump begin to produce NGF (Heumann et al. 1987). NGF administered to the proximal stump of axotomized ganglion cells is able to prevent a number of the changes described above, such as depletion of FRAP and substance P, the receptive field expansion (Fitzgerald et al. 1985), and the ganglion cell death (Rich et al. 1987). Thus, it appears that exogenous NGF creates a condition which strongly mimics that which meets the outgrowing axons after a crush.

A most important question arising from these findings is whether the transection-induced degenerative and regressive changes can be prevented or reversed by early nerve repair, a procedure which might bring the regenerating axons in rapid contact with NGF-producing cells in the distal stump or in a graft. Along the same line, it would seem from these findings that a delay in the interaction between the regrowing axons and the environment of the distal stump might lead to irreversible changes, such as ganglion cell death and central degeneration.

The Possibility of Central "Regeneration"

As described above, crushing the nerve appears to be followed by restoration of many of the initial central effects, such as return of staining for FRAP and substance P in the dorsal horn, and a reversal of previously altered primary sensory terminals to a normal state (Knyihar-Csillik and Csillik 1981). The normalization of dorsal horn chemistry could easily be explained by a resumption of perikaryal synthesis and axonal transport of the substances in questions. A morphological recovery, as suggested by some ultrastructural findings, will of course require at least some limited process of growth. The capacity for sensory ganglion cells to express growth of their central process is indicated in experiments where a peripheral nerve graft was implanted into the injured dorsal column in order to stimulate the lesioned ascending primary sensory processes to extend into the graft (Richardson and Issa 1984). Significant ingrowth into the graft occurred only by ganglion cells in which the peripheral process had been injured as well, suggesting that a peripheral nerve lesion – under certain conditions – could uncover a central growth potential. To elucidate this possible potential nerve injuries might be of great importance for the development of new directions in the treatment of peripheral nerve injuries.

Summary and Conclusions

Following peripheral nerve transection a significant number of neurons in the affected sensory ganglia are lost. It is presently not quite clear whether this cell loss is in any way selective with regard to the morphological and/or functional type of neuron. The cell loss is accompanied – and perhaps even preceded – by degenerative axonal alterations and glial cell changes in central termination areas of the injured neurons. Concomitantly with these morphological changes, alterations take place in central synaptic transmission. The precise correlations between the morphological and physiological changes are not yet determined. Lesions which allow the regenerating axons to gain rapid access to the distal stump – such as crushing the nerve – prevent at least some of the central changes. Likewise, administration of NGF to the proximal stump of the lesioned nerve prevents ganglion cell death and at least some of the central changes. It is still an open question, however, whether central degeneration might occur without ganglion cell death.

The central changes may be viewed as opening up a possibility for some central reorganization after peripheral nerve injury. It is not clear, however, to what extent such a reorganization might occur, and whether it would be useful for the individual. Preventing degenerative changes – and in particular the loss of ganglion cells – might be more useful in a long-term perspective. In this respect, attempts to aid the injured axons to interact effectively with Schwann's cells which have recently lost axonal contact, such as those in the distal stump or a graft, appear to be a logical measure.

Acknowledgements. Secretarial assistance was provided by Ms. Siv Blomquist and Ms. Marianne Rapp.

References

Aldskogius H, Arvidsson J, Grant G (1985) The reaction of primary sensory neurons to peripheral nerve injury with particular emphasis on transganglionic changes. Brain Res 10:27–46

Arvidsson J (1986) Transganglionic degeneration in vibrissae innervating primary sensory neurons of the rat: a light and electron microscopic study. J Comp Neurol 249:392–403

Arvidsson J, Ygge J, Grant G (1986) Cell loss in lumbar dorsal root ganglia and transganglionic degeneration after sciatic nerve resection in the rat. Brain Res 373:15–21

Austin L, Langford CJ (1980) Nerve regeneration: a biochemical view. Trends in Neurosci, May:130–132

Castro-Lopes JM, Coimbra A, Grant G (1987) Ultrastructural changes of primary afferent endings in the spinal cord substantia gelatinosa during transganglionic degeneration. Neurosci 22:S713

Csillik B, Knyihar-Csillik, E (1981) Regenerative synaptogenesis in the mammalian spinal cord: dynamics of synaptochemical restoration in the Rolando substance after transganglionic degenerative atrophy. J Neural Transm 53:303–317

Devor M (1983) Plasticity of spinal cord somatotopy in adult mammals: involvement of relatively ineffective synapses. Birth Defects: Original Article Series 19:287–314

Fields HL, Emson PC, Leigh BK, Gilbert RFT, Iversen LL (1980) Multiple opiate receptor sites on primary afferent fibres. Nature (Lond) 284:351–353

Fitzgerald M, Wall PD, Goedert M, Emson PE (1985) Nerve growth factor counteracts the neurophysiological effects of chronic sciatic nerve section. Brain Res 332:131–141

Gilmore SA, Leiting JE (1984) Immunostaining of astrocytes following sciatic axotomy. Anat Rec 208:61A

Heumann R, Korshing S, Bandtlow C, Thoenen H (1987) Changes of nerve growth factor synthesis in nonneuronal cells in response to sciatic nerve transection. J Cell Biol 104:1623–1631

Horch KW, Lisney SJW (1981) Changes in primary afferent depolarization of sensory neurones during peripheral nerve regeneration in the cat. J Physiol (Lond) 313:287–299

Hunt SP, Rossor MN, Emson PC, Clement-Jones V (1982) Substance P and enkephalins in spinal cord after limb amputation. Lancet 8279:1023

Jessell T, Tsunoo A, Kanawawa I, Otsuka M (1979) Substance P: depletion in the dorsal horn of rat spinal cord after section of the peripheral processes of primary sensory neurons. Brain Res 168:247–259

Knyihar-Csillik E, Csillik B (1981) FRAP: histochemistry of the primary nociceptive neuron. Progr Histochem Cytochem, Vol 14. G. Fischer, Stuttgart New York

Markus H, Pomeranz B, Krushelnycky D (1984) Spread of saphenous somatotopic projection map in spinal cord and hypersensitivity of the foot after chronic sciatic denervation. Brain Res 296:27–39

McGregor GP, Gibson SJ, Sabate IM, Blank MA, Christofides ND, Wall PD, Polak JM, Bloom SR (1984) Effect of peripheral nerve section and nerve crush on spinal cord neuropeptides in the rat: increased VIP and PHI in the dorsal horn. Neurosci 13:207–216

McQuarrie IG (1983) Role of the axonal cytoskeleton in the regenerating nervous system. In: Seil F (ed) Nerve, organ, and tissue regeneration. Academic Press, London New York, pp 51–88

Persson J, Arvidsson J, Aldskogius H (1987) Changes in dorsal root ganglion neurons projecting to the gracile nucleus after sciatic nerve transection in the rat. Neurosci 22:S251

Peyronnard JM, Messier A, Charron L, Lavoie J, Bergouignan FX, Dubreuil M (1986) Carbonic anhydrase activity in the normal and injured peripheral nervous system. Exp Neurol 93:481–499

Redshaw JD, Bisby MA (1985) Comparison of the effects of sciatic nerve crush or resection on the proteins of fast axonal transport in rat dorsal root ganglion cell axons. Exp Neurol 88:437–446

Rich KM, Luszczynski JR, Osborne PA, Johnson EM Jr (1987) Nerve growth factor protects adult sensory neurons from cell death and atrophy caused by nerve injury. J Neurocytol 16:261–268

Richardson PM, Issa VMK (1984) Peripheral nerve injury enhances central regeneration of primary sensory neurons. Nature (Lond) 309:791–793

Sjöberg J, Kanje M (1987) Incorporation of (32 P) phosphate into nucleoteides of the dorsal root ganglia of regenerating rat sciatic nerve. Brain Res 415:270–274

Skene JHP, Willard M (1981) Axonally transported proteins associated with axon growth in rabbit central and peripheral nervous system. J Cell Biol 89:96–103

Wall PD, Devor M (1981) The effect of peripheral nerve injury on dorsal root potentials and on transmission of afferent signals into the spinal cord. Brain Res 209:95–111

Woolf CJ, Wall PD (1982) Chronic peripheral nerve section diminishes the primary afferent A-fibre mediated inhibition of rat dorsal horn neurones. Brain Res 242:77–85

Ygge J, Aldskogius H (1984) Intercostal nerve transection and its effect on the dorsal root ganglion. A quantitative study on ganglion cell numbers and sizes. Exp Brain Res 55:402–408

Pathomorphology of Regenerating Peripheral Nerves

J. M. SCHRÖDER, Aachen/FRG

Regeneration of peripheral nerve fibers following various lesions (see Sunderland 1978) and restitution of peripheral nerve structure after severance of a nerve are followed by a number of changes. These are considered below.

Neuroma Formation

Following transection of a peripheral nerve, neuroma formation ensues. Neuromas are microscopically characterized by regenerating myelinated and unmyelinated nerve fibers that are oriented at random ("heteromorphous or neuromatous neurotisation," Hiller 1951) and grouped within small bundles, surrounded by a well-differentiated perineurial and epineurial connective tissue ("minifascicles," Schröder and Seiffert 1970). The perineurial cells are covered by a basement membrane and may be formed by fibroblasts, as has recently been shown by Bunge et al. (1987), who used viral markers for identifying either Schwann's cells or fibroblasts before adding them to tissue culture.

Neuromatous Type of Regeneration

A similar pattern of regeneration as in neuromas may be seen in nerve grafts when the original fascicles have become ischemic and fibrotic. A certain degree of neuroma formation is always seen at the proximal and distal site of a reinnervated nerve graft. Along the intermediate portion of the graft, however, the newly formed minifascicles are usually not oriented at random but may be arranged in a more regular proximodistal direction causing an "isomorphous" pattern of neuromatous neurotization (Schröder and Seiffert 1972).

Dimensions of Regenerated Nerve Fibers

The largest regenerated nerve fibers do not reach the dimensions of the largest normal nerve fibers. The difference was clearly apparent in regenerated nerve fibers distal to various autologous and homologous nerve grafts 18–24 months after implanting nerve grafts into sciatic nerves of dogs (Schröder and Seiffert

1972). The axons, however, reach better values than the myelin sheaths (Schröder 1972; Friede and Bischhausen 1980; Smith et al. 1982; Beuche and Friede 1985). Also, internodal lengths are reduced. The number of Schmidt-Lanterman incisures, on the other hand, increases compared to normal myelin sheaths of equal thickness. Two-dimensional reconstructions of myelin lamellae simultaneously illustrate changes of internodal length, number of myelin lamellae as counted on electron micrographs, and axonal perimeters, also measured on electron micrographs (Schröder 1974, 1987; Schröder et al. 1988). Three-dimensional reconstructions of bundles of regenerated nerve fibers from serial semithin and ultrathin sections revealed uneven myelination of subsequent internodes as well as defective myelination of presumably supernumerary axons that were myelinated in other planes of section (Schröder 1975).

Although we were able to study more than 1500 sural nerve biopsies we rarely had the chance to investigate successfully regenerated nerve fibers in human nerves following severance and subsequent nerve grafting or nerve suture. Usually these happened to be inefficient grafts or sutures at rather early stages of regeneration, i.e., several weeks or months after surgery, but not 1–2 years after the lesion representing the final state of regeneration. In one instance a child was autopsied at the age of 12.9 months after it had had a fascicular sural nerve biopsy (four fascicles) at the age of 3 months (Fig. 1). Reinnervation of the distal portion (Figs. 1d, 2d) is here shown in comparison to the biopsy (Figs. 1a, 2a), the contralateral normal side (Figs. 1b, 2b), and the proximal portion (Figs. 1c, 2c) of the sural nerve that had been biopsied further distally. Reinnervation was remarkably good (Figs. 1d, 2d) although neither the axonal calibers nor the myelin sheaths of the largest regenerated nerve fibers reached the dimensions of the normal contralateral nerve (Figs. 1b, 2b) of the same individual. The presence of some preexisting fibers however, cannot be excluded since a fascicular, not a complete biopsy had been performed. This confirms our earlier findings in dogs and rats that large nerve fibers do not reach the proportions seen in large normal nerves. The regression line for the ratio between axonal perimeter and the number of myelin lamellae as measured on electron micrographs, however, did not deviate significantly from that in the contralateral control although there was considerably more scatter among values. Correspondingly, the correlation coefficient was lower in the reinnervated than in the normal nerve ($r = 0.62$ versus 0.87, respectively) as well as in the previous biopsy ($r = 0.82$), indicating increased variability between axon caliber and myelin sheath thickness.

At another rare occasion, we were able to study a human dorsal root ganglion following trauma of the brachial plexus with root avulsion about 3 months after the lesion. The ganglion cells were well preserved. Distal nerve fiber regeneration at this early stage appeared to be unimpaired although there was no connection of neurons to the spinal cord, i.e., to the central nervous system (Schröder 1985).

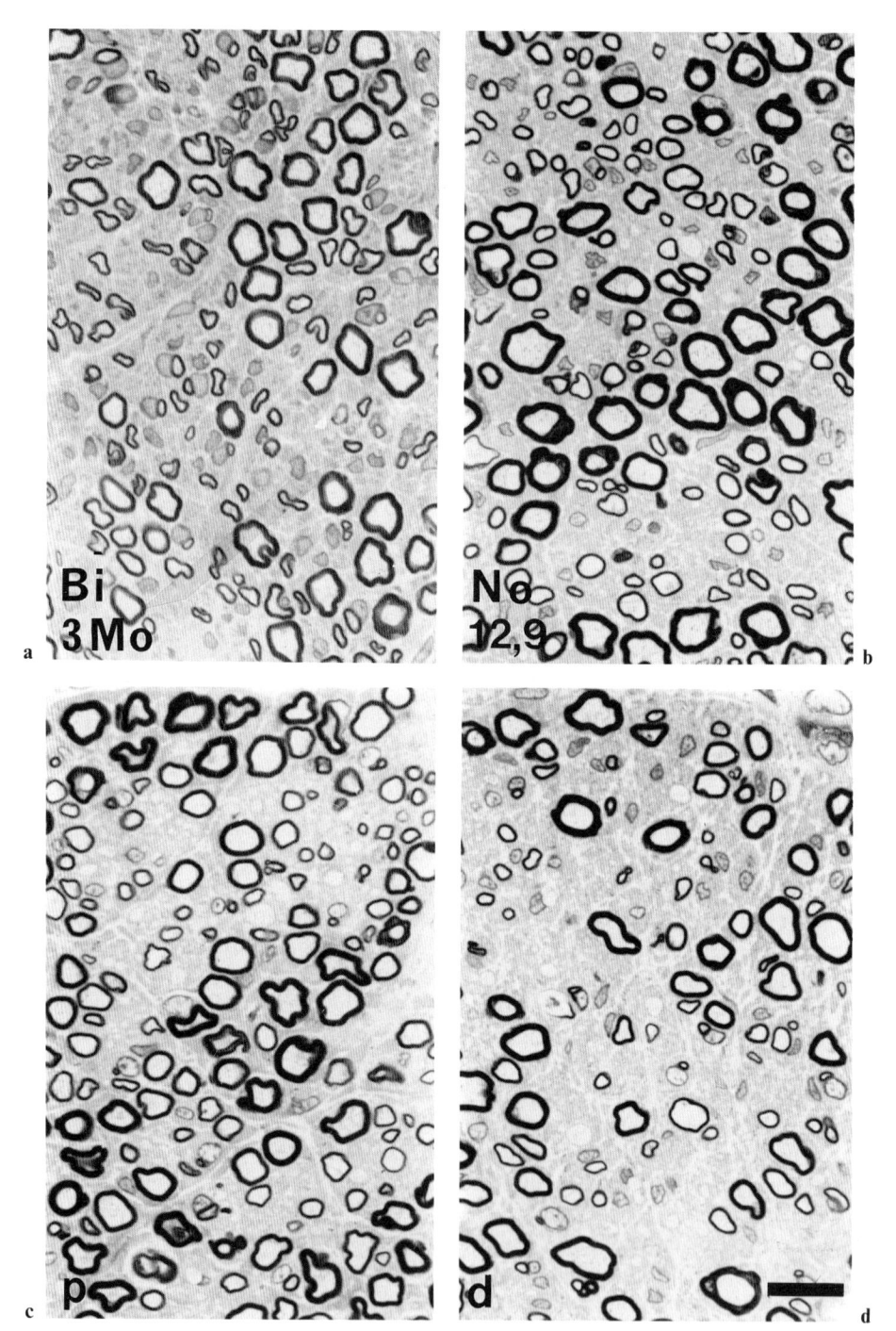

Fig. 1. a Sural nerve biopsy in a 3-month-old boy. **b** Contralateral sural nerve at autopsy of the same patient, then at the age of 12.9 months. Reinnervated nerve (**c**) proximal and (**d**) distal to the site of the biopsy, both also at autopsy. Morphometric data concerning these nerve portions are illustrated in Fig. 2. *Bar*, 27 µm

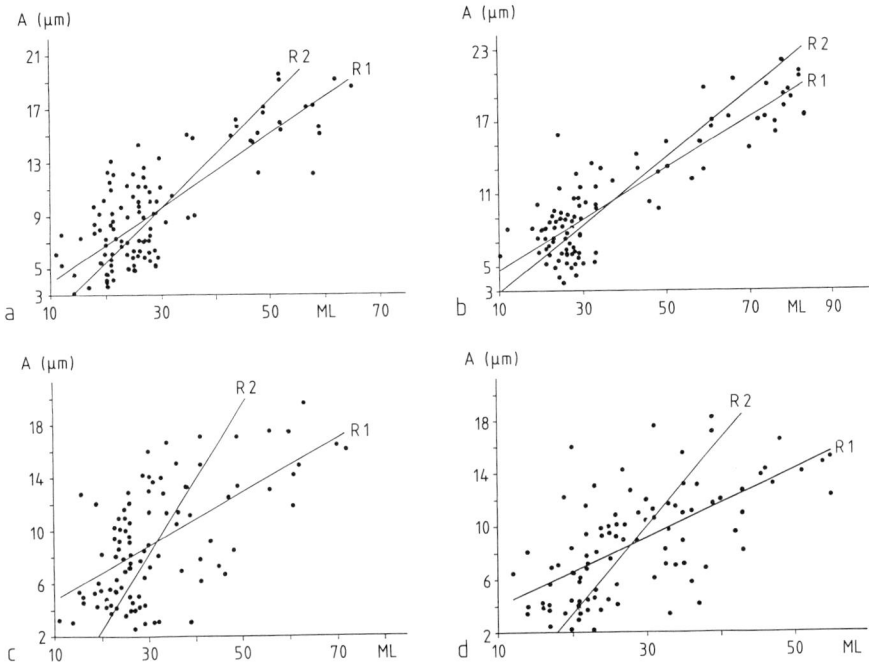

Fig. 2a–d. Measurements of axonal perimeters (A in μm at the oridinate) in relation to counts of the number of myelin lamellae (ML at the abscissa) of the sural nerve segments illustrated in Fig. 1. The diagrams are arranged in the same sequence as in Fig. 1, yet the scaling of axonal and myelin values is different in each diagram. Axonal perimeters and number of myelin lamellae in the reinnervated nerve (**d**) are significantly smaller at a probability of 95% than the values in the contralateral control nerve (**b**). In addition, there is considerably more scatter of individual values around the regression line in the regenerated than in the control nerve. Nevertheless, the corresponding regression lines which were calculated both for the x/y ($R1$) and the y/x ($R2$) relationships do not differ significantly

Retrograde Fiber Atrophy and Degeneration

Nerve fibers proximal to inefficient long (8.5–10.0 cm) homologous grafts 6 months after surgery showed a characteristic pattern of retrograde atrophy: axonal perimeter and myelin sheath thickness appeared to be rather normal, but the axonal cross sectional areas were severely reduced (Schröder and Müller 1982; Schröder 1987). This had been studied morphometrically also by Dyck et al. (1981). But the essential finding was already apparent from earlier light microscopic measurements of axonal caliber and myelin sheath thickness in the largest nerve fibers proximal to sciatic nerve grafts in dogs (Schröder and Seiffert 1972). The circularity of axons was reduced; it was also noted, thus confirming observations of others, that in normal nerve fibers circularity is lower in smaller than in larger nerve fibers.

Proximal to an amputation neuroma, 42 years after leg amputation following a traffic accident at the age of 4 years, there was not only axonal atrophy but almost total loss of large nerve fibers, with only some small regenerated myelinated nerve fibers remaining (Schröder 1985). This confirms the observation of Kawamura and Dyck (1981) on the loss of motor neurons following permanent axotomy by amputation.

Sectorial, Presumably Ischemic Necrosis

There was conspicuous change in occasional proximal nerve stumps after surgery, i.e., sectorlike areas with loss of large nerve fibers comprising small regenerated fibers only. This change was thought to be caused by focal traumatic arterial occlusion and incomplete microinfarcts immediately proximal to the site of transection of the nerve trunk with subsequent regeneration after restoration of blood supply.

Surgical Maneuvers to Prevent Neuroma Formation

To prevent neuroma formation and other complications seen in central portions of transected peripheral nerves surgical maneuvers have been proposed, such as centro-central anastomosis (Samii 1981). Similar reflection of a nerve into or through itself was initially performed by Bardenheuer as early as in 1908 (see Guttmann and Medawar 1942). We reinvestigated this method experimentally in rats and found very little evidence for endoneurial innervation of proximal stumps (Schröder 1985). The nerve fiber bundles deviated laterally. Some small regenerated nerve fibers more proximally were obviously caused by preexisting fibers degenerating and regenerating within the proximal stump. Since fat tissue showed strong inhibitory effects on regenerating nerve fibers in regeneration chambers (Weis and Schröder 1989a) we studied the effect of fat tissue on neuroma formation in sciatic nerves of rats in situ (Weis and Schröder 1989b). Neuroma formation could not be totally prevented, but the size of the neuromas appeared to be reduced (Weis and Schröder 1989b, and this volume).

Distal and Proximal Sites for Possible Functional Disturbances

In the peripheral sensory nervous system 12 different sites were defined where functional disturbances could occur following nerve lesions (Wall and Devor 1978). This includes alterations within the central nervous system (see Kreutzberg and Graeber, this volume) as well as changes at the motor endplates (e.g., collateral reinnervation and fiber type grouping). In addition, there may be changes in muscle spindles that are usually not considered as a source of functional disturbances following regeneration, although experimental reinnervation resulting in various abnormalities has been documented by light and electron microscopy (Schröder et al. 1979; Dieler and Schröder

1990). In man, however, following severance of peripheral nerves, reinnervation of muscle spindles is said not to occur (Struppler and Ochs, this volume).

It is well known that de-efferentation has severe effects on extrafusal muscle fibers. Yet deafferentation also results in some degree of atrophy, although to a much smaller extent (Bohl et al. 1981). Thus it is obvious that not only motor innervation is of importance in maintaining skeletal muscles. The afferent innervation via muscle spindles is also necessary for maintaining structural integrity, and this, presumably, comprises motor function and performance as well.

Acknowledgement. The assistance of Gerhard Braun in morphometric evaluation of nerve fibers illustrated in Fig. 1 is appreciated.

References

Bardenheuer E (1908) Behandlung der Nerven bei Amputationen zur Verhütung der Amputationsneurome und zur Heilung der bestehenden Neurome durch die sogenannte Neurinkampsis. Dtsch Z Chir 96:126–135

Beuche W, Friede RL (1985) A new approach toward analyzing peripheral nerve fiber populations. II. Foreshortening of regenerated internodes corresponds to reduced sheath thickness. J Neuropathol Exp Neurol 44:73–84

Bohl J, Wallenfang T, von Bardeleben U, Schröder JM (1981) Kapselveränderungen an experimentell denervierten Muskelspindeln. In: Fortschritte der Myologie, Bd VI. Gutenbergdruckerei; Freiburg i. Br. 199–209

Bunge MB, Sanes JR, Wood PM, Tynan LB, Bates ML (1987) The cellular source of perineurium determined with a retroviral marker. Abstract, p. 79 8th Meeting of the Lake Couchiching Peripheral Nerve Study Group, Orsillia, Ontario, Canada, August 24–27, 1987

Dieler R, Schröder JM (1990) Abnormal sensory and motor reinnervations of rat muscle spindles following nerve transection and suture. Acta Neuropathol (Berl): in press

Dyck PJ, Lais AC, Karnes JL, Sparks M, Hunder H, Low PA, Windebank AJ (1981) Permanent axotomy, a model of axonal atrophy and secondary segmental demyelination and remyelination. Ann Neurol 9:575–583

Friede RL, Bischhausen R (1980) The precise geometry of large internodes. J Neurol Sci 48:367–381

Guttmann L, Medawar PB (1942) The chemical inhibition of fibre regeneration and neuroma formation in peripheral nerves. J Neurol Psychiat 5:130–141

Hiller F (1951) Nerve regeneration in grafts. J Neuropathol Clin Neurol 1:5–25

Kawamura Y, Dyck PJ (1981) Permanent axotomy by amputation results in loss of motor neurons in man. J Neuropathol Exp Neurol 40:658–666

Samii M (1981) Centrocentral anastomosis of peripheral nerves: A neurosurgical treatment of amputation neuromas. In: Siegfried J, Zimmermann M (eds) Phantom and Stump Pain. Springer, Berlin Heidelberg New York, 123–125

Schröder JM (1972) Altered ratio between axon diameter and myelin sheath thickness in regenerated nerve fibers. Brain Res 45:49–65

Schröder JM (1974) Two-dimensional reconstruction of Schwann cell changes following remyelination of regenerated nerve fibers. In: Hausmanova-Petrusewicz I, Jedrzejowska H (eds) Proceedings of the symposium on structure and function of normal and diseased muscle and peripheral nerve, in Kazimierz upon Vistula, Poland, May 18–20. Polish Medical Publ, pp 299–304

Schröder JM (1975) Quantitative evaluation of regenerated nerve fibers. In: Kunze K, Desmedt JE (eds) Studies on neuromuscular diseases. Proceedings of the international symposium on quantitative methods of investigations in the clinic of neuromuscular diseases. Gießen, April 8–10, 1973. Karger, Basel, pp 206–210

Schröder JM (1985) Degeneration und Regeneration nach Plexus-brachialis-Verletzungen. In: Hase U, Reulen H-J (Hrsg) Läsionen des Plexus brachialis. De Gruyter, Berlin New York, 65–70

Schröder JM (1987) Pathomorphologie der peripheren Nerven. In: Neundörfer (Hrsg.) Polyneuritiden und Polyneuropathien. In: Neundörfer B, Schirmig K, Soyka D (Hrsg) Praktische Neurologie, Bd 2 Edition Medizin VCH, Weinheim, 11–104

Schröder JM, Müller E (1982) Fine structural morphometric evaluation of secondary myelin changes in retrograde axonal atrophy. Abstract. Arch. Suisses de Neurologie, Neurochirurgie et de Psychiatrie 131:254

Schröder JM, Seiffert KE (1970) Die Feinstruktur der neuromatösen Neurotisation von Nerventransplantaten. Virch Arch Abt B Zellpath 5:219–235

Schröder JM, Seiffert KW (1972) Untersuchungen zur homologen Nerventransplantation. Morphologische Ergebnisse. Zbl Neurochir 53:103–118

Schröder JM, Kemme PT, Scholz L (1979) The fine structure of denervated and reinnervated muscle spindles: morphometric study of intrafusal muscle fibers. Acta neuropathol (Berl) 46:95–106

Schröder JM, Bohl J, von Bardeleben U (1988) Changes of the ratio between myelin thickness and axon diameter in human developing sural, femoral, ulnar, facial and trochlear nerves. Acta Neuropathol (Berl) 76:471–483

Smith KJ, Blakemore WF, Murray JA, Patterson RC (1982) Internodal myelin volume and axon surface area. J Neurol Sci 55:231–245

Sunderland S (1978) Nerves and nerve injuries. 2nd edn. Churchill Livingstone, Edinburgh London New York, p 1046

Wall PD, Devor M (1978) Physiology of sensation after peripheral nerve injury, regeneration, and neuroma formation. In: Waxmann SG (ed) Physiology and pathobiology of axons. Raven Press, New York, pp 377–388

Weis J, Schröder JM (1989a) Differential effects of nerve, muscle, and fat tissue on regenerating nerve fibers in vivo. Muscle & Nerve 12:723–734

Weis J, Schröder JM (1989b) The influence of fat tissue on neuroma formation. J Neurosurg 71:588–593

Role of Neurotrophic Factors in Peripheral Nerve Regeneration

D. Lindholm and H. Thoenen, Martinsried/FRG

A peripheral nerve injury leads to a number of changes in the metabolism of the injured neurons and of the non-neuronal cells surrounding their axons. Some of these changes are directly related to the trauma itself and occur rapidly in the non-neuronal cells close to the site of injury; others are characteristic of neurons which depend on a proper interaction with their target for their normal function. Thus, a nerve transection interrupts the axoplasmic transport which carries molecular information from the periphery to the centrally located neuronal cell body and can result in nerve atrophy and ultimately in death of specific populations of neurons. In this context, neurotrophic factors providing trophic support play an essential role in counteracting the deleterious effects of the nerve injury.

Neurotrophic factors are proteins which regulate the survival of specific types of neurons during limited periods of development. They also influence the differentiation of these neurons and maintain their specialized functions, for example, regulating synthesis of enzymes involved in transmitter production (Thoenen and Edgar 1985). Of the many factors described, nerve growth factor (NGF) is by far the best characterized neurotrophic molecule whose physiological role is well established (Thoenen and Barde 1980; Levi-Montalcini 1987). That NGF regulates the survival and differentiation of peripheral sympathetic and neural crest derived sensory neurons was shown using neutralizing anti-NGF antibodies administered into neonatal animals, which led to the degeneration of the responsive neurons (Levi-Montalcini 1987). Surgical (peripheral nerve transection) and chemical (e.g., colchicine treatment) interruption of the retrograde transport of NGF produced similar changes in the sympathetic and some sensory neurons, showing that NGF acts as a retrogradely transported signal from the periphery. Naturally occurring cell death in the developing nervous system is regarded as a normal process resulting from the competition by a surplus of neurons for a limiting quantity of trophic molecules produced in the target tissues. Moreover, the results of recent studies have shown that NGF also affects central cholinergic neurons of the basal forebrain nuclei (Korsching 1986; Thoenen et al. 1987).

In the adult animal NGF is required for the maintenance of specialized functions of the mature sympathetic and of some sensory neurons in the dorsal root ganglia (DRG). Thus, NGF regulates the synthesis of enzymes which are involved in production of neurotransmitters, such as tyrosine hydroxylase and dopamine β-hydroxylase in sympathetic neurons and substance P in some sensory neurons (Otten 1984; Thoenen et al. 1987). Although mature DRG sensory neurons respond to NGF under normal circumstances, they do not seem to depend on NGF for their survival (Johnson et al. 1986). Moreover, only a part of adult sensory neurons (about 50%; Lindsay 1988) contain high-affinity receptors for NGF, which are thought to mediate the biological effect of NGF on target cells (Sutter et al 1979; Riopelle et al. 1987). However, it has been shown that a long-lasting deficiency of NGF (such as in the autoimmune model for NGF deprivation; see Johnson et al. 1986) results in a marked atrophy and possibly degeneration of the adult, fully mature sympathetic neurons. Available data also indicate that a peripheral axotomy, for example, of the sciatic nerve, results in a small but significant decrease (15%–30%) in the number of adult DRG neurons within 1 month after the lesion (Aldskogius et al. 1985; Rich et al. 1987).

In contrast to the extent of our knowledge of the distribution and physiological function of NGF in the peripheral nervous system, relatively little is known as to how NGF synthesis is regulated during development or under pathophysiological conditions. It has recently been shown that an axotomy of the rat sciatic nerve results in a dramatic increase in NGF production by the non-neuronal cells, suggesting an important role for endogenous NGF in nerve regeneration (Heumann et al. 1987a). The increase in NGF messenger RNA (NGF-mRNA) was maximally 15-fold in the nerve distal to the transection site and was accompanied by an appearance of NGF receptors on Schwann cells in the distal nerve segments (Taniuchi et al. 1986; Heumann et al. 1987b). In situ hybridization experiments revealed that all non-neuronal cells in the sciatic nerve (mainly Schwann cells and fibroblast-like cells) have the capability to synthesize NGF (Bandtlow et al. 1987).

Interestingly, proximal to the cut the changes were confined to the nerve segment adjacent to the transection site, which in a neuroma structure contains the regenerating axons. However, since the NGF protein level in the proximal segments reached only 40% of the control values, it is clear that the local production of NGF following the injury is too small to compensate fully for the lacking supply of NGF from the periphery (Heumann et al. 1987a). Moreover, previous studies have shown that the administration of exogenous NGF (applied locally to the sciatic nerve stump) ameliorates some of the neurochemical and neurophysiological alterations in adult DRG neurons observed after a nerve transection (Fitzgerald et al. 1985). It has recently been reported that the attachment of silicone tubes filled with NGF to the proximal nerve stump prevents nerve cell death in the lumbar DRG caused by a sciatic lesion (Rich et al. 1987; Otto et al. 1987). In these experiments it was also found that NGF partially counteracts the injury-induced neuronal atrophy in DRG, but that NGF has no effect on chromatolysis (Rich et al. 1987).

It is important to remember that sensory DRG neurons receive trophic support both from their peripheral and their central target fields, and that the factors involved are most probably different molecules. Thus, it has been shown that there is very little NGF in the spinal cord (see Thoenen et al. 1987), and that another molecule from the central nervous system, namely brain-derived neurotrophic factor, influences the survival of some early DRG cells (Kalcheim et al. 1987).

Comparing the changes in NGF-mRNA found in vivo following an axotomy with those observed in sciatic nerve segments placed into culture, it was found that activated macrophages are involved in the regulation of NGF synthesis (Heumann et al. 1987b). Moreover, interleukin 1 was identified as the responsible agent stimulating NGF-mRNA levels in the non-neuronal cells (Lindholm et al. 1987). Since macrophages are known to infiltrate the injured nerve following a peripheral nerve injury, they play an important role in nerve regeneration by stimulating NGF synthesis, which provides trophic support for the regenerating axons. It remains to be established whether following axotomy other neurotrophic factors are also produced by the non-neuronal cells. Previously it has been shown that the injured sciatic nerve contains other molecules than NGF (Richardson and Ebendal 1982), but their molecular characterization remains to be established. It would be very important to know whether molecules are present in the peripheral nerve which support motoneurons. Furthermore, the clinical use of NGF in various peripheral nerve injuries must also await the successful production of sufficient amounts of recombinant human NGF.

Acknowledgements. The authors wish to thank all their colleagues at the Department of Neurochemistry involved in the work discussed here. D.L. is a recipient of a fellowship from EMBO.

References

1. Aldskogius H, Arvidsson J, Grant G (1985) Brain Res Reviews 10:27–46
2. Bandtlow C, Heumann R, Schwab ME, Thoenen H (1987) EMBO J 6:891–899
3. Fitzgerald M, Wall PD, Goedert M, Emson PC (1985) Brain Res 332:131–141
4. Heumann R, Korsching S, Bandtlow C, Thoenen H (1987a) J Cell Biol 104:1623–1632
5. Heumann R, Lindholm D, Bandtlow C, Meyer M, Radeke MJ, Misko TP, Shooter E, Thoenen H (1987b) Proc Natl Acad Sci USA 84:8735–8739
6. Johnson EM, Rich KM, Yip HK (1986) Trends Neurosci 9:33–37
7. Kalcheim C, Barde Y-A, Thoenen H, Le Douarin NM (1987) EMBO J 2871–2873
8. Korsching S (1986) Trends Neurosci 9:570–573
9. Levi-Montalcini R (1987) EMBO J 6:1145–1154
10. Lindholm D, Heumann R, Meyer M, Thoenen H (1987) Nature 330:658–659
11. Lindsay R (1988) personal communication
12. Otten U (1984) Trends Pharmacol 7:307–310
13. Otto D, Unsicker K, Grothe C (1987) Neurosci Lett 83:156–159
14. Rich KM, Luszczynski JR, Osborne PA, Johnson EM (1987) J Neurocyt 16:261–268
15. Richardson PM, Ebendal T (1982) Brain Res 246:57–64
16. Riopelle RJ, Verge VMK, Richardson PM (1987) Mol Brain Res 3:39-43
17. Sutter A, Riopelle RJ, Harris-Warrick RM, Shooter EM (1979) J Biol Chem 254:5972–5982
18. Taniuchi M, Clark HB, Johnson EM (1986) Proc Natl Acad Sci USA 83:4094–4098
19. Thoenen H, Barde YA (1980) Physiol Rev 60:1284–1335
20. Thoenen H, Edgar D (1985) Science 229:238–242
21. Thoenen H, Bandtlow C, Heumann R (1987) Rev Physiol Biochem Pharmacol 109:145–178

Electrophysiological Changes Due to Motor Nerve Injury

H. C. Hopf, Mainz/FRG

The peripheral nerve lesions dealt with in clinical practice may be classified into four distinct categories: (a) block of impulse conduction without destruction of the axon, as observed in acute nerve compression; (b) axonal discontinuation followed by Wallerian degeneration due to nerve transection or severe traction of nerves; (c) axon stenosis, the common condition in entrapment neuropathies; and (d) double crush by two separate lesions at different levels, as may be found after nerve suture if the nerve is exposed to constriction by scar tissue. Electrophysiologically the reactions of motor nerves to such lesions cover a wide range of characteristic abnormalities that may be of diagnostic relevance. There is a well-defined basis for the coexistence of conduction block, slowing of conduction velocity, and axon degeneration in peripheral nerve compression (Gilliatt 1980). Precise analysis of each component is of clinical importance.

Significance of Conduction Block

Conduction block is usually estimated from the difference in amplitude of the evoked compound muscle response (ECMR) by comparing proximal and distal stimulation (Fig. 1). A decrease in the proximal response to below 69% of the distal response is thought to indicate conduction block by demyelination (Sedal et al. 1983). This may hold true for inflammatory neuritis of the Guillain-Barré type but obviously does not for entrapment neuropathy. Olney and Miller (1984) have shown that the area of the ECMR is a more reliable parameter than amplitude. Area better discriminates between response decreases due to conduction block and to slowing of conduction with temporal dispersion. The overestimation of conduction block measuring amplitude only may be up to 30%. Posttraumatic conduction block was reported to persist over 3–56 months (Miller and Olney 1982), and it may yet turn into axon degeneration (Perticoni and Mauro 1982), although most frequently full recovery is achieved. Distal to conduction block the nerve fibers conduct normally (Brown and Feasby 1984; Esslen 1977; Fig. 2). Conduction through a demyelinated region is regained before the axon is remyelinated but may remain slow indefinitely (Smith et al. 1982).

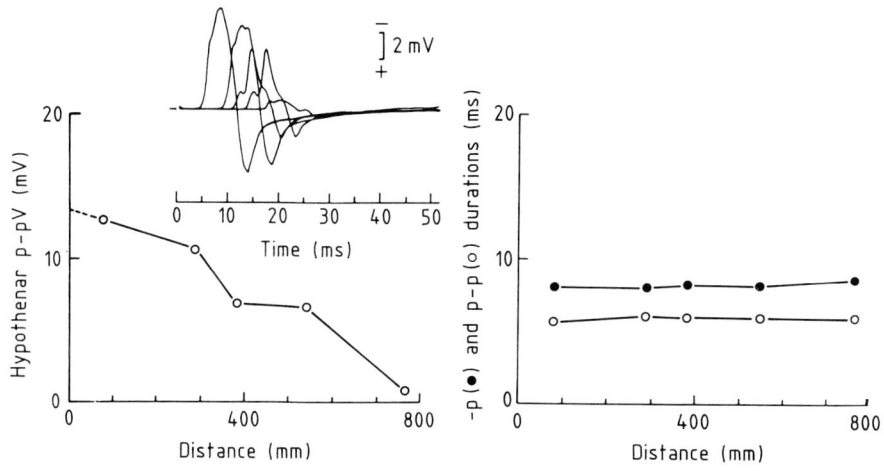

Fig. 1. Demonstration of conduction block in Guillain-Barré syndrom. *Left,* peak to peak amplitude $(p-pV)$ changes of the hypothenar muscle response elicited from wrist, distal cubital tunnel, proximal to elbow proximal upper arm, and Erb's point. *Inset,* the recorded potentials. *Right,* corresponding changes of the negative phase $(-p)$ and total potential $(p-p)$ duration. (From Brown and Feasby 1984)

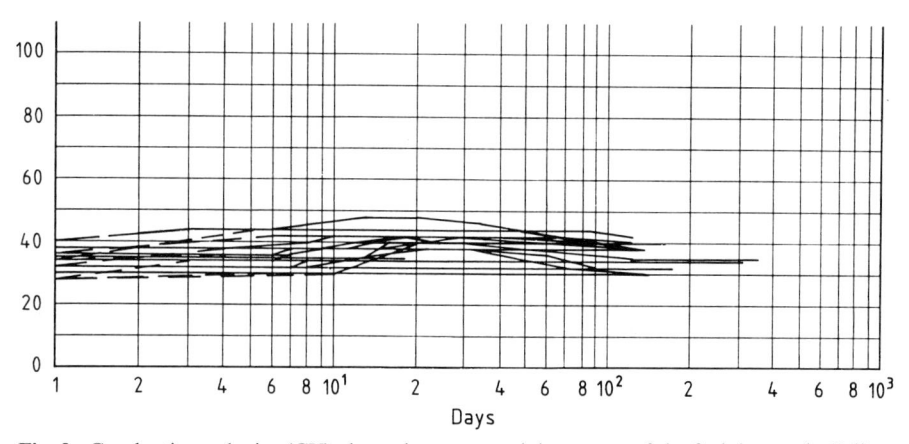

Fig. 2. Conduction velocity (CV) along the extracranial segment of the facial nerve in Bell's palsy with paralysis of facial muscles. CV (m/s) plotted against time (days). (From Esslen 1977)

Excitability and Impulse Conduction Following Axonotmesis

Wallerian degeneration after transection of the axon develops slowly. Regarding the distal axon segment the excitability ceases after approximately 2–4 days (Fig. 3). These changes coincidentally affect nerve divisions that are adjacent to (5–10 cm apart) or remote from (25–30 cm apart) the site of transection

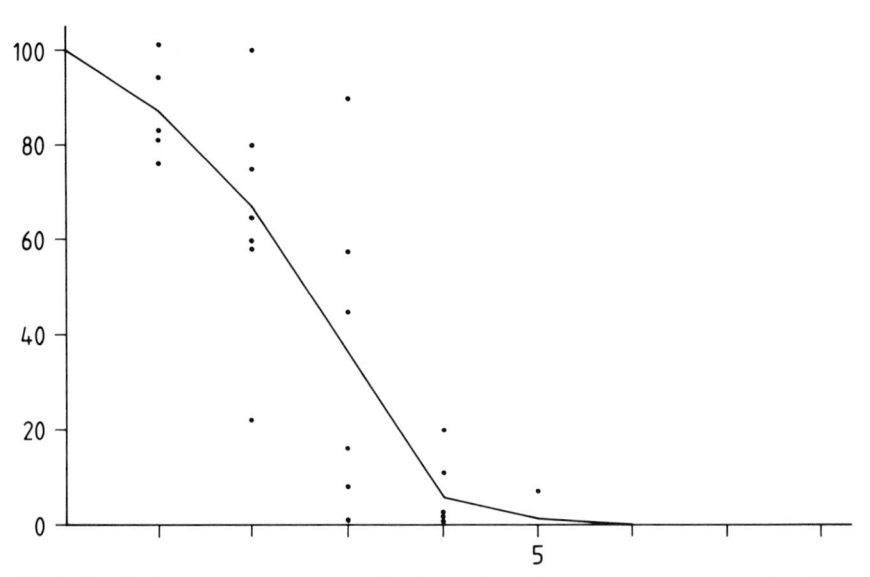

Fig. 3. Decline in motor response amplitude to stimulation below nerve transection. (From Gilliatt and Hjort 1972)

(Gilliatt and Hjort 1972). The ability of the separate axon segment to propagate action potentials remains unimpaired for a slightly longer period of 1–8 days (Rosenblueth and Dempsey 1939; Gutmann and Holubar 1950). During this time impulse conduction is kept at normal velocity (Gilliatt and Taylor; Fig. 4).

In vivo, motor nerves comprise a large number of axons. Thus, with incomplete nerve lesions the decrease in ECMR due to inexcitability of degenerating axons is related to the number of diseased axons (Bigland et al. 1953; Brown and Matthews 1959). In other words, the residual amplitude or area of the muscle response to nerve stimulation in vivo can be taken as a measure of the number of surviving axons (Esslen 1977). There is no difference in the muscle response whether the nerve is stimulated distally or proximally to a partial transection. In this respect such lesions behave differently from lesions causing conduction block, as was demonstrated above.

As a diagnostic aid, nerve stimulation was applied mainly to the facial nerve to predict the outcome of Bell's palsy. This procedure is called the nerve excitability test (Mamoli 1976) or the evoked electromyography (May et al. 1983). A decrease in the evoked response by up to 70% as compared to the contralateral side still indicates a good prognosis. The findings in Bell's palsy demonstrate that this condition in some aspects differs from uncomplicated nerve transection. In Bell's palsy the axons obviously do not expire simultaneously but within a range of several days. This can be concluded from the fact that in Bell's palsy the evoked response declines much more slowly than after transection (from day 2 to day 12; Fig. 5), suggesting a diphasic deterioration in individual cases (Esslen 1977). In addition, conduction velocity along the

Electrophysiological Changes Due to Motor Nerve Injury 35

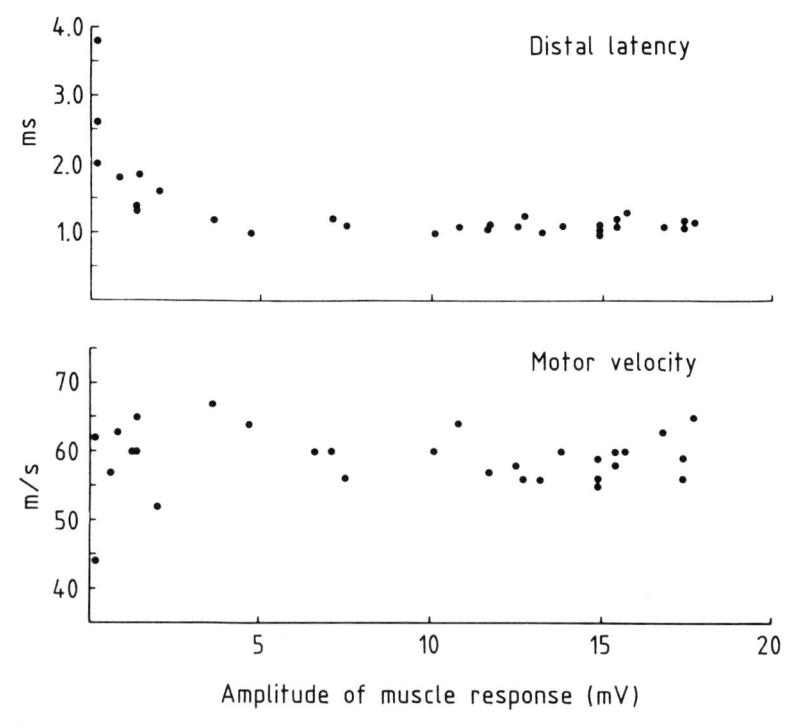

Fig. 4. Motor conduction velocity and distal latency on successive days after nerve section, plotted against amplitude of the evoked response. (From Gilliatt and Hjort 1972)

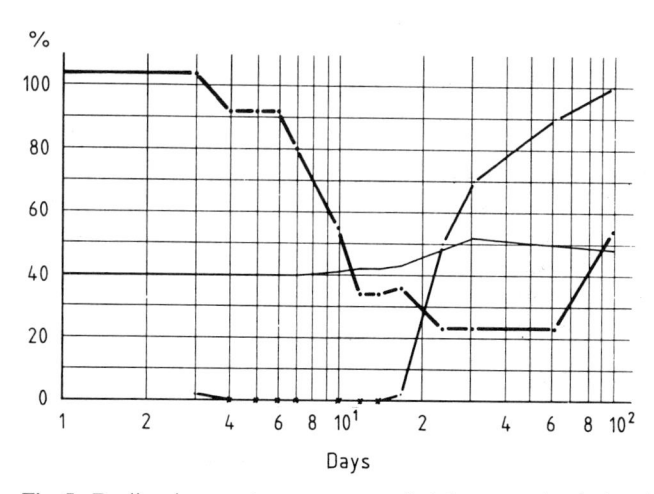

Fig. 5. Decline in muscle response to facial nerve stimulation in Bell's palsy from the beginning to recovery. *Thick line*, amplitude; *medium line*, estimated degree of innervation (in percentage); *thin line*, latency of muscle response (in ms). (From Esslen 1977)

segment below the lesion is definitely slowed in many cases of Bell's palsy, and the stimulus threshold is considerably increased (Olsen 1975; Esslen 1977).

Along the segment proximal to nerve transection conduction velocity decreases moderately. This decrease may be up to 10 m/s (for the 80% of maximum velocity fiber pool in cat tibial nerve; Milner and Stein 1981; Gillespie and Stein 1983). These electrophysiological changes are closely related to changes in axon diameter or circumference (Cragg and Thomas 1961; Arbuthnott et al. 1980; Gillespie and Stein 1983). They proceed more quickly, are more pronounced in fast fibers than in slow fibers, and progress over time, as has been shown over a period of 30 to almost 300 days postsurgery (Milner and Stein 1981). Conduction velocity of the proximal segment may recover completely in adults but possibly not in the growing subject (Cullheim et al. 1984). A significant loss of motor axons above transection was not observed (Carlson et al. 1979), and, as could be argued, muscle disuse per se does not cause a decline in conduction velocity of the supplying axons (Czeh et al. 1978). These figures, however, are from short-term observation.

After the nerve has been resutured, conduction velocity and axon diameter recover to a varying extent (see below: Davis et al. 1978; Milner and Stein 1981).

Effects of Axon Stenosis on Impulse Conduction

In man as well as in the animal, experimental long-standing compression or ligation of peripheral nerves causes damage of varying degree to fibers of different diameters. Regeneration of such compound nerves was found to be impaired only if many large myelinated fibers evolve to axon death and subsequent Wallerian degeneration (Baba et al. 1982). As in other types of nerve injury (Gilliatt 1981), part of the surviving fibers develop axon blocking at the site of ligation but recover after several days (Baba and Matsunaga 1984).

Propagation of impulse trains seems to be the most sensitive measure for detecting minor impairment of nerve function at the site of nerve stenosis (Jewett et al. 1985), like in other types of nerve disorder (Lowitzsch and Hopf 1973; Hopf and Lowitzsch 1974; Hopf and Eysholt 1978). Distal to nerve stenosis conduction velocity decreases progressively – by 17% after 1 week to 28% after 3 weeks (Baba et al. 1982). Again, the decrease is related to the reduction in axon diameter rather than to fiber diameter (Friede and Miyagishi 1972; Minwegen and Friede 1984). Proximal to nerve stenosis conduction velocity may also be slowed, depending on the number of severely diseased nerve fibers. The amount of slowing may be one-half of that found distal to nerve constriction (18% as compared to 33%; Baba et al. 1983).

Disorders of the vascular supply, which is a possible accompanying factor in human tunnel syndromes, results in focal conduction block and slowed impulse conduction of the ischemic region (Parry and Linn 1986).

Properties of Nerves Subjected to Double Crush

Double crush conditions occur frequently in peripheral nerve injuries. They have recently been studied in the rabbit. Severe continuing axon stenosis by ligation of the nerve trunk proximal to crush and preceding it by 1 week (Reiners et al. 1987) delays or inhibits recovery of impulse conduction, i.e.,

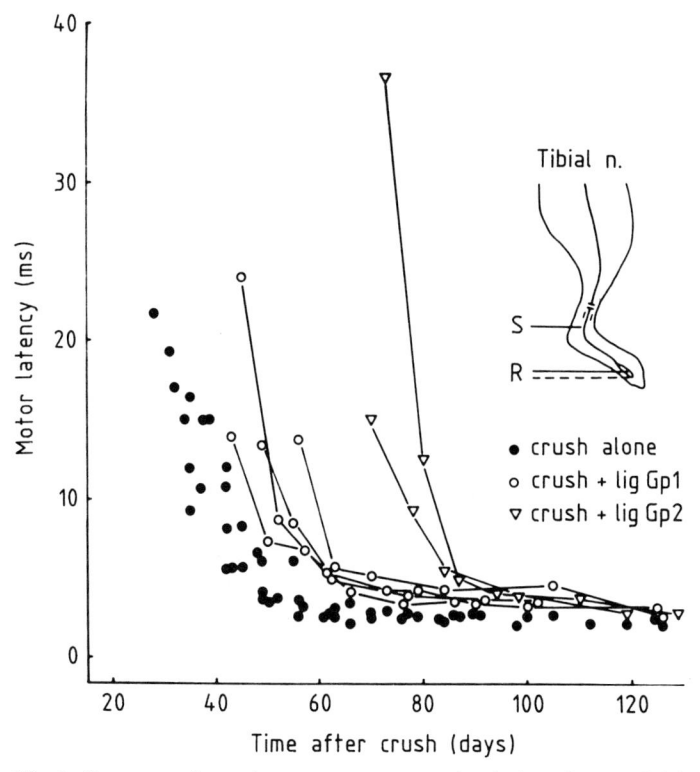

Fig. 6. Recovery of muscle response to nerve stimulation after crush (●) and after crush plus ligature of more (▽) and less (○) affected nerves. (From Krarup and Gilliatt 1985)

keeps the velocity at low levels. But after early relief from nerve constriction recovery is not delayed (Williams and Gilliatt 1977). If ligation is applied distal to nerve crush, impulse conduction is restored even later than with proximal ligation but once begun improves more rapidly than after crush alone (Krarup and Gilliatt 1985; Fig. 6). The evoked muscle response, however, remains at remarkably low aplitudes, which is difficult to explain. Preexisting neurotoxic influences act roughly in the same way as preexisting axon stenosis (Baba et al. 1984; Shiraishi et al. 1985).

Muscle Reactions to Nerve Injury

Regardless of disuse atrophy the muscle reacts only to interruption of the nerve-muscle continuity. Thus, only axon transection induces electrophysiological changes of skeletal muscle, not so conduction block or axon stenosis. Denervated muscle fibers show a decreased resting membrane potential (Ludin 1977), delayed rise in potassium membrane conductance, and fall in chloride conductance (Klaus et al. 1960; Bryant and Camerino 1976; Lorkovic and Tomanek 1977). Spontaneous rhythmic oscillations of the membrane potential (Li et al. 1957) are responsible for the generation of spontaneous muscle fiber discharging.

These changes following nerve transection occur with a delay which is roughly related to the distance between the site of transection and the muscle endplate (Luco and Eyzaguirre 1955). Correspondingly, spontaneous muscle fiber activity (muscle fiber action potentials) occurs 2–3 weeks after severe motor nerve lesions. There are two types of spontaneous muscle fiber discharges. Propagated muscle fiber action potentials which pass the recording electrode show a triphasic shape starting with a positive deflection; these are called fibrillations. If propagation of the muscle fiber potential stops at the site of the recording electrode, only a more or less monophasic positive deflection results; this discharge is called a positive sharp wave. Both fibrillation and positive waves discharge with rather constant frequency. The density on these two reflects the number of denervated muscle fibers.

Denervated muscle fibers slowly become atrophic. Impulse conduction along the fiber decreases (Buchthal and Rosenfalck 1958; Gruener et al. 1979), as with muscle atrophy of other origin (Hopf 1974) or with changes of contraction speed (Hopf et al. 1974). With numerical reduction of active motor units following axon degeneration the surviving units discharge at higher rates during voluntary contraction (Fuglsang-Frederiksen et al. 1987). Such changes are of diagnostic relevance, mainly in chronic neurogenic lesions.

Conclusions

The electrophysiological criterion of conduction block is definite reduction in the area of the ECMR to proximal as compared to distal stimulation. With axonotmesis conductivity along the distal segment is kept at normal velocity until axon death occurs after some days. Along the proximal nerve segment conduction velocity is moderately slowed. For diagnostic purposes it is important that with partial nerve lesions the amplitude and/or area of the ECMR is closely related to the number of surviving/conducting axons.

Axon stenosis due to nerve compression leads to slowing of conduction velocity below and above the lesion. However, the most sensitive measure for detecting diseased function at the stenosis is the propagation of impulse trains.

The electrophysiological muscle fiber changes following denervation are spontaneous rhythmic discharges and slowing of spike propagation in relation to the decrease in muscle fiber diameter. An increase in motor unit discharge rates is a sensitive measure of a decreased number of motor units within a given muscle.

References

1. Arbuthnott ER, Boyd IA, Kalu KU (1980) Ultrastructural dimensions of myelinated peripheral nerve fibres in the cat and their relation to conduction velocity. J Physiol (Lond) 308:125–157
2. Baba M, Fowler CJ, Jacobs JM, Gilliatt RW (1982) Changes in peripheral nerve fibres distal to a constriction. J Neurol Scien 54:197–208
3. Baba M, Gilliatt RW, Jacobs JM (1983) Recovery of distal changes after nerve constriction by a ligature. J Neurol Scien 60:235–246
4. Baba M, Gilliatt RW, Harding AE, Reiners K (1984) Demyelination following diphtheria toxin in the presence of axonal atrophy. J Neurol Scien 64:199–211
5. Baba M, Matsunaga M (1984) Recovery from acute demyelinating conduction block in the presence of prolonged distal conduction delay due to peripheral nerve constriction. Electromyogr Clin Neurphysiol 24:611–617
6. Bigland B, Hutter OF, Lippold OC (1953) Action potentials and tension in mammalian nerve-muscle preparations. Proc Physiol Soc 121:1–121
7. Brown MC, Matthews PBC (1959) A possible explanation of the different contraction of muscle produced by synchronous and asynchronous motor volleys. J Physiol (Lond) 150:27–28
8. Brown WF, Feasby TE (1984) Conduction block and denervation in Guillain-Barré polyneuropathy. Brain 107:219–239
9. Bryant SH, Camerino D (1976) Chloride conductance of denervated gastrocnemius fibers from normal goast. J Neurobiol 7:229–240
10. Buchthal F, Rosenfalck P (1958) Rate of impulse conduction in denervated human muscle. Electroenceph. Clin Neurophysiol 10:521–529
11. Carlson J, Lais A, Dyck PJ (1979) Axonal atrophy from permanent peripheral axotomy in adult cat. Neuropath Exo Neurol 38:579–585
12. Cragg BG, Thomas PK (1961) Changes in conduction velocity and fibre size proximal to peripheral nerve lesion. J Physiol (Lond) 157:315–327
13. Cullheim S, Risling M, Berglund S, Linda H (1984) Conduction velocities of nerve fibres proximal to muscle nerve transection in kittens and adult cats. Experimental Neurology 84:484–487
14. Czeh G, Gallego R, Kudo N, Kuno M (1978) Evidence for the maintenance of motoneurone properties by muscle activity. J Physiol (Lond) 281:239–252
15. Davis LA, Gordon T, Hoffer JA, Jhamandas J, Stein RB (1978) Compound action potentials recorded from mammalian peripheral nerves following ligation or resuturing. J Physiol 285:543–559
16. Esslen E (1977) The acute facial palsies. Springer, Berlin Heidelberg New York
17. Friede RL, Miyagishi T (1972) Adjustment of the myelin sheath to changes in axon caliber. Anat Rec 172:1–13
18. Fuglsang-Frederiksen A, Smith T, Hogenhaven H (1987) Motor unit firing intervals and parameters of electrical activity in normal and pathological muscle. J Neurol Scien 78:51–62
19. Gillespie MJ, Stein RB (1983) The relationship between axon diameter, myelin thickness and conduction velocity during atrophy of mammalian peripheral nerve. Brain Research 259:41–56
20. Gilliatt RW, Taylor JC (1959) Electrical changes following section of the facial nerve. Proc Royal Soc Med 52:1080–1083
21. Gilliatt RW, Hjort RJ (1972) Nerve conduction during Wallerian degeneration in the baboon. J Neurol Neurosurg Psychiat 35:335–341

22. Gilliatt RW (1980) Acute compression block. In: Sumner AJ (ed) The physiology of peripheral nerve disease, chapter 9, Saunders, Philadelphia, pp 287–315
23. Gilliatt RW (1981) Physical injury to peripheral nerves – physiologic and electrodiagnostic aspects. Proc Mayo Clin 56:361–370
24. Gruener R, Stern LZ, Weisz RR (1979) Conduction velocities in single fibres of diseased human muscle. Neurology 29:1293–1297
25. Gutmann E, Holubar J (1950) The degeneration of peripheral nerve fibres. J Neurol Neurosurg Psychiat 13:89–105
26. Hopf HC (1974) Conduction velocity of skeletal muscle fibres under various pathological conditions. In: Hausmannowa-Petrusewicz H, Jedrzejoswska H (eds) Structure and function of normal and diseased muscle and peripheral nerve. Polish Medical Publ, Warsaw, pp 165–168
27. Hopf HC, Herbort RL, Gnass M, Günther H, Lowitzsch K (1974) Fast and slow contraction times associated with fast and slow spike conduction of skeletal muscle fibres in normal subjects and in spastic hemiparesis. Z Neurol 206:193–202
28. Hopf HC, Lowitzsch K (1974) Methoden zur Erkennung leichter Funktionsstörungen peripherer Nerven. Z EEG-EMG 5:142–150
29. Hopf HC, Eysholdt M (1978) Impaired refractory periods of peripheral sensory nerves in multiple sclerosis. Am Neurol 4:499–501
30. Jewett DL, Walden Colene A, Chimento TC, Morris JH (1985) Effects of acute nerve compression on conduction of impulse trains of increasing frequency. J Neurol Scien 67:187–199
31. Krarup C, Gilliatt RW (1985) Some effects of prolonged constriction on nerve regeneration in the rabbit. J Neurol Scien 68:1–14
32. Klaus W, Lüllmann H, Muscholl E (1960) Der Kaliumflux des normalen und denervierten Rattenzwerchfells. Pflügers Arch ges Physiol 271:761
33. Li ChL, Shy MG, Wells J (1957) Some properties of mammalian skeletal muscle fibres with particular references to fibrillation potentials. J Physiol (Lond) 135:522
34. Lorkovic H, Tomanek RJ (1977) Potassium and chloride conductances in normal and denervated rat muscle. J Gen Physiol 61:1–23
35. Lowitzsch K, Hopf HC (1973) Refraktärperioden und frequente Impulsfortleitung im gemischten N. ulnaris des Menschen bei Polyneuropathien. Z Neurol 205:123–144
36. Luco JV, Eyzaguirre C (1955) Fibrillations and hypersensitivity to ACh in denervated muscle: effect of length of degenerating nerve fibres. J Neurophysiol 18:65
37. Ludin HP (1977) Pathophysiologische Grundlagen elektromyographischer Befunde bei Neuropathien und Myopathien, 2. Aufl. Thieme, Stuttgart
38. Mamoli B (1976) Zur Prognoseerstellung peripherer Fazialisparesen unter besonderer Berücksichtigung der Elektroneurographie. Wien Klin Wschr 88 (Suppl. 53):1–85
39. May M, Blumenthal FS, Klein SR (1983) Acute Bell's palsy: prognostic value of evoked electromyography, maximal stimulation, and other electrical tests. Am J Otol 5:1–121
40. Miller RG, Olney RK (1982) Persistent conduction block in compression neuropathy. Muscle & Nerve 5:154–156
41. Milner TE, Stein RB (1981) The effects of axotomy on the conduction of action potentials in peripheral sensory and motor nerve fibres. J Neurol Neurosurg Psychiat 44:485–496
42. Minwegen P, Friede RL (1984) Conduction velocity varies with osmotically induced changes of the area of the axon's profile. Brain Research 297:105–113
43. Olsen PZ (1975) Prediction of recovery in Bell's palsy. Acta Neurol Scand 55 (Suppl. 61):1–121
44. Olney RK, Miller GR (1984) Conduction block in compression neuropathy: recognition and quantification. Muscle & Nerve 7:662–667
45. Parry, GJ, Linn, Diana J (1986) Transient focal conduction block following experimental occlusion of the vasa nervorum. Muscle & Nerve 9:345–348
46. Perticoni G, Mauro LM (1982) Prolonged conduction blocks: late evolution in axonal degeneration. Electromyogr Clin Neurophysiol 22:591–604
47. Reiners K, Gilliatt RW, Harding AE, O'Neill JH (1987) Regeneration following tibial nerve crush in the rabbit: the effect of proximal constriction. J Neurol Neurosurg Psychiat 50:6–11

48. Rosenblueth A, Dempsey EW (1939) A Study of Wallerian degeneration. Am J Physiol 128:19–30
49. Sedal L, Ghabriel MN, Fensheng HE, Allt G, LeQuesne Pamela M, Harrison MJG (1983) A combined morphological and electrophysiological study of conduction block in peripheral nerve. J Neurol Scien 60:293–306
50. Shiraishi S, LeQuesne Pamela M, Gajree T (1985) The effect vincristine on nerve regeneration in the rat. J Neurol Scien 71:9–17
51. Smith KJ, Bostock H, Hall SM (1982) Saltatory conduction precedes remyelination in axons demyelinated with lysophosphatidyl choline. J Neurol Scien 54:13–31
52. Williams IR, Gilliatt RE (1977) Regeneration distal to a prolonged conduction block. J Neurol Scien 33:267–273

Somatosensory Regeneration Following Peripheral Nerve Injury[*]

A. STRUPPLER and G. OCHS, München/FRG

Introduction

A variety of regenerative processes are known to occur in the peripheral and central nervous system after nerve trauma (Devor and Wall 1981; Dykes and Terzis 1979; Horch and Lisney 1981; McGregor et al. 1984). As a consequence, typical positive and negative symptoms occur during recovery, even in the chronic situation, when plastic reorganization has reached a steady state (Sunderland 1978; Merle et al. 1986; Noordenbos 1979). Nevertheless, many questions remain to be answered concerning sensory disturbances encountered in patients.

The aim of this investigation was to obtain detailed information on somatosensory restitution, i.e., to gather data on the regeneration of single units, the various modalities represented, and to quantify the total degree and quality of recovery in consideration of the different sensory performances. The clinical testing of sensory experience provides an overall estimate of the integrity of both the peripheral and central pathways.

Degeneration and regeneration are dynamic processes in bridging peripheral and central lesions and establishing central reorganization. This makes time dependence crucial in assessing the degree of recovery and in determining therapeutic strategies.

A number of possibilities can be offered in order to quantify such deficits clinically and electrophysiologically (Tables 1, 2). These include detailed

Table 1. Phenomena that can be investigated with clinical or electrophysiological procedures in the examination of the sensory system (bilaterally tested)

Stimulus parameters and sensation	Quality
	Intensity
	Area
Somesthetic modalities	Touch-pressure
	Position sense
	Warmth-cold
	Pain
Synesthesias	

---

[*] This research was supported by the Deutsche Forschungsgemeinschaft (grant Str 11/29-4).

Table 2. Suggested experimental procedures (unilaterally tested)

Microneurography	
Single-fiber recordings	Receptor identification
	Discharge characteristics
	(SA, RA, uni-/bidirectional, static, dynamic)
	Neural response and sensation
Multifiber recordings	Estimation of total afferent input

sensory testing, differential block, and investigation of single receptor properties by use of microneurography and microstimulation. The following summarizes our present knowledge of the normal and pathological sensory integration and perception on the basis of such clinical and neurophysiological procedures.

Clinical Findings

Figure 1 A illustrates patterns of sensory disturbance frequently encountered in these patients. The terms used to describe the sensory disturbances are adapted from the definitions recommended by the International Society for the Study of pain (Lindblom et al. 1985). Depending on the actual state of recovery, various deficit symptoms, such as anesthesia or hypoesthesia are usually combined with paresthesia or dysesthesia. The terms hyperpathia (dull, delayed, irradiating pain syndrome) or allodynia (pain due to stimuli usually not painful) describe painful sensations that may be spontaneous or evoked. The findings in a median nerve lesion examined 7 months after suture are summarized in Fig. 1 B. There are still hypoesthetic and dysesthetic areas, typically in the most distal part of the reinnervated region. The proximal part, however, exhibits minor deficits in terms of paresthesia. The sympathetic functions semiquantitatively substantiated from the Ninhydrin finger printing test (Aschan and Moberg 1962) reveal an efferent deficit in the second finger, corresponding to the areas of poor recovery.

Mislocalizations, as exemplified in Fig. 1C, are a frequent phenomenon after recovery from nerve transection; mechanical stimuli are mislocalized within the corresponding innervation region. Obviously, fibers sprout to cutaneous sites apart from the original receptors, probably regenerating through another fascicle, whereas the proximal part of the fiber remains, including its central connections. Pressure on a muscle (interosseus I) can also be mislocalized. Such patients report dysesthesia in the cutaneous innervation zone of the corresponding nerve. Probably cross-reinnervation from sensory to motor fascicles occurs; thus former cutaneous sensory fibers sprouting to muscle end as deep, unspecific units. Pressure on such units elicits a sensation localized in the original site of the receptive corpuscle (Fig. 1D).

After complete transection of median or ulnar nerve more than 90% of the allodynia patients had most severe clinical deficits at the same time. Patients with dysesthesia had similar deficits but to a much less degree; in those qualities

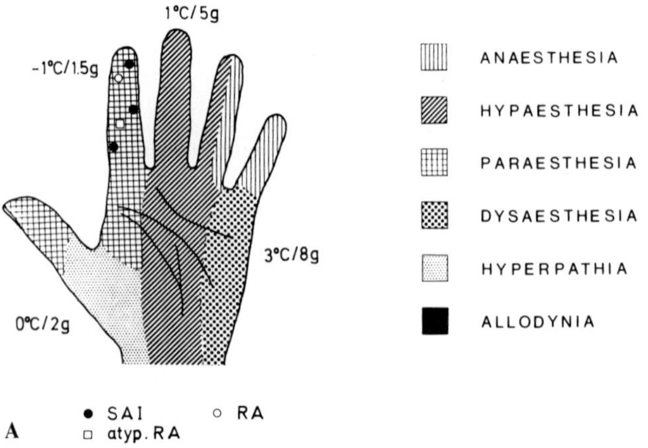
1°C/5g
-1°C/1.5g
3°C/8g
0°C/2g
ANAESTHESIA
HYPAESTHESIA
PARAESTHESIA
DYSAESTHESIA
HYPERPATHIA
ALLODYNIA
SAI
RA
atyp. RA

A

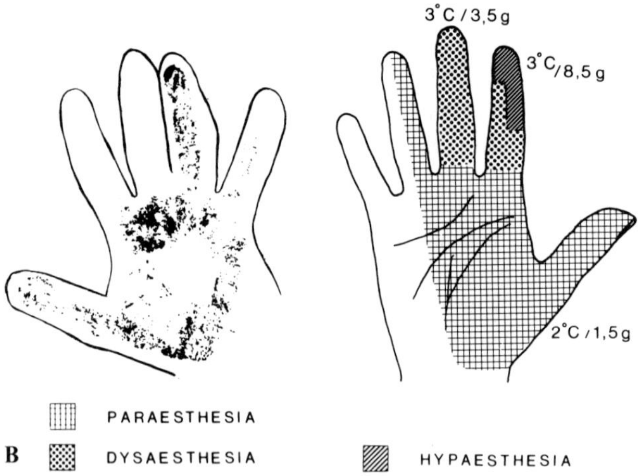
3°C/3,5g
3°C/8,5g
2°C/1,5g
PARAESTHESIA
DYSAESTHESIA
HYPAESTHESIA

B

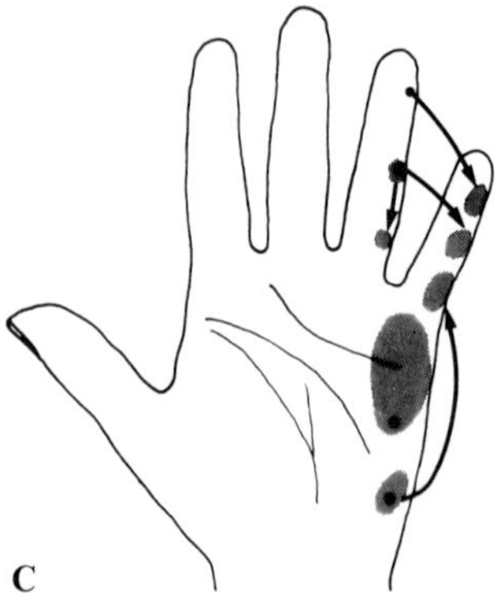

C

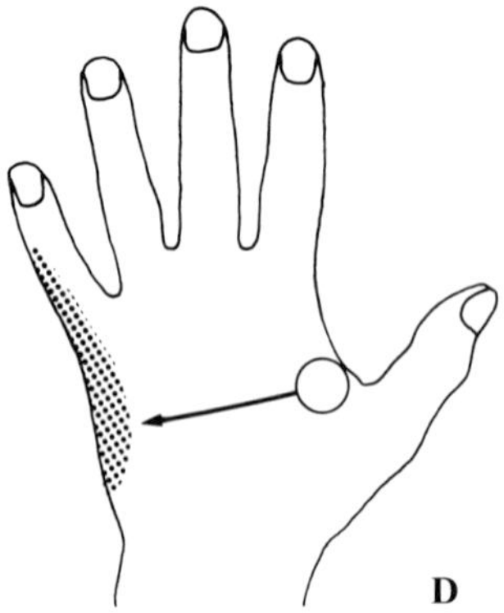

D

that are mediated mainly by thin, essentially unmyelinated fibers, only 20% – 30% of patients had comparable sensory loss. Among the paresthesia patients without painful sequelae, only 25% had similar severe sensory deficits. These findings support the concept that painful symptoms are highly correlated to poor recovery.

The cuff test has provided further information of the mechanisms underlying painful sensory disturbances. After 20–40 min of ischemia, allodynia and dysesthesia disappeared completely, whereas hyperpathia remained unchanged. Since fast-conducting, myelinated fibers are thought to be preferentially blocked by this procedure, allodynia (and dysesthesia) appears to be related to intact myelinated fiber function. Hyperpathia, on the other hand, seems to depend on C fiber mediated processes. Perception delayed and persists for minutes subsequent to the stimulus, irradiating far over the area of mechanical or thermal stimulation. This concept is supported by the persistence of this painful condition after ischemia.

Peripheral Nerve

In the periphery, unmyelinated or thin myelinated fibers (C and A-delta fibers) developed quite early in phylogenesis account for unspecific and basic functions of CNS, such as nociception, thermoreception, visceral sensation, and probably the control of muscle tone. In contrast, fast-conducting, myelinated fibers (A-alpha and A-beta fibers) are involved in highly differentiated tasks. The specific cutaneous sensibility mediated by a variety of mechanoreceptors or sensory corpuscles is mediated by these fibers. Skillful movements require fast-conducting systems using cutaneous and muscle spindle afferents.

Even after completed recovery a considerable loss of connections across the site of the nerve transection persists, leaving recovery always imperfect. All patients exhibit more or less pronounced deficits, in particular in respect to the performance of skillful fine movements (precision grip) and highly evaluated sensory tasks (Brink and Mackel 1987). The latter is in part due to imperfect reunion to specific end-organs which are subject to progressive atrophy after deafferentation. For example, muscle spindles, although shown to be morphologically reinnervated in animal experiments, remain functionally de-

---

Fig. 1 A–D. Clinical findings in patients with ulnar or median nerve lesions after suture or grafting of the transection. Mechanical sensitivity and thresholds were tested by Frey bristles. Threshold values are quantified in grams. Heat sensation tested by a calibrated radiant heat source detects deficits in unmyelinated (C fiber) or thin myelinated (A-delta fiber) sensory modalities. Autonomic dysfunction was found in some of the patients objectivated by the Ninhydrin finger printing test. **A** Replanted hand of a 21-year-old man, 6 years after suture of the ulnar and median nerve. **B** Median nerve transection in a 20-year-old man, 7 months after suture of the nerve (*right panel*). Sudomotor activity qualitatively shown in the Ninhydrin test (*left panel*). **C, D** Mislocalizations due to misdirected fiber outgrowth. Cutaneous and muscle belly stimuli are mislocalized

nervated, which becomes most obvious clinically from the lost tendon jerk. However, the quality of regeneration is highly dependent on the patient's age, the kind of surgical intervention, if any, and the nerve injured (Thomas et al. 1987).

Reinnervation of Cutaneous Receptors in Man

The discharge properties of a variety of cutaneous receptors have been investigated and classified as rapidly adapting (RA) and slowly adapting (SA I and II). Their distribution in human glabrous skin, their density, receptive field size, and thresholds have been determined (Vallbo and Hagbarth 1968; Johansson and Vallbo 1979; Knibestöl and Vallbo 1979; Vallbo and Johansson 1984). Although much information on intact human cutaneous receptors is available in the literature, data on the regenerating nerve in animals (Dykes and Terzis 1979; Horch 1979; Sanders and Zimmermann 1986) and humans (Hallin et al. 1981) are still rare. However, some recent studies on the reinnervation of human cutaneous mechanoreceptors are available from complete nerve transection in man (Mackel et al. 1983, 1985; Mackel 1985; Ochs et al. 1989). The patients were examined by means of various thorough clinical tests. Thereafter, microneurographic recordings and microstimulation were performed using well-elaborated techniques. The latter methods, although ambiguously discussed in the literature, offer the unique opportunity to correlate sensory disturbances and subjective sensory experience encountered in the patient with the recordings from corresponding single units.

Standard microneurographic techniques were used in recordings from the regenerated units illustrated in Fig. 2 encountered in a median nerve 3 years

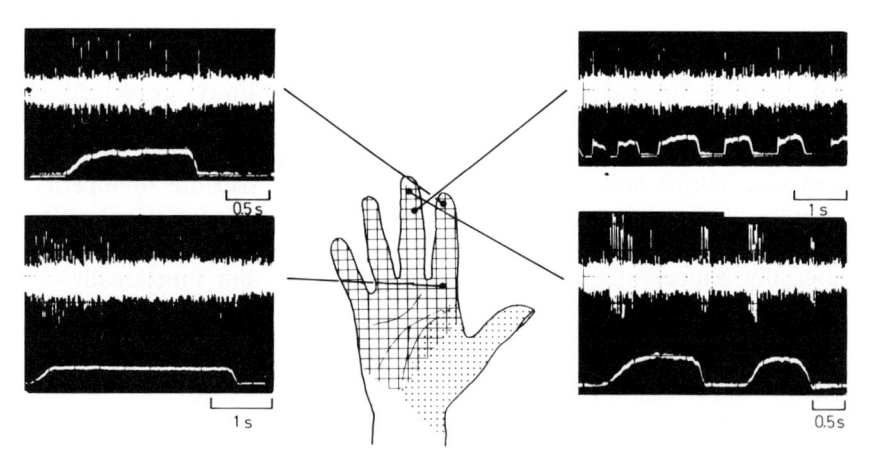

Fig. 2. Typical single-fiber recording with microelectrode technique (details, see text). In this example four individual receptors could be identified by discharge properties, receptive field size, and threshold behavior. They exhibited essentially normal properties compared to normal controls investigated prior to the patients by the same method. *Left upper*, SA I unit, manually applied mechanical stimulus, measured by the force transducer (*lower trace*). *Left lower*, SA II receptor. *Right upper*, atypical RA unit. *Right lower*, typical RA unit. Three years after primary suture of both nerves

after suture. The traumatically amputated hand had been replanted, suturing both median and ulnar nerves. SA receptors are shown in the left and RA units in the right row. Receptive field size, threshold, and discharge characteristics were similar or equal to normal controls in most regenerated units. We therefore were able to classify more than 80% of the regenerated receptors. Some of these, however, exhibited atypical properties. An example of this is presented on the right side. Only one on-spike was elicited in this recording, suggesting an atypical pacinian receptor. Nevertheless, vibration by a tuning fork did not cause any discharge (not shown), probably due to the high mechanical threshold. We assume that some of the abnormal receptors from which the recordings were made were localized in deep tissue, tendinous tissue, or muscles. On the other hand, approximately 5% of the units encountered in normal skin have also been shown to exhibit abnormal properties, suggesting that the relative portion of atypical units is increased in the regenerated nerve. Similar numbers have been reported elsewhere (Mackel et al. 1985).

Microstimulation

The stimulation of single afferent fibers has been evaluated in a considerable number of volunteers (Ochoa and Torebjörk 1983; Schady et al. 1983; Schady and Torebjörk 1983). The intrafascicular microstimulation was also performed in a subgroup of our patients and compared with the projected sensation in normal controls. Although tentative results could be obtained (summarized in Fig. 3), the procedure cannot be judged as very reliable. Obviously, one major

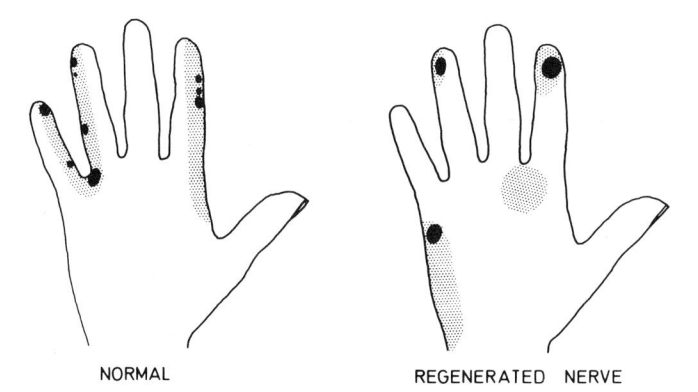

Fig. 3. Microstimulation. Single nerve fibers were preferentially stimulated using the recording needle immediately after an individual receptor was identified. *Black spots*, projected fields at low stimulation intensities; *shaded areas*, expanded zones at high stimulation. The voluteers (*left*) and the patients (*right*) were able to characterize projected sensations according to localization, intensity, and quality as indicated. The patients (data from two patients shown: one ulnar and one median nerve lesion) were unable to localize projected sensation in the typical spotlike distribution pattern surrounded by the fascicular boundaries. However, the procedure was not very reliable, especially in the patients, and was very dependent on the degree of cooperation which the individual was able to give

difference consists in discontinuous projected fields and singular fascicular projections; some are apart from the projection maximum.

Discussion

The central question in the interpretation of microstimulation data is whether mislocalizations arise due to peripheral sprouting or to central reorganization on the cortical, subcortical, or spinal level. Of course, the stimulation-induced sensation definitely depends on the actual surrounding of the stimulating electrode, i.e., whether myelinated or unmyelinated fibers are preferentially affected, and whether surrounding intrafascicular tissue impedance or stimulation thresholds are adequate. However, tentative conclusions may be derived from such data, leading to the assumption of potentially central (dorsal horn or cortical) reorganization taking place and probably playing an essential role for pathologic sensory integration. This appears to be substantiated by animal data (Wall et al. 1986; Knyhar and Csillik 1976; Merzenich et al. 1984).

In conclusion, it remains an open question to what extent peripheral changes are responsible for the clinical symptoms. From animal work, there is accumulated evidence that transsynaptic plasticity takes place in CNS after a peripheral lesion. Merzenich and Kaas (1978) were among the first to demonstrate cortical reorganization after complete median nerve transection. The dynamic process of reorganization of cortical receptive fields occurs early and later after deafferentation (Renehan and Munger 1986; Terzis and Dykes 1980). We wonder whether similar changes do not take place in the human somesthetic cortex as well, at least in the case of adequately large denervated areas.

The functional significance of these changes remains a matter of discussion regarding the kind of sensory disturbance, (unpleasant or painful) and the role which they may play in mislocalization and sensory recovery. They must certainly be taken into account at all levels of the neuraxis if sequelae of peripheral lesions are discussed. Microneurography, on the other hand, shows clearly that the changes at the peripheral termination are not the only explanation.

References

Aschan W, Moberg E (1962) The Ninhydrin finger printing test used to map out partial lesions to hand nerves. Acta Chir Scand 123:365–370
Brink EE, Mackel R (1987) Sensorimotor performance of the hand during peripheral nerve regeneration. J Neurolog Sci 77:249–66
Devor M, Wall PD (1981) Plasticity in the spinal cord sensory map following peripheral nerve injury in rats. J Neurosci 7:679–684
Dykes RW, Terzis JK (1979) Reinnervation of glabrous skin in baboons: properties of cutaneous mechanoreceptors subsequent to nerve crush. J Neurophysiol 42:1461–78

Hallin RG, Wiesenfeld Z, Lindblom U (1981) Neurophysiological studies on patients with sutured median nerves: faulty sensory localization after nerve regeneration and its physiological correlates. Exp Neurology 73:90–106

Horch K (1979) Guidance of regrowing sensory axons after cutaneous nerve lesions in the cat. J Neurophysiol 5:1437–49

Horch KW, Lisney SJW (1981) Changes in primary afferent depolarisation of sensory neurons during peripheral nerve regeneration in the cat. J Physiol (Lond) 313:287–99

Johansson RS, Vallbo AB (1979) Tactile sensibility in the human hand: relative and absolute densities of 4 types of mechanoreceptive units in glabrous skin. J Physiol 286:283–300

Knibestöl M, Vallbo AB (1979) Single unit analysis of mechanoreceptor activity from the human glabrous skin. Acta Physiol Scand 44:178–195

Knyihar E, Csillik B (1976) Effect of peripheral axotomy on the fine structure and histochemistry of the rolando substance: degenerative atrophy and central processes of pseudounipolar cells. Exp Brain Res 26:73–87

Lindblom U, Merskey H, Mumford JM, Nathan PW, Noordenbos W, Sunderland S (1985) Pain terms – a current list with definitions and notes on usage with definitions and notes on usage. Pain, Suppl. 3:215–221

Mackel R (1985) Human cutaneous mechanoreceptors during regeneration: physiology and interpretation. Ann Neurol 18:165–72

Mackel R, Kunesch E, Waldhör F, Struppler A (1983) Reinnervation of mechanoreceptors in the human glabrous skin following peripheral nerve repair. Brain Res 268:49–65

Mackel R, Brink EE, Wittkowsky G (1985) Properties of cutaneous mechanosensitive afferents during the early stages of regeneration in man. Brain Res 329:49–69

McGregor GP, Gibson SJ, Sabate IM, Blank MA, Christofides ND, Wall PD, Polak JM, Boom SR (1984) Effect of peripheral nerve section and nerve crush on spinal cord neuropeptides in the rat: increased VIP and PIH in the dorsal horn. Neurosci 13:207–216

Merle M, Amand P, Cour C, Foucher G, Michon J (1986) Microsurgical repair of peripheral nerve lesions – a study of 150 injuries of the median and ulnar nerve. Periph Nerve Rep Reg 2:17–26

Merzenich MM, Kaas JH, Sur M, Lin CS (1978) Double representation of the body surface within the cytoarchitectonic area 3b and 1 in "S-I" in the owl monkey. J Comp Neurol 181:41–73

Merzenich MM, Nelson RJ, Stryker MP, Cynader MS, Schoppmann A, Zook JM (1984) Somatosensory cortical map changes following digit amputation in adult monkeys. J Comp Neurol 224:591–605

Noordenbos W (1979) Sensory findings in painful traumatic nerve lesions. Advances in pain Research and Therapy, Vol. 3. Raven Press, New York

Ochoa J, Torebjörk HE (1983) Sensations evoked by intraneural microstimulation of single mechanoreceptor units innervating the human hand. J Physiol 342:33–54

Ochs G, Schenk M, Struppler A (1989) Painful dysaesthesias following peripheral nerve injury: a clinical and electrophysiological study. Brain Res 496, 1–2:228–240

Renehan WE, Munger BL (1986) Degeneration and regeneration of peripheral nerve in the rat trigeminal system. II. Response to nerve lesion. J Comp Neurol 249:429–59

Sanders KH, Zimmermann M (1986) Mechanoreceptors in rat glabrous skin: redevelopment of function after nerve crush. J Neurophysiol 55:644–659

Schady WJL, Torebjörk HE (1983) Projected and receptive fields: a comparison of projected areas of sensations evoked by intraneural stimulation of mechanoreceptive units and their innervation territories. Acta Physiol Scand 119:267–285

Schady WJL, Ochoa J, Torebjörk HE, Chen LS (1983) Peripheral projections of fascicles in the human median nerve. Brain 106:745–760

Struppler A, Mackel R, Besinger U, Waldhör F (1981) Electromyography and Microneurography following Peripheral Nerve Transplantations. In: Gorio A, Millesi H, Mingrino S (eds) Posttraumatic Peripheral Nerve Regeneration. Raven Press, New York, 581–589

Sunderland S (1978) Nerve and nerve injuries, 2nd ed. Churchill Livingston, London

Terzis JK, Dykes RW (1980) Reinnervation of glabrous skin in baboons: properties of cutaneous mechanoreceptors subsequent to nerve transection. J Neurophysiol 44:1214–25

Thomas CK, Stein RB, Gordon T, Lee RG, Elleker MG (1987) Patterns of reinnervation and motor unit recruitment in human hand muscles after complete ulnar and median nerve section and resuture. J Neurol Neurosurg Psychiat 50:259–268

Vallbo AB, Hagbarth KE (1968) Activity from skin mechanoreceptors recorded percutaneously in awake human subjects. Exp Neurol 21:270–89

Vallbo AB, Johansson RS (1984) Properties of cutaneous mechanoreceptors in the human hand related to touch sensation. Human Neurobiology 3:3–14

Wall JT, Kaas JH, Sur M, Nelson RJ, Fellmann DJ, Merzenich MM (1986) Functional reorganization in somatosensory cortical areas 3b and 1 of adult monkeys after median nerve repair: possible relationships to sensory recovery in humans. J Neurosci 6:218–233

The Contribution of Both the Peripheral and Central Nervous Systems to the Pain that Follows Peripheral Nerve Injury

C. J. WOOLF, London/England

Pain, as a sensory state, is not simply the inevitable consequence of the activation of a defined set of sensory pathways in the periphery. Rather, pain is a descriptor that we choose to identify a variety of different unpleasant, uncomfortable and distressing sensations that may be elicited in quite a number of different ways. It is useful to look at pain in terms of its pathogenesis as consisting of three different types: physiological, inflammatory and neuropathic pain (the latter two constituting clinical pain; Woolf 1987a). Physiological pain is that sensation elicited by transient non-tissue-damaging noxious stimuli that activate high threshold A-delta and C nociceptors. This type of pain, which we commonly experience as pin prick, pinch, or excessive heat or cold, has a distinct threshold and a quantifiable stimulus-response relationship. These properties of physiological pain have led to the idea that there are specific pain pathways in the peripheral and central nervous systems that are similar to the specific pathways that are considered to mediate the innocuous somatosensations such as touch, pressure, vibration, hot or cold. However, what this analysis fails to take account of is that physiological pain is very different from inflammatory and neuropathic pain. Clinical pain is not simply excessive or prolonged 'physiological' pain; it is a qualitatively different sensory experience with different neural mechanisms.

Inflammatory pain is that pain which accompanies tissue damage and is associated with the inflammatory response. It is distinguishable from physiological pain not only in the intensity of the stimuli that are required to initiate it but also in its duration. Two interesting features of inflammatory pain are that there is spontaneous pain in the absence of external stimuli, and that pain can be elicited by innocuous stimuli. The reduction in the intensity of stimuli required to produce pain, which we call hyperalgesia, operates by two mechanisms. In the periphery there is a reduction in the threshold of primary afferents, peripheral sensitization (Meyer et al. 1985). Centrally, C afferent fibre inputs have recently been shown to have the capacity to sensitize dorsal horn neurones by increasing their excitability (Woolf 1983; Woolf and Wall 1986). Following such input the receptive fields of dorsal horn neurones expand, and those neurones that initially responded only to noxious stimuli begin to respond to innocuous stimuli (Cook et al. 1987). This latter change means that information in channels that formerly signalled exclusively low-intensity stimuli is now interpreted by the altered central nervous system as being painful. It is this aberrant convergence which distinguishes clinical pain from other types of sensation.

Neuropathic pain represents that pain which is generated by a disturbance in the nervous system, peripheral or central. Although lesions to the nervous system may be associated with inflammation, as with neuritis, vasculitis and physical injury, neuropathic pain differs from inflammatory pain in that the pain is the consequence of an abnormality in the functioning of the nervous system rather than the sensory detection of tissue damage inducing changes in the nervous system. Although there are similarities between inflammatory and neuropathic pains, notably the presence of aberrant convergences in both, neuropathic pain is much more long lasting, severe and refractory to treatment.

Peripheral nerve lesions are amongst the commonest sources of neuropathic pain, and in this chapter I attempt to establish what factors contribute to this pain.

Pain and Peripheral Nerve Injury

Peripheral nerve injury does not inevitably lead to lasting pain although permanent dysfunction is common. The pain may follow complete nerve section, as in amputation; it may accompany neuroma formation or follow regeneration with the development of hyperpathia after reinnervation. Most devastatingly, partial nerve injury may produce the causalgic syndrome in which both hyperpathic pain and a reflex sympathetic dystrophy is present.

Why one patient with peripheral nerve injury develops painful sequelae to the injury and another with apparently very similar injuries does not, remains baffling. It is not possible from the site, extent or nature of the injury to predict accurately who will suffer pain. Our failure to provide an explanation for this is a powerful reflection of our ignorance concerning the mechanisms that operate to produce neuropathic pain. The key to this issue is likely, however, to be the development of maladaptive compensatory changes in both the peripheral and central nervous systems. The nervous system has at its disposal a variety of mechanisms to compensate for the effects of disruption of its normal functioning. In the periphery this includes the capacity to regenerate with the potentiality of restoring function (Sunderland 1968). In the adult central nervous system the capacity for regrowth is highly limited although it can occur in appropriate circumstances (Aguayo 1985). More important is the capacity for central neurones that do not degenerate following a lesion to alter their function (Woolf 1987b). This alteration or plasticity appears to operate by changes in intrinsic membrane properties (Gustafsson 1979) and by alterations in synaptic efficacy (Kuno and Llinas 1970; Mendell 1984). In the majority of patients with peripheral nerve lesions, the combination of the peripheral and central compensating mechanisms assists in maximizing the recovery of function. In a minority of patients, however, these same mechanisms appear to become maladaptive and instead of contributing to restoration of function actually generate alterations in function that manifest as pain or altered sympathetic reflexes. Certain individuals may have a propensity to maladaptive changes.

There are three general features of the pain that follows peripheral nerve lesions. The first is spontaneous pain. The second is a mismatch between afferent input and sensation, so that, for example, innocuous inputs typically begin to be capable of generating pain, and stimuli that would normally be expected to produce mild transient pain produce severe and disturbing pain (dysesthesia and hyperpathia). Finally, although not always present, there is an abnormal sympathetic outflow. In analysing the mechanisms responsible for producing these disturbances one must look both at the peripheral and the central nervous systems.

Peripheral Changes Following Nerve Injury

Peripheral nerve injury can produce both positive and negative influences on the central nervous system. The positive influences relate to the abnormal afferent input that follows nerve injury with the development of ectopic excitability at sprouts in the neuroma (Wall and Gutnick 1974) and within dorsal root ganglia (Wall and Devor 1983), altered mechanosensitivity (Wall and Gutnick 1974), altered chemosensitivity (Scadding 1981) and ephaptic connections (Seltzer and Devor 1979). The possibility that hyperactive sympathetic efferents make ephaptic connections with abnormally sensitive afferent fibres has been used to explain the pathogenesis of causalgia (Devor 1983; Janig 1985).

However, in addition to these changes in the amount and patterns of electrical activity that are carried by the central branches of damaged primary afferent neurones into the spinal cord, there are more subtle changes as well. Peripheral nerve section, for example, produces profound metabolic alterations in the cell bodies and central terminals of the axotomized afferent neurones. A potentially most important change is the alteration in the amounts of neuropeptides, such as substance P, vasoactive intestinal polypeptides or somatostatin in axotomized C afferent neurones (Barbut et al. 1981). The reason why this is important is simply that these neuropeptides appear to act not as fast transmitters, producing brief excitation of dorsal horn neurones, but by modulating the activity of the dorsal horn over much more prolonged periods. Removal of these neuromodulators following nerve section (due to the interruption of the trophic influence of nerve growth factor, which is transported from the periphery to the dorsal root ganglion, resulting in abnormal gene expression) is likely to induce complex central changes (Wall and Woolf 1986). Every time an action potential reaches the central terminal of a damaged C primary afferent neurone it now evokes the release of an abnormal combination of fast transmitters (such as the excitatory amino acid glutamate) and neuromodulators.

Neurotransmitters and neuromodulators in addition to altering the membrane potential of dorsal horn neurones by acting on ion channels also have the capacity to alter second messenger systems (Woolf et al. 1985) and gene expression (Hunt et al. 1987). Because of this, disturbances and alterations in the chemical signals released by afferents may have prolonged and profound effects on their target neurones.

The third type of alteration in afferent input consequent upon a lesion in the periphery is due to cell death. Up to one-third of dorsal root ganglion cells die in experimental animals following peripheral nerve section (Aldskogius et al. 1985). Apart from reducing the total number of input lines, the presence of degenerating afferent terminals leading to vacant synaptic sites in the dorsal horn is likely to be a potent trigger for inducing changes in the neuronal circuitry of the dorsal horn (Gobel 1984). Following nerve injury transganglionic degenerative changes can be seen at central terminals (Aldskogius et al. 1985). Whether these are present in all axotomized neurones, including those that survive or only in those that are in the process of dying, is not clearly established yet.

Central Changes Following Peripheral Nerve Injury

The sensory disturbances, including pain, that may accompany or are consequent on peripheral nerve lesions may arise both from changes in the periphery and in the central nervous system. The changes in primary afferent function and chemistry discussed in the previous section clearly lead to an abnormal input into the central nervous system. This abnormal input may be sufficient in its own right, by altering the signal processing of central sensory pathways that are themselves unchanged, to produce the abnormal sensations. For example, spontaneous activity in or abnormal mechano- and chemosensitivity of a C afferent fibre in a damaged nerve could produce pain simply by activating the pathways that a nociceptor C fibre normally would.

If such changes were the only ones that occurred with nerve injury, then naturally maximum effort should be devoted at preventing peripheral changes, or, if they occur, all therapeutic interventions should be aimed at the periphery. However, if peripheral nerve injury induces alterations in the structure and function of second and higher order neurones, such alterations could result in the inappropriate processing of both abnormal and normal afferent input. In this case attempting to modify the peripheral input would not necessarily reduce the sensory disorder if disturbed functioning of central pathways persists.

Although the relative importance of peripheral and central sites for producing the sensory changes following peripheral nerve lesions may differ from patient to patient (Ochoa et al. 1985), what is clear, as a result of recent experimental work, is that the sensory disturbances due to peripheral nerve lesions cannot be accounted for exclusively by the alterations that are known to occur in primary afferent neurones. The pioneer in this field has been Wall, who together with Devor has demonstrated that peripheral nerve section induces dramatic alterations in the functional performance of dorsal horn cells (Devor and Wall 1981; Wall and Devor 1981). Essentially what they have demonstrated is that following nerve section, the area of cord that is functionally deafferented begins, with time, to respond to distant intact inputs. This plasticity cannot be explained by collateral sprouting of afferent fibres and must represent changes in synaptic efficacy (Wall 1983). Such changes could occur by activating previously 'silent synapses' by removing inhibition (Woolf and Wall 1982) or by increasing the excitability of deafferented cells. What is of great interest is that changes similar to those found in the spinal cord have also been found in the somatosensory cortex following nerve lesions (Wall and Kaas 1986). What has emerged from these experiments is the concept that the nervous system is not organized in a rigid, hard-wired hierarchical fashion but instead displays considerable plasticity in response to changes in its input (Cook et al. 1987; Juliano and Whitsel 1987). The clinical significance of central plasticity following peripheral nerve lesions is shown by two studies that have demonstrated that the dysaesthesias and hyperalgesias due to peripheral nerve injury are due, in the majority of cases, to signals carried to the central nervous system in the large myelinated A-beta afferents (Cambell et al. 1987; Ochs et al. 1987). Since these fibres never normally signal pain, this indicates a profound disruption in the sensory interpretive properties of the central nervous system.

Disturbances in sympathetic outflow are a prominent feature of peripheral nerve lesions (Janig 1985), whether the abnormal sympathetic reflexes are the consequences of increases in the excitability of sympathetic preganglionic motoneurones or the interneurones that feed onto them is not known (Blumberg and Janig 1983). The disturbances in autonomic function are nevertheless a clear indication that central changes have occurred. Because of the possible excitatory action of postganglionic sympathetic efferents on damaged axons (Devor 1983) a positive feedback circle of pain may be set up (Livingstone 1948); injured afferents send abnormal signals into the spinal cord producing abnormal excitability of dorsal horn neurones, these directly or indirectly act on sympathetic motoneurones increasing their output, and these in turn via the postganglionic fibres increase activity in the primary afferents.

Conclusion

Injury to a peripheral nerve results in direct and indirect changes in primary afferent neurones. These may lead to an altered pattern of input to the spinal cord, changes in the chemical signals of the afferents or even in cell death. While these alterations in the primary afferent are clearly of great importance in the pathogenesis of the sensory disturbances that accompany peripheral nerve lesions, there are in addition compensatory changes within central neurones. These include changes in the excitatory and inhibitory influences on the neurones in somatosensory circuits, leading to alterations in response properties with the recruitment of novel inputs. The plasticity may be adaptive in most patients, aiding restoration of function, but in others could be maladaptive, resulting in abnormal sensory states. In particular the generation of pain by low intensity stimuli that activate A-beta afferents (aberrant convergence) represents a substantial disturbance in the sensory processing properties of the central nervous system. Effective treatment of peripheral nerve lesions must take into account the complex and subtle interactions between primary afferent neurones and higher order neurones within the central nervous system. Disorder in one element in a neuronal chain can induce transynaptic changes in the next element.

References

Aguayo AJ (1985) Capacity for renewed axonal growth in the mammalian central nervous system. In: Bignani A, Bloom FE, Breis CL, Adelaye A (eds) Central nervous system plasticity. Raven Press, New York
Aldskogius H, Arvidsson J, Grant G (1985) The reaction of primary sensory neurones to peripheral nerve injury with particular emphasis on transganglionic changes. Brain Res Reviews 10:27–40
Barbut D, Polak JM, Wall PD (1981) Substance P in the spinal cord dorsal horn decreases following peripheral nerve injury. Brain Res 205:289–298
Blumberg H, Janig W (1983) Changes of reflexes in vasoconstrictor neurons supplying the cat hindlimb following chronic nerve lesions: a model for studying mechanisms of reflex sympathetic dystrophy? J Auton Nerv Syst 7:399–411
Cambell JN, Raja SN, Mayer RA (1987) Painful sequelae of nerve injury. Pain, Suppl 4:S334
Cook AJ, Woolf CJ, Wall PD, McMahon SB (1987) Dynamic receptive field plasticity in rat spinal dorsal horn following C-primary afferent input. Nature 325:151–153
Devor M (1983) Nerve pathophysiology and mechanisms of pain in causalgia. J Auton Nerv Syst 7:371–384
Devor M, Wall PD (1981) Plasticity in the spinal cord sensory map following peripheral nerve injury in rats. J Neurosci 1:679–684
Gobel S (1984) Trans-synaptic effects of peripheral nerve injury. J Neurosci 4:2281–2290
Gustafsson B (1979) Changes in motoneurones electrical properties following axotomy. J Physiol (Lond) 293:197–215
Hunt SP, Pini A, Evan G (1987) Induction of C-*fos*-like protein in spinal cord neurones following sensory stimulation. Nature 328:632–634
Janig W (1985) Causalgia and reflex sympathetic dystrophy: in which way is the sympathetic nervous system involved. TINS 8:471–477
Juliano SL, Whitsel BL (1987) A combined 2-deoxyglucose and neurophysiological study of primate somatosensory cortex. J Comp Neurol 263:515–528
Kuno M, Llinas R (1970) Enhancement of synaptic transmission by dendritic potentials in chromatolysed motoneurones of the cat. J Physiol (Lond) 210:807–821
Livingstone K (1948) The vicious circle in causalgia. Ann NY Acad Sci 50:247–258
Mendell LM (1984) Modifiability of spinal synapses. Physiol Rev 64:260–324
Meyer RA, Cambell JN, Raja SN (1985) Peripheral neural mechanisms of cutaneous hyperalgesia. Adv Pain Res & Ther 9:53–72
Ochoa JL, Torebjork E, Marchetti P, Swok M (1985) Mechanisms of neuropathic pain: cumulative observations, new experiments and further speculation. Adv Pain Res & Ther 9:431–450
Ochs G, Schenk M, Struppler A (1987) Painful states following peripheral nerve injury: clinical and electrophysiological data. Pain, Suppl. 4:S200
Scadding JW (1981) Development of ongoing activity, mechanosensitivity and adrenaline sensitivity in severed peripheral nerve axons. Exp Neurol 73:345–364
Seltzer M, Devor M (1979) Ephaptic transmission in chronically damaged peripheral nerves. Neurology (Minneap) 29:1061–1064
Sunderland S (1968) Nerves and nerve injuries. Churchill Livingstone, Edinburgh
Wall JT, Kaas JH (1986) Long-term cortical consequences of reinnervation errors after nerve regeneration in monkey. Brain Res 372:400–404

Wall PD (1983) Alterations in the central nervous system after deafferentation: connectivity control. Adv Pain Res & Ther 5:677–689

Wall PD, Devor M (1981) The effects of peripheral nerve injury on dorsal root potentials and transmission of afferent signals into the spinal cord. Brain Res 209:95–111

Wall PD, Devor M (1983) Sensory afferent impulses originate from dorsal root ganglia as well as from the periphery in normal and nerve injured rats. Pain 17:321–339

Wall PD, Gutnick M (1974) Ongoing activity in peripheral nerves: the physiology and pharmacology of impulses originating from a neuroma. Exptl Neurol 43:580–593

Wall PD, Woolf CJ (1986) The brief and the prolonged facilitatory effects of unmyelinated afferent input on the rat spinal cord are independently influenced by peripheral nerve section. Neuroscience 17:1199–1205

Woolf CJ (1983) Evidence for a central component of postinjury pain hypersensitivity. Nature 308:686–688

Woolf CJ (1988) Neuroplasticity and injury to the spinal cord. In: Illis L (ed) Dysfunction after spinal injury. Oxford University Press, pp 129–147

Woolf CJ (1988) Physiological, inflammatory and neuropathic pain. In: Symon L (ed) Advances and technical standards in neurosurgery, vol. 15. Springer-Verlag, Heidelberg, 39–62

Woolf CJ, Wall PD (1982) Chronic peripheral nerve section diminishes the primary afferent A-fibre mediated inhibition of rat dorsal horn neurones. Brain Res 242:77–85

Woolf CJ, Wall PD (1986) The relative effectiveness of C primary afferent fibres of different origins in evoking a prolonged facilitation of the flexor reflex in the rat. J Neurosci 6:1433–1443

Woolf CJ, Chong MS, Rashdi TA (1985) Mapping increased glycogen phosphorylase activity in dorsal root ganglia and in the spinal cord following peripheral stimuli. J Comp Neurol 234:60–76

Clinical Symptoms, Electrophysiological and Morphological Findings in Traumatic Lesions of the Ischiadic Nerve in Domestic Fowl

H.-E. NAU, M. BLANK, M. A. KONERDING, P. WENZEL, and R. WERNER, Essen/FRG

Introduction

In 1938, electrophysiological investigations after nerve compression in rats were conducted by Allen. Since then, various models of nerve compression have been described by Aguayo et al. (1971), Bentley and Schlapp (1943), Denny-Brown and Brenner (1944a, b), Duncan (1948), Dyck (1969), Lehmann and Pretschner (1966), Mayer and Denny-Brown (1964), and Weiss and Davis (1943). The investigations generally had no comparable clinical, electrophysiological, or morphological findings in a single animal. In addition, pressure neuropathies have been examined in quadrupeds. The hen with its two legs seemed to be not only a simple model for pressure neuropathy studies and comparison with man but also a cheap one. In 1958, Henschler used hens for testing neurotoxic substances, and in 1961 Glees and White did so in experimental fiber studies. In 1955, Koch and Heim pointed to the high body temperature and the higher rate of metabolism. The quick appearance of clinical and morphological alterations were described by Blank in 1966. Therefore clinical symptoms, electrophysiological, and morphological findings following nerve compression should be described in these animals.

Animals and Methods

Studies were done in HLA-Leghorn hens (females and males; Lohmann Tierzucht, Cuxhaven, FRG) aged 14–16 weeks. The animals were taken care of and observed by the Central Animal Laboratory of the University Clinic of Essen. The cocks were kept in individual cages, hens in chicken runs.

The ischiadic nerve derives from four roots of the sacral plexus. On the medial side of femor, proximal to the knee joint, the ischiadic nerve divides into the femoral and tibial nerves. The tibial nerve also supplies the gastrocnemius muscle. This muscle consists of three parts and extends the tarsometatarsal joint and bends the digits and the knee joint. In all the animals the left ischiadic nerve in the middle of the femor was compressed under local anesthesia after the feathers were removed. The nerve was prepared and clipped. For nerve compression we used Haifetz and Yasargil clips with different grades of pressures (70, 90, 130 p). The clip remained in situ for 5 min, 2, 6, 24, 72, 96, and 120 h (Table 1). Wound closure was done with resorbable sutures.

Table 1. Listing of animals, pressure of clips, duration of compression, and survival time after compression

Animal number	Sex	Clip in situ (hours)	Pressure of clip	Training (+yes/−no)	Survival time (days)
1	M	24	70	−	10
2	M	2	70	−	30
3	M	2	70	+	30
4	M	2	70	+	23
5	M	24	70	+	61
6	M	24	70	+	61
7	M	2	90	+	48
8	M	2	90	−	79
9	M	6	90	+	63
10	M	6	90	+	63
11	M	6	90	−	56
12	M	6	90	+	79
13	M	6	90	−	63
14	M	6	90	−	79
15	M	24	90	+	79
16	M	24	90	+	56
17	M	24	90	−	56
18	M	24	90	−	79
19	M	6	90	−	48
20	M	6	90	−	48
21	M	6	90	−	62
22	M	6	90	−	2
23	M	6	90	−	2
24	M	6	90	−	49
25	M	6	90	−	100
26	M	6	90	−	98
27	M	6	90	−	100
28	M	6	90	−	100
29	F	6	90	−	42
30	F	6	90	−	82
31	F	6	90	−	82
32	F	6	90	−	67
33	F	6	90	−	82
34	F	6	90	−	78
35	F	6	90	−	82
36	F	6	90	−	22
37	F	6	90	−	20
38	F	6	90	−	40
39	F	6	90	−	40
40	F	6	90	−	82
41	F	96	130	−	100
42	F	96	130	−	100
43	F	120	130	−	100
44	F	120	130	−	100
45	F	72	130	−	102
46	F	72	130	−	102
47	F	120	130	−	102
48	F	120	130	−	102
49	F	96	130	−	102
50	F	96	130	−	100

Table 2. The development of body weight in a group of animals with and without training

Animal number	Training (+yes/−no)	Increase in body weight	
		Absolute (grams)	Relative (percentage)
7	+	−	−
8	−	500	34.5
9	+	630	47.2
10	+	445	29.9
11	−	555	37.0
12	+	330	25.0
13	−	270	19.5
14	−	305	21.6
15	+	350	22.2
16	+	345	23.1
17	−	345	21.9
18	−	420	25.3

Ten animals were trained. The body weight was controlled and the femoral temperature was taken. The reflexes, the degree of trophic disorders, and the degree of paresis were clinically examined. Electromyographic and neurographic controls were done by measurements of distal motor latency, nerve conduction velocity, and the F reflex. These investigations were done with steel needle electrodes (DISA) from the gastrocnemius muscle and with the nerve root stimulation electrode (DISA) and electromyograph 2000 (Schwarzer). Supramaximal rectangular impulses with a duration of 0.1 ms and a rate of 1/s were employed. The morphological investigations were done after fixation and staining (modification of Karnovsky's method; Blank et al. 1978). Light and scanning electron microscopic (stereoscan 180, Cambridge, UK) studies were carried out.

Table 3. Temperature of healthy and operated legs

Animal number	Temperature (°C)	
	Operated leg	Healthy leg
7	41.0	41.0
8	40.5	41.0
9	40.5	41.0
10	41.5	41.5
11	40.5	40.5
12	41.0	41.0
13	40.5	41.0
14	40.5	41.0
15	40.5	41.0
16	40.5	40.5
17	40.5	41.0
18	41.0	41.5

The training did not influence the body weight (Table 2). The temperature (Table 3) was 40.5°–41.5 °C, with a significant diminution on the operated side (confirmed by Wilcoxon and t tests).

Results

Clinical Examinations. When the hen is taken by the wings, there is a light antetorsion in the hip joint and light flexion in the knee and of the claws. If the shank is hit, the claws extend and splay. The same reflex can be obtained by dropping the animal. These reflexes disappeared directly after the nerve was clipped. They returned between the 32nd and 52nd days (Fig. 1), in most animals between the 36th and 41st days after operation. There was no difference in the time in which the reflexes disappeared and returned in the same animal. An edematous swelling of the feathered distal part of the operated leg was seen at the tarsometatarsocrural joint. In only two animals were ulcerations observed. These alterations also disappeared without any therapeutic procedures with reinnervation.

Electromyoneurography. Electromyographic potentials were similar to those in man (Fig. 2): amplitudes of about 1 mV and duration of the potentials 1–2 ms. No spontaneous activity was found in the healthy animal. The distal motor latencies (calculated by the method of Denny-Brown and Brenner 1944a) and values of 50 ± 10 m/s. The values did not change in the non-operated legs. The nerve conduction velocity of the ischiadic nerve was 80 ± 10 m/s in the femoral region.

After nerve compression pathological spontaneous activity (Fig. 2), such as fibrillation potentials and positive denervation potentials, was usually found in all animals. Fibrillation potentials had amplitudes of about 0.5 mV and a

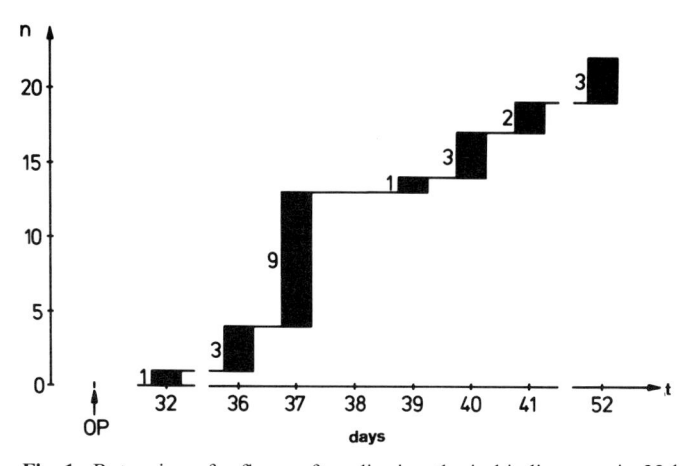

Fig. 1. Returning of reflexes after clipping the ischiadic nerve in 22 hens

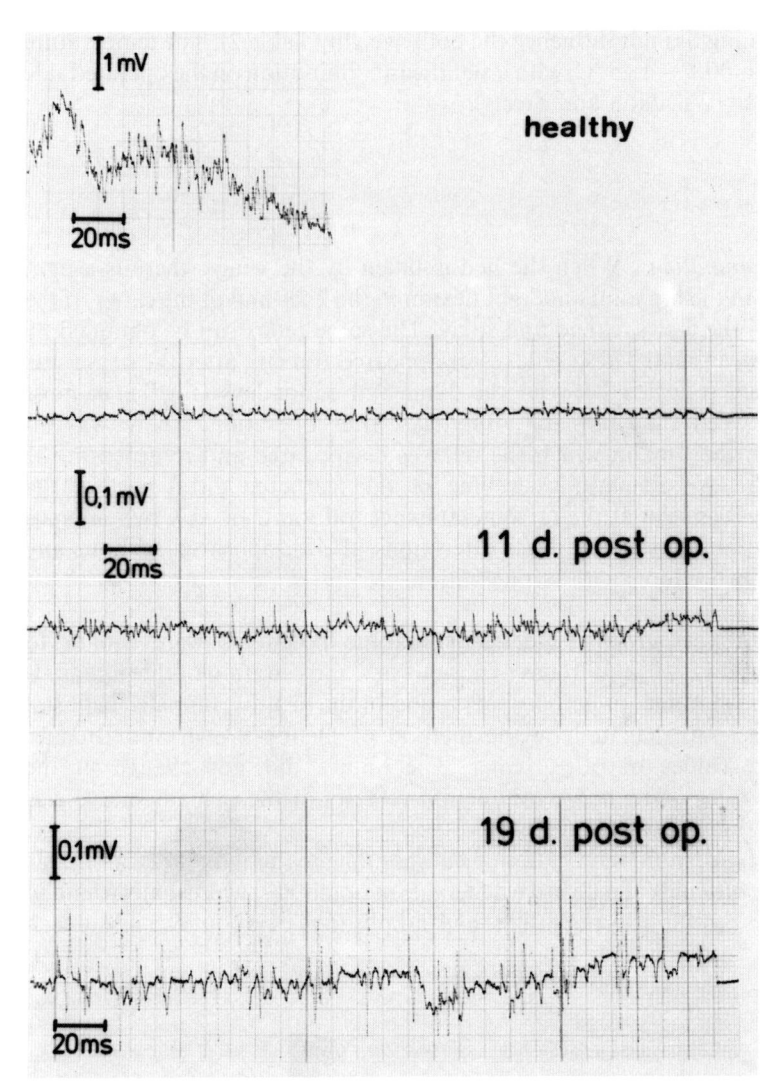

Fig. 2. Normal electromyogram and that after nerve compression (spontaneous activity and signs of reinnervation)

duration of 1–2 ms. They are biphasic with a positive reflection. Some weeks after the clipping of the nerve, pseudomyotonic discharges were observed in some cases. The first pathological signs of denervation (Fig. 3) were found on the 4th day, at first fibrillation potentials and after some days also positive denervation potentials. The maximum of spontaneous acivity was found from the 10th to 22nd postoperative days and ended on the 52nd day. During the reinnervation period at first small bi-, tri-, and polyphasic potentials with amplitudes of 0.1–0.5 mV were seen. The degree of polyphasic potentials diminished and the height of the amplitudes increased.

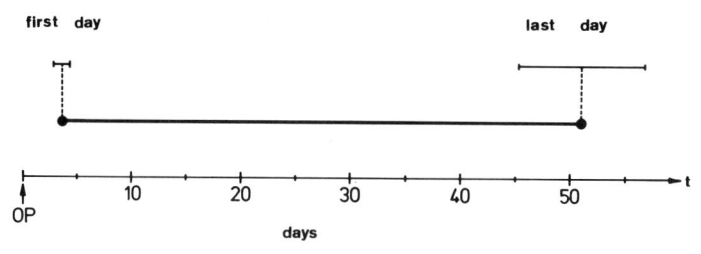

Fig. 3. Duration of spontaneous activity after nerve compression

In the first period after clipping, the distal motor latency increased and disappeared within 24 h. Between the 35th and 40th days the excitability reappeared with a marked diminution in distal velocity (Fig. 4). Training did not influence the temporal course of returning to normal. There was no difference between the animals with different clips from 70 to 130 p and no difference in the animals with a different duration of clipping. The nerve conduction velocity was slow and slowly returned to normal. After the 85th–90th days the normal conduction velocity was reached, but the preoperative values were hardly reached. In some hens the F reflex (Fig. 5) could be seen with a latency of 16–19 ms.

Morphological Investigations. The normal anatomy and the pathological findings in these hens are described by in detail by Blank et al. (this volume). The first pathological finding was the alteration of the impregnation of the myelin sheath, which was found even some minutes after clipping. This was followed by a worse impregnation of the axons themselves. The diameter of the nerve fibers and axons were greater proximally than distally. In scanning

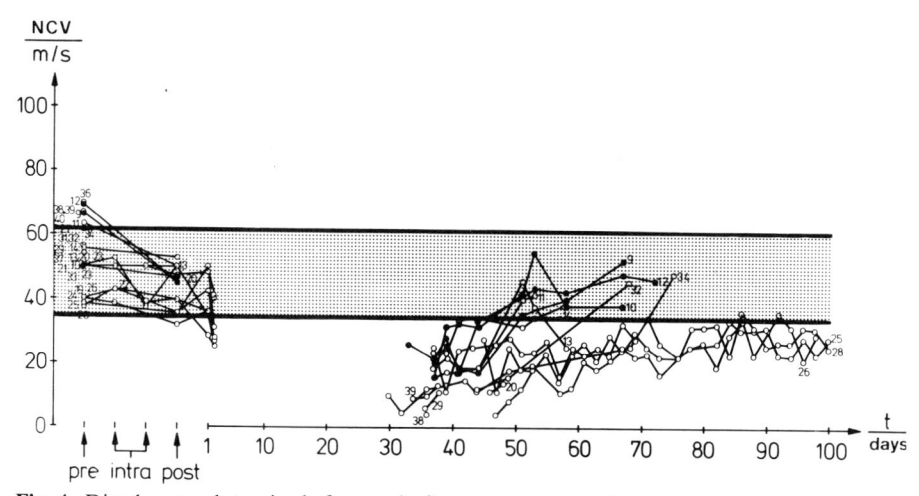

Fig. 4. Distal motor latencies before and after nerve compression

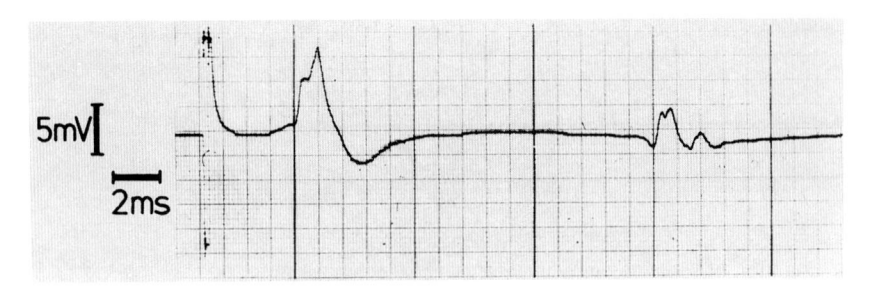

Fig. 5. F-reflex

electron microscopy we found an augmentation of reticular fiber structures, fibrocytes and a thickening of the perineurium and the basal membrane, and alterations of the endothelium of the neural vessels.

Discussion

The acute pressure model serves different purposes, not only to demonstrate electrophysiological and morphological findings but also to perform clinical examinations, e.g., reflex studies and observation of trophic disorders. The quick temporal development of alterations in denervation and reinnervation in the hen seemed to be due to the high temperature and metabolic rate. The excitability of the nerve disappeared after pressure was applied to the nerve, but not at once, which corresponds to findings in other animals (Denny-Brown and Brenner 1944). The time required for the effects to disappear was different in the study by Krücke (1974). The disappearance of electrical excitability corresponded to the alterations of silver impregnation of myelin sheath and axons. Proximal and distal to the site of compression, intrafascicular edema developed, leading to a swelling at the site of compression. Nerve excitability disappeared at the same time as the reflexes. This was independent of the pressure of the clips, which may be due to the fact (morphologically verified) that all clips produced axonotmesis. Therefore it did not matter how long compression lasted. The great alterations in morphological structures demonstrated in microscopy seem to explain why the nerve conduction velocity does not return to preoperative values. The augmentation of connective tissue and the lesions of the vessels thus seem to limit the restitutio ad integrum. The alterations of the perineural basal membrane may contribute to a different diffusion. Training does not influence the results except for its positive effect on the motility of the joints. This is an accepted fact in man (Grote 1987). Nevertheless, the discrepancy between the degree of morphological and electrophysiological changes is very astonishing and contrary to the excellent result of reinnervation.

Summary

In the domestic fowl the ischiadic nerve was compressed by aneurysm clips with different pressures and duration. Proximal to the lesion there was no electrical excitability after clipping, below the lesion splitting of the potential and disappearance of the excitability in 24 h. Motor function and reflexes disappeared at once after clipping. Excitability returned independently of the duration of clipping and the pressure of the clips. The nerve conduction velocities normalized more quickly in the proximal parts than in the distal ones. They did not reach the preoperative values. The disappearance of reflexes and motor function corresponds to morphological alterations in staining. At later stages the normal function contrasts with the electrophysiological and morphological findings.

References

Aguayo A, Nair CPV, Midgley R (1971) Experimental progressive compression neuropathy in the rabbit. Arch Neurol 24:358–364
Allen FM (1938) Effects of ligations on nerves of the extremities. Ann Surg 108:1088–1093
Bentley FH, Schlapp W (1943) The effects of pressure on conduction in peripheral nerve. J Physiol 102:72–82
Blank M (1966) Intrazelluläre Strukturveränderungen der Motoneurone des Haushuhns, gallus domesticus, nach peripherer Nervendurchtrennung. J Hirnforsch 8:103–109
Blank M, Lehmann M, El-Hifnawi ES (1978) Eine Modifikation der Kodousek'schen Silberimprägnationsmethode, die für elektronenmikroskopische Vergleichsuntersuchungen geeignet ist. Beitr. elektronenmikroskop. Direktabb Oberfl 11:263–268
Denny-Brown D, Brenner C (1944a) Paralysis of nerve induced by direct pressure and by tourniquet. Arch Neurol Psychiat 51:1–26
Denny-Brown D, Brenner C (1944b) Lesion in peripheral nerve resulting from compression by spring clip. Arch Neurol Psychiat 52:1–19
Duncan D (1948) Alterations in the structure of nerves caused by restricting their growth with ligatures. J Neuropath exp Neurol 7
Dyck PJ (1969) Experimental hypertrophic neuropathy. Arch Neurol 21:73–95
Glees R, White WG (1961) The absorption of tri-ortho-cresylphosphate through the skin of hens and its neurotoxic effects. J Neurol Neurosurg Psychiat 24:271–274
Grote W (1987) Neurochirurgie. Thieme, Stuttgart
Henschler D (1958) Die Trikresylphosphatvergiftung. Klin Wschr 36:663–774
Koch W, Heim G (1955) Die Haltung und Zucht von Versuchstieren. Enke, Stuttgart
Krücke W (1974) Pathologie der peripheren Nerven. In: Olivecrona H, Tönnis W, Krenkel W (Hrsg) Handbuch der Neurochirurgie, Bd VII/3. Springer, Berlin Heidelberg New York
Lehmann HJ, Pretschner DP (1966) Experimentelle Untersuchungen zum Engpaßsyndrom peripherer Nerven. Dtsch Z Nervenheilk 183:308–330
Mayer RF, Denny-Brown D (1964) Conduction velocity in peripheral nerve during experimental demyelination in the cat. Neurology 14:714–726
Weiss P, Davis H (1943) Pressure block in nerves provided with arterial sleeves. J Neurophysiol 6:269–286

Regeneration of Peripheral Nerves by Means of Muscle and Nerve Transplants

M. Sparmann, G. Friedebold, and T. Meyer, Berlin/FRG

Introduction

The bridging of nerve defects remains a clinical problem. Despite the development of nerve transplants (Millesi 1975; Millesi et al. 1982) the search continues for alternatives to the defect bridging of nerve injuries.

Experimental investigations by Lundborg and coworkers (Lundborg and Hansson 1979, 1980; Lundborg et al. 1981, 1982a, b, c) and Rigoni et al. (1983) have shown that, at least in animals, a free neuromatous neurotization is possible over short defective nerve segments. These findings were confirmed under similar experimental conditions of our own. However, the qualitative results of free neuromatous neurotization are considerably poorer than those after nerve transplantations (Sparmann et al. 1987). The electrophysiological and quantitative analyses in the target muscle have shown that these methods cannot be regarded as an alternative to free nerve transplantation.

Findings on the process of peripheral nerve regeneration after complete severance, as reported by Schröder and Seifert (1970), confirm that nerve replacement requires a substance that imitates the ultrastructural architecture of the nerve. Only in this way is it possible to achieve specific growth in a peripheral direction, as in the endoneural tube.

Since, within certain limits, the skeletal muscles show an ultrastructure similar to that of peripheral nerve tissues, i.e., parallel arrangement of tube systems (sarcolemmic tubes) with basement membranes, the question arose whether an interpositioning of muscle can fulfill the contact guidance principle just as well as nerve transplants. The encouragement for this investigation was derived from studies by Glasby et al. (1986), who published the first favorable results after animal experiments of this kind.

Methods

In our clinic surgery was performed bilaterally on the peroneal nerve of 20 female rabbits. A length of 1 cm of the nerve was resected, and the nerve defect was concurrently bridged with muscle and nerve transplants. After 6 and 12 months, an electrophysiological examination of the nerves involved was performed as well as light- and electron-miscroscopic analyses of the muscle and nerve transplants. The quality of nerve regeneration was determined by histomorphometric evaluations of the target muscle (anterior tibial muscle).

Results

Light-Microscopic Examination of the Transplants. On the side of the nerve transplants there was specific growth in a peripheral direction. On the side of the muscular implant, it was possible after 6 and 12 months to detect intact myofibrils with typical transverse striation interspersed with individual nerve fibers showing specific growth in a peripheral direction (Figs. 1, 2). Neuromatous alterations could be found only in the area of the muscles to an insignificant degree. The regeneration of the nerve by means of muscle was specific.

Neurophysiological examinations. The relative nerve conduction velocity of the peroneal nerve distal to the implant was 60.3% for the control side and 48.3% for the side of the muscle implant after one-half year. There was an approximation of the values after 1 year with 73.1% on the side of the nerve transplant and 66.1% on that of the muscle transplant. These results were markedly better than those obtained in comparative investigations dealing with free neuromatous neurotization.

In addition, the maximal amplitudes of the distally recorded action potential were measured. This yielded a ratio of 1.7:3.4 mV after 6 months and

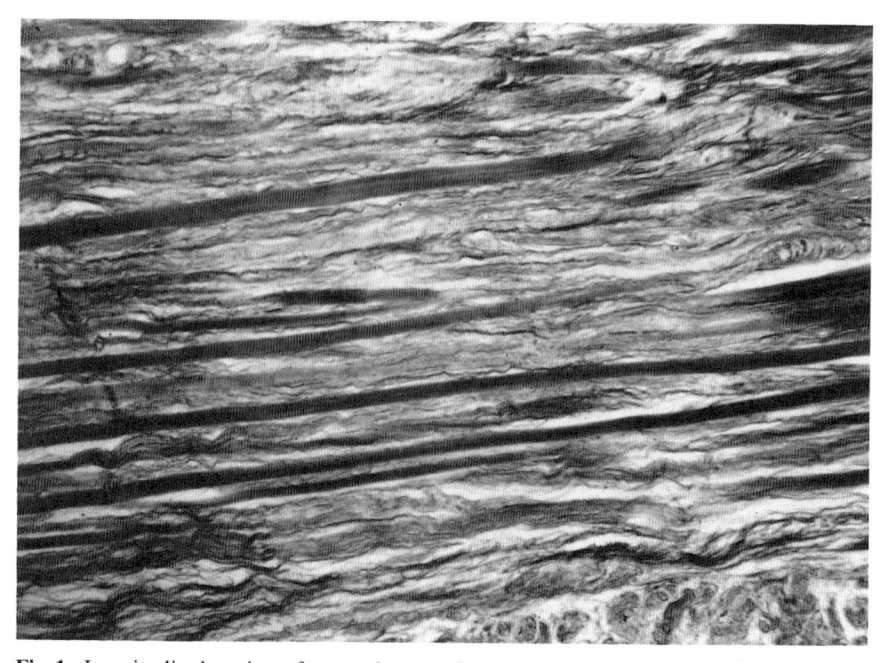

Fig. 1. Longitudinal section of a muscle transplant, 1 year after implantation. Some muscle fibers are still visible, between many axonal structures without neuromatous changes. (Masson-Goldner, ×210)

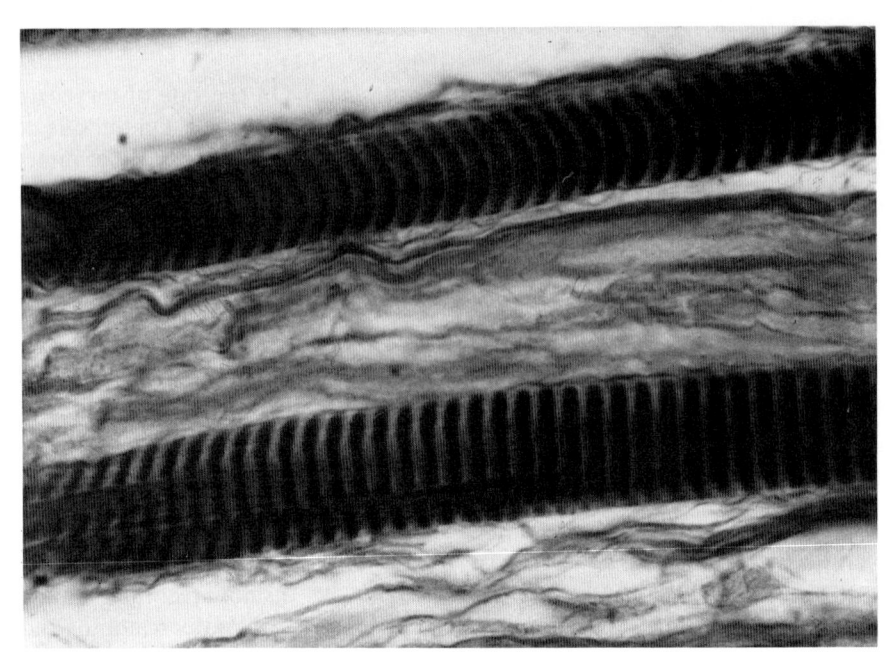

Fig. 2. Longitudinal section of a muscle transplant 1 year after implantation. Striated muscle fibers, myelinated axonal structures growing in a peripheral direction. (Palmgreen, × 860)

2.07:3.45 mV after 12 months for the two sides. Although the muscle transplants were slightly poorer here than the nerve transplants, a better result could also be achieved in these cases for the muscle transplants than with free neuromatous neurotizations. These neurophysiological results emphasize the importance of the guide-rail effect for nerve regeneration.

Planimetry. Planimetric analyses of the regenerated target muscle were also carried out for quantitative evaluation of the investigation. This involved the measurement of the total areas that actually regenerated. It was found that the muscle regeneration achieved for the muscle transplants after both 6 and 12 months was far superior to the free neuromatous neurotizations.

The qualitative histochemical examinations of the muscles confirmed these results, revealing a matured fiber type of distribution in the regeneration products of the musculature.

Summary

In the light of these results nerve regeneration appears to be dependent to a significant degree upon the ultrastructural architecture with which the defective segment is to be bridged. Although skeletal muscles cannot completely replace nerve transplants in animal experiments, the results of nerve regeneration are nevertheless markedly better than after free neuromatous neurotizations and approach those achieved with nerve transplants.

In view of the different regenerative potencies of peripheral nerves in animals and humans, no consequences for human medicine can presently be derived from these findings.

References

1. Glasby MA, Gschmeissner SE, Hitchcock RJI, Huang CLH et al. (1986) A comparison of nerve regeneration through nerve and muscle grafts in rat. Neuro-Orthop 2:21–28
2. Lundborg G, Hansson HA (1979) Regeneration of peripheral nerve through a performed tissue space. Preliminary observations on the reorganization of regenerating nerve fibres and perineurium. Brain Res 179:573–576
3. Lundborg G, Hansson HA (1980) Nerve regeneration through performed pseudosynovial tubes. A preliminary report of a new experimental model for studying the regeneration and reorganization capacity of peripheral nerve tissue. J Hand Surg 5:35–38
4. Lundborg G, Dahlin LB, Danielsen N, Hansson HA, Larsson K (1981) Reorganization and orientation of regenerating nerve fibres perineurium and epineurium in performed mesothelial tubes – an experimental study in sciatic nerve of rats. J Neurosci 6:265–281
5. Lundborg G, Dahlin LB, Danielsen N, Gelbermann R et al. (1982a) Nerve regeneration in silicone chambers: influence of gap length and presence of distal stump components. Exp Neurol 76:361–375
6. Lundborg G, Dahlin LB, Danielsen N, Hansson HA et al. (1982b) Nerve regeneration across an extended gap: a neurobiological view of neurotropic factors. J Hand Surg 7:580–587
7. Lundborg G, Gelbermann RH, Longo FM, Powell H et al. (1982c) In vivo regeneration of cut nerves encased in silicone tubes: growth across a six millimeter gap. J Neuropath Exp Neurol 4:412–422
8. Millesi H (1975) Bedeutung der Nerventransplantation in der Chirurgie der peripheren Nerven. Zbl Chir 100:1537–1546
9. Millesi H, Meissl G, Berger A (1982) Nerve sutures and nerve grafting. Scand J Plast Reconstr Surg 19:25–37
10. Rigoni G, Smahel J, Chiu DTW, Meyer VE (1983) Veneninterponat als Leitbahn für die Regeneration peripherer Nerven. Handchirurgie 15:227–231
11. Schröder JM, Seifert KE (1970) Zur Feinstruktur der neuromatösen Neurotisation von Nerventransplantaten. Virch Arch Abl B Zellpath 5:219
12. Sparmann M, Mellerowicz H, Meyer T, King B (1987) Die Bedeutung des Nerventransplantates für die Nervenregeneration. Das Transplantat in der Plastischen Chirurgie, S 240–244

Motor Recovery After Delayed Nerve Suture

H.-P. RICHTER, Fulda/FRG

Introduction

The degree of skeletal muscle recovery and the restitution of motor function which can be achieved by nerve suture decreases with increasingly late nerve repair. Early repair leads to a qualitatively good recovery, whereas very late repair is regularly followed by no or only minor recovery. The best achievable function therefore decreases with an increase in the delay of nerve suture. This knowledge is based on clinical and experimental evidence. Morphological structures responsible for a gradual decline in the quality of motor recovery can be the anterior horn cells within the spinal cord, the peripheral nerve fibers, the motor endplates or the muscle cells themselves.

Experiments dealing with the results after delayed nerve repair are rare. Only Gutmann and Young (1944) presented a systematic study in the rabbit. We extended their experiments and used modern electrophysiological and morphological methods for the evaluation of motor restitution (Richter 1980, 1982; Richter and Ketelsen 1982).

Materials and Methods

In a first operation, rabbit peroneal nerve was cut at the distal thigh. In a second operation, we removed the neuroma and reanastomosed proximal and distal stumps by microsurgical epineurial sutures. The various groups of animals differed in respect to the interval between nerve transection and repair: the shortest presuture interval was only minutes, because primary suture was performed in this group of animals. In the group with the longest presuture denervation period, this interval was 12 months. Six months after nerve suture, the toe-spreading reflex was tested semiquantitatively and investigated electrophysiologically (needle recordings, conduction studies), before nerve and muscle material was removed for light and electron microscopic evaluation. The animals were then killed. A total of 75 nerve and muscle specimens from 47 animals were examined.

Results

With increasing denervation periods, the strength of the toe-spreading reflex diminished, the amplitude of the evoked muscle action potential decreased, and the structural abnormalities within the peroneus longus muscles increased. These findings were statistically significant.

Even in the animals with a denervation period of 11–12 months, there was a good neurotization of the peroneal nerve distal to the suture site, although motor function was highly insufficient, measured in terms of the strength of the toe-spreading reflex and the amplitude of the evoked muscle action potential. The spectrum of myelinated nerve fibers showed a shift towards smaller diameters. Such a shift already occurs after primary nerve suture and did not change considerably among the groups of increasing presuture denervation invervals.

The motor endplates showed important alterations in those animals with very late nerve repair (11–12 months after severance). The contact between axon terminal and sarcolemma or muscle cell surface was imperfect. The width of the normally narrow primary synaptic cleft was irregular. Basal lamina duplications and Schwann's cell processes were found within this cleft, thus causing an insufficient neuromuscular contact.

The enzymatic pattern of certain muscle fibers within the muscle changes after successful reinnervation, even after primary nerve suture. The mosaic pattern of a normal muscle is lost, and a grouping of enzymatically identical muscle fibers is seen instead. This is a sign of reinnervation of neighboring muscle cells by collateral sprouts of one motor neuron. With later nerve suture, the capacity of muscle fibers to form groups decreases, and degenerative processes become prominent. This is, for example, increased fibrosis of the muscle, which is more and more replaced by fat tissue.

Discussion

When discussing the relationship between the quality of motor recovery and the interval between nerve transection and nerve repair, attention is focused mainly on the nerve. This may contribute to a bad functional result owing to endoneural fibrosis. This again impedes the outgrowth of regenerating axons. Very little attention, on the other hand, is paid to the neuromuscular junction and the end-organ or target – the muscle cells themselves. But these are also important components of the motor system.

Although endoneural fibrosis is said to increase with later nerve repair, we found a good neurotization distal to the suture site even in those animals in which the severed nerve was reanastomosed only after 11–12 months. The degree of neurotization did not appear to differ considerably among the various groups of animals. The reason for a bad motor restitution after late nerve suture may also be located within the motor endplates and the muscle fibers. Structural abnormalities at the motor endplates, such as invaginations of the basal lamina or interposition of Schwann's cell processes into the primary synaptic cleft between nerve fiber terminal and muscle cell membrane, are certainly not induced by the regenerating axon. They are simply the expression of an insufficient recovery of motor endplate structure.

On the way to the target, many fibers lose contact, and others – such as sensory axons – are incapable of establishing functional contact with muscle cells. After a longer time without innervation and without neurotrophic influences the muscle may be degenerated to such an extent that regenerating axons arrive at a target which cannot be reinnervated because there are no viable muscle cells left. This critical denervation period is difficult or impossible to define precisely, although in rabbit the quality of motor recovery deteriorated when the presuture denervation had lasted 8–9 months or longer. Such a statement can only be valid for the rabbit's peroneal nerve and cannot be extrapolated to primates and to man. For patients with peripheral nerve transection it has been virtually impossible up to now to define the interval beyond which nerve suture would be meaningless because the muscles are – irreversibly – degenerated.

According to Wechsler and Hager (1961), skeletal muscle can be reinnervated up to its afibrillar state. This statement by neuropathologists does not help the clinician very much. The clinician needs a predictive test which tells him whether a nerve repair may still be useful, or whether it is too late. Many peripheral nerve surgeons follow the hypothesis that a muscle is capable of reinnervation as long as fibrillation potentials are recorded during electromyography. Others think that a muscle denervated for 18 months or longer rarely has a chance to recover to a useful function.

Conclusion

There is no question that it is not the – reversible – atrophy alone but also irreversible degenerative changes which become of increasing significance with longer intervals between nerve transection and nerve repair. The structure responsible for such a worsened motor restitution is certainly not the nerve alone but also the motor endplates and muscle cells. The critical denervation interval cannot be defined precisely. From a statistical point of view, this question is a regression problem with gradual decrease of function with time. Intervals determined in animals cannot be extrapolated to animals of higher phyla and not to humans. Because motor function becomes worse the longer the muscle remains denervated, these experimental data support the demand for an early repair of a severed peripheral nerve.

References

Gutmann E, Young JZ (1944) The re-innervation of muscle after various periods of atrophy. J Anat (Lond) 78:15–43
Richter HP (1980) Tierexperimentelle Untersuchungen über die Restitution der Skelettmuskulatur nach Nervennaht – mit besonderer Berücksichtigung der späten Sekundärnaht. Habilitationsschrift, Universität Ulm
Richter HP (1982) Impairment of motor recovery after late nerve suture: experimental study in the rabbit. I. Functional and electromyographic findings. Neurosurg 10:70–74
Richter HP, Ketelsen UP (1982) Impairment of motor recovery after late nerve suture: experimental study in the rabbit. II. Morphological findings. Neurosurg 10:75–85
Wechsler W, Hager H (1961) Elektronenmikroskopische Befunde bei Muskelatrophie nach Nervendurchtrennung bei der weißen Ratte. Beitr Pathol Anat 125:31–53

Stimulation of Nerve Axon Outgrowth by Means of Fibrin Adhesive with Added Melanotropic Neuropeptide *

O. OSGAARD, Glostrup/Denmark and N. H. DIEMER, Copenhagen/Denmark

In nerve grafting today a biological two-component tissue adhesive is commonly used to fixate the nerve grafts to the nerve stumps. Several reports have shown that this technique offers the same functional results as the microsuturing technique but is easier to apply and considerably more time saving. Several factors have been described to promote nerve regeneration by increasing the number of outgrowing nerve fibers. These substances include nerve growth factor [1], the peptide hormones $ACTH_{4-10}$ [2], $ACTH_{4-9}$, and alpha-melanocortine [3]. In several experimental studies from the University of Utrecht [3–5], the melanotropic neuropeptides have been shown to stimulate the nerve axon outgrowth, both by systemic and local application.

The aim of the present study was to determine whether an addition of $ACTH_{4-9}$ to the fibrin adhesive might stimulate an increased or faster outgrowth of nerve axons in repaired sciatic nerve lesions in the rat.

Methods

In male Wistar rats (200 g) anesthetized with ketamine (10 mg/100 g, intraperitoneally) both sciatic nerves were exposed and cut a few millimeters below the sciatic notch. The nerve stumps were then immediately approximated with one or two microvascular sutures under microscope. The anastomosis was then coated, on one side with fibrin adhesive alone and on the other with fibrin adhesive, with 5 µm peptide added to the calcium chloride part of the solution. In this way, each animal served as its own control. A total of 18 rats were operated on. On the 10th, 20th, and 30th day, six rats were killed by decapitation and both sciatic nerves removed. The specimens were stretched between pins on a wooden spatula to prevent shrinkage, fixed in 2.5% glutaraldehyde in 0.1 M phosphate buffer, washed in the buffer and post-fixed in 1% OsO_4. After dehydration with alcohol, the specimens were embedded in epon. Cross-sections were cut above and below the anastomosis, as close as possible, stained with toluidine blue, and examined by the neuropathologist (N. H. D) who was blinded as to which nerve had been treated with the peptide. The counting of the myelinated fibers was done under 1000 × magnification in a light microscope, linked to a videocamera and a Leitz TAS plus video-based image analyzer. On the image-analyzed screen, all dark figures (myelin,

---

* This research was supported by a grant from Immuno A/S, Denmark.

macrophages, and vessels) were detected, and the image was stored in the video memory. After this, all holes in the picture were closed, and the picture was stored in the video memory. Finally, an exclusive or transformation was performed between the two foregoing pictures and the holes counted. Four to six representative sections per specimen were counted.

Results

After 10 days the proximal stumps of the peptide-treated nerves displayed a tendency of more myelinated nerve fibers than did the non-treated nerves, thus indicating an increased sprouting activity. There were 52% more outgrowing nerve fibers in the treated group than in the non-treated group (14.6% versus 9.6%; $p < 0.05$). After 20 days the pattern changed, displaying no difference between the treated and non-treated proximal stumps. In the distal stumps, however, the difference had become more pronounced than after 10 days, with 74% more outgrowing nerve fibers in the treated nerves (33.7% versus 14.2%; $p < 0.05$). After 30 days, the difference had disappeared completely, with an outgrowth of 52% versus 49.7%.

Conclusion

These findings closely resemble those reported by the Utrecht group; however, the maximal sprouting in the present study comes a little later. One may conclude that the beneficial effect of the neuropeptides seems linked to an increased sprouting activity from the proximal stump rather than to an increased outgrowth velocity.

Acknowledgements. The fibrin adhesive (Tisseel) used in this study was provided by Immuno A/S, Denmark, and the $ACTH_{4-9}$ (Org 2766) by Organon, The Netherlands.

References

1. Richardson PM, Ebendal T, Riopelle RJ (1985) Nerve growth and nerve growth factor within peripheral nervous tissue. In: Björklund A, Stenevi U (eds) Neural grafting in the mammalian. Elsevier Science Publishers, pp 319–327
2. Bijlsma WA, Jennekens FGI, Schotman P, Gispen W-H (1983) Stimulation by $ACTH_{4-10}$ of nerve fiber regeneration following sciatic nerve crush. Muscle & Nerve 6:104–112
3. Edwards PM, Van der Zee CEEM, Verhagen J, Schotman P, Jennekens FGI, Gispen W-H (1984) Evidence that the neurotrophic actions of α-MSH may derive from its ability to mimic the actions of a peptide formed in degeneration nerve stumps. J Neurol Sci 64:333–340
4. Bijlsma WA, Schotman P, Jennekens FGI, Gispen W-H, Wied D (1983) The enhanced recovery of sensimotor functions in rat is related to the melanotropic moiety of ACTH/MSH neuropeptides. Europ J Pharmacol 92:231–236
5. Verhagen J, Edwards PM, Jennekens FGI, Schotman P, Gispen W-H (1986) α-Melanocyte-stimulating hormone (α-MSH) stimulates the outgrowth of myelinated nerve fibers after peripheral nerve crush. Exp Neurol 92(2):451–454

Nerve Regeneration in the Centrocentral Anastomosis

J. M. GONZÁLEZ-DARDER, J. BARBERÁ, J. L. GIL- SALÚ, and F. GARCIA-VÁZQUEZ, Cadiz/Spain

The centrocentral anastomosis (CCA) can be defined as an end-to-end microsuture among the fascicles of the central stump of a severed peripheral nerve, with an interposed autologous nerve graft between each pair of fascicles. This technique was developed by Samii [4, 5] in an attempt to reduce the size of terminal neuromas and subsequentely to achieve control of neuroma and postamputation pain.

Clinical and Experimental Studies

Some clinical studies, involving small groups of patients, have shown the disappearance or alleviation of chronic pain in cases of stump pain with a CCA performed after resection of amputation neuromas and also when the CCA is carried out following resection of painful terminal neuromas if functional motor or sensory recuperation is not the objective. Centrocentral anastomosis has been used in the prevention of painful neuromas after emergency or elective amputations. In the event of limb amputation CCA can be performed among fascicles of the main nerves of the extremity. In hand surgery, following finger amputations, CCA is carried out between dorsal and palmar collateral nerves. However, these encouraging clinical results [2–6] should be carefully evaluated, taking into consideration that one-third of patients with painful neuromas can be cured or improve in the long term with a simple neuroma resection, and that only a small percentage of patients develop some type of postamputation pain, even years after surgery.

On the other hand, experimental studies have shown that CCA reduces the size of terminal neuromas resulting from transection of sciatic nerves in rats and rabbits [1–4]. We have examined the role of CCA on the time course of autotomy following experimental transection of sciatic nerves in rats [1], considered by many authors as a valid experimental model of chronic pain. We found that CCA significantly reduces the autotomy behavior in rats when the procedure is performed immediately after nerve transection or following neuroma resection.

With these clinical and experimental data it is tempting to speculate that the decrease of autotomy score in chronic pain animal models and pain control in patients with neuroma or postamputation pain is achieved by reducing the size of terminal neuroma. These kinds of pain have been related to many physiopathological causes, but we believe that peripheral factors may play a major role in their pathogenesis. In fact, electroneurophysiological studies have shown aberrant properties in axon sprouts of rat sciatic neuromas as the result of sprout growing into a foreign chemical and cellular environment. Thus, the results of CCA could be explained if we consider that regenerated axon sprouts which cross the suture line penetrate into the nerve graft where they grow freely isolated and protected from the scar. If the graft is not interposed, and the terminal stumps of fascicles are sutured end-to-end, the axon sprouts of the fascicles cannot penetrate into the contralateral, occupied endoneural tubes, and a true neuroma in continuity is formed.

Regeneration in the Centrocentral Anastomosis

In addition to this clinical interest, the CCA itself is an interesting experimental model to study the peripheral nerve regeneration as the regenerating axons grow into the nerve graft from both ends lacking peripheral motor or sensory targets to reach. With the aim of investigating this, a simple model of CCA was developed in rats by suturing the peroneal and sural branches of the sciatic nerve. A 5-mm nerve portion taken from the peroneal branch was used as interposed graft (Fig. 1). The animals were operated on using a microsurgical technique. In most animals 10/0 Ethilon was used as suture material, but

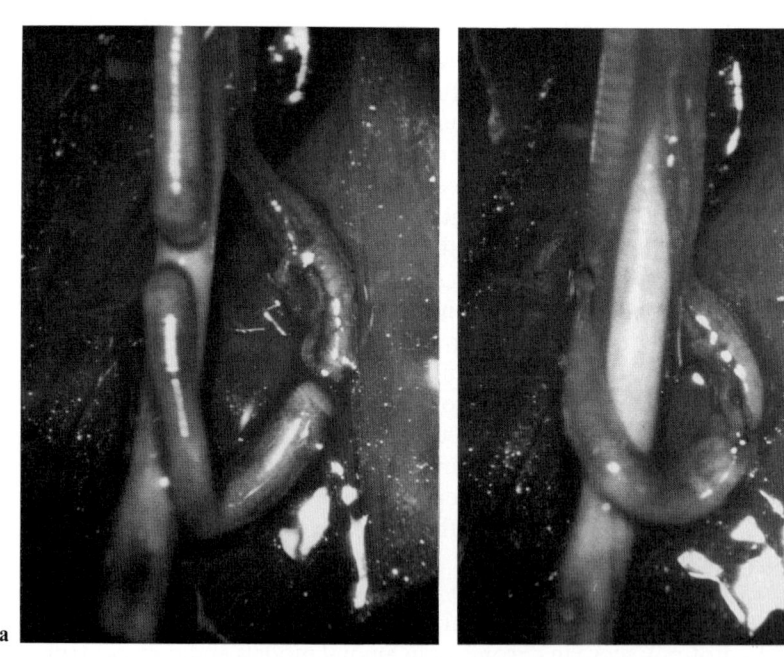

Fig. 1 a, b. Operative photographs of a completed simple centrocentral anastomosis. The sural and peroneal branches of the sciatic nerve of the rat are anastomosed. A nerve graft taken from the peroneal nerve is interposed

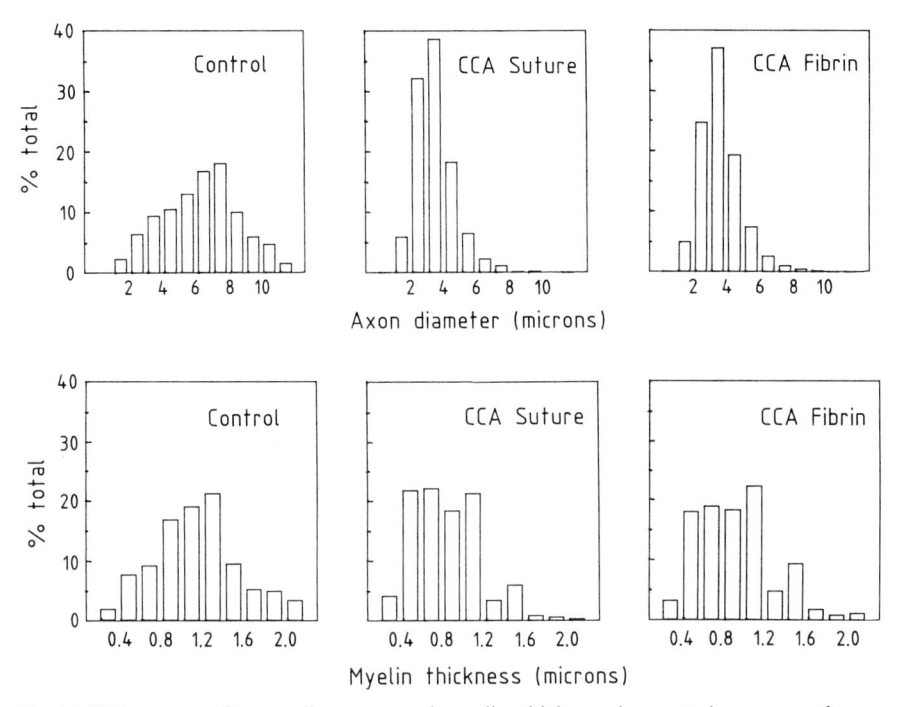

Fig. 2. Histograms of axon diameters and myelin thickness in control nerves and centrocentral anastomosis grafts at 90 days of regeneration in control, suture, and fibrin groups

in a few cases a non-suture technique was carried out using Tissucol, a fibrin adhesive glue. After killing, the CCA were carefully removed from each animal and the specimens processed for pathological study, obtaining semithin cuts stained by toluidine blue technique.

One group of animals was killed 45 or 90 days after surgery. For the purpose of quantitative analysis transverse sections at the midpoint of the nerve graft were cut, stained, and examined under light microscope. Microphotographs were taken and enlarged at 1000 and 1600 times real magnification. Montages of nerve sections were made from prints for morphometric analysis of myelinated fibers. Each nerve cross-section was divided into fields of $10\,823\,\mu m^2$. Measurements were made of the number of fibers per field, diameter of axons, and myelin thickness. The study was done manually using a digitalized graphic table attached to a microcomputed Apple II working with a "four points" software program for calculations. Normal contralateral peroneal nerves were used as control group.

The results show that the number of axons per field increases with postoperative time. The mean number of axons per field was 137 in the suture group and 122 in the fibrin group at 45 days of regeneration, reaching 208 and 200, respectively, at 90 days. The mean number of fibers per field was 128 in control nerves. Size-frequency histograms for axon diameters and myelin thickness are presented for control and experimental groups in Fig. 2. After 90

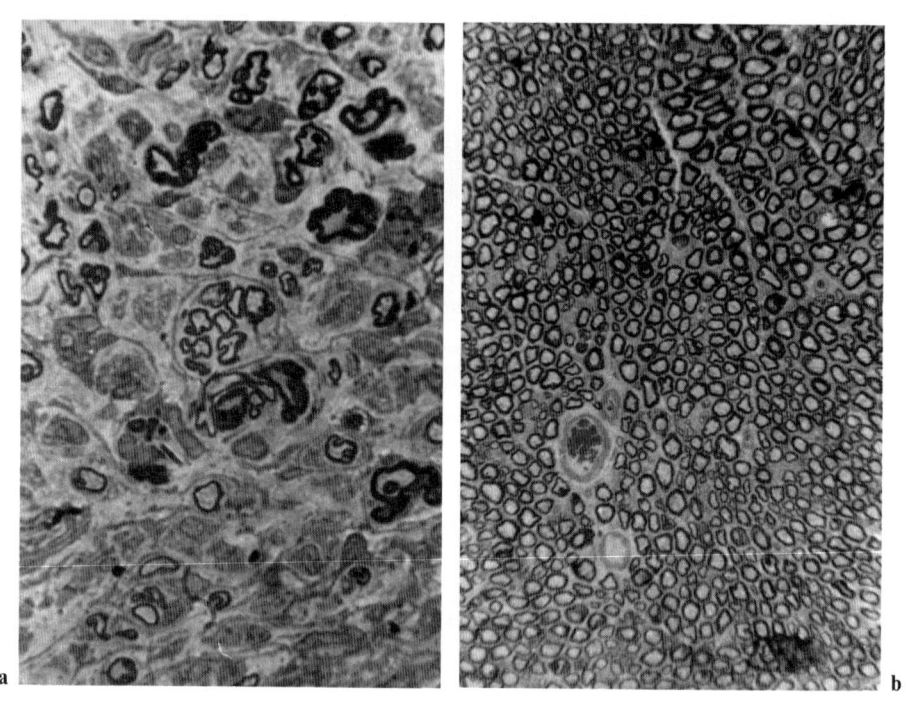

Fig. 3. a Microphotograph of the nerve graft of centrocentral anastomosis showing a mixed degenerative-regenerative pattern. **b** The parent nerve has no degenerative changes, showing the normal features of a peripheral nerve

days of regeneration the mean size of myelinated axons into the graft was 3.6 µm in the suture group, 3.5 µm in the fibrin group, and 6.4 µm in control nerves. The thickness of myelin was 0.9 µm in both experimental groups, compared with 1.2 in normal nerves. Finally, the ratio of total fiber diameter to axon diameter was 0.80 in the suture group, 0.78 in the fibrin group, and 0.84 in normal nerves.

A different experiment, using a technique of anterograde degeneration, was designed in a second group of rats to determine the distal points reached by regenerated axon sprouts. After 60 days of regenerating period following CCA the grafts were carefully cut in their midpoint to allow an anterograde wallerian degeneration in the fibers which had crossed the midpoint of the graft. Both stumps were fixed to neighboring tissues with a perineurial suture. We left 10 days for degeneration. The animals were then killed, removing the stumps of the grafts and the parent peroneal and sural nerves. The specimens were identified, orientated, and cut each 500 µm for histological examination in the search for nerve degeneration features. The nerve graft below the suture contained fascicles of fibers in a stage of recent wallerian degeneration mixed with fascicles containing fibers in different stages of regeneration (Fig. 3a). Some occasional fascicles housing simultaneously regenerated and degenerated fibers were found. This mixed degenerative-regenerative pattern was also observed in the portion of graft near the suture line, but in the parent nerves above the suture area there was no evidence of wallerian degeneration, and the nerves showed a normal pattern (Fig. 3b).

The results of our experimental studies show that axon sprouts grow into the interposed nerve graft, and although they are able to cross the first suture line penetrating into the graft, they cannot jump over the contralateral suture line. The morphometric study indicates an increase in number of axons with small myelinated fibers predominant, as would be expected in a regenerated nerve. However, the relationship between myelin thickness and fiber diameter is within the normal range of 0.5–0.9, meaning that regenerated axons in the nerve graft are fully myelinated in relation to their diameters. This phenomenon should occur, because it appears related only to the presence of Schwann's cells surrounding a nerve fiber.

However, the main issue to be explained is why the fibers are not able to cross the contralateral suture line stopping their regenerative activity. The first factor to be considered is related to the mechanical barrier developed by the scar in the suture line. An additional factor should be the lack of free Büngner's band on the other side of the suture line attracting and guiding fibers in the event of an axon sprout crossing the suture line. Another mechanical element was pointed out by Gorkisch et al. [2], who suggested that the blockage of regeneration in CCA should be due to an alteration in axonal flow produced by an increase of the intraperineurial pressure in the nerve graft. However, it is attractive to consider as the cause of this phenomenon that axon sprouts in CCA are confined to a non-target environment and perhaps isolated from contact with nerve growth factor action. In this way, further pathological studies using silicone chambers interposed between distal stumps of peroneal and sural nerves have been designed in rats to answer these questions.

Conclusions

Following centrocentral anastomosis axon sprouts grow into the interposed nerve graft crossing the first suture line. The sprouts remain confined and become myelinated in the graft. They are also protected against the irritating perineurial scar. We consider that all these pathological findings could explain the role of centrocentral anastomosis in the control of neuroma pain. However, the mechanisms blocking nerve regeneration in centrocentral anastomosis are not yet completely understood.

References

1. González-Darder JM, Barberá J, Abellán MJ, Mora A (1985) Centrocentral anastomosis in the prevention and treatment of painful terminal neuromas. An experimental study in the rat. J Neurosurg 63:754–758
2. Gorkisch K, Boese-Landgraf J, Vaubel E (1984) Treatment and prevention of amputation neuromas in hand surgery. Plast Reconstr Surg 74:293–296
3. Lagarrigue J, Chavoin JP, Belahovari L, Savazza R (1982) Traitment des neuromes doloreux par anastomoses nerveuse en anse 'piege a neurone'. Neurochirurgie 28:91–92
4. Samii M (1975) Modern aspects of peripheral nerve surgery. Advances and technical standards in neurosurgery, vol. 2. Springer, Berlin Heidelberg New York, pp 3–84
5. Samii M (1981) Centrocentral anastomosis of peripheral nerves: a neurosurgical treatment of amputation neuromas. In: Siegfried J, Zimmermann M (eds) Phantom and stump pain. Springer, Berlin Heidelberg New York, pp 123–125
6. Slooff ACJ (1978) Microsurgical possibilities in the treatment of peripheral pain. Clin Neurol Neurosurg 80:107–111

Biochemical Manipulation of the Microenvironment in Experimental Nerve Regeneration Chambers *

H. MÜLLER, Lübeck/FRG

Despite improved microsurgical techniques, the results of peripheral nerve repair very often remain unsatisfactory [1–4]. Therefore, studies aimed at a better identification and potential manipulation of the cellular and molecular events in PNS regeneration are still meaningful to both scientists and clinicians [5].

In the early 1980s Lundborg and Varon developed an in vivo chamber model for such investigations [6–8], following earlier attempts at entubation nerve repair techniques by other investigators [9–14]. In this model, the proximal and distal stumps of a transected rat sciatic nerve are sutured into the ends of a silicone tube, leaving a defined gap between the nerve stumps. So far, the model has been used to define the spatiotemporal progress of cellular regeneration [15, 16], to compare entubation repair with autologous grafting [17–20], to elicit the influence of neuronotrophic and neurite-promoting factors such as extracellular matrix components [21, 22], and to begin with delicate approaches to eventually manipulate the "spontaneous" sequence of events by increasing the chamber volume and subsequently filling it with either phosphate-buffered saline (PBS) or a preformed matrix [23, 24].

A long list of potentially "neurotrophic" biochemical agents can be derived from either in vitro cell culture studies or in vivo experiments reported in the literature. Of these, we have chosen 12, shown in Table 1, to be introduced into our regeneration chambers by means of multiple, direct injection in situ. Because of the necessity to screen them over a wide range of concentrations, we have chosen to group them arbitrarily into three mixtures of agents – recognizing the possibility of missing individual properties. Chambers of 25 µl volume were injected with 70 µl biochemical agents (25 µl/min) at the time of implantation and again 6 and 10 days thereafter. The excess fluid was allowed to leak out of a second, distally placed microneedle. All operations were performed under sterile conditions and with the aid of the operating microscope. The animals were killed at day 16. Details on materials and methods are given elsewhere [25].

The first series of these screening experiments showed a tendency towards a stimulatory effect only in group 2, i.e., the mix containing laminin, testosterone, ganglioside GM_1, and catalase (LTGC; Table 2). Moreover, the effect on

---

* This work was supported by a grant from the Deutsche Forschungsgemeinschaft (Mu 699/1–2).

Table 1. Grouping and molarity of agents (10)[a]

Group 1	
Pyruvate	1×10^{-3}
Forskolin	1×10^{-5}
Potassium	4×10^{-2}
TPA	1×10^{-8}
Group 2	
Laminin	1×10^{-3}
Testosterone	1×10^{-6}
Ganglioside GM_1	1×10^{-6}
Catalase	2×10^{-2}
Group 3	
L-Phosphatidyl-serine	1×10^{-6}
Insulin	1×10^{-6}
Fibronectin	3×10^{-7}
L-Triiodothyronine (T_3)	1×10^{-6}

[a] Given as a median concentration. Threefold ($=30$) and tenfold ($=100$) lower and higher concentrations were also administered, i.e., three to five different concentrations in each group of agents.

Table 2. Screening series of agents injected versus controls

	n	n_{ev}	S_3					S_5				
			C	V	Sc	Ax	M	C	V	Sc	Ax	M
PBS-injected controls	12	8	7	4	4	3	1	7	2	2	1	–
Group 1												
3	4	3	2	–	–	–	–	2	–	–	–	–
10	4	4	3	1	–	–	–	2	1	–	–	–
30	4	4	2	1	–	–	–	1	1	–	–	–
Group 2												
1	4	3	2	2	2	2	2	2	2	2	2	–
3	4	1	1	–	–	–	–	1	–	–	–	–
10	4	3	2	–	–	–	–	1	–	–	–	–
30	4	4	4	4	4	3	1	3	3	2	1	–
100	4	2	2	2	2	1	–	2	–	–	–	–
Group 3												
1	4	3	3	2	1	1	–	2	1	–	–	–
3	4	3	3	2	2	2	–	2	1	1	–	–
10	4	2	1	1	1	–	–	1	–	–	–	–
30	4	4	3	2	1	–	–	2	1	–	–	–
100	4	1	1	1	1	1	–	1	1	1	–	–
	64	45										

C, Circumferential cells; V, blood vessels; Sc, Schwann's cells; Ax, axons; M, myelin.

Table 3. Extended study of numerical LTGC effects

	Percentage of Chambers			LTGC $\times 30$ (16)
	Not injected (13)	Injected (19)	Averages (32)	
S_3				
Vessels	69	58	64	81
Schwann's cells	54	53	54	81
Axons	23	21	22	50
Myelin	8	5	7	31
S_5				
Vessels	38	37	38	75
Schwann's cells	23	21	22	70
Axons	0	5	3	31
Myelin	0	0	0	6

Figures in parentheses, number of chambers evaluated.

the presence of defined cellular elements in the center of the chambers (S_3 and S_5, respectively) was pronounced in a concentration of $30 \times$ (of a predefined basal level, see Table 1). The results obtained in group 1 could cautiously be interpreted as being inhibitory, and in group 3 as "indifferent."

An extended series was then undertaken with the LTGC mixture, another control group – with PBS prefilling but no further injection – now being included (Table 3). No difference was found between the two control groups. At S_3 the occurrence frequency in treated chambers was about twofold for axons and fourfold for myelin. At S_5 it appeared to be twofold for vessels (75% versus 38%), threefold for Schwann's cells (70% versus 22%), and tenfold for axons (31% versus 3%). Figure 1 illustrates these results. Perineurial-like

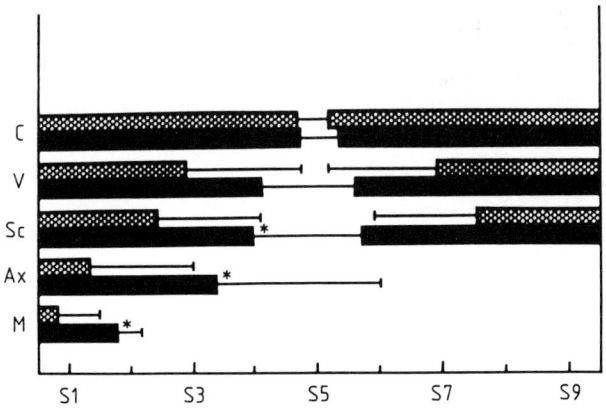

Fig. 1. Spatial progression across 16-day chambers injected with either PBS alone (▢▢▢; $n = 19$) or PBS containing the LTGC mixture (■■■; $n = 16$). C, Circumferential cells; V, blood vessels; Sc, Schwann's cells; Ax, axons, regardless of myelination; M, myelin. * $p < 0.02$, Mann-Whitney U test

Table 4. Quantitative analyses of S_3 cross-sections from control and LTGC-treated chambers, selected for the presence of axons

	Control (4)	Experimental (8)	E/C
Cross-sectional areas (mm² × 10³)			
Nerve regenerate	280 ± 7	490 ± 97[a]	1.7
Endoneurium	210 ± 17	420 ± 94[a]	2.0
Vessels	8 ± 2	18 ± 4[a]	2.2
Total numbers/cross-section			
Axons	650 ± 460	600 ± 570	0.9
Schwann's cells	980 ± 450	1030 ± 930	1.0
Vessels	27 ± 2	51 ± 10[a]	1.9

Figures in parentheses, number of S_3 chambers evaluated.
[a] $p < 0.01$ (Mann-Whitney U test).

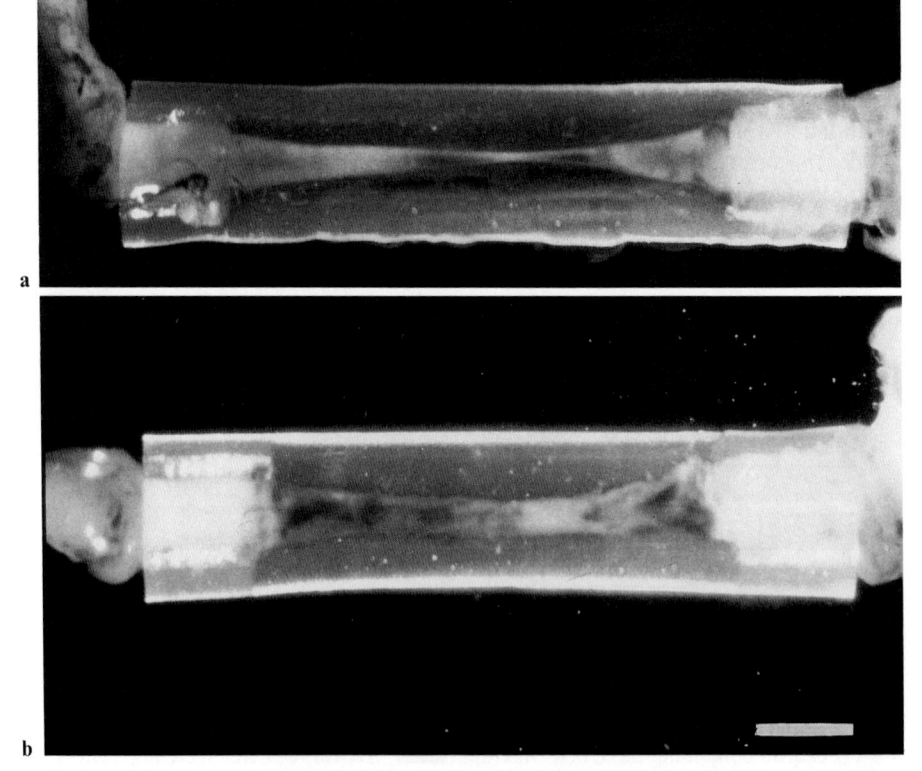

Fig. 2. 16-day nerve regenerates within silicone chambers subjected to PBS (controls) (**a**) or LTGC injection (**b**). *Scale bar*, 2 mm

circumferential cells had migrated over the entire length of the chamber matrix in both control and treated chambers. Vessels and Schwann's cells occupied only about the proximal and distal one-third of 16-day control chambers and had nearly doubled their advance in LTGC-treated chambers. Axons lagged behind Schwann's cells in controls but were nearly as advanced as the latter in treated chambers. Lastly, myelin was barely detected in the most proximal part of control chambers but significantly further advanced in treated ones.

Some computer-aided morphometric measurements on S_3 cross-sections were additionally done. We selected only those chamber regenerates that had been scored positive for the presence of axons (at S_3) to determine whether there were quantitative numerical differences beyond the mere presence or absence of the various cellular elements. The results are presented in Table 4. Values for cross-sectional areas of the whole nerve regenerate, endoneural space, and the area occupied by vessels all yielded about twofold greater numbers in LTGC-treated chambers. No significant differences were found concerning the total number of axons and Schwann's cells, whereas there were 2.5-fold more vessels in LTGC chambers.

Figure 2 shows two representative examples of control (Fig. 2a) and treated (Fig. 2b) nerve regenerates. The proximal part is to the left. Note the obvious differences in shape and calibers. The experimental investigations reported here demonstrate that nerve regeneration can be manipulated on a cellular level by various molecules, or at least by one or more agents used in combination. All of them, namely laminin [26–32], testosterone [33–36], gangliosides [37–42], and catalase [43] have been reported to elicit effects on the behaviour of neurons and/or neurites during development or regeneration – most of them, however, being studied under in vitro conditions. Further in vivo experiments are currently being evaluated [44] to clarify the respective roles of the substances used in our combinations. It is the working hypothesis that each component may well address different aspects of the regenerative process and hence may not be able "to do the job" by itself – or not to a fully recognizable extent.

Acknowledgements. The author is indebted to Drs. S. Varon and L. R. Williams for very helpful discussions and to Ms. E. Hewitt and Mr. H. L. Vahlsing for technical support.

References

1. Müller H (1978) Dokumentation und Analyse klinischer Resultate nach Nervennähten. Doct. Thesis. University of Hamburg
2. Müller H, Grubel G (1981) Long-term results of peripheral nerve sutures – a comparison of micro- and macrosurgical techniques. Adv Neurosurg 9:381–387
3. Müller H, Grubel G (1982) Periphere Nervenverletzungen: Indikation und Ergebnisse der frühen Sekundärversorgung. Hefte Unfallheilkd 158:453–459
4. Müller H, Grubel G (1983) Factors influencing peripheral nerve suture results. Arch Orthop Trauma Surg 102:51–55
5. Lundborg G (1988) Nerve injury and repair. Churchill Livingstone, New York
6. Lundborg G, Gelberman RH, Longo FM, Powell HC, Varon S (1982) In vivo regeneration of cut nerves encased in silicone tubes. J Neuropath Exp Neurol 41:412–422

7. Lundborg G, Dahlin LB, Danielsen N, Gelberman RH, Longo FM, Powell HC, Varon S (1982) Nerve regeneration in silicone chambers: influence of gap length and of distal stump components. Exp Neurol 76:361–375
8. Lundborg G, Longo FM, Varon S (1982) Nerve regeneration model and trophic factors in vivo. Brain Res 232:157–161
9. Weiss P (1944) Sutureless reunion of severed nerves with elastic cuffs of tantalum. J Neurosurg 1:219–225
10. Weiss P (1944) The technology of nerve regeneration: a review. Sutureless tubulation and related methods of nerve repair. J Neurosurg 1:400–450
11. Campbell JB, Bassett CAL, Husby J, Thulin CA, Feringa ER (1961) Microfilter sheaths in peripheral nerve surgery. J Trauma 1:139–155
12. Kline DG, Hayes GJ (1964) The use of a resorbable wrapper for peripheral-nerve repair. Experimental studies in chimpanzees. J Neurosurg 21:737–750
13. Lehmann RAW, Hayes GJ (1967) Degeneration and regeneration in peripheral nerve. Brain 90y:285–296
14. Midgley RD, Woolhouse FM (1968) Silastic sheating technique for the anastomoses of nerves and tendons. Canad Med Ass J 98:550–551
15. Williams LR, Longo FM, Powell HC, Lundborg G, Varon S (1983) Spatial-temporal progress of peripheral nerve regeneration within a silicone chamber: parameters for a bioassay. J Comp Neurol 218:460–470
16. Williams LR, Müller H, Margolin L, Varon S (1985) The rat as a model for the study of peripheral nerve regeneration within a silicone chamber. Abstract. 36th Ann Bess Amer Assoc Lab Animal Sci, Baltimore
17. Müller H, Shibib K, Friedrich H, Modrack M (1987) Evoked muscle action potentials from regenerated rat tibial and peroneal nerves: synthetic versus autologous interfascicular grafts. Exp Neurol 95:21–33
18. Müller H, Shibib K, Modrack M, Friedrich H (1987) Nerve regeneration in synthetic and autologous interfascicular grafts. II. Morphometric analysis. Exp Neurol 98:1, p 161–169
19. Jenq CB, Coggeshall RE (1986) The effects of an autologous transplant on patterns of regeneration in rat sciatic nerve. Brain Res 364:45–56
20. Molander H, Engkvist O, Haaglund J, Olsson Y, Torebjörk E (1983) Nerve repair using a polyglactin tube and nerve graft: an experimental study in the rabbit. Biomaterials 4:276–280
21. Longo FM, Skaper SD, Manthorpe M, Williams LR, Lundborg G, Varon S (1983) Temporal changes of neuronotrophic activities accumulating in vivo within nerve regeneration chambers. Exp Neurol 81:756–769
22. Longe FM, Hayman EG, Davis GE, Ruoslahti E, Engvall E, Manthorpe M, Varon S (1984) Neurite-promoting factors and extracellular matrix components accumulating in vivo within nerve regeneration chambers. Brain Res 309:105–117
23. Williams LR, Varon S (1985) Modification of vibrin matrix formation in situ enhances nerve regeneration in silicone chambers. J Comp Neurol 231:209–220
24. Williams LR, Danielsen N, Müller H, Varon S (1987) Exogenous matrix precursors promote functional nerve regeneration across a 15 mm gap within a silicone chamber in the rat. J Comp Neurol 231
25. Müller H, Williams LR, Varon S (1987) Nerve regeneration chamber: evaluation of exogenous agents applied by multiple injections. Brain Res 413:320–326
26. Davis G, Manthorpe M, Engvall E, Varon S (1985) Isolation and characterization of rat schwannoma neurite-promoting factor: evidence that the factor contains laminin. J Neurosci 5:2662–2671
27. Ide C, Tohyama K, Yokota R, Nitatori T, Onodera S (1983) Schwann cell basal lamina and nerve regeneration. Brain Res 288:61–75
28. Manthorpe M, Engvall E, Ruoslahti E, Longo FM, Davis GE, Varon S (1983) Laminin promotes neuritic regeneration from cultured peripheral and central neurons. J Cell Biol 97:1882–1890

29. Madison R, Silva CF da, Dikkes P, Sidman RL, Chiu TH (1985) Increased rate of peripheral nerve regeneration using bioresorbable nerve guides and a laminin-containing gel. Exp Neurol 88:767–772
30. Patterson PH (1985) On the role of proteases, their inhibitors and the extracellular matrix in promoting neurite outgrowth. J de Physiol 80:207–211
31. Lander AD, Fujii DK, Gospodarowisz D, Reichardt LF (1984) Neurite outgrowth-promoting factors in conditioned media are complexes containing laminin. Abstract. Soc Neurosci 10:1614
32. Timpl R, Rohde H, Robey PG, Rennard SI, Foidart JM, Martin GR (1979) Laminin – a glycoprotein from basement membranes. J Biol Chem 254:9933–9937
33. Hannouche N, Samperez S, Jouan P (1980) Accumulation of 5 alpha-dihydrotestosterone in purified plasma membranes and in the myelin of male rat hypothalamus. CR Soc Biol 174:963–968
34. Sar M, Stumpf WE (1977) Androgen concentration in motor neurons of cranial nerves and spinal cord. Science 197:77–79
35. Snyder EY, Kim SU (1979) Hormonal requirements for neuronal survival in culture. Neurosci Lett 13:225–230
36. Yu WHA (1982) Effect of testosterone on the regeneration of the hypoglossal nerve in rats. Exp Neurol 77:129–141
37. Facci L, Leon A, Toffano G, Sonino S, Ghidoni R, Tettamanti G (1984) Promotion of neuritogenesis in mouse neuroblastoma cells by exogenous gangliosides. Relationship between the effect and the cell association of ganglioside GM_1. J Neurochem 42:299–305
38. Ferrari G, Fabris M, Gorio G (1983) Gangliosides enhance neurite outgrowth in PC 12 cells. Dev Brain Res 8:215–222
39. Gorio A, Carmignoto G, Facci L, Finesso M (1980) Motor nerve sprouting induced by ganglioside treatment. Possible implications for gangliosides on neuronal growth. Brain Res 197:236–241
40. Gorio A, Marini P, Zanoni R (1984) Muscle reinnervation. III. Motoneuron sprouting capacity, enhancement by exogenous gangliosides. Neuroscience 8:417–429
41. Katoh-Semba R, Skaper SD, Varon S (1984) Interaction of GM_1 ganglioside with PC 12 pheochromocytoma cells: serum- and NGF-dependent effects on neurite growth (and proliferation). J Neurosci Res 12:299–310
42. Skaper SD, Katoh-Semba R, Varon S (1985) GM_1 ganglioside accelerates neurite outgrowth from primary peripheral and central neurons under selected culture conditions. Dev Brain Res 23:19–26
43. Walicke P, Varon S, Manthorpe M (1986) Purification of a human red blood cell protein supporting the survival of cultured CNS neurons, and its identification as catalase. J Neurosci 6:1114–1121
44. Müller H (1988) Further evaluation of the effects of laminin, testosterone, ganglioside GM_1, and catalase on early growth in rat nerve regeneration chambers. Exp Neurol 101:2, p 228–233

Experimental Repair of Peripheral Nerve Injury Using Venous Autograft

A. LEVENTIS, A. MAILLIS, E. SINGOUNAS, P. DAVAKI, and N. KARANDREAS, Athens/Greece

Introduction

The problem of peripheral nerve injuries and their repair has been of great concern to those practicing medicine since the times of Galen (130–200 A. D.) and Paul of Aegina (seventh century A. D.) [1, 2] and continues to be so in our era of modern microsurgical techniques [3, 4].

One of the major obstacles to methods of nerve repair has been the development of connective tissue between the stumps [5]. Epineural [6] and perineural [7] suture techniques as well as sutureless methods of agglutination [8] and tubulization [9] of the stumps, either alone or in combination [10], have all been employed, but each has had its own drawbacks. Autografting methods using veins [11, 12, 13], arteries, or fasciae have also been employed, alone or combined [14] with agglutination techniques, to protect the anastomosis from surrounding tissue reactions and to stabilize more effectively the contact between the stumps. However, the inability of the venous grafts and fasciae to hold the stumps in contact and the development of arterial spasm with subsequent neural necrosis have been among the major disadvantages leading to abandonment of these techniques.

Materials and Methods

Adult rabbits weighing 3.0–3.5 kg were used in this study. In all our experiments general anesthesia was administered intraperitoneally, using 30–40 mg/kg Nembutal Sodium. A 5–32 × magnification was employed, and Prolene 10–stitches were used. Antibiotics were not administered locally or systemically. It should be mentioned that six animals that developed infections were excluded from the study. The animals were kept in special cages under standard conditions.

Surgical Procedure. In all animals the right common peroneal nerve was exposed. A venous segment 2 cm long was cut from the ipsilateral saphenous minor vein and kept in normal saline. The common peroneal nerve was freed from its epineurium at a distance of 5 mm (Fig. 1). To facilitate this procedure, a small quantity of normal saline was injected below the epineurium through a 33-gauge needle. The common peroneal nerve was then cut transversely at the

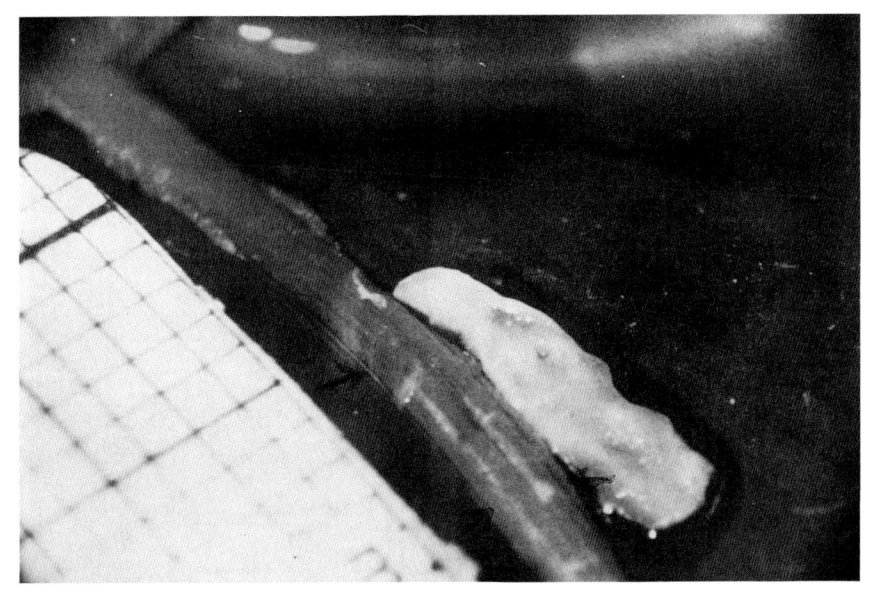

Experimental Repair of Peripheral Nerve Injury Using Venous Autograft

Fig. 1. The common peroneal nerve of a rabbit, with the epineurium removed. The venous graft is opened up

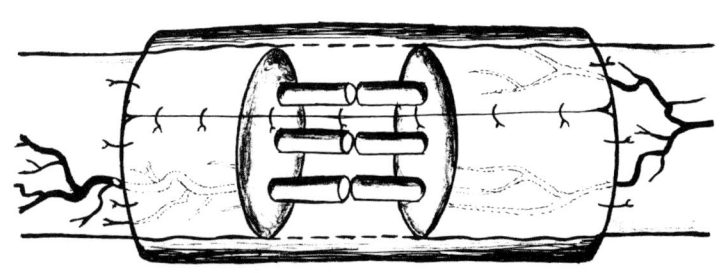

Fig. 2. The technique of neural anastomosis using the venous graft. The epineurium has been removed from the anastomotic surface, the venous graft fixed on to the epineurium, and the wall of the venous graft stitched up, creating a sleeve around the whole anastomotic area

middle portion of its freed segment and at approximately 2 cm from its entrance into the peroneus longus muscle. The two stumps were kept in close proximity with the help of an approximator. The venous graft was opened alongside, put beneath the nerve, stretched along its longitudinal axis to exceed 3 cm length, wrapped around the stumps of the nerve and fastened by interrupted prolene 10–0 stitches at a distance of approximately 1.5 cm from the anastomotic surfaces of the nerve bilaterally (Fig. 2).

The longitudinal opening of the vein was closed up by stitches including a small part of epineurium (Fig. 3). This supports the cut ends of the nerve at close proximity and reduces rotational movements of the opposed fascicles (Fig. 4).

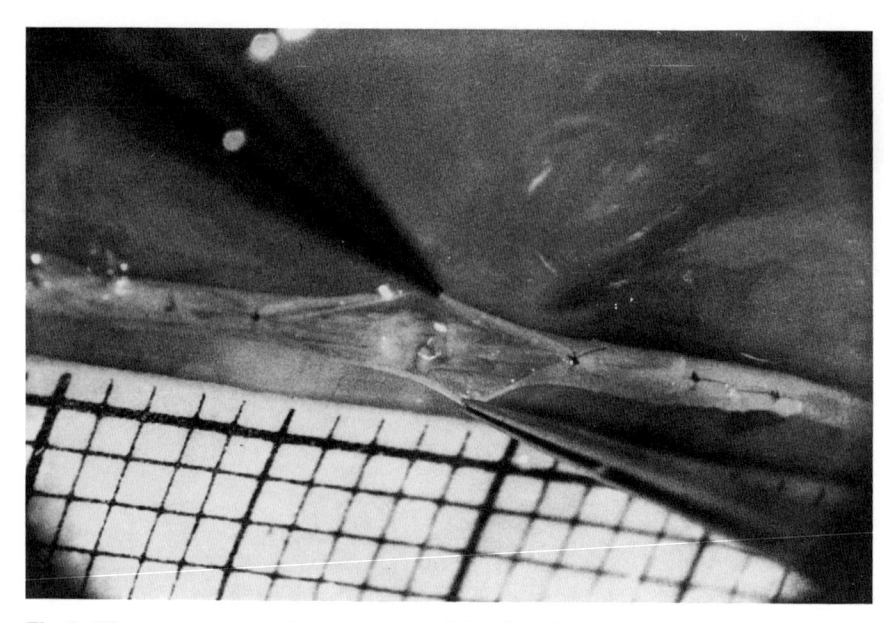

Fig. 3. The anastomosis and the venous graft holding the stumps in contact

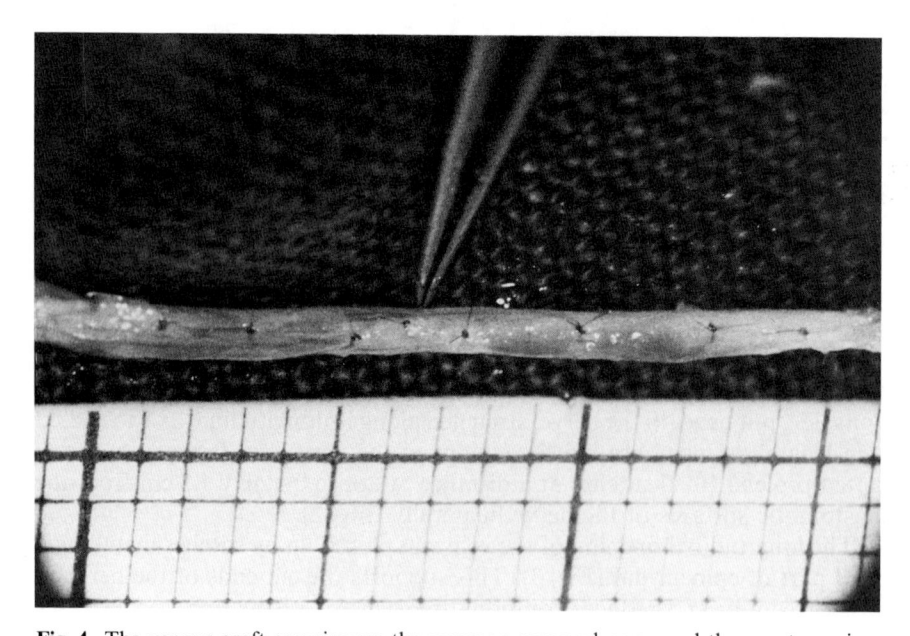

Fig. 4. The venous graft covering up the common peroneal nerve and the anastomosis

An alternative approach to that above was to use the venous graft as a sleeve without cutting its wall and to insert both ends of the nerve into the venous canal. Apart from the venous graft technique the epineural and perineural (fascicular) anastomoses were also employed. These two conventional methods were applied for comparison in two similar animal groups of 50 rabbits and under the same surgical conditions.

Neurophysiological and Morphological Studies. The neurophysiological activity of the tibialis anterior muscle was studied by means of concentric needle electrodes coupled with the Medelec electromyograph. Conduction velocities were also measured from both common peroneal nerves in all animals studied, under slight general anesthesia using the same apparatus. At the end of each experiment both common peroneal nerves and the anterior tibial muscles were removed. Nerves were divided at equal distances proximal and distal to the anastomosis. The central segment including the anastomosis was immersed in 10% buffered formalin solution while the more distal segments were cut at 1 cm distance bilaterally from the anastomosis and put into Fleming's solution. Paraffin sections were taken subsequently and stained with hemotoxylin-eosin or by the Weigert-Pal method. Anterior tibial muscles were also taken and fixed in 10% buffered formalin solution. Fixed muscles were cut in half at approximately the same level, and both transversee and longitudinal paraffin sections were taken and stained with hematoxylin-eosin, phosphotungstic acid-hematoxylin, and van Gieson's trichrome methods.

Results

The anastomosis with venous graft clearly provided earlier and better results, leading to rapid neural regeneration in the first 6 months (Table 1). This was confirmed by neurophysiological and histological studies. Statistical analysis showed the difference to be statistically significant ($p < 0.05$). Comparison with conventional methods (peri- and epineural sutures) shows that the perineural suture is slightly superior to the epineural, but the difference here is not statistically significant.

Clinical evaluation of the three animal groups showed no clear difference between those operated on by epineural and by perineural suture techniques, but there was an obvious difference between these and those of the venous graft group. Dystrophic skin lesions and those produced by dragging the leg were less pronounced and showed faster healing and recovery. Mobilization of the leg and particularly that of the toes was faster compared to the animals in the other two groups. The same was true for walking ability and for the restoration of muscle bulk. Thus, the reinnervation process in the venous graft group was faster and superior compared to that in the other two groups.

More objectively, the following neurophysiological criteria for a successful anastomosis have been used for evaluation: (a) the absence of automatic degenerative potentials in EMG; (b) an amplitude of the induced muscle

Table 1. Neurophysiological and histological results

Groups	Months after anastomis	Neurophysiological results			Histological results in nerves				Histological results in muscles			
		Very good	Satis-factory	Poor	Very good	Good	Mod-erate	Poor	Very good	Good	Mod-erate	Poor
Venous graft anastomosis												
A	1	1	2	7	0	1	2	7	0	1	2	7
B	2	3	2	5	2	3	1	4	1	2	2	5
C	4	4	2	4	3	2	3	2	3	2	3	2
D	6	5	3	2	4	3	1	2	4	3	1	2
E	12	6	3	1	5	3	1	1	5	2	1	2
Epineural suture												
A	1	0	2	8	0	1	1	8	0	0	1	9
B	2	1	3	6	1	2	1	6	0	1	2	7
C	4	2	3	5	2	2	3	3	1	2	3	4
D	6	4	3	3	3	2	2	3	3	2	1	4
E	12	4	4	2	4	2	2	2	4	1	3	2
Perineural (fascicular) suture												
A	1	1	3	6	0	0	1	9	0	0	1	9
B	2	2	3	5	1	2	2	5	0	2	2	6
C	4	3	2	5	2	3	2	3	2	1	3	4
D	6	4	3	3	3	2	3	2	3	2	2	3
E	12	5	3	2	4	3	1	2	4	2	2	2

Ten nerves were operated on in each of the 15 groups.

potential under 8 mV; and (c) return of the motor conduction velocities to normal levels (70–100 m/s for the common peroneal nerve of the rabbit). Results were classified as being very good if measurements were within these limits and as satisfactory if there were some spontaneous degenerative muscle potentials, the amplitude of the evoked muscle response was reduced (4–8 mV), and the conduction velocities were in the range of 40–70 m/s. The outcome was characterized as poor if substantial spontaneous fibrillatory potentials were present, the evoked muscle potential was further reduced (below 4 mV in amplitude), and the conduction velocities were below 40 m/s.

The histological criteria for a successful anastomosis were the number of myelinated nerve fibers which passed into the peripheral stump and their degree of remyelination (i.e., the thickness of myelin sheath as compared with the diameter of the neuraxis). The specimen for measurement was taken at a distance of 1 cm from the anastomotic surface of each stump. If the number of fibers of the distal (peripheral) stump was over 75% of the number in the proximal stump, the result was considered as very good, 50%–75% as good, 25%–50% as moderate, and below 25% as poor.

Transverse and longitudinal paraffin sections were evaluated for the degree of muscle degeneration and recovery. In these sections we examined the architecture of the muscle fiber grouping, muscle diameter histograms, presence of central nucleus, degree of connective tissue, and presence of lipid. For muscle diameter histograms we usually measured 100 individual consecutive muscle fibers from the best part of the muscle in transverse sections. The result was considered as very good if over 75% of the muscle fibers were normal, good if 50%–75% were normal, moderate if 25%–50%, and poor if less than 25% of the fibers were normal.

Discussion

The success of peripheral nerve anastomosis is inhibited by numerous factors, among which the development of reactive connective tissue plays a predominant role. The newly formed connective tissue interferes with the anastomosis process by distorting the proper morphological and functional fiber-to-fiber bridging and by strangulating the nerve itself. The epineurium, and to a much lesser degree the perineurium, are considered major sources for the development of connective tissue.

In order to overcome this problem, commonly seen in epineural anastomosis, the technique of perineural (or fascicular) anastomosis has been developed. The main advantages of this technique are that the epineurium is removed, and that individual nerve fascicles are bridged together, held in close end-to-end contact with the help of surgical sutures. However, again the main disadvantage with this technique is the development of intra- and perineural connective tissue septa due to the surgical trauma and the presence of sutures. Perineuronal tissue trauma is also responsible for the development of extraneuronal connective tissue which, if in excess, strangulates the nerve trunk. In an effort to overcome these obstacles, we have used venous autografts for the support and protection of the anastomosis. The main advantage of this technique is that it reduces the development of connective tissue because the epineurium is removed, and there are no sutures or other foreign materials present across or around the anastomosing surfaces.

The comparative study of three groups of animals operated on with the venous autograft technique, the epineurial, and the perineurial suture, shows clearly the superiority of the venous graft technique. It is of particular interest that with this method the development of the connective tissue at the anastomosis of the nerve was significantly slower and quantitatively much less around the freed portion of the nerve. The stumps of the nerve were maintained in close proximity due to the elastic properties of the stretched wall of the supporting vein. The proximal and distal epineural cuts being at a distance from the anastomotic point seems to offer adequate time for the regeneration process to occur, much before the development of reactive connective tissue obstructs this process.

The venous sleeve also protects the anastomosis by interposing itself between the nerve and the extraneuronal connective tissue. The cut-opposing fascicles of the nerve can be maintained at a proper distance without being held in position by foreign materials such as sutures or agglutinins. In the venous graft technique the sutures are always applied to the epineurium 1.5 cm away from the anastomotic area. In only a few cases was neuronal recovery delayed or unsuccessful due to the development of connective tissue.

In conclusion, although the venous graft technique does not seem to retard completely the development of connective tissue, it seems safer for peripheral nerve anastomosis. It protects the opposing ends of nerve fibers during the critical early stages of anastomosis and produces much better functional and morphological results, as shown by our clinical, neurophysiological, and histological observations.

References

1. Ochs S (1980) A brief history of nerve repair and regeneration. Nerve repair and regeneration, pp. 1–8
2. Paulus Aegeneta (Paul of Aegina) (1844–1847) The seven books (Translated by F. Adams), Vol. II, Sydenham Society, London, pp 132–137
3. Millesi H (1982) Peripheral nerve injuries. Nerve sutures and grafting. Scand. J Plast Reconst Surg (Suppl.) 19:25–37
4. Samii M (1975) Use of microtechniques in peripheral nerve surgery. Experience with over 300 cases in hand. Microneurosurgery: 85–93
5. Sunderland S (1978) Nerves and nerve injuries. Churchill Livingstone, London
6. Omer G (1980) Past experience with epineural repair: primary, secondary and grafts. Nerve repair and regeneration: 267–276
7. Orgel M, Terzis J (1977) Epineurial vs. perineurial repair: an ultrastructural and electrophysiological study of nerve regeneration. Plast Reconstr Surg 60:80–91
8. Metz R, Seeger W (1969) Collagen wrapping of nerve homotransplants in dogs. Eur Surg Res 1:157

9. Rosen JM et al. (1979) Fascicular sutureless and suture repair on peripheral nerves. A comparison study in laboratory animals. Orthop Rev 8:85
10. Gibby W, Koerber R, Horch K (1983) A quantitative evaluation of suture and tubulization nerve repair techniques. J Neuros 58:574–579
11. Ramon y Cajal S (1968) Degeneration and regeneration of the nervous system (Translated by R. M. May) (2 Vols) 1928. Reprint by Hafner, New York
12. Godard J, Monnier G, Rouillon D, Jaquet G, Bourchi A, Steimle R (1983) Regenerescence nerveuse à travers un greffon veineux chez le rat. Calendrier Scientifique de la Societé de Neurochirurgie de Langue Francaise, Paris, 28–30 Nov
13. Hirasawa Y, Marmor L (1967) The protective effect of irradiation combined with sheathing methods on experimental nerve heterografts: silastic, autogenous veins and heterogenous arteries. J Neuros 27:489
14. Hurwitz PJ (1974) Microsurgical techniques and the use of tissue adhesive in the repair of peripheral nerves. J Surg Res 17:245

Experimental Nerve Regeneration Under a Vein Graft in the Rat

J. Godard, G. Coulon*, G. Monnier, D. Rouillon, G. Jacquet, and R. Steimle, Besançon/France

Following the section of a nerve, suture is either immediate or secondary and sometimes makes use of nerve grafts. It is the problem of establishing a bridge between two nerve ends which has particularly attracted our attention. Our experimental study involved the section of 8 mm of common fibular nerve, with the interposition of a 10-mm venous graft replacing the missing portion of nerve. Electrophysiological, histological, and immunological evaluations were carried out over a period ranging from 4 to 12 weeks of nerve regeneration.

Material and Methods

Wistar strain rats were used, aged 5 months to 1 year and weighing between 250 and 300 g. A total of 15 rats underwent surgery, generally on both sides. All rats were anesthetized with an injection of 1.4 cc ketamine per 50 mg. Mean

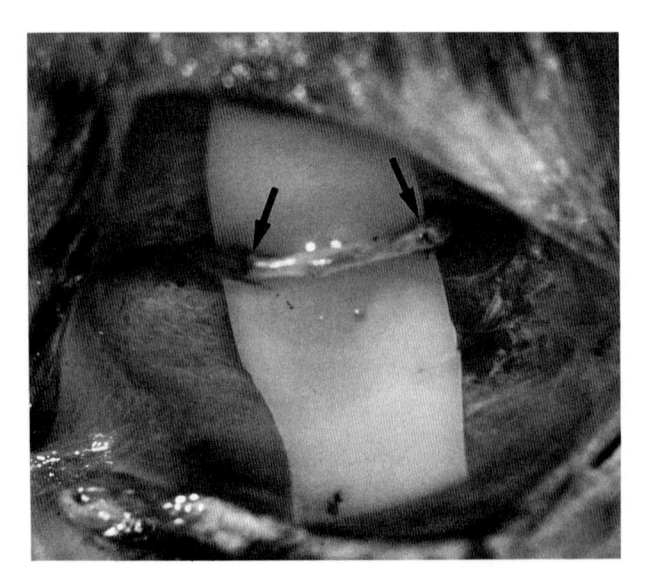

Fig. 1. The graft in situ immediately postoperative

---

* Deceased.

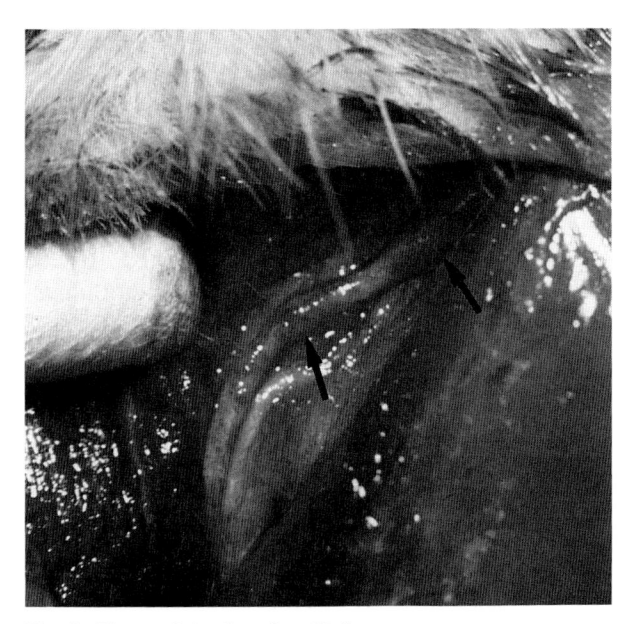

Fig. 2. The graft in situ after 75 days

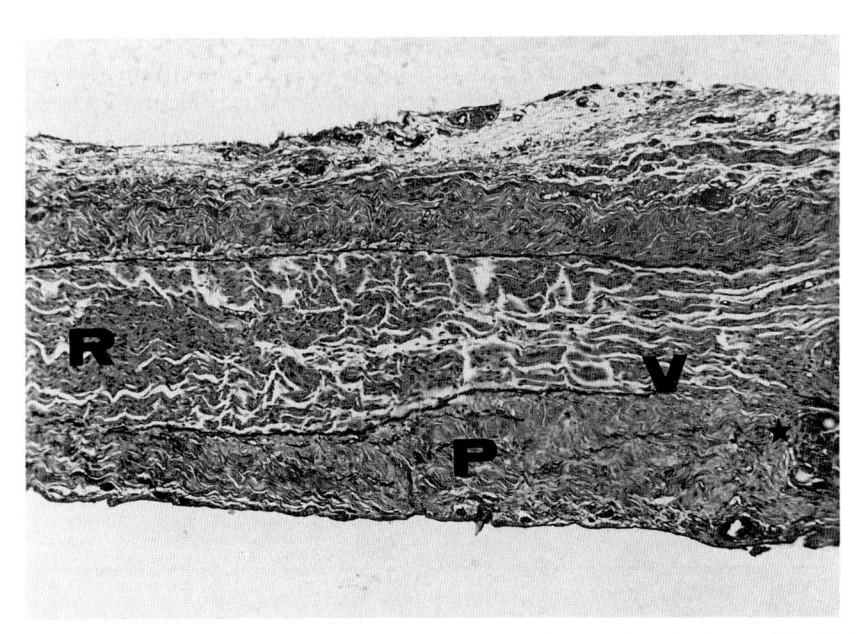

Fig. 3. On day 81, the nerve regeneration (*R*) totally fills up the vein lumen (*V*) which is outlived by the internal lamina elastics. No inflammatory reactions were observed apart from a granuloma which developed on the nylon suture (★). *P*, Vein Wall. (Orcéine; × 100)

anesthesia duration was 4 h, and there were no peri- or postoperative accidents during the 38 surgical procedures performed. The common peroneal nerve was selected since it is easily isolated on the posterolateral side of the thigh. The nerve was dissected under microscopic control, and 8 mm of nerve was removed. Previously, the external jugular vein had been dissected and 10 mm removed. This vein fragment was rinsed with heparinized saline. The vein was then used as a graft between the two nerve ends (Fig. 1). This vein graft was subjected to a certain degree of tension. Of the 25 vein grafts inserted, 16 were studied histologically, 12 electrophysiologically, and 16 by immunofluorescence at different times of regeneration (Figs. 2, 3).

Results

After a few weeks, there was wasting of the posterolateral portion of the thigh due to muscular scarring and partial inactivity of the operated limb. When the graft was removed, there was sometimes evidence of fibrous tissue around the zone of healing, but generally the appearance of the graft was smooth. Nerve potential and muscle potential were recorded from the common peroneal nerve isolated in vivo. Previously, records had been obtained from five healthy nerves with a mean of 1.5–1.6 ms for muscular latent period and 1–1.2 ms for nerve latent period (Table 1). There was neither nerve nor muscle potential immediately after the graft (Fig. 4).

Electrophysiological results are summarized in Table 2. The first responses were recorded by the 25th day. There was no proportional relationship between the duration of recovery and conduction times. Light microscopic study of vein grafts and their contents in transverse or longitudinal sections showed that the nerve response was constant.

Histological results were evaluated in terms of four groups, depending on the timing of graft insertion. In the first group, four grafts aged 25–33 days were studied. The venous lumen was occupied by loose material, rich in Schwann's cells and collagen fibers separated by edema. Myelin sheaths, few in

Table 1. Electromyographic study of healthy nerves in vivo

	Muscle potential			Nerve potential		
	Latent period (ms)	Amplitude (mV)	No. of phases	Latent period (ms)	Amplitude mV)	No. of phases
1	1.6	1.5	3	1	1	3
2	1.5	1.2	3	1	0.850	2
3	1.6	1.5	Polyphasic	1.2	1	3
4	1.5	2.5	3	1	0.8	2
5	1.5	3	2	1	0.8	2

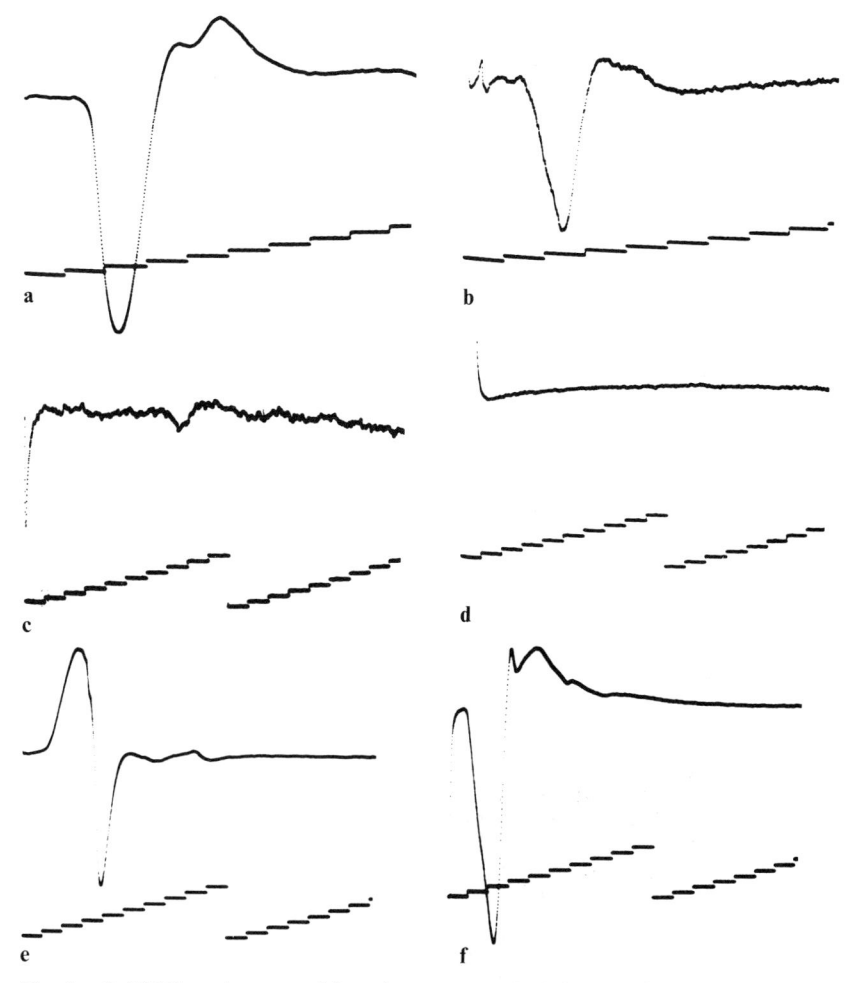

Fig. 4a–f. EMG study. **a, c, e** Muscular response. **b, d, f** Nerve potential. **a, b** Before the nerve section. Muscular response: latency 1.5 ms, amplitude 30 mV (**a**); nerve potential: latency 1 ms, amplitude 0.8 mV (**b**). **c, d** Immediately after the graft, lack of muscular response (**c**) and nerve potential (**d**). **e, f** After 25 days. Muscular response: latency 1.8 ms, amplitude 2.5 mV (**e**); nerve potential: latency 1.3 ms, amplitude 1 mV (**f**)

number and of small caliber, were revealed by staining with luxol fast blue. In the second group, grafts ranged in age from 65 to 75 days. Myelin sheaths were more easily visible. There was endoneural fibrosis with early fasciculation, while minimal interstitial edema persisted. In the third group, grafts were aged 82–84 days. Endoneural fibrosis was very clearly evident, forming pseudofasciculation, grouping together four to eight myelinized nerve fibers in a transverse section. Neurites were regular in caliber on longitudinal sections, although of smaller caliber than that of neurites of the normal nerve. Finally, in the last group grafts were in place for more than 100 days. Myelin sheaths were

Table 2. Electromyographic study of grafts in vivo

	Time (days)	Muscle potential			Nerve potential		
		Latent period (ms)	Amplitude (mV)	No. of phases	Latent period (ms)	Amplitude (mV)	No. of phases
Group 1							
6	25	1.8	2.5	2	1	1	2
Group 2							
7	65	3.5	0.25	Polyphasic	1.8	0.6	2
8	63	1.8	3	2	1	0.7	2
9	75	2.1	0.5	2	1.5	0.15	3
Group 3							
10	81	2.5	0.75	2	1.2	0.5	3
11	84	2.1	1.6	2	1	1.2	3
12	85	1.8	1.5	Polyphasic	1.5	0.7	2
13	85	2.2	1.3	2	1.9	0.25	2
Group 4							
14	101	1.5	1.5	Polyphasic	11	1	2
15	109	1.4	3	2	0.9	1.7	2
16	120	3.3	0.4	3	1.6	0.05	2
17	123	2	1	2	1.5	0.05	2

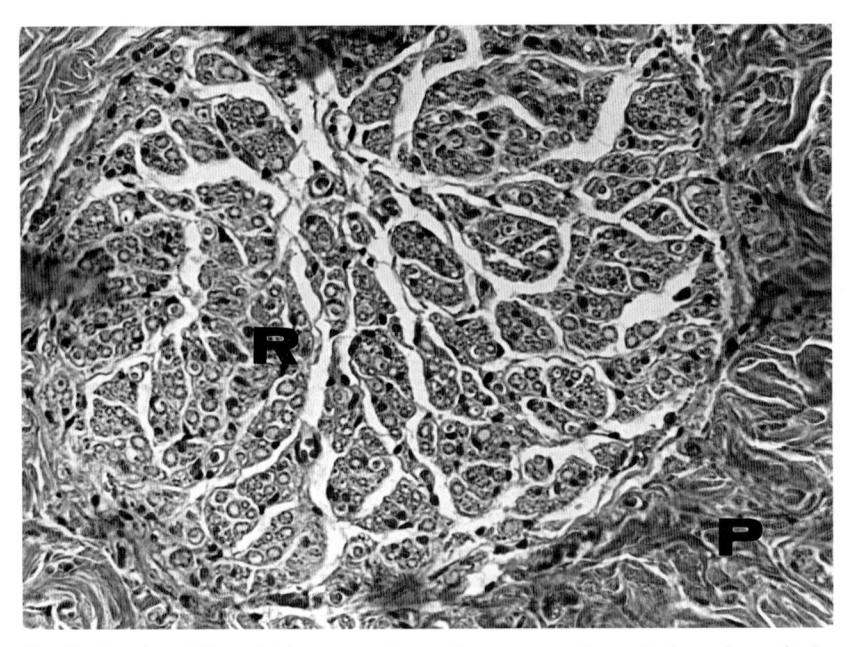

Fig. 5. On day 103, a high-power view of a cross-section of the vein-grafted nerve demonstrates the presence of myelin sheaths. *P*, Vein wall; *R*, nerve regeneration. (H & E; ×300)

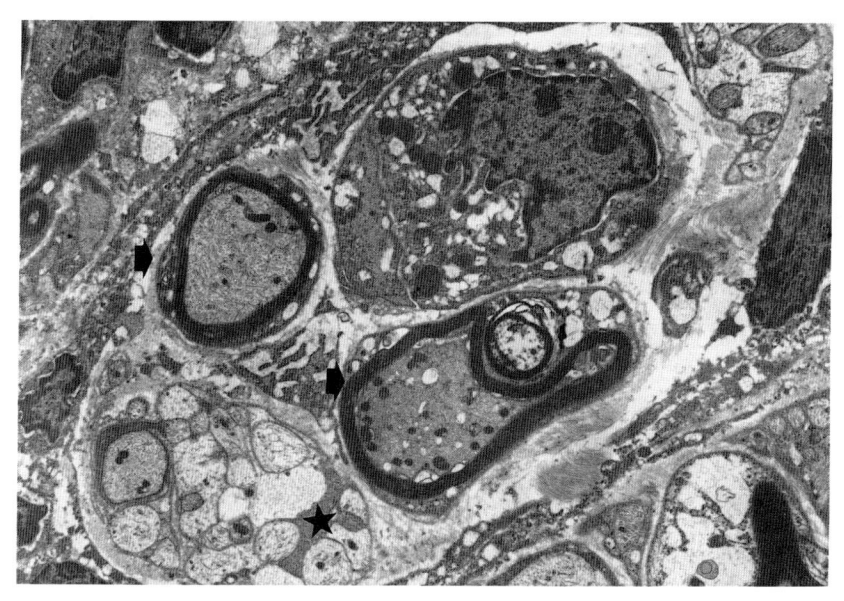

Fig. 6. On day 25, electron microscopy. Cross-section showing myelinated (*arrow*) and amyelinated fibers (*asterisk*). (ur. Pb; × 7000)

more regular and thicker. Axons were sinuous and smaller than normal in caliber (Fig. 5). In each group the venous lumen was found to be filled with nerve fibers of varying degrees of myelinization. A few small nerve filaments had actually penetrated into the thickness of the venous wall. Electron microscopic study confirmed the presence of myelinized and amyelinized nerve fibers. There was no any evidence of thrombosis of the vein. Complete absence of any inflammatory infiltrate in the graft and its surroundings was noted (Fig. 6).

Several *immunohistochemical* labeling techniques were applied to control nerves and then to nerve grafts at the different stages of nerve response. Among the immune sera (IS) selected, two were felt to be worthy of interest: those of alpha-MSH (melanocyte-stimulating hormone) and enolase. These two IS are present in normal nerve fibers. They were found during regeneration after 20 days and 40 days. Fluorescence with enolase IS was weak in comparison with the control nerve and appeared after about 40 days. With alpha-MSH IS, labeling was more marked in the proximal portion of the graft starting from 20 days, with better distribution after approximately 40 days.

Discussion

Experimental studies of nerve regeneration have been carried out for many years. Since the neurite response occurs very rapidly (1.5–3 mm in the rat), it is hardly surprising to note the rapid occupation of the graft by nerve fibers.

Appearance of myelin sheaths was delayed in time. This was dependent upon proliferation of the Schwann's cells, the latter probably able to migrate from the proximal nerve end. The mechanism of colonization of the graft by axons and Schwann's cells is difficult to define. The fibrous canal formed by the vein graft no doubt acts as a mold penetrated by the nerve fibers in the course of regeneration. In the absence of proper coadaptation between the graft and the proximal nerve end, the formation of an amputation neuroma could be avoided. However, in certain cases nerve fibers followed the graft stuck to its outer surface and appeared to progress regularly and in parallel with it, without forming a neuroma of an anarchic nature. The vein graft could thus act not only as a mold but also as a guide for neurites on both its inner and outer surfaces.

Certain authors such as Chiu et al. (1982) have discovered that nerve regrowth in the graft lumen is more rapid peripherally in contact with the venous wall than in the center of the lumen, as if the wall played a facilitating role.

The thickness of myelin sheaths increased with time, as did their caliber. This reflects the quality of nerve regrowth and is an essential factor in terms of functional potential. However, endoneural fibrosis resulting in fasciculation probably inhibits nerve conduction. It would be of great interest to analyze the proportion of myelinized fibers in relation to fibrosis as well as the thickness of myelin sheaths by histomorphometric methods to which we do not currently have access.

The vein graft itself showed no evidence of any inflammatory reaction. This absence of local inflammatory reaction is hardly surprising insofar as an autograft was used. Only suture material induced a minimal inflammatory reaction in its immediate surroundings. Absence of thrombosis is probably explained by rinsing with physiological saline combined with heparin. In some cases, there was evidence of regional fibrosis making graft dissection somewhat more difficult. It was felt during recordings that this fibrosis interfered with nerve conduction by decreasing amplitude and increasing latent period. Venault 1981 has described similar findings in the dog. Comparison of results in our three groups showed evidence of a correlation between increase in myelin sheaths and electrophysiological response in time.

The immunohistochemical study provided valuable additional information using two types of IS: anti-enolase and anti-alpha-MSH. The presence of enolase in the central nervous system and the peripheral system is known and appears to be specific to neurones. Its actual site and mode of action are not yet known. Our experience confirmed the presence of enolase, which appeared to play a late role during regeneration since it was found at the proximal end of the graft only after 40 days. More recently, an alpha-MSH-like peptide has been isolated which appears to have a trophic action on the axon. The more the axon grows, the more alpha-MSH-like fluorescence takes on a regular form and becomes more intense. Further knowledge of the activity of this alpha-MSH-like protein would be necessary to prevent drawing overly hasty conclusions.

References

1. Boedts D (1982) Nerve anastomosis by a fibrinogen tissue adhesive. J Head and Neck Pathol 3:86–89
2. Büngner OV (1981) Die Degenerations- und Regenerationsvorgänge am Nerven nach Verletzungen. Beith Path Anat 10:321–393
3. Capo SR, Fernandez CN, Obiols LM, Soler RR (1982) Greffe nerveuse prédégénérée "in situ" et egreffe nerveuse fraîche. Etude comparative chez le lapin. Rev Chir Orthop 68:291–297
4. Chiu DTW, Janecka I, Krizek TJ, Wolff M, Lovelace RE (1982) Autogenous vein graft as a conduit for nerve regeneration. Surgery 91(2):226–233
5. Dolenc V, Janko M (1976) Nerve regeneration following primary repair. Acta Neurochir 34:223–234
6. Duncan D, Jarvis WH (1943) Observation on repeated regeneration of the facial nerve in cats. J Comp Neurol 79:315–327
7. Eden R (1916) Untersuchungen über spontane Wiedervereinigung durchtrennter Nerven im strömenden Blut und im leeren Gefässrohr. Arch Klin Chir 108:344–357
8. Gibby WA, Koerber HR, Horch HW (1983) A quantitative evaluation of suture and tubulization nerve repair techniques. J Neurosurg 58:574–579
9. Gordon L, Buncke H, Jewett DL, Muldowney B, Buncke G (1979) Predegenerated nerve autografts as compared with fresh nerve autografts in freshly cut and precut motor nerve defects in the rat. J Hand Surg 4:42–77
10. Greenee L (1963). The anatomy of the rat. Hafner, New York
11. Guegan Y, Pecker J (1979) Les greffes nerveuses. Etude expérimentale. Intérêt du nombre de points de suture. Neurochir 25:232–238
12. Gueuning C, Graff GLA, Ploncard P (1982) Récupération métabolique du muscle de rat après microchirurgie réparatrice du nerf périphérique en fonction des techniques de suture. Neurochir 28:207–212
13. Hatand, E (1981) A comparative study on primary and secondary nerve repair. Plast Reconst Surg 68(5):760–767
14. Lundborg G, Gelberman RH, Longo FM, Powell HC, Varon S, Eng D (1982) In vivo regeneration of cat nerves encased in silicone tubes. J of Neuropathol and Experimental Neurology 41(4):412–422
15. Mackinnon S, Hudson A, Falk R, Bilbao J, Kline D, Hunter D (1982) Nerve allograft response: a quantitative immunological study. Neurosurg 10(1):61–69
16. Mira JC (1981) Le nerf périphérique. Int J Microsurg 3(2):5–10
17. Mira JC (1981) Dégénérescence et regénération des nerfs périphériques: observations ultrastructurales et électrophysiologiques. Aspects quantitatifs et conséquences musculaires. Int J Microsurg 3(2):30–47
18. Mira JC (1976) Etudes quantitatives sur la régénération des fibres nerveuses myélinisées dans les nerfs de rats normaux. Arch Anat Micr Morph Exp 65:209–229
19. Molander H, Olsson Y, Engkvist O, Bowald S, Ericksson I (1982) Regeneration of peripheral nerve through a polyglaction tube. Muscle & Nerve 5:54–57
20. Nageotte J (1915) Le processus de la cicatrisation des nerfs. Cr Soc Biol (Paris) 78:249–254
21. Richter HP, Ketelsen UP (1982) Impairment of motor recovery after late nerve suture, experimental study in the rabbit. Neurosurg 10(1):75–85
22. Sebille A (1981) Méthodes expérimentales d'évolution de la régénération axonale des nerfs périphériques axotomisées. Int J Microsurg 3(2):75–79
23. Van Beek A, Glover JL, Zook E (1975) Primary versus delayed. Primary neurorrhaphy in rat sciatic nerve. J Surg Research 18:335–339
24. Venault B, Roffe JL, Magalon G, Chrestian M, Bureau H (1981) Régénération nerveuse. Etude expérimentale chez le chien. Trois techniques de sutures nerveuses. Ann Chir 35(6):441–446

Rejection of Allogenic Nerve Grafts in a Genetic Model of the Rat

E. Schaller, P. Mailänder, M. Becker, G. F. Walter, and A. Berger, Hannover/FRG

Introduction

The major problem in reconstructive operations on the peripheral nerve is the lack of a sufficient number of autologous nerve grafts. In the past 10 years the number of transplantations of allogenic organs has increased as new immunosuppressive drugs and knowledge of genetic and immunological backgrounds have made possible better results in transplantation surgery. Therefore the demand for transplantations of other tissues such as nerves is becoming more interesting and important.

The major problem in allogenic transplantations is the genetic difference between donor and recipient and the immunological response of the recipient and the graft. The genetic responsibility for rejection and for interactions between donor and recipient is found principally in the major histocompatibility complex (MHC) and the major histocompatibility system. The MHC system lies in the cytomembranes and consists of all transplantation antigens. These antigens of the cytomembranes are controlled by a genetic region on some alleles which are called MHC. These antigens are responsible for rejection. The MHC of the rat corresponds to the HLA system of humans.

Besides the MHC there exists a minor system called non-MHC. The aim of our study was to demonstrate the different forms of rejection in disparities of the MHC and non-MHC systems in allogenic nerve grafts.

Material and Methods

A panel of congenic strains of rats type LEW 1A and 1U were used for allogenic transplantations of the right sciatic nerve in 39 cases. These rats differ only in terms of MHC and possess the same non-MHC background. The regeneration, degeneration, and rejection phases were compared with autologous transplantations between strains of rats type LEW 1A or LEW 1U in 72 cases. Animals weighed between 390 and 410 g. Under Nembutal anesthesia the graft was taken distally from the branches of the ischiocrural muscles up to separation for the femoral and tibial muscles over a length of 2.5 cm (Fig. 1). The nerve graft was coapted in the recipient with 10–0 sutures (Ethilon) after preparation under microscope (Carl Zeiss). Transplantations were practiced in both directions, LEW 1A ↔ LEW 1U.

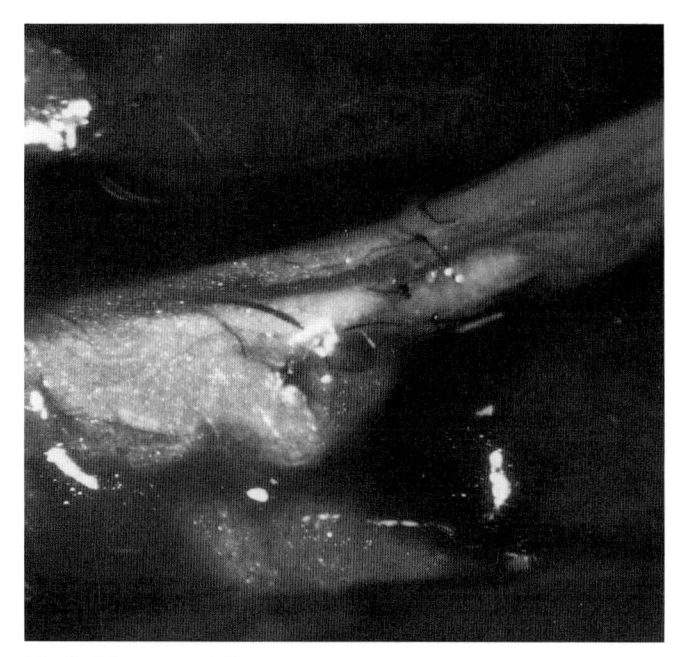

Fig. 1. Distal coaptation

Nerve regeneration was studied in three main groups:

group 1, autologous transplantations, LEW 1 A or LEW 1 U, $n = 72$; group 2, allogenic transplantations, LEW 1 A ↔ 1 U (MHC disparity), $n = 39$; and group 3, allogenic transplantations, MHC disparity plus cyclosporin A, $n = 36$.

In the third group cyclosporin A was fed by oral tube in a dosage of 15 mg/kg body weight every day for 2 weeks followed by a dose given every 2nd day.

After 2, 3, 4, 6, 9, 12, and 16 weeks animals were anesthetized, the situs was prepared, and the nerve was stimulated. Animals were killed, and the regeneration and forms of rejection were studied histologically in a longitudinally split graft and in a vertically taken excision proximal of the distal coaptation. The number of animals studied at 2, 3, 4, 6, 9, 12, and 16 weeks was as follows: group 1: 10, 10, 11, 11, 10, 10, 10; group 2: 7, 7, 7, 8, 0, 5, 5; group 3: 6, 6, 6, 6, 6, 6, 0. Histological slides were stained with hemalaune-eosin and Masson trichrome and impregnated with silver in the Bodian method. Semithin sections were stained with toluidine blue.

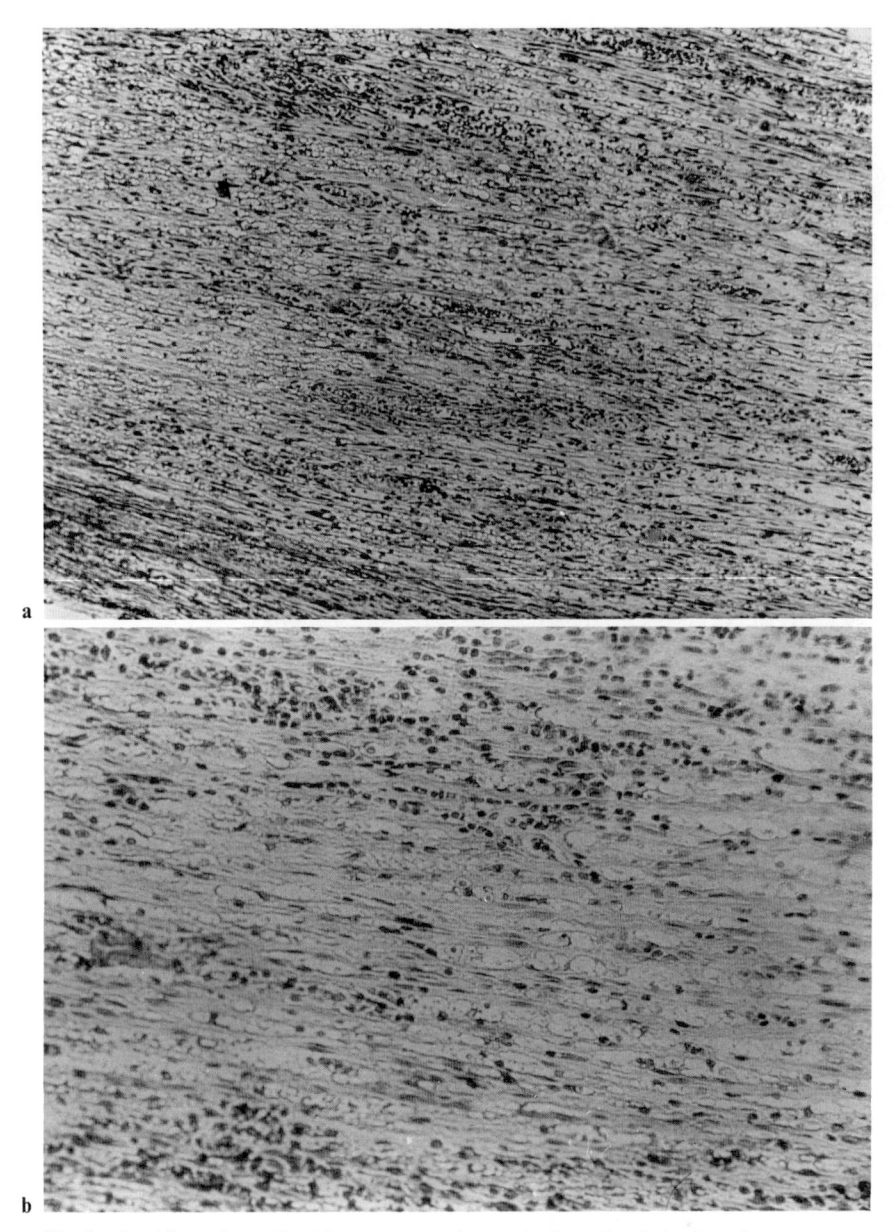

Fig. 2a, b. Allogenic graft without suppression. **a** At 3 weeks. **b** At 4 weeks

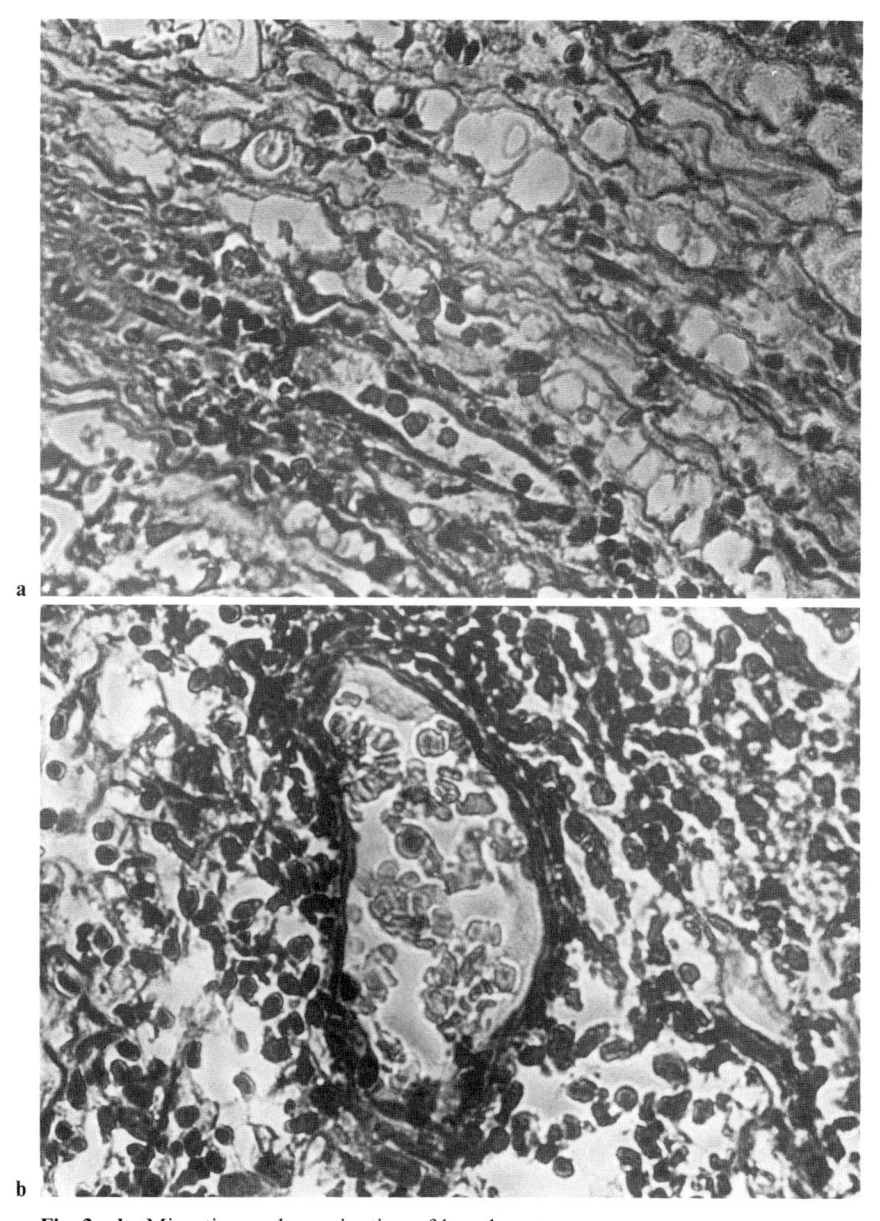

Fig. 3a, b. Migration and margination of lymphocytes

Results

As Millesi et al. (1972) showed in their studies of autologous grafts in rabbits, we observed that autologous nerve grafts show all signs of wallerian degeneration after 2 and 3 weeks along the whole length of the graft. After 4 weeks signs of regeneration could be recognized mixed with areas of wallerian degeneration, which diminished from week to week.

Allogenic nerve grafts differing in MHC showed a severe degeneration with proliferation of connective tissue after 6 weeks. Only very few axons or myelin sheaths could be found at this time.

Lymphocytic infiltration and degeneration increased from the 2nd to the 4th week and then decreased (Fig. 2). In all these groups one sees infiltration from peripheral vessels to the central areas of the graft. Migration and margination of lymphocytes are typical signs of mild rejection (Fig. 3). In all cases lymphocytes were distributed along the myelin sheaths (Fig. 4). The degree of rejection was one of mild graduation. After 16 weeks axonal growth could be found resembling that in autologous grafts after 9 weeks (Figs. 5, 6).

In the cyclosporin A treated group we saw axonal growth as fast as in the autologous group (Fig. 7). However, there were few regenerating fibers, and these did not seem to differ substantially from those of allogenic nerve grafts after 16 weeks without treatment. Until the 9th week lymphocytic infiltration was as high as in untreated animals; after 12 weeks we saw fewer lymphocytes.

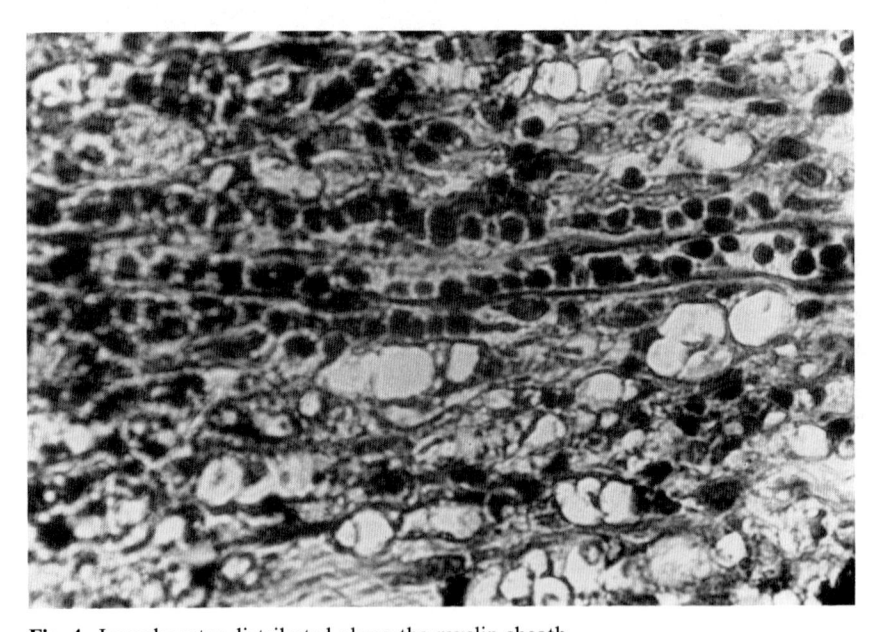

Fig. 4. Lymphocytes distributed along the myelin sheath

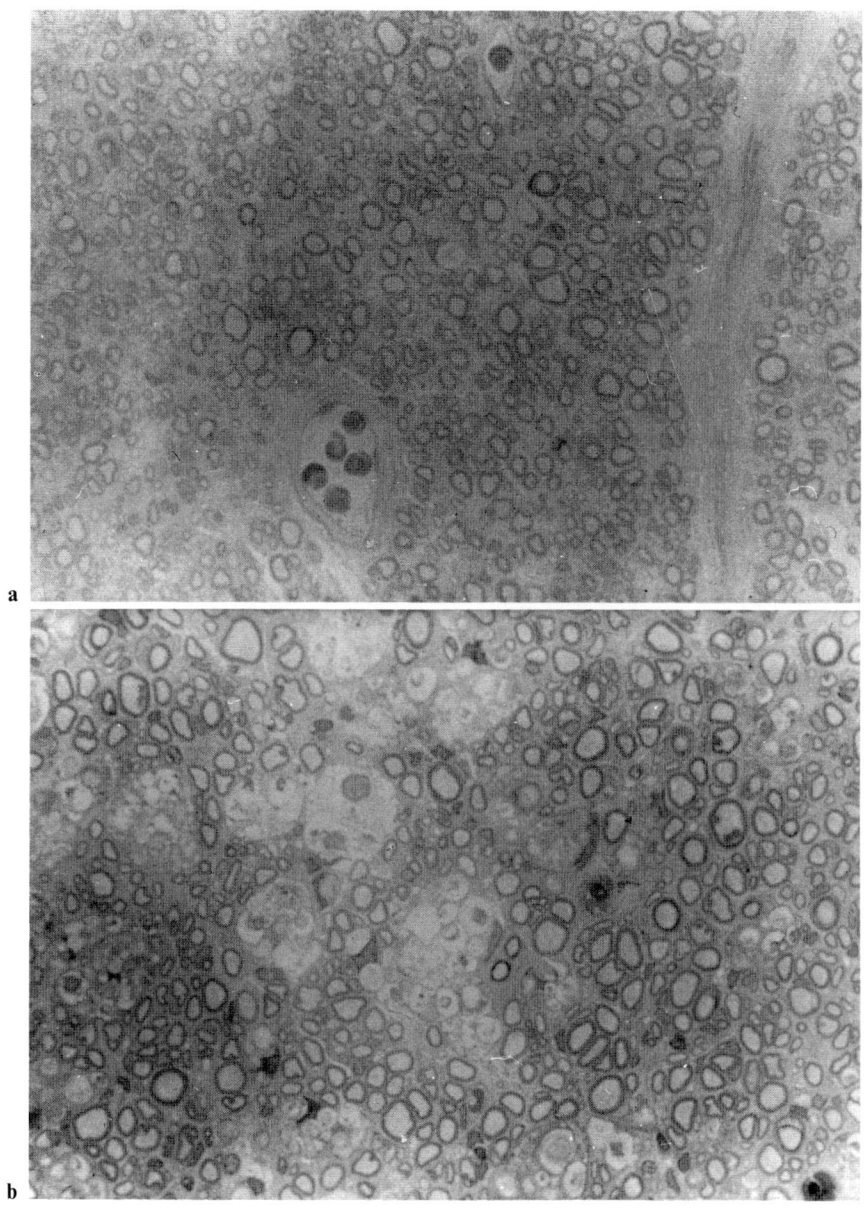

Fig. 5. a Autologous graft at 9 weeks. **b** Allogenic graft without immunosuppression at 16 weeks

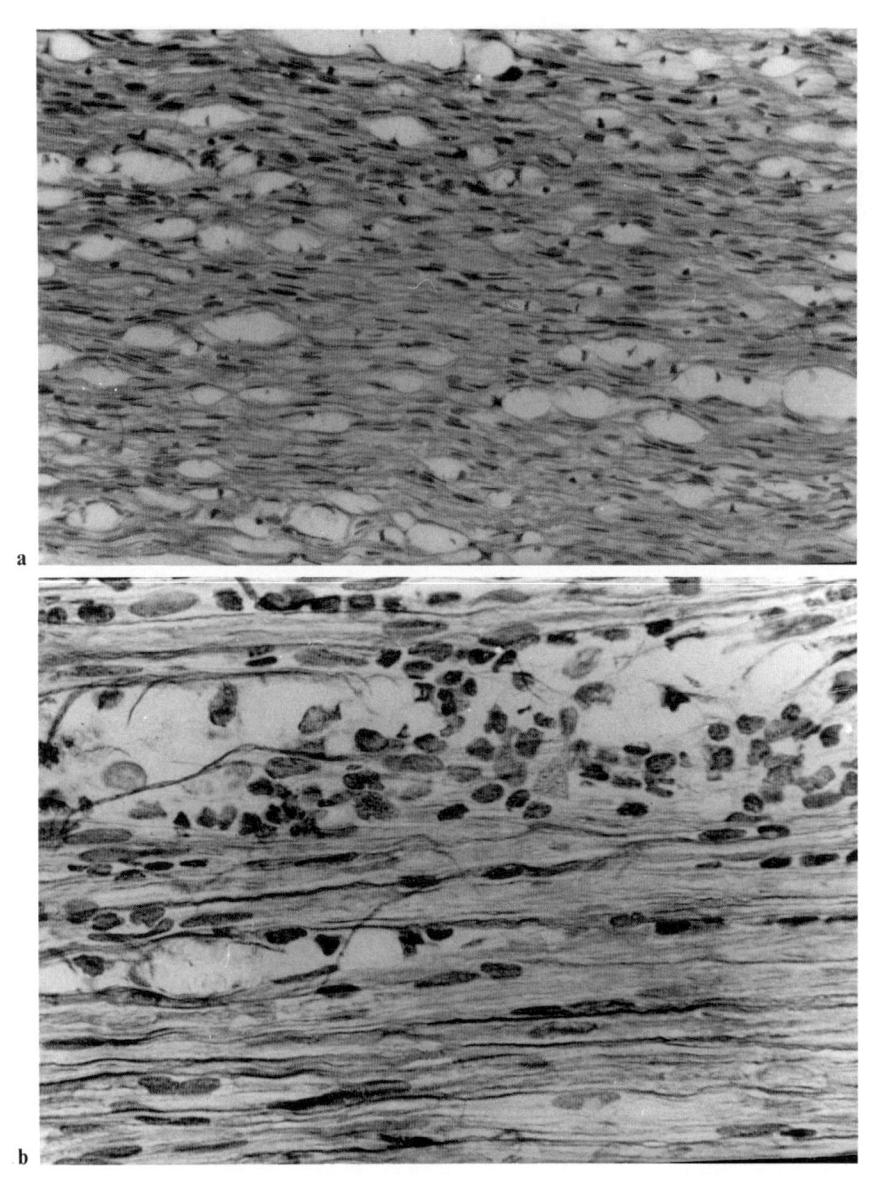

Fig. 6. a Autologous graft at 9 weeks. **b** Allogenic graft without immunosuppression at 16 weeks

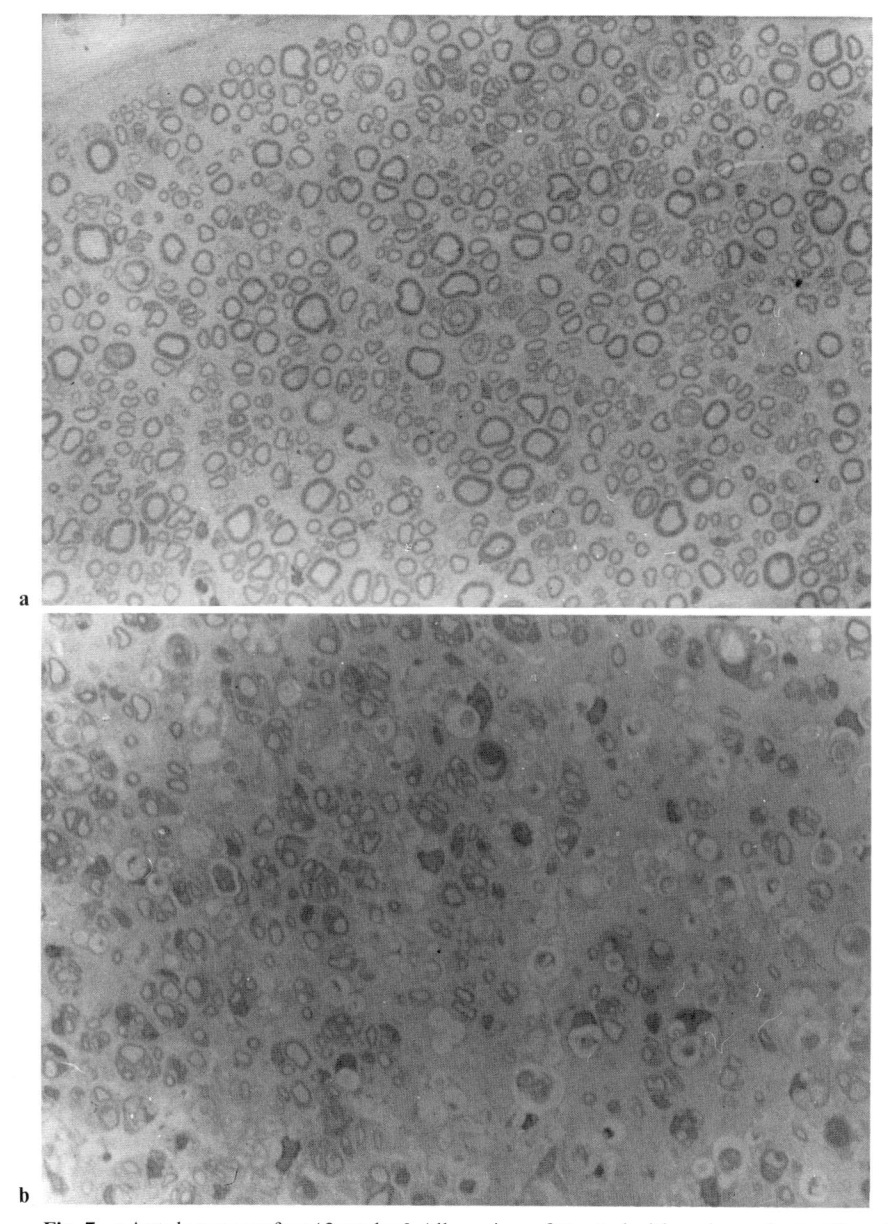

Fig. 7. a Autologous graft at 12 weeks. **b** Allogenic graft treated with cyclosporin A at 9 weeks

Discussion

Our results show that no severe rejection can be recognized in full MHC disparities. Regeneration in the allogenic nerve graft is possible in MHC disparities with the same non-MHC background, but it is slower and shows more areas of degeneration than in autologous nerve grafts. This demonstrates that the MHC system does not play the major role in rejection of allogenic nerve grafts that had been suspected.

Zalewski et al. (1981, 1982, 1983, 1984) and Mackinnon et al. (1985, 1986, 1987) have shown full rejection of allografts in a full disparity of MHC and non-MHC systems. We have investigated whether the non-MHC system bears a major responsibility for rejection of nerve allografts and plan to examine the role which subgroups of the MHC system play in allogenic reactions to nerve grafts.

Literature remains to the author.

Spinal Nerve Lesion and its Regeneration with and without Nerve Suture: An Experimental Study in Rats

T. WALLENFANG, J. BOHL, J. P. JANTZEN, and B. WALLESCH, Mainz/FRG

Introduction

Lesions in close proximity to the perikaryon – anterior horn or spinal ganglion – have a poor prognosis. Apparently, neuronal traumatization is more severe the closer the lesion of the peripheral nerve fiber is to the perikaryon. A subsequent retrograde degeneration may lead to nerve cell destruction [8]. This type of lesion is frequently seen in injuries involving neck and shoulder, mainly those resulting from motor cycle accidents in which the brachial plexus is exposed to major traumatic force [7, 8, 9]. Another group are primary irritations of the brachial and lumbosacral plexus following surgical intervention.

In an experimental setting we have investigated two forms of treatment of nerve lesions in close proximity to the spinal ganglion. It was the aim of this study to elucidate whether suturing of nerve stumps could provide better results functionally and morphologically with respect to regeneration of peripheral nerves and reinnervation of skeletal muscles.

Material and Methods

Twenty female Wistar rats were randomly allocated to two groups of ten rats each. Under general anesthesia (ether inhalation followed by peritoneal administration of 1 ml chloralhydrate 4% per 100 g body weight) the operation was performed microsurgically: hemilaminectomy of L5 with subsequent transection of the right spinal nerve of the corresponding segment distal from the spinal ganglion. In one experimental group the nerve stumps were repositioned to their original site without suture, in the second group the nerves were sutured by one or two threads through the epi- and perineurium. Seven months later the animals were killed by cardiac perfusion with 3.9% buffered glutaraldehyde under chloralhydrate anesthesia.

Sciatic and spinal nerves, dorsal and ventral roots of segment L5 as well as the corresponding skeletal muscles (gastrocnemius, tibialis cranialis, extensor digitorum longus) were examined histologically and morphometrically. Homologous nerves and muscles from the unaffected side served as control. Fixation, embedding, slice thickness, and staining method were the same in all nerves. The preparations were postfixed in 2% osmium tetroxide, embedded in epon and transversely sectioned in slices of 1.5 µm. The myelin sheaths were stained with 1% paraphenylene diamine for light microscopy. This procedure is described by Schröder [10].

The profile of the spinal nerve of the ventral and dorsal root and the muscles were subjected to histological work-up. Histological analysis was performed with a Zeiss photomicroscope (Optovar 1.25, projective 3.2, objective 100 for nerve slices and objective 10 for muscle slices) and was confined to randomly drawn samples. The final enlargement was 3000 × for nerves and 300 × for muscles. By morphometric examination with a Kontron videoplan computer we measured the circumference of the nerve fibers and axons and the thickness of the myelin sheaths. In the case of muscle fibers, the calculations referred to the smallest diameter. Histograms were selected to represent absolute frequencies with one column every 2 µm for fiber and axon circumferences, one column every 0.5 µm for myelin sheath thickness, and one column every 1 µm for muscle fiber diameters.

Results

Sciatic Nerve. In the sciatic nerve, fiber circumference of the control side ranged from 0 to 70 µm, including three minor peaks near 20, 30, and 46 µm. In the nerves of both the non-sutured and sutured groups, only one high peak was found near 12 µm with almost identical mean values of 17.4 and 17.6 µm, respectively. In both operated groups there was a distinct increase in numbers of fibers of smaller circumference. Axon circumference and myelin sheath thickness were not different between the treated groups, but both were smaller than those of the control group (Table 1).

Spinal Nerve. The distribution of fiber circumferences in the control group ranged between 4 and 64 µm, with minor peaks near 13, 28, and 41 µm. The nerves of the treated groups showed an increase in smaller fibers with a peak between 10 and 12 µm. Despite a second peak near 35 µm in the sutured group, no significant difference between the operated groups was found. Axon circumferences and myelin sheath thickness were similar in treated groups but smaller than in the control group (Table 1; Fig. 1).

Ventral Root. The distribution of fiber circumferences from 0 to 70 µm in control ventral roots showed three peaks (near 15, 31, and 47 µm). Non-sutured nerves showed an increase of smaller fibers in charge of larger ones. The remaining peaks lay near 9 and 41 µm. Ventral roots of sutured nerves showed also two peaks (near 11 and 35 µm), but fiber circumferences were greater ($p = 0.01$) – although still below control. Axon circumferences and myelin sheath thickness showed similar significant intergroup differences (Table 1; Fig. 2).

Dorsal Root. The fiber circumferences in the control dorsal root – ranging from 0 to 64 µm – included two peaks, with the smaller fibers near 11 µm

Table 1. Morphometric data, µm, $\bar{X} \pm SD$

	Control	Non-sutured	Sutured	Significance[a]
Sciatic nerves				
Fiber circumference	28.46 ± 11.94	17.43 ± 9.93	17.61 ± 10.28	$p \leq 0.06$
Axon circumference	17.97 ± 8.32	10.72 ± 6.98	11.15 ± 7.36	$p \leq 0.01$
Myelin sheath thickness	1.76 ± 0.70	1.19 ± 0.60	1.22 ± 0.58	*$p \leq 0.01$*
Spinal nerves				
Fiber circumference	25.40 ± 12.62	17.36 ± 9.60	17.40 ± 9.40	$p \leq 0.01$
Axon circumference	16.02 ± 9.06	10.81 ± 7.06	10.81 ± 6.97	$p \leq 0.01$
Myelin sheath thickness	1.71 ± 0.79	1.18 ± 0.61	1.21 ± 0.57	$p \leq 0.01$
Ventral roots				
Fiber circumference	27.50 ± 15.32	20.86 ± 14.38	21.38 ± 11.66	$p \leq 0.01$
Axon circumference	17.41 ± 11.01	13.16 ± 9.92	13.67 ± 7.99	$p \leq 0.01$
Myelin sheath thickness	1.75 ± 0.77	1.42 ± 0.80	1.36 ± 0.75	$p \leq 0.01$
Dorsal roots				
Fiber circumference	23.18 ± 11.71	14.35 ± 8.11	11.07 ± 4.32	$p \leq 0.49$
Axon circumference	14.25 ± 8.22	8.87 ± 5.41	6.47 ± 3.28	$p \leq 0.34$
Myelin sheath thickness	1.58 ± 0.71	0.98 ± 0.51	0.90 ± 0.50	$p \leq 0.06$

[a] Mann-Whitney U test for intergroup differences (non-sutured versus sutured).

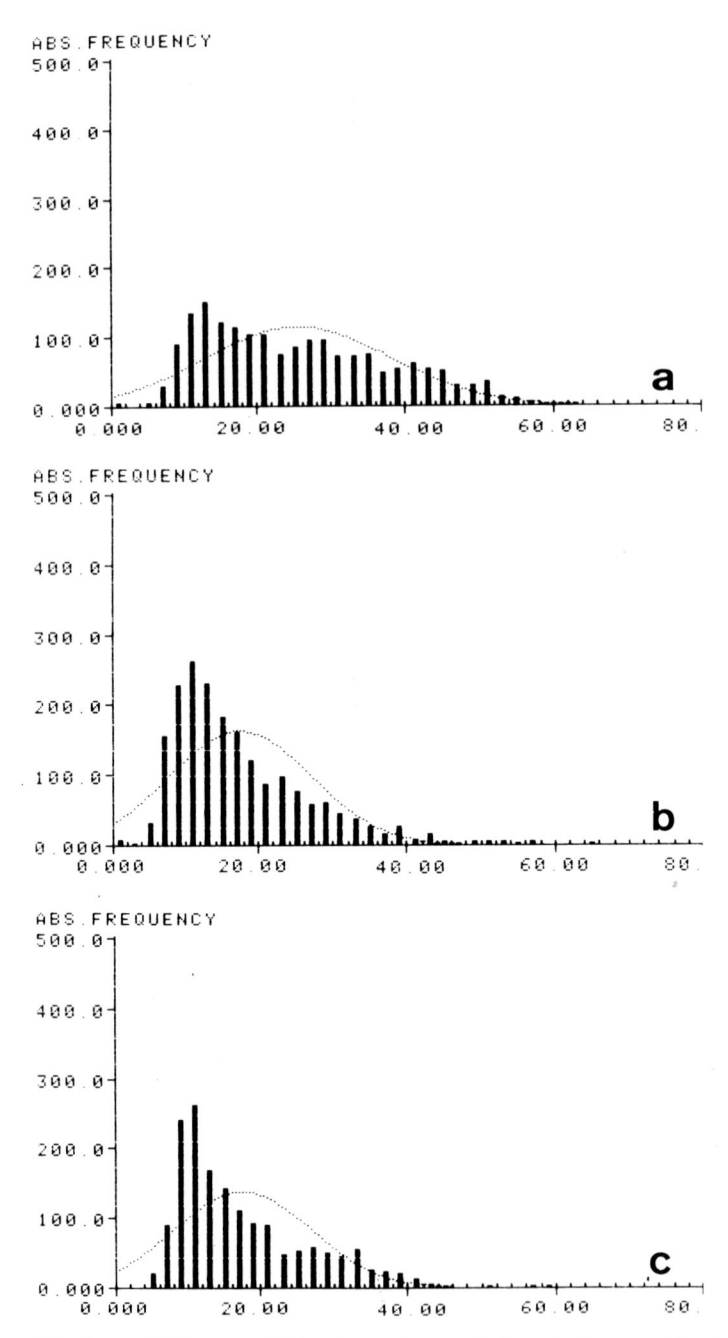

Fig. 1a–c. Histograms of fiber circumferences in the spinal nerve. **a** Control. **b** Non-sutured. **c** Sutured

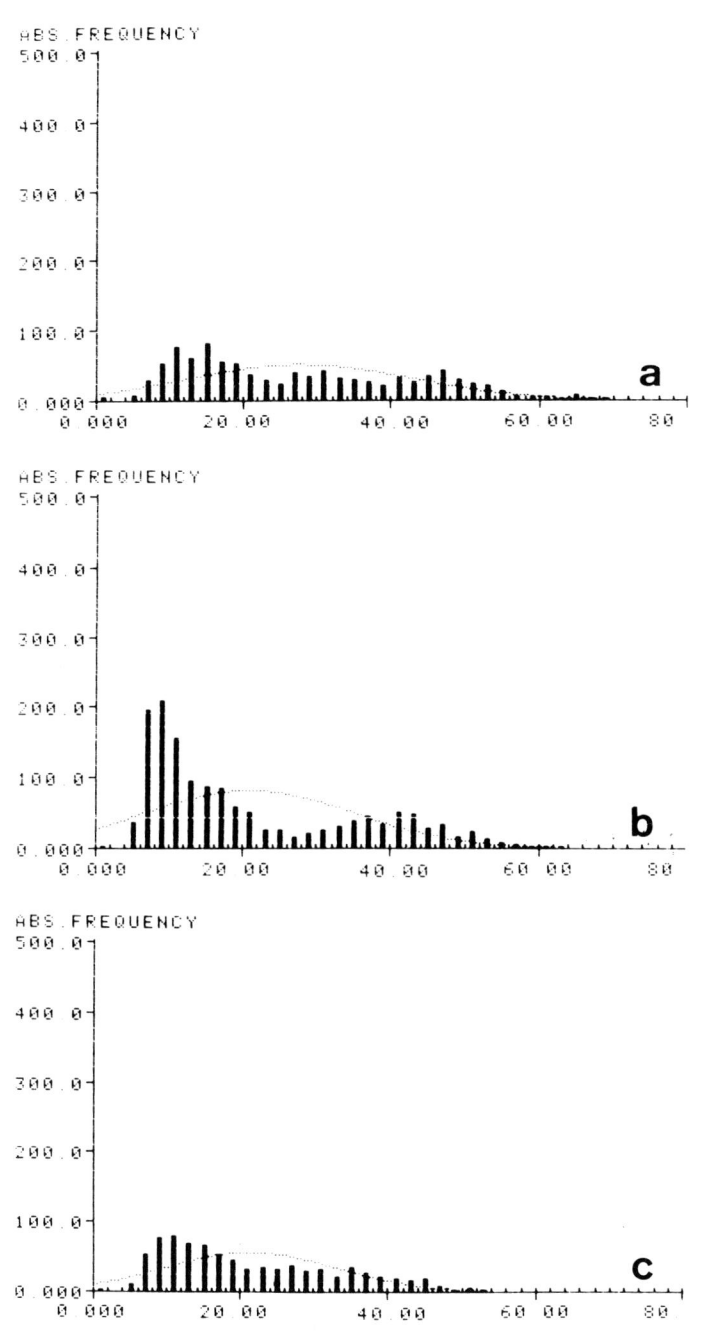

Fig. 2a–c. Histograms of fiber circumferences in the ventral root of L5. **a** Control. **b** Non-sutured. **c** Sutured

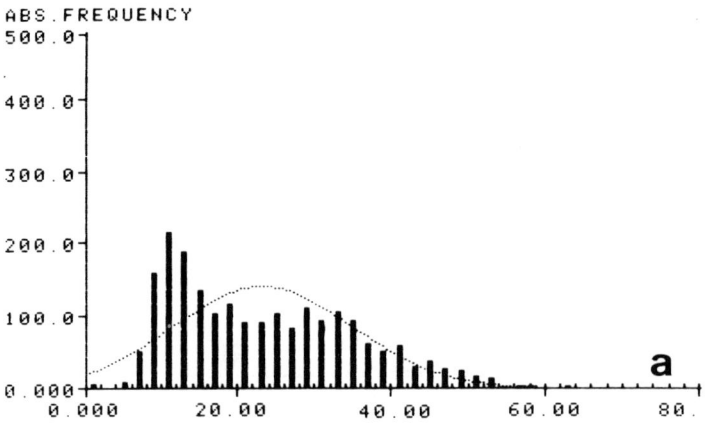

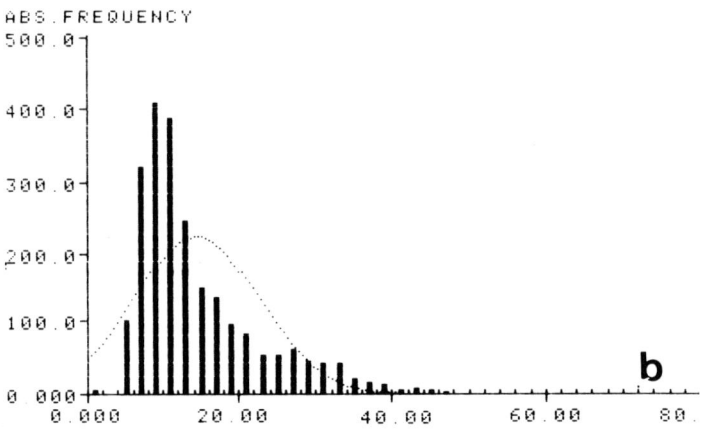

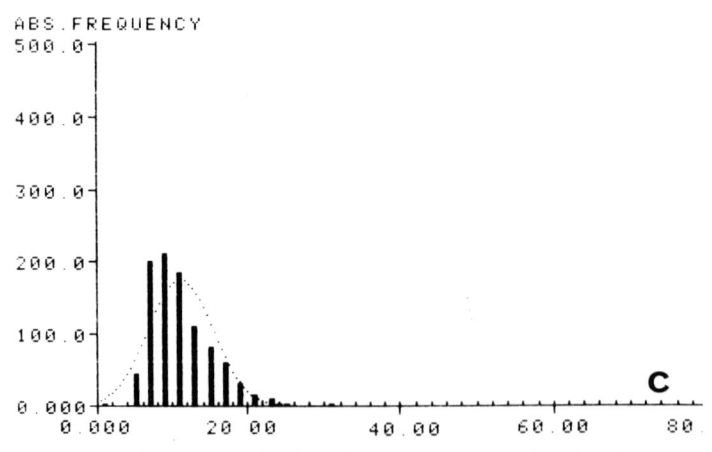

Fig. 3a–c. Histograms of fiber circumferences in the dorsal root of L5. **a** Control. **b** Non-sutured. **c** Sutured

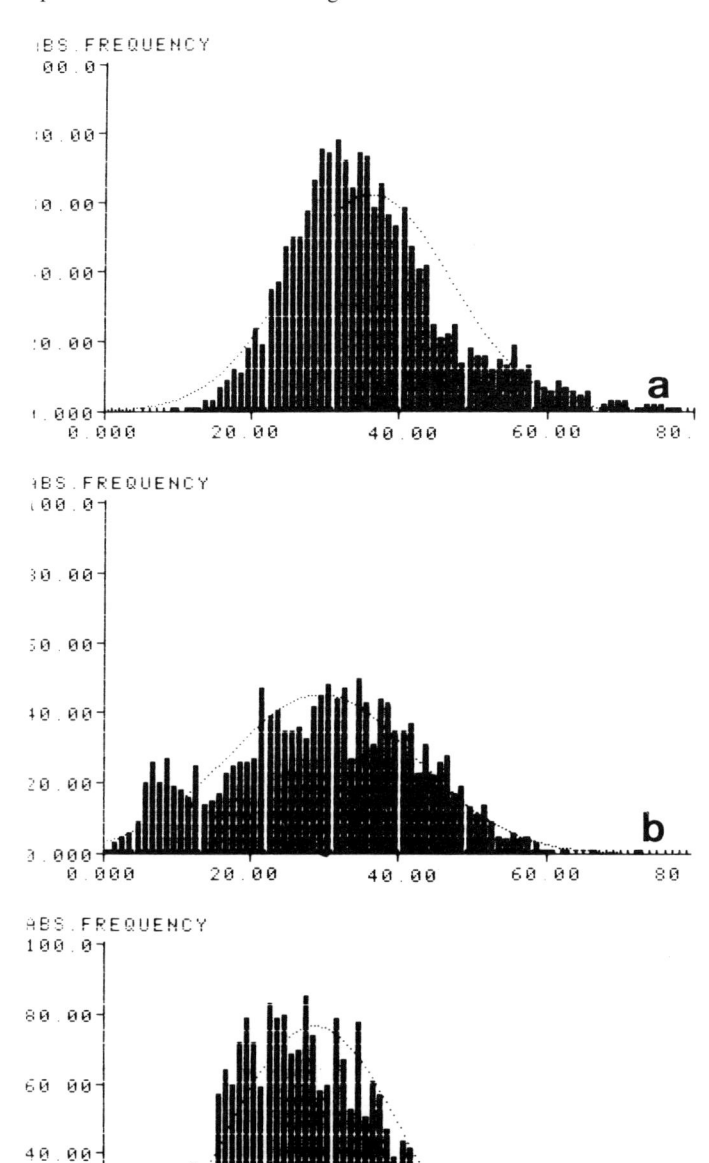

Fig. 4a–c. Histograms of fiber diameters in gastrocnemius muscle. **a** Control. **b** Non-sutured. **c** Sutured

prevailing over those near 30 µm. Transection resulted in a significant loss of fibers with larger circumferences. Sutured nerves showed smaller values in fiber circumference – ranging from 0 to 32 µm with a peak near 9 µm – than those in the non-sutured group. For the latter a distribution from 0 to 48 µm was found with two peaks, one near 9 µm and a second near 27 µm.

This unfavorable effect of suturing the transected spinal nerves on the dorsal root was also indicated by an increased frequency of smaller axon circumference and myelin sheath thickness in the sutured group (Table 1; Fig. 3).

Gastrocnemius Muscle. The calculated smallest diameter of skeletal muscle fibers in the rat gastrocnemius muscle of the control side ranged from 9 to 78 µm (mean, 36 ± 10.9 µm). In transected non-sutured nerves the measured data of muscle fibers ranged between 0 and 66 µm with two peaks. The first increase in small muscle fibers below normal values (varying between 5 and 13 µm) represented atrophic muscle fibers. The second peak near 35 µm suggested a large number of hypertrophic fibers, which was not seen after nerve suture. Nerve suture led to significantly smaller muscle fibers, as seen in the one-peaked histogram. Results ranged from 0 to 68 µm (mean, 28.7 ± 11.9 µm). This suggests that nerve suture prevented compensatory hypertrophy. The distribution of muscle fiber diameter consequently resembled that of control muscles (Table 2; Fig. 4).

Table 2. Morphometric data (smallest diameters, µm, $\bar{X} \pm SD$)

	Control	Non-sutured	Sutured	Significance[a]
Gastrocnemius muscles	35.98 ± 10.88	29.42 ± 12.79	28.68 ± 11.91	$p \leq 0.01$
Tibialis cranialis muscles	29.66 ± 9.20	23.18 ± 10.18	24.20 ± 8.02	$p \leq 0.01$
Extensor digitorum longus muscles	26.12 ± 7.07	20.76 ± 7.04	26.15 ± 9.60	$p \leq 0.01$

[a] Mann-Whitney U test for intergroup differences (non-sutured versus sutured).

Tibialis Cranialis and Extensor Digitorum Longus Muscles. The distribution of muscle fiber diameters in tibialis cranialis and extensor digitorum longus muscles showed a shift in the histogram towards lower values in both transected groups, with a one-peaked formation. In contrast to the gastrocnemius muscle neither compensatory hypertrophy nor atrophic fibers were found in the non-sutured spinal nerve stumps. Muscle histograms indicated more favorable results in the sutured group, but the muscle fiber diameters in both treatment groups were smaller than in the control group (Table 2).

Discussion

Damage to peripheral nerves is a severe complication of traffic injuries and sometimes also a result of surgical treatment [6, 8]. Recovery of nerve function is improved when the proximal regenerating nerve stump of a transected nerve obtains close contact to the distal degenerated nerve stump. This may be achieved by a microsurgically performed epineural or perineural fascicular nerve suture, distal from the spinal ganglion or the anterior horn [1, 2, 5]. If the lesion is adjacent to perikaryon, the additional stress of suturing and foreign body irritation may worsen the injury and interfere with regeneration.

To elucidate such mechanisms, an experimental study was performed with special interest in nerve regeneration near the spinal ganglion and recovery of motor function. This study confirms finding of other authors [3, 10] that the myelin sheath of regenerating nerve fibers is thinner than normal, and unaffected by suture techniques. Distal from the lesion in the sciatic and spinal nerve all investigated parameters showed significantly smaller values when compared to control.

Distal from the lesion the examined parameters did not show a different course of regeneration in the two treatment groups. Nerve fiber circumference, axon circumference, and myelin sheath thickness were similar in both operated groups, but were significantly smaller than in the control group. This absence of significant treatment differences during the course of recovery of sciatic and spinal nerves may be ascribed to the fact that conditions for the nerve fibers are the same in both groups as soon as the site of lesion has been overcome. The metabolic activity of the motoric soma is not affected by the presence or absence of a suture on the spinal nerve. Nor could we observe an improved or depressed activity of Schwann's cells ascribable to the additional intervention on the spinal nerve. In the ventral root of sutured nerves all parameters (fiber and axon circumferences, myelin sheath thickness) showed greater values than without suture. These were, however, still far below control. Since the examined ventral root lies proximal to the lesion, the changes may be due either to regenerating motoric fibers in the case of a retrograde degeneration exceeding the site of lesion or motoric and sensitive fibers showing retrograde growth [4].

The differences between the two operated groups are probably due to fibers germinating retrogradely from the site of lesion. Following mere adaptation of nerve stumps a false conduction of germinating nerve fibers in centripetal direction is likely, since the epineurium remains interrupted and does not act as a guiding sheath any more. This could explain the shift towards smaller mean values in the non-sutured group, i.e., an increase of smaller fibers in the ventral root population. The impression that retrogradely germinating neurites are favored without suture is also supported by the observation that nerve fibers in the ventral root lie closer together than in the ventral root of the sutured group. Nerve suture obviously favors orthograde growth of regenerating axons, i.e., the risk of neuroma formation is reduced.

In the dorsal root suturing was associated with poorer outcome, i.e., the fibers were significantly smaller when the nerve stumps were sutured in close proximity to the spinal ganglion. This is due either to a damage of the bipolar neuron and its peripheral process which is regenerating again or to the result of misled fibers growing retrogradely out of the spinal ganglion or the ventral root [6]. The latter possibility assumes, however, that such fibers surmount the barrier of the spinal ganglion. Retrograde growth of motor and sensor neurons is, however, the more likely course, since otherwise similarly directed and more distinct changes in the ventral roots should be expected, since there the spinal ganglion does not pose a barrier.

In all examined muscles of the operated groups we found fibers significantly decreased in diameter as compared to control. It must, however, be considered that the leg of the control side was conditioned due to the paresis on the contralateral side. Although the tibialis cranialis and extensor digitorum longus muscles in the sutured group compared favorably (i.e., significantly larger fiber diameter) to those in the non-sutured group, and both were significantly worse than control, there were neither signs for compensatory hypertrophy nor peaks in the histogram indicating atrophy. Obviously muscle fiber reinnervation took place in both operated groups. Pronounced inhomogenity in muscle fiber diameter was observed in the gastrocnemius muscle when the nerve stumps were not sutured. This may be due to the large number of atrophic fibers and to compensatory hypertrophy of the fibers of non-injured segments. The effect is that – despite worse reinnervation – the mean diameter shifts toward larger fibers in the non-sutured group. The homogeneous smaller muscle fiber diameter without atrophic and hypertrophic fibers in the sutured group resembles that of control muscle and represents the better surgical result. Probably in sutured nerves a greater number of motor fibers reaches the target organ earlier, thus favoring the restoration of function.

Conclusions

It can be concluded that nerve suturing does not lead to morphologic differences in the nerve fiber population distal to the lesion. As soon as the site of lesion has been overcome – whether by scar tissue or foreign body – the further development is dependent on the metabolic potency of the perikaryon, the ramification of the peripheral processes, and the function of Schwann's cells. Positive effects of nerve suture include a limiting effect on axon sprouts, reduction of neuroma formation, faster normalization of the fiber count distal to the lesion, and improved morphology of the muscle fibers. The nerve suture, even in close proximity to the spinal ganglion, yields better recovery of motor function, even though deterioration in sensory qualities by additional damage to the perikaryon remains possible.

As a clinical conclusion, we suggest microsurgical nerve suture as the preferable treatment for neurotmesis. The close proximity to the spinal ganglion in the case of plexus lesion is not necessarily a contra-indication to a surgical approach. Surgical intervention establishes and substantiates the diagnosis and results in improved motor function.

References

1. Brunelli G (1980) Nerve suture. Intern Surg 65, 6:499–501
2. Cabaud HE, Rodkey WG (1976) Epineural and perineural fascicular nerve repair: a critical comparison. J Hand Surg 1/2:131–137
3. Feasby TE, Pullen AH, Seass TA (1981) A quantitative ultrastructural study of dorsal root regeneration. J Neurol Sci 49:363–386
4. Meier C, Sollmann H (1977) Regeneration of cauda equina fibers after transection and end-to-end suture. J Neurol 215:81–90
5. Millesi H (1981) Neurorrhaphy. In: Gorio A, Millesi H, Mingrino S (eds) Posttraumatic peripheral nerve regeneration, experimental basis and clinical implications. Raven Press, New York
6. Narakas AO (1980) The surgical treatment of traumatic brachial plexus lesions. Intern Surg 65, 6:522–527
7. Samii M (1974) Verletzungen der Hirnnerven und des Plexus brachialis. Hefte der Unfallheilkunde 117:372–376
8. Samii M (1982) Funktionswandel und Funktionsverlust der oberen Extremität durch isolierte Lähmung. Z Orthop 120:424–428
9. Sunderland J (1968) Nerve and nerve injuries. Williams & Wilkins, Baltimore
10. Schröder JM (1972) Altered ratio between axon diameter and myelin sheath thickness in regenerated nerve fibers. Brain Res 45:49–66

Limitation of Neuroma Formation by Fat Tissue

J. WEIS and J. M. SCHRÖDER, Aachen/FRG

Introduction

Various methods have been proposed for limiting axonal growth at the proximal stump of a transected peripheral nerve to prevent neuroma formation. These include coagulation of the proximal nerve stump by heat (Hedri 1921) or freezing (Läwen 1925), ligation (Battista and Cravioto 1981), centrocentral anastomosis (Bardenheuer 1908; Samii 1981), and injection of various chemicals (Petropoulos and Stefanko 1961) as well as capping the nerve end with silicone rubber (Evans et al. 1968) or histoacryl (Martini 1985).

Another approach to the management of painful neuromas is the implantation of the proximal nerve stump into bone (Boldrey 1943; Petropoulos and Stefanko 1961; Goldstein and Sturim 1985) or muscle (Tenneff 1949). Dellon and Mackinnon (1986) reported good or excellent results in 82% of the nerve stumps treated by neuroma resection and implantation of the nerve end into muscle. In four cases of otherwise intractable pain following nerve injuries of the hand, Brown and Flynn (1973) replaced the scar tissue by an abdominal pedicle flap. If the nerves were completely dissected, they were embedded in muscle or bone and then covered by the flap.

Some of the methods cited above were discussed critically by Tupper (1986), who could not find a superior effect of these approaches compared to the resection of the neuroma together with the adjacent parts of the distal nerve stump followed by retraction of the nerve end into the injured tissue.

The present study is based on the results of experiments using the nerve tubulation system designed by Forssmann (1900) and Cajal (1928) and reestablished by Lundborg et al. (1982). In Lundborg's system, a silicone tube connected the proximal and the distal stumps of a transected nerve leaving a gap of 10 mm. The studies suggested that successful regeneration occurs only if both the proximal and the distal nerve segments are inserted into the tube. In our experiments (Weis and Schröder 1989a), the distal nerve stump was compared to preatrophied muscle or to abdominal fat tissue. Not only distal nerve stumps but also, as would be suggested, preatrophied muscle was well innervated 6 and 8 weeks after surgery, indicating a "neurotrophic" effect to both tissues on regenerating nerve fibers. However, only a few regenerating axons, if any, were found in the connective tissue surrounding the implanted distal fat tissue, and no nerve fibers were found between fat cells. These observations suggested that fat tissue could have an inhibiting or even "antineurotrophic" influence on the outgrowth of nerve fibers from the proximal nerve stump. In order to further test the possibly inhibitory effect of fat tissue on nerve regeneration and, especially, on neuroma formation, proximal nerve stumps were implanted into fat tissue without interposition of a tube (Weis and Schröder 1989b).

Material and Methods

A total of 47 adult female Wistar rats weighing 200–270 g were used for the study, 27 for the implantation of the proximal nerve stump into fat tissue and 20 for controls. The animals were held according to the 1986 law on protection of animals.

The rats were deeply anesthetized by intraperitoneal injection of chloralhydrate (35 mg/ml) following ether anesthesia. The left sciatic nerve was exposed by a dorsal incision in the midthigh. To create an abdominal pedicle flap, fat tissue was mobilized by Z-shaped incisions. The flap was incised at the apex to form a fat tissue bed for the nerve stump. The sciatic nerve was transected close to the knee, and the proximal end was implanted into the fat tissue flap by two or three stitches (9.0 Prolene) so that it was completely covered by fat. Sciatic nerves that had been transected without implantation served as controls.

Anesthetized rats of each group were sacrificed 4, 8, and 24 weeks after surgery, by intraaortal perfusion of 3.9% glutaraldehyde with 0.1 M phosphate buffer at pH 7.4. The proximal stump of the left sciatic nerve was transected shortly behind the lumbar plexus and removed together with the pedicle fat flap. The nerve ends with the main part of fat tissue were embedded in paraffin. Serial sections were stained with hematoxylin-eosin or were silver impregnated by the method of Bodian. Segments of neuromas, 8 and 24 weeks after implantation into fat tissue, were embedded in epoxy resin and stained with toluidine blue or paraphenylenediamine. Ultrathin sections were stained with uranyl acetate and lead citrate and examined with a Philips EM 400 T electron microscope.

Results

The resulting neuromas in the control group and in the fat implantation group were solid end bulbs consisting of nerve fibers, Schwann cells, perineurial and connective tissue cells. There was an increase in size of the neuromas by massive outgrowth of regenerating nerve fibers during the observation period of 24 weeks in both groups. A macroscopically significant difference in size between the two groups could not be detected. In most of the control animals, however, a widespread outgrowth of nerve fibers beyond the outer margins of the solid neuroma bulb rich in collagen fibers was observed (Fig. 1). In the fat implantation group, infiltration of fat tissue by regenerating nerve fibers was apparent to a minor degree or – in several experimental animals – nearly absent

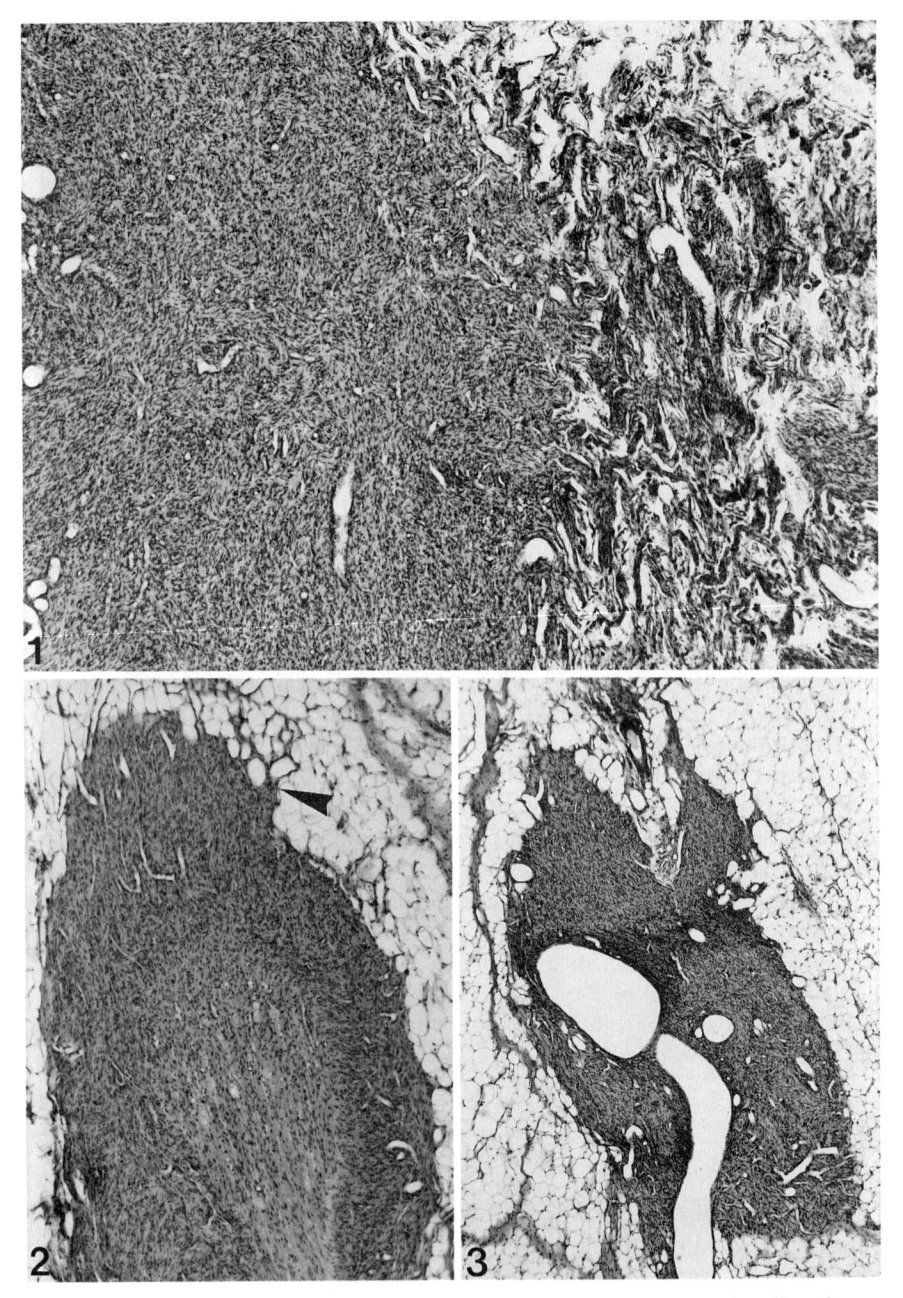

Fig. 1. Proximal end of a control nerve, 24 weeks after surgery. Numerous bundles of nerve fibers (*right side*) extend from the solid part of the neuroma (*left side*). (H & E; ×55)

Fig. 2. Nerve stump implanted into fat tissue, 24 weeks after surgery. Between fat cells only minimal outgrowth of nerve fibers is apparent (*arrowhead*). (H & E; ×45)

Fig. 3. Nerve stump implanted into fat tissue, 24 weeks after surgery. The fat tissue is infiltrated mainly along (perfused, empty) blood vessels or connective tissue septa. (H & E; ×30)

Limitation of Neuroma Formation by Fat Tissue

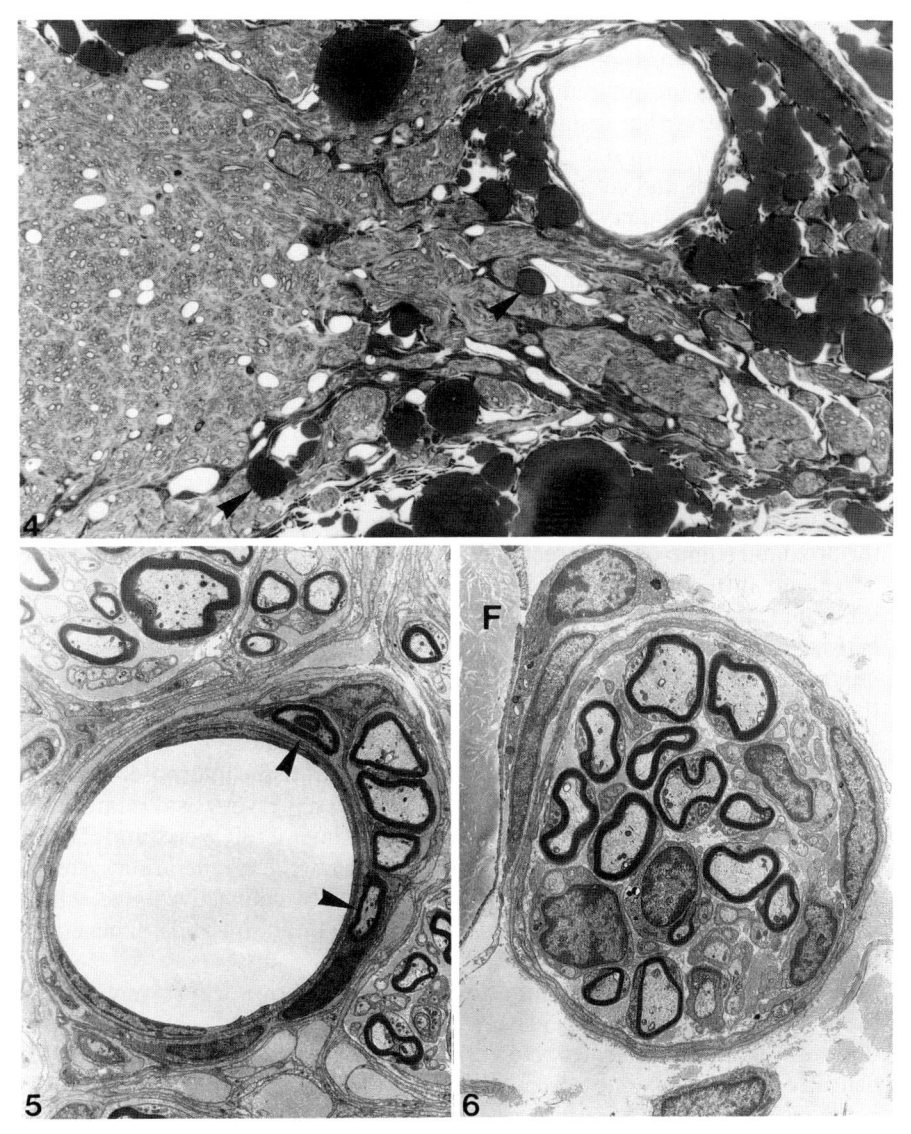

Fig. 4. Distal part of a neuroma implanted into fat tissue, 24 weeks after surgery. Only at the margins of the neuroma are some fat cells (*arrowheads*) surrounded by minifascicles. (Paraphenylendiamine; ×150)

Fig. 5. Capillary in a neuroma, 24 weeks after surgery. Five regenerated myelinated nerve fibers are extending along the vessel. Two myelinated nerve fibers (*arrowheads*) are found in close proximity to the endothelial cells or their basement membranes. (×3300)

Fig. 6. Minifascicle with several myelinated and unmyelinated nerve fibers, 24 weeks after surgery. The nerve fibers are separated from the fat cell (*F*) by intervening perineurial cells, a fibroblast, and a macrophage. (×2700)

(Fig. 2). Minifascicles were seen to extend mainly from the solid neuroma along connective tissue cords or blood vessels (Fig. 3). Between fat cells, infiltrating minifascicles were found only in close proximity to the proximal nerve stump (Fig. 4) but not farther distally. In several control animals, adjacent muscles were extensively infiltrated by regenerating nerve fibers.

Semithin sections and electron microscopy revealed the characteristic pattern of neuromatous reinnervation in both groups. Regenerating axons followed pioneer fibers mainly along connective tissue cords and blood vessels. Later these hypomyelinated or unmyelinated axons were grouped in minifascicles that were enclosed by perineurial cells and epineurial connective tissue rich in collagen fibers at the center of neuromas (Fig. 5). Nerve fibers between fat cells were isolated by intervening perineurial cells and collagen fibers (Fig. 6).

Discussion

This study has revealed that widespread outgrowth of regenerating axons from the proximal stump of a transected nerve can be limited by implantation of the nerve end into fat tissue. At the margins of the neuroma, fat tissue was infiltrated along perivascular strands of connective tissue but usually not between fat cells, indicating that blood supply is a prerequisite for nerve fiber outgrowth. Fat tissue, however, did not prevent formation of solid neuromas at the site of the proximal nerve stump (Weis and Schröder 1989b).

In a nonsystematic histological study on the effect of fat tissue on regenerating nerve fibers, Cajal (1928) noted that fat tissue interposed between the proximal and distal stumps of a transected nerve was "retardedly" penetrated by regenerating axons. In the experiments of Weiss and Taylor (1944), arteries served as the tubes in distally open nerve regeneration systems. After surgery, the distal end of the tube was closed by connective tissue, which was replaced by fat tissue afterwards. The regenerating axons did not penetrate this fat tissue.

From the experimental findings of others cited above, which were not the results of systematic experiments and evaluations, and the results presented in this study, no "antineurotrophic" effect of fat tissue could be elicited. The neurotrophic activity, however, that promotes nerve fiber regeneration in nerve-nerve and nerve-muscle regeneration chambers (Weis and Schröder 1989a) is obviously not present in fat tissue.

Fat tissue ensheathing the proximal nerve end might meet the requirements of Sunderland (1978) to "provide a suitable soft pressure-free bed for the central stump of the nerve severed at amputation."

References

Bardenheuer E (1908) Behandlung der Nerven bei Amputationen zur Verhütung der Amputationsneurome und zur Heilung der bestehenden Neurome durch die sogenannte Neurinkampsis. Dtsch Z Chir 96:126–135

Battista A, Cravioto H (1981) Neuroma formation and prevention by fascicle ligation in the rat. Neurosurg 8 (2):191–204

Boldrey E (1943) Amputation neuroma in nerves implanted in bone. Ann Surg 118 (6):1052–1057

Brown H, Flynn JE (1973) Abdominal pedicle flap for hand neuromas and entrapped nerves. J Bone Joint Surg 55-A (3):575–579

Cajal SR (1928) Degeneration and regeneration of the nervous system. Hafner, New York (reprint 1959)

Dellon AL, Mackinnon SE (1986) Treatment of the painful neuroma by neuroma resection and muscle implantation. Plast Reconstr Surg 77:427–436

Evans LH, Campbell JB, Pinner-Poole B, Jenny J (1968) Prevention of painful neuromas in horses. JAVMA 153 (3):313–324

Forssmann J (1900) Zur Kenntnis des Neurotropismus. Beitr Path Anat 27:407–430

Goldstein SA, Sturim HS (1985) Interosseus nerve transposition for treatment of painful neuromas. J Hand Surg (Am) 10:270–274

Hedri A (1921) Ein einfaches Verfahren zur Verhütung der Trennungsneurome. Arch Klin Chir 117:842–854

Läwen A (1925) Über Nervenvereisungen bei Amputationen, Amputationsneuromen, Angiospasmen, Erythromelalgie, seniler Gangrän und Ulcus cruris varicosum. Beitr Klin Chir 133:405–428

Lundborg G, Longo FM, Varon S (1982) Nerve regeneration and trophic factors in vivo. Brain Res 232:157–161

Martini AK (1985) Neurombehandlung mit Histoacryl im Tierversuch. Handchir 17:78–80

Petropoulos PC, Stefanko S (1961) Experimental observations on the prevention of neuroma formation. J Surg Res 1 (3):241–248

Samii M (1981) Centrocentral anastomosis of peripheral nerves: a neurosurgical treatment of amputation neuromas. In: Siegfried J, Zimmerman M (eds) Phantom and stump pain. Springer, Berlin Heidelberg New York, pp 123–125

Sunderland S (1978) Nerves and nerve injuries. 2nd edn. Churchill Livingstone, Edinburgh London

Tenneff S (1949) Prevention of amputation neuroma. J Int Coll Surg 12:16–20

Tupper JW (1986) Discussion of the study of Dellon and Mackinnon (1986). Plast Reconstr Surg 77:437–438

Weis J, Schröder JM (1989a) Differential effects of nerve, muscle, and fat tissue on regenerating nerve fibers in vivo. Muscle & Nerve 12:723–734

Weis J, Schröder JM (1989b) The influence of fat tissue on neuroma formation. J Neurosurg 71:588–593

Weiss P, Taylor AC (1944) Further experimental evidence against "neurotropsin" in nerve regeneration. J Exp Zool 95:233–257

The Blood-Nerve Barrier in Peripheral Nerve Injury, Repair, and Regeneration

J. R. Bain, A. R. Hudson, S. E. Mackinnon, F. Gentili, and D. Hunter, Toronto/Canada

Introduction

The endoneurial environment of the peripheral nervous system is a physiologically specialized site, analagous to the central nervous system and other sites with specialized function that have been in some sense separated from the systemic circulation. The reasons for the phylogenetic development of a specialized endothelial barrier and relative impermeability of the perineurium have not been fully elucidated, nor has been the full understanding of the importance of this barrier in normal physiological function, peripheral nerve regeneration following injury, and effects of dysfunction or its role in peripheral neuropathy.

The terminology must also be carefully employed. The term "barrier" is a relative one. Certainly, essential nutrients, low molecular weight macromolecules, electrolytes, and water move through this barrier at rates and by mechanisms determined by numerous factors [4]. The main body of investigation, as well as the major physiological significance, appears to surround the movement of proteins and larger macromolecules. In addition, this "barrier" should not be viewed as a static mechanical barrier, but rather as structures that can respond to various physiological and pathophysiological processes to effect changes in permeability to these proteins. Some of the structures composing the blood-nerve barrier as well as the methods by which to assess the blood-nerve barrier are discussed here. In addition, a review of the clinically relevant conditions that lead to blood-nerve barrier dysfunction and the sequence of events that lead to its reconstitution are discussed.

Anatomy and Morphology

The vasculature of the peripheral nerve has been reviewed by several authors [24, 14]. The majority of peripheral nerves receive their major segmental supply from regional arteries that provide feeding branches. These major branches anastomose with a plexus of vessels in three overlapping anatomical locations: the epineurium, perineurium, and endoneurium.

In the epineurium there is a rich plexus of vessels of varying sizes supplied by branches of regional vessels [14]. This plexus is primarily longitudinally oriented, but many anastomoses exist supplying epineurial vessels throughout the nerve, including extensive branches located in the internal epineurium between fascicles.

The perineurial vessels are also primarily of longitudinal orientation, with the majority of vessels traveling in the outer layers of the perineurial connective tissue. Some vessels are noted to course in the internal lamellae of the perineurium. The connections between the perineurial and epineurial plexuses are vast, as are the connections with the endoneurial vessels.

The caliber of the endoneurial microvessels is generally smaller than the aforementioned plexuses, but occasionally a larger vessel is identified. The longitudinal orientation is most common with some loop formations. There is a larger preponderance of vessels located immediately subperineurially, which communicate extensively with the perineurial vessels.

This extensive longitudinal vascular network of the perineurium and endoneurium has been demonstrated to maintain blood flow when the epineurial vessels are damaged, as seen in extensive mobilization of the nerve

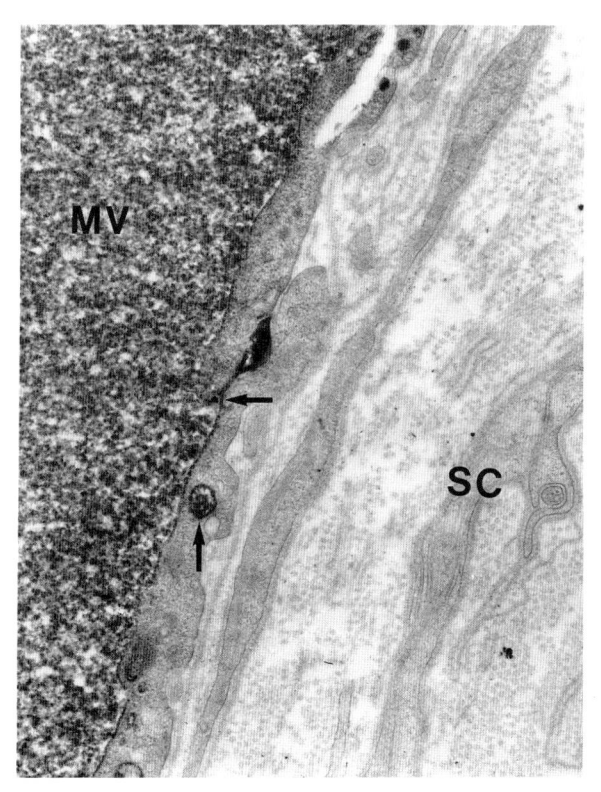

Fig. 1. Electron micrograph of endoneurium. *MV*, Microvessel containing HRP reaction product; ↑, HRP reaction product within pinocytotic vesicle of endothelial cell; ←, tight junction; *SC*, Schwann's cell. Note that the tracer is maintained within the lumen of the microvessel in the normal state. (× 36 400)

[15]. It was also noted that the blood flow in the venules of all three vascular networks of the nerve were able to change direction if damage to part of the plexus occurred.

The two sites at which the endoneurial environment is separated from the surrounding tissue, as discerned by the inability of certain plasma proteins or tracers to freely equilibrate, are the inner layers of the perineurium and the endothelial cells of the endoneurial vasculature [28, 29]. These sites are defined collectively as the blood-nerve barrier and are subsequently described.

The components of the wall of the endoneurial vessels are histologically similar to many other organs and tissues except at an ultrastructural level. The endothelial cells of the endoneurial vessels are not fenestrated and have tight junctions (zonulae occludentes) between the cells (Fig. 1). It appears that this is the site of limitation of many macromolecular substances. In the epineurium, however, the endothelial cells have open junctions between the cells, as in many other organs, and may have some fenestrated cells. The perineurial vessels that pierce the perineurium to become endothelial vessels take on the characteristics of tight junctions as they traverse this barrier [25].

Perineurium

The perineurium with the modified intercellular connections, tight junctions in the innermost layers [5], forms a continuous impermeable barrier to many large macromolecules in a similar fashion to the tight junctions of the endoneurial vessels (Fig. 2). This is the second structure which contributes to the blood-nerve barrier. The thickness of the perineurium varies with the size of the fascicle, but even 1 or 2 layers of cells with these tight intercellular connections appear to be impermeable to tracers except in the most terminal portions of the peripheral nerve. As the vessels pass through the perineurium, the endothelial cells acquire this relatively impermeable characteristic.

Assessment Techniques

The assessment of the blood-nerve barrier has been achieved largely by qualitative methodologies, however quantitative studies have been attempted. The major difficulty in the quantitative technique is the inability to separate the epineural components from the perineurium and endoneurium. The standard qualitative methodology to assess the blood-nerve barrier involves either (a) the application of a microscopically identifiable macromolecule (directly or indirectly) to the external surface of the nerve if assessing the perineurial integrity alone or (b) administering the tracer intravenously and subsequently viewing the distribution in the various intravascular and extravascular compartments. The critical characteristic of these tracers is that they do not cross the blood-nerve barrier in the normal situation but do leave the intravascular compartment in both extraneural vessels and some abnormal

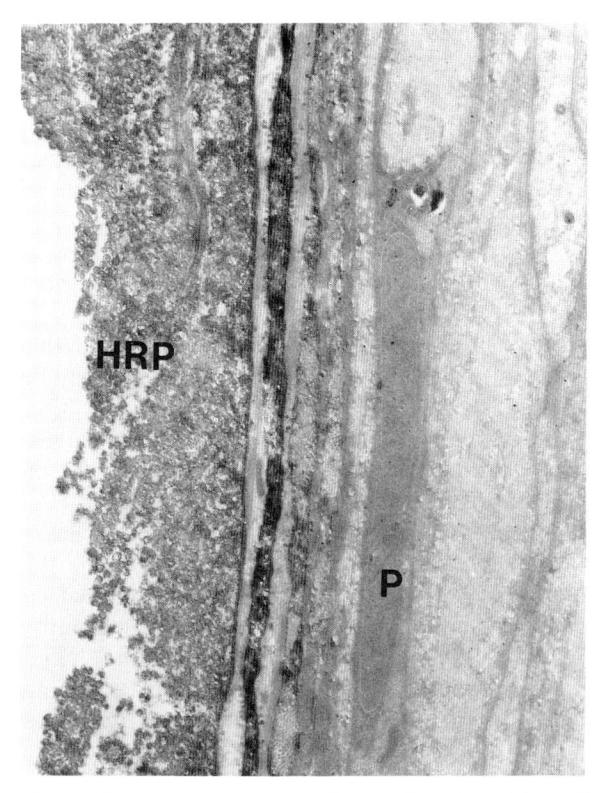

Fig. 2. Electron photomicrograph of perineurium, 1.5 cm distal to a cut and sutured nerve, 3 months postrepair. *HRP*, Tracer reaction product; *P* perineurial cell. Note that the barrier function of the perineurium has been restored so that the HRP tracer, which has leaked through the epineurial vessels, is prevented from entering the endoneurium of the fascicle. ($\times 12740$)

situations. The various substances that have been used to investigate the blood-nerve barrier include: albumin labeled with Evans blue (EBA) or trypan blue [34], dextrans labeled with fluorochrome [12], sodium fluoroscein [20], diaminocridine [2], ferritin, ^{131}I-labeled albumin [23], and horseradish peroxidase (HRP) [11]. The two methodologies utilized extensively include examination of the permeability of a fluorescent protein tracer (EBA) described by Steinwall and Klatzo [34] and HRP described by Graham and Karnovsky [11]. One methodology utilizing fluorescence microscopy (EBA) that allows examination of light microscopy morphometric characteristics, and another utilizing electron microscopy (HRP) that permits examination of the ultrastructural morphology, are outlined below.

EBA is prepared by mixing in vitro bovine albumin (5% solution Cohn Fraction V, molecular weight 60 000; Nutritional Biochemical, Cleveland, Ohio) with 1% Evans blue (Fischer Scientific, Toronto, Ontario). After thorough mixing, the EBA solution is passed through a Sephadex column

(Sephadex G-25 M; Pharmacia Chemical, Uppsala, Sweden) to remove any unbound fluorescent tracer. The EBA solution is slowly injected intravenously (50 ml/100 mg body weight). After EBA perfusion, the animal is killed, and the nerve to be studied is dissected out utilizing the operating microscope, fixed in 5% formalin for 24 h. Frozen longitudinal sections 10–15 μm thick are cut and mounted in 50% glycerin and examined under fluorescence microscope utilizing a N 2 filter system (Leitz SM-Lux, Wild Leitz Canada, Willowdale, Ontario). EBA produces a bright red fluorescence when this filter system is utilized allowing the investigator to localize and assess the extent of tracer movement into the tissues.

Although HRP is extensively used in studies of axonal transport, this methodology utilizes HRP as an intravenously administered tracer that can be indirectly visualized in the tissues by localization of reaction product after processing. Briefly, HRP (Type II, 100 mg, MW 40 000; Sigma Chemical, St. Louis, Missouri) is dissolved in 1 ml normal saline. Animals should be pretreated with atropine sulphate (0.05 mg/kg) and diphenhydramine HCl (Benadryl; Parke-Davis, Brockville, Ontario) to prevent the histamine release mediated by intravenous administration of HRP. After circulation, the animal is killed and the nerve to be studied is removed and fixed in Karnovsky's fixative prepared in a sodium cacodylate buffer. Subsequently, the tissue must be cut into 1-mm sections and incubated at 37 °C for 3 h in a solution consisting of 20 mg 3,3'-diaminobenzidine (Sigma Chemical), 0.49 mg sucrose, 0.2 ml 1% magnesium chloride, 0.2 ml 1% hydrogen peroxide in a 0.05-M tris buffer (pH 8.1). The tissue is then washed in a 1-M cacodylate buffer. Incubation of the tissue in the solution results in the formation of a brown reaction product at the sites of HRP infiltration. This product can be visualized on light microscopy and is electron dense after osmification, permitting the more precise localization of the tracer by electron microscopy. Several additional points should be emphasized regarding this technique. Firstly, although localization of the reaction product is excellent, the processing technique is not ideal for membrane preservation, and hence morphometry of axons, myelin, and Schwann's cells is compromised. In addition, the sections are stained with lead citrate only, not uranyl acetate, hence endoneurial collagen is not stained. Darkening in the endoneurial space therefore indicates the penetration of HRP and subsequent formation of the reaction product.

Examination of Blood-Nerve Barrier in Clinical Applications

Nerve Injection Injuries

Substances frequently given by hypodermic injection such as antibiotics [7], major tranquilizers [7], steroids [19], chymopapain [16], local anesthetic agents [8], or bovine collagen [18] can lead to iatrogenic peripheral nerve injury arising from inadvertent extrafascicular or intrafascicular administration of such drugs [6]. These agents have been investigated in this laboratory to determine the pathology in the peripheral nerve arising from these injuries.

The rat sciatic nerve was employed with administration of active drug or an equal volume of saline as control, into either an intrafascicular or extrafascicular location with a 30-gauge needle [7].

The control nerves injected with normal saline in the extrafascicular position showed no signs of increased permeability of the blood-nerve barrier by either assessment technique. However, with the intrafascicular administration there was a slight increase in the leakage of tracer in the immediate site of the intraneural injection presumably due to the local trauma of the perineurium and adjacent vessels by the 30-gauge needle. At 2-week assessments there was no leakage. The administration of most agents in the extrafascicular position did not result in an alteration of the perineurial or endoneurial vessel permeability to the tracers with the exception of: benzylpenicillin, diazepam, chlordiazepoxide, chlorpromazine, dimenhydrinate, and tetracaine. Most local anesthetics, common antibiotics, and parenteral analgesics did not produce any alteration in permeability when administered extrafascicularly, attesting to the integrity of the perineurium with this local insult.

In the study of the local anesthetics, it was evident that the nature and severity of the neural pathology following intrafascicular injection was dependent upon the type of anesthetic employed. The more toxic local anesthetic agents caused a marked disruption of the blood-nerve barrier, as demonstrated by extensive leakage of the tracers up to 1 cm proximal and distal to the site of administration. It was apparent that the agents that caused marked early disruption of the blood-nerve barrier were subsequently found to cause the most extensive damage when examined histologically.

Nerve Compression Injuries

Acute Compression. Rydevik et al. investigated the effects of graded compression injuries on the peripheral nerve in the rabbit tibial nerve model [30, 31]. Included in these studies was an investigation of the effects on the integrity of the blood-nerve barrier. It was determined that both the amount of pressure and the duration of the compressive force affected the ability of the endoneurial vessels to maintain the EBA intravascularly. While 50 mm Hg for 2 h caused some increase in the epineurial leakage, none was noted in the endoneurium until 4 h of compression. When the pressure was increased to 200 or 400 mm Hg, there was a marked increase in the extravasation of the tracer, more marked with a prolonged period of compression. When animals were investigated 2–7 days postcompression with 400 mm Hg for 2 h, there was still evidence of leakage of the tracer. In most of these studies, the effect of the compression was most marked at the edge of the compression chamber [30].

Chronic Compression. The pathophysiology of chronic peripheral compression neuropathy is thought to be substantially different from that of acute compression. Mackinnon et al. described a model of chronic nerve com-

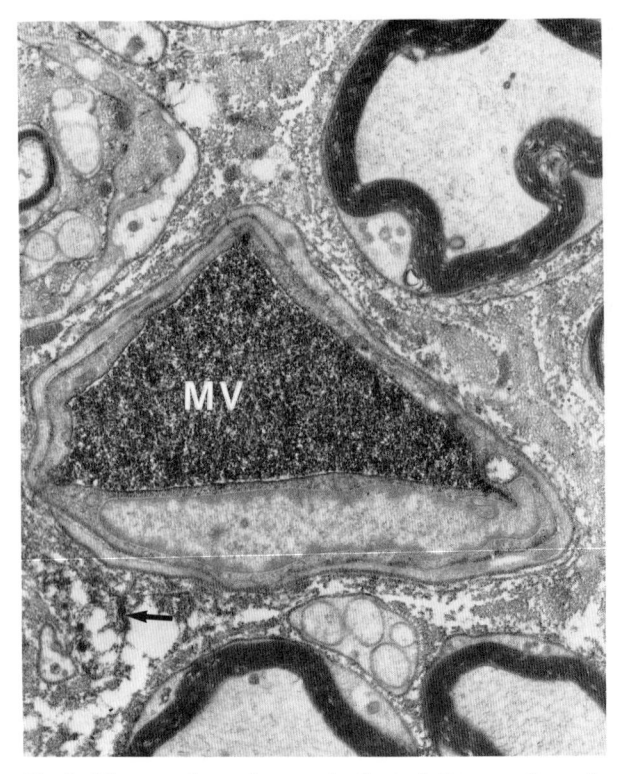

Fig. 3. Electron photomicrograph of rat sciatic nerve, 3 months after compression with a 0.6-mm internal diameter cuff. *MV*, Microvessel containing tracer; ←, HRP reaction product in the endoneurium of the damaged nerve. (× 15 600)

pression in which the sciatic nerve of the rat was entubulated with a 1 cm silastic cuff of varying diameters. A silastic tube with an internal diameter slightly larger (1.5 cm) than the sciatic nerve (1.2 cm) reproduced the histological and electrophysiological characteristics of chronic nerve compression. The first changes noted were the disruption of the blood-nerve barrier. Utilizing the EBA and HRP tracer techniques, after 2 months of compression there was marked extravasation of the tracers into the endoneurial compartment in the area of compression (Figs. 3–5). These changes were noted prior to any histological or electrophysiological signs of nerve compression [17].

Given the fact that the endoneurial compartment is devoid of lymphatics, the extravasation of plasma proteins into the endoneurial space would increase the osmotic and likely the hydrostatic pressure of this compartment. Accomodation in such a closed compartment results in either progressive ischemia, a decrease in the cellular components of that compartment, or the loss of large myelinated fibers and thinning of the myelin in the area of compression. This simplistic hypothesis expresses the importance of maintenance of the blood-nerve barrier.

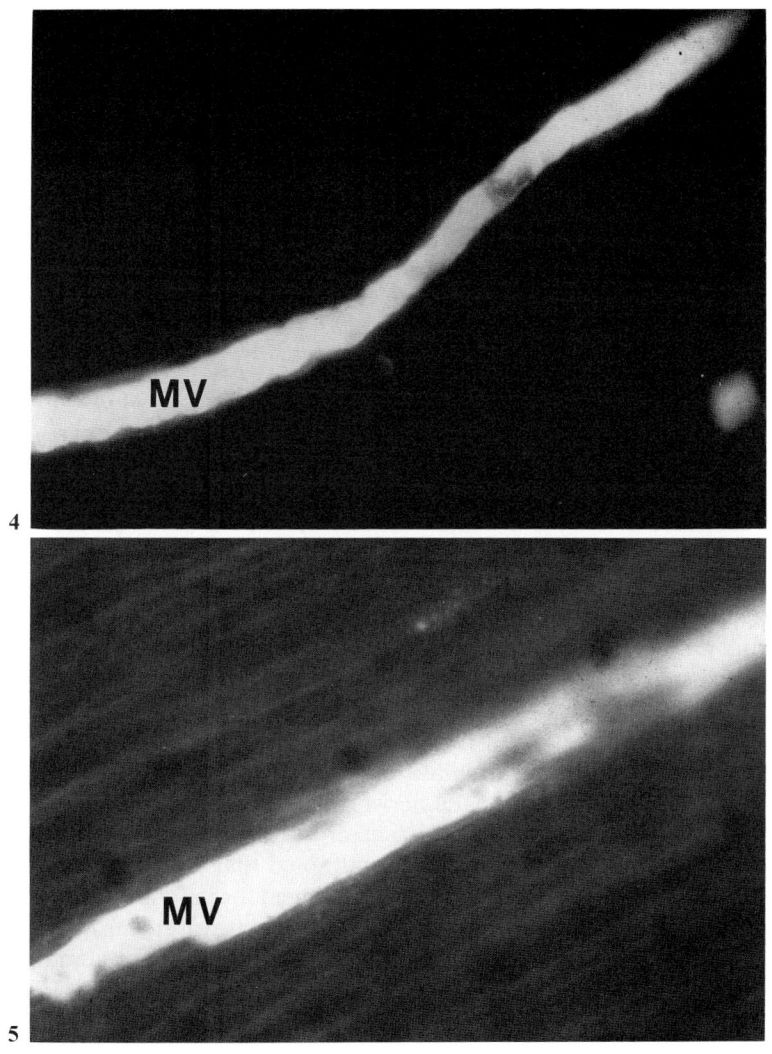

Fig. 4. Fluorescent light photomicrograph. *MV*, Microvessel containing EBA tracer. Section taken proximal to a sciatic nerve compressed for 1 month. Note that the tracer is confined to the microvessel

Fig. 5. Fluorescent light photomicrograph. Sciatic nerve section through level of compression 1 month after cuff application. *MV*, Microvessel. Note the tracer has leaked into the endoneurial space and is now outlining the parallel nerve fibers

Internal Neurolysis. Many authors have advocated internal neurolysis as a treatment for chronic nerve compression; this is required for some reconstructive procedures in order to determine fascicular organization prior to grafting or repair. The effect of internal neurolysis on the short and long term integrity of the blood-nerve barrier was investigated by Gentili et al. in a rat model [10].

Rats without previous pathology were subjected to internal neurolysis utilizing appropriate magnification ($6-25 \times$) and microinstruments. It was shown that there was extravasation of the protein tracers EBA and HRP at 1 and 24 h following internal neurolysis both at the level of perineurium and vascular endothelium in the endoneurium. The amount of leakage was rated as minimal at the endoneurial vessel and moderate at the perineurium. The integrity of both barriers was reconstituted by 7 days. This transient increase in the plasma protein permeability caused by the procedure was not associated with long-term electrophysiological or histological changes (except in the occasional animal in which the perineurium was violated, i.e., endoneurial herniation) [10].

Axonotmesis and Neurotmesis. Several investigators have attempted to determine the sequence of alterations in the blood-nerve barrier, both at the perineurium and endoneurial vessels in peripheral nerves subjected to crush, transection and proximal stump ligature, and transection and repair. These studies have sought to determine the various contributions of initial injury, the process of wallerian degeneration, and regenerating units on this barrier function [9, 24, 26, 27, 28, 32, 33]. With either a crush injury or transection of the nerve, an immediate and severe disruption of the barrier function is noted at the area of injury, both in the perineurium and endoneurial vasculature extending for a short distance both proximal and distal to the primary injury site [9, 28].

The reported changes that occur in the perineurium and the endoneurial vasculature distal to the site of injury have been variable. Olsson noted that animals with crush injuries of the sciatic nerve displayed leakage only at the crush site over the first 24 hours. Olsson also described the changes occurring over 12 weeks following a nerve transection and noted that the endoneurial vessels displayed some leakage in the entire distal segment for the entire period. Over the entire 12-week assessment period protein tracer extravasated from the region of the scar [28]. He also investigated the integrity of the perineurium to directly applied EBA in the rodent with a crush injury of the sciatic nerve. He demonstrated that the perineurium permitted entrance of the tracer into the endoneurium at the crush site for up to 4 months, however the distal segment of the nerve was impervious to the tracer [26].

Sparrow and Kiernan investigated the effect of the regenerating growth cone on the endoneurial vascular permeability of vessels in the nerve segment distal to either a crush injury or a proximally ligated and transected nerve for 21 days following nerve injury. They found that the increased permeability of endoneurial vessels paralleled the advancing edge of regenerating fibers in the crushed nerve group. In contrast, the ligated and transected group demonstrated no increased leakage until day 6 posttransection in the distal segment, at which time sustained but less intense fluorescent tracer was present in the distal nerve segment. They hypothesized that the presence of plasma proteins is essential for the ongoing regeneration of peripheral neurons [33].

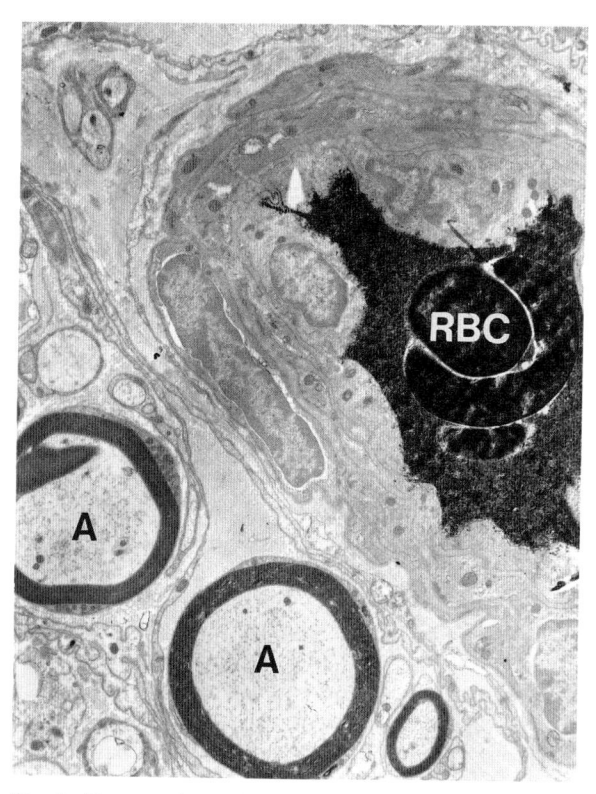

Fig. 6. Electron photomicrograph rat sciatic nerve at suture line 4 months after nerve suture. *RBC*, Red blood corpuscle surrounded by HRP reaction product; *A*, regenerating axons traversing the suture line. Note that the blood-nerve barrier has been restored, and that the reaction product is once again confined to the lumen of the microvessel. ($\times 10400$)

Gentili et al. demonstrated similar findings in the rat with neurotmesis of the sciatic nerve primarily repaired with 10-O sutures utilizing microsurgical technique. The distal nerve segment showed progressive leakage to protein tracers in a proximal-to-distal segment followed by restoration of the normal barrier function with maturation of the regenerative process. The neurorrhaphy site was impervious to EBA and HRP by 3 months after repair (Fig. 6). It was also noted that the breakdown of the blood-nerve barrier extended up to 5 mm proximal to the transection site when tested at 24 h [9].

Nerve Grafting: Autografts. The nerve grafting situation adds an additional factor to the transection and neurorrhaphy condition, that of a nerve graft that in the process of procurement and placement is devascularized and must be revascularized. Therefore, the process of ingrowth of vessels from the proximal and distal nerve stumps as well as from the surrounding soft tissue bed may additionally affect barrier function as well as the presence of two repair sites. Using a sural neve graft model in the rat, Ahmed and Weller investigated the influence of regenerating axons on the barrier function of a 1-cm graft held in place of a 0.5-cm deficit by gel foam and thrombin over a 24-week period. They described the formation of "compartments" in the gap between the proximal nerve segment and the graft which contained a few axons and were impermeable to HRP. However, the perineurium in the area of the "junction" was not reconstituted [1]. At 6 months, they found that the perineurium was still permeable to the protein tracer HRP. In contrast to Sparrow and Kiernan [32], they found that the perineurium of the distal nerve segment was permeable to HRP while the endoneurial vessels were not. Curiously, they reported that the perineurium of the graft was impermeable to tracer.

Nerve Grafting: Allografts. Our laboratory has investigated the potential role of both pretreated peripheral nerve allografts [21] and fresh allografts in immunosuppressed recipients [22, 3]. Recent investigations have demonstrated excellent regeneration across such grafts in animals immunosuppressed with cyclosporin A (CsA) comparable to that of autografts [3]. Investigation of the blood-nerve barrier in CsA-treated and untreated recipients of allogenic nerve grafts has yielded some interesting preliminary results. As would be expected, the process of foreign tissue rejection causes a marked disruption of the blood-nerve barrier of the allograft in the untreated recipient. CsA therapy, in a dosage regimen effective in preventing nerve allograft rejection has several interesting effects. Not only is the prolonged and extensive disruption of the blood-nerve barrier of the allograft as compared with the autograft prevented, but the reconstitution of the barrier function in both autografts and allografts in CsA-treated recipients is accelerated. The mechanism by which this immunosuppressive agent affects the blood-nerve barrier has not been determined.

Summary

The properties of the perineurium and vascular endothelium in the endoneurial compartment that restrict the passage of plasma proteins have been outlined both in the normal and traumatized peripheral nerve. While it is obvious that physical violation of these structures results in breakdown of their barrier function, the extent of disruption of the blood-nerve barrier both proximal and distal to the injury site, the time course of this breakdown and restoration thereof, and the effect of regenerating axons on the distal nerve are less intuitive. The ability to pharmacologically modify the integrity of the blood-nerve barrier may provide the neurobiologist and peripheral nerve surgeon further understanding in peripheral nerve regeneration and improved clinical results.

References

1. Ahmed AM, Weller RO (1979) The blood-nerve barrier and reconstitution of the perineurium following nerve grafting. Neuropath Appl Neurobiol 5:469–483
2. Aker FD (1972) A study of hematic barriers in peripheral nerves of albino rabbits. Anat Rec 174:21–38
3. Bain JR, Mackinnon SE, Hudson AR, Falk RE, Falk JA, Hunter DA (1988) The peripheral nerve allograft: an assessment of regeneration across nerve allografts in rats immunosuppressed with cyclosporin A. Plast Reconstr Surg 82:1052–1064
4. Bradbury M (1979) The concept of a blood-brain barrier. Wiley, New York
5. Burkel WE (1967) The histological fine structure of perineurium. Anat Rec 158:177–190
6. Gentili F, Hudson AR, Hunter D (1980) Clinical and experimental aspects of injection injuries of peripheral nerves. Can J Neurol Sci 7:143–151
7. Gentili F, Hudson AR, Kline DG, Hunter D (1979) Peripheral nerve injection injury: an experimental study. Neurosurgery 4:244–253
8. Gentili F, Hudson AR, Hunter D, Kline DG (1980) Nerve injection injury with local anesthetic agents: a light and electron microscopic, fluorescent microscopic and horseradish peroxidase study. Neurosurgery 6:263–272
9. Gentili F, Hudson AR, Hunter D, Knapp C (1982) Alterations in the microcirculation and blood-nerve barrier during degeneration and regeneration in the sciatic nerve of the rat. Surgical Forum 33:498–500
10. Gentili F, Hudson AR, Kline DG, Hunter D (1981) Morphological and physiological alterations following internal neurolysis of the normal rat sciatic nerve. In: Gorio A et al. (eds) Posttraumatic peripheral nerve regeneration; experimental basis and clinical implications. Raven Press, New York, pp 183–196
11. Graham RC, Karnovsky MJ (1966) The early stages of absorption of injected horseradish peroxidase in the proximal tubules of mouse kidney: ultrastructural cytochemistry by a new technique. J Histochem Cytochem 14:291–302
12. Hulstrom D, Malmgren L, Gilstring D, Olsson Y (1983) FITC-dextrans as tracers for macromolecular movements in the nervous system. Acta Neuropathol (Berl) 59:53–62
13. Lundborg G, Myers R, Powell H (1983) Nerve compression injury and increased endoneurial fluid pressure: a "miniature compartment syndrome". J Neurol Neurosurg Psych 46:1119–1124
14. Lundborg G (1979) The intrinsic vascularization of human peripheral nerves: structural and functional aspects. J Hand Surg (Am) 4:34–41
15. Lundborg G (1970) Ischemic nerve injury. Experimental studies on intraneural microvascular pathophysiology and nerve function in a limb subjected to temporary circulatory arrest. Scand J Plast Reconstr Surg Supple 6
16. Mackinnon SE, Hudson AR, Llamas F, Dellon AL, Kline DG, Hunter DA (1984) Peripheral nerve injury by chymopapain injection. J Neurosurg 61:1–8
17. Mackinnon SE, Dellon AL, Hudson AR, Hunter DA (1984) Chronic nerve compression – an experimental model in the rat. Ann Plast Surg 13:112–120
18. Mackinnon SE, Hudson AR, Bojanowski V, Hunter DA, Maraghi E (1985) Peripheral nerve injection injury with purified bovine collagen – an experimental model in the rat. Ann Plast Surg 14:428–436
19. Mackinnon SE, Hudson AR, Gentili F, Kline DG, Hunter DA (1982) Peripheral nerve injection injury with steroid agents. Plast Reconstr Surg 69:482–489
20. Mackinnon SE, Hudson AR, Falk RE, Kline D, Hunter D (1984) Peripheral nerve allograft: an assessment of regeneration across pretreated nerve allografts. Neurosurgery 15:690–693
21. Mackinnon SE, Hudson AR, Bain JR, Falk RE, Hunter DA (1987) The peripheral nerve allograft: an assessment of regeneration in the immunosuppressed host. Plast Reconstr Surg 79:436–444
22. Malmgren LT, Olsson Y (1980) Differences between the peripheral and the central nervous system in permeability to sodium fluorescein. J Comp Neurol 191:103

23. Mellick RS, Cavanagn JB (1968) Changes in blood vessel permeability during degeneration and regeneration in peripheral nerves. Brain 91:141, 160
24. Olsson Y (1984) Vascular permeability in the peripheral nevous system. In: Dyck PJ et al. (eds) Peripheral neuropathy. Saunders, Philadelphia, pp 579–597
25. Olsson Y (1971) Studies on vascular permeability in peripheral nerves. IV. Distribution of intravenously injected protein tracers in the peripheral nervous system of various species. Acta Neuropathol (Berl) 17:115–126
26. Olsson Y, Kristensson K (1973) The perineurium as a diffusion barrier to protein tracers following trauma to nerves. Acta Neuropathol (Berl) 23:105–111
27. Olsson Y (1968) Topographical differences in the vascular permeability of the peripheral nervous system. Acta Neuropathol 10:26–33
28. Olsson Y (1966) Studies on vascular permeability in peripheral nerves. I. Distribution of circulating fluorescent serum albumin in normal, crushed and sectioned rat sciatic nerve. Acta Neuropathol 7:1–15
29. Olsson Y, Reese TS (1971) Permeability of vasa nervorum and perineurium in mouse sciatic nerve studied by fluorescence and electron microscopy. J Neuropath Exper Neurol 30:105–119
30. Rydevik B, Lundborg G (1977) Permeability of intraneural microvessels and perineurium following acute, graded experimental nerve compression. Scand J Plast Reconstr Surg 11:179–187
31. Rydevik B, Lundborg G, Bagge U (1981) Effects of graded compression on intraneural blood flow – an in vivo study on rabbit tibial nerve. J. Hand Surg (Am) 6:3–12
32. Sparrow JR, Kiernan JA (1979) Uptake and transport of proteins by regenerating axons. Acta Neuropathol (Berl) 47:39–47
33. Sparrow JR, Kiernan JA (1981) Endoneurial vascular permeability in degenerating and regenerating peripheral nerves. Acta Neuropathol (Berl) 53:181–188
34. Steinwall O, Klatzo I (1966) Selective vulnerability of the blood-brain barrier in chemically induced lesions. J Neuropathol Exp Neurol 25:542–559

Revascularization of Free Autologous Nerve Grafts

G. PENKERT and M. SAMII, Hanover/FRG

Introduction

It is known today that regeneration in nerve grafts requires "isomorphic" conditions, i.e., a preserved endoneural architecture and the survival of the Schwann's cells within the graft. Only the preserved vitality of Schwann's cells offers the essential precondition for the breakdown of the myelin and subsequent final removal of degenerated axons by macrophages [1]. Furthermore, the Schwann's cells form a new and, as is well-known, indispensable myelin sheath along the newly formed axon sprouting.

In the case of preserved endoneural structures a so-called rail is provided for the regenerative axon sprouts; otherwise a neuromatous axon sprouting results. These concepts were introduced into the literature by Hiller in 1949 [2] and were electronmicroscopically confirmed by Schröder and collaborators at the beginning of the 1970s [3]. Both these preconditions for "isomorphic" regeneration are found only in autologous nerve grafts.

The Schwann's cells are extremely sensitive and are easily in danger of losing their vitality, i.e., their capability for pseudopodic spreading, if not sufficiently nourished. Since the report of Weiss and Taylor in 1946 it has been known that they survive without nutrition for only 2 days and by maintained nutrition through diffusion for approximately 1 week, with a tendency to decrease beginning on the 3rd day [4]. Consequently nerve grafts must be revascularized during this time, if possible independently of the length of the defect. Our aim was to address two issues, the one relating to the timing of revascularization and the other relating to its independence of graft length.

Material and Methods

Tests were performed on rabbits. Of 40 animals 37 could be operated on, and in 35 microangiography could be performed. Two cases were not included due to technical failures in the microangiographic procedure. Separate experiments were conducted on two sets of animals.

Group 1. Exposure of the sciatic nerve of one side was followed by an incision at two points. The ends of the transplant thus obtained were wrapped in a sterile membrane and replaced into musculature (Fig. 1). After 2, 3, 4, 5 and

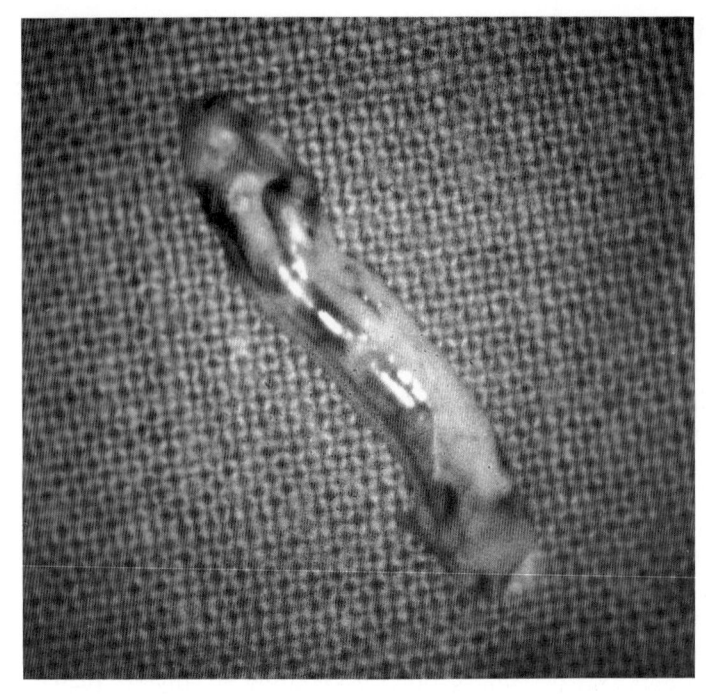

Fig. 1. Nerve graft ends wrapped in a sterile membrane. Only strictly lateral revascularization is possible

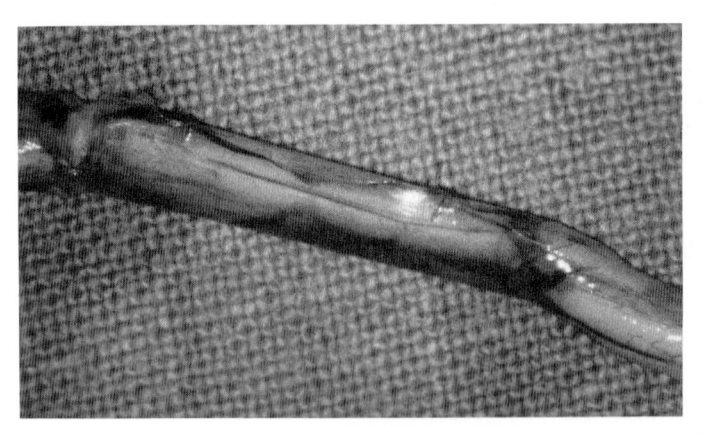

Fig. 2. Nerve graft enclosed in a dialysis membrane. Nutrition by diffusion maintained. Revascularization only in longitudinal direction

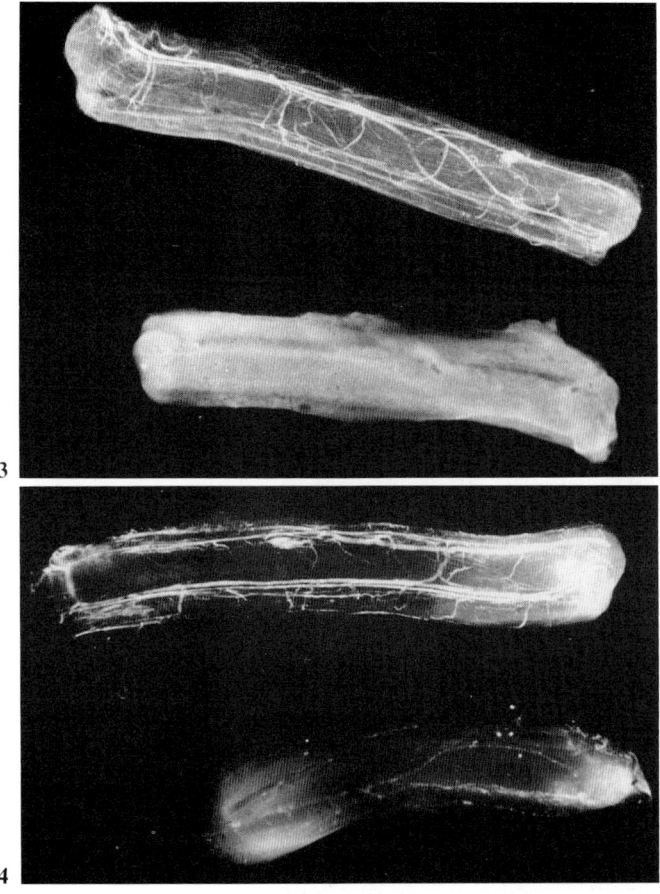

Fig. 3. Group 1 experiment. Angiography 2 days postoperatively shows no sign of revascularization in the graft (control nerve of the opposite side above)

Fig. 4. Group 1 experiment. Angiography 3 days postoperatively shows a very fragile vessel filling in the graft

6 days laparotomy was performed, cannulation of the aorta to distal, proximal ligature of the aorta, high-pressure perfusion with 25% barium sulfate roentgen contrast medium under heparinization for 1 h, then the transplant was removed together with a piece of the sciatic nerve of the opposite side as control nerve. Graft and control nerve were placed on a fine-grained photo-coated glass plate and irradiated with 15 kV_p for 1 h. Finally, the plates were developed and photo-enlarged showing revascularization through (regional) vascular sprouting from the recipient bed.

Group 2. Exposure of the sciatic nerve on one side was followed by an incision at two points. The sciatic nerve of the opposite side was exposed,

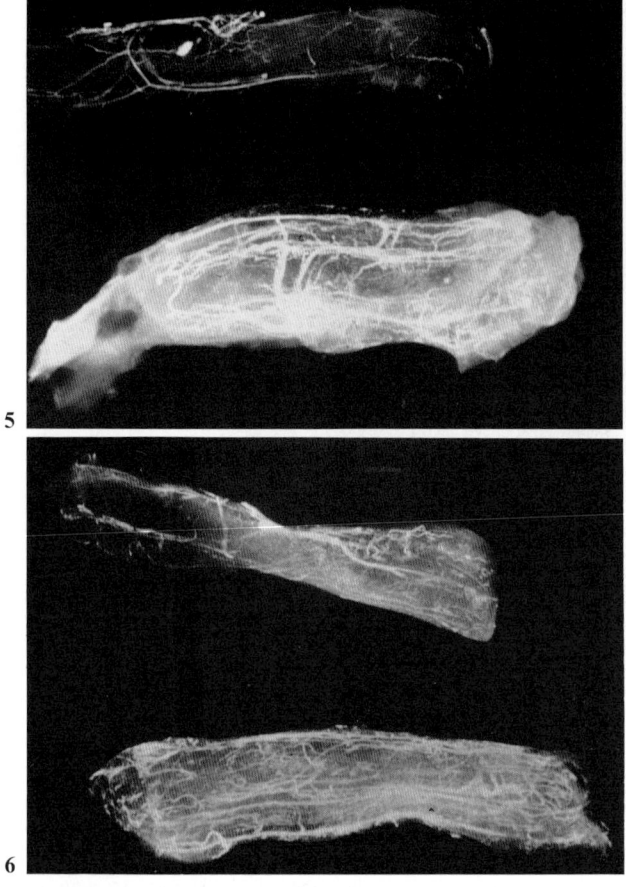

Fig. 5. Group 1 experiment. Angiography on 4th day shows all vessels filled indicating a hyperemic situation

Fig. 6. Group 1 experiment. Angiography on the 5th postoperative day is comparable to that on the day before

followed by interposition here without tension of the previously obtained transplant, circularly wrapped in a dialysis membrane fixed by microsutures (Fig. 2). After 2–6 days the graft was removed and microangiography was performed. Here the nutrition was maintained by diffusion; revascularization is possible through the anastomosis only longitudinally.

Results

Group 1 Experiments. In six transplants, angiographically examined 2 days postoperatively, there were no signs of revascularization from the side (Fig. 3).

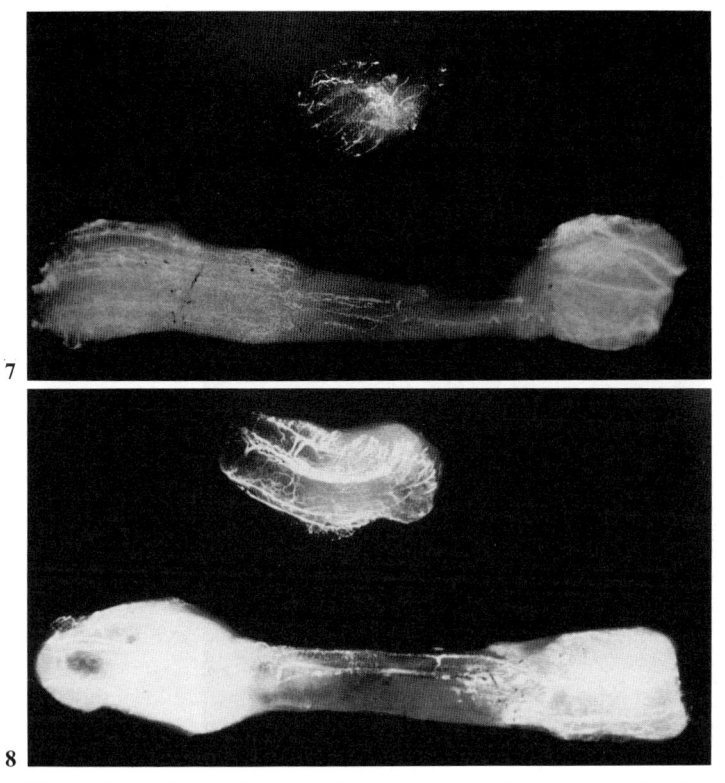

Fig. 7. Group 2 experiment. Angiography on the 3rd postoperative day shows very fragile longitudinal vessel filling within the graft

Fig. 8. Group 2 experiment. Angiography on the 4th postoperative day again shows an insufficient vessel filling

After 3 days, in all examined cases – six grafts – there was a partial and beginning vessel filling (Fig. 4). On the next day, we observed a hyperemic situation, persisting the following days (Figs. 5, 6).

Group 2 Experiments. Based on the results in group 1, we began our first angiography on the 3rd day postoperatively. This showed a very fragile vessel filling through the longitudinal vessel system (Fig. 7), persisting on the 4th and 5th day (Figs. 8, 9). On the 6th day, a beginning hyperemic situation could be traced (Fig. 10).

Conclusion

We can summarize our findings as follows. (a) Revascularization of the autologous transplant clearly begins on the 3rd postoperative day. (b) Through

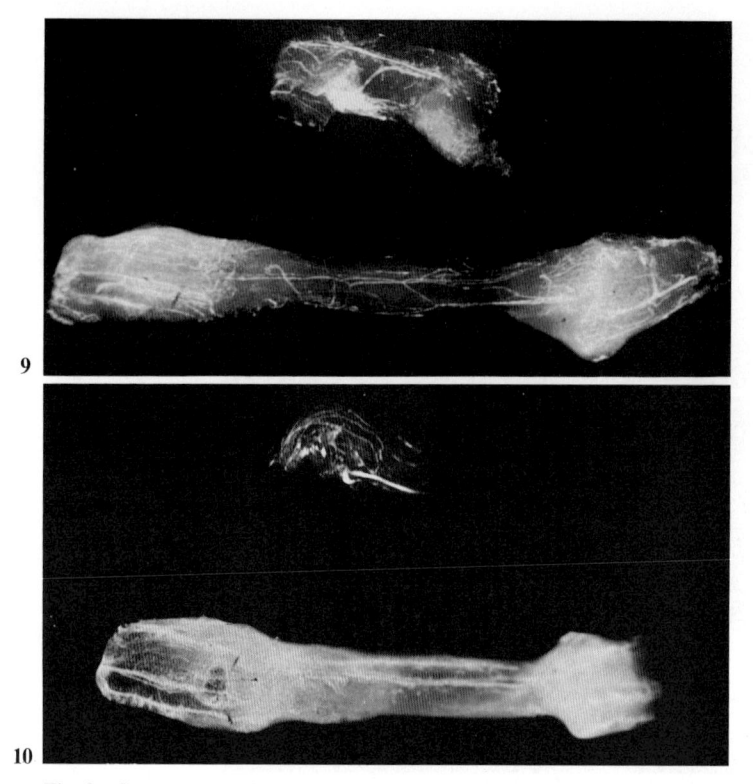

Fig. 9. Group 2 experiment. Angiography on the 5th day still shows a thin and precarious vessel filling

Fig. 10. Group 2 experiment. Angiography after 6 days now shows a beginning hyperemic situation within the graft – still not comparable to the 4th day experiment of group 1

regional sprouting a hyperemia develops on the 4th postoperative day. (c) The longitudinal revascularization is insignificant. This demonstrates that the length of a nerve graft in itself does not hinder its timely reconnection to the blood circulation.

References

1. Asbury AK (1975) The biology of Schwann cells. In: Dyck PJ, Thomas PK, Lambert EH (eds) Peripheral neuropathy. Saunders, Philadelphia London Toronto, pp 201–212
2. Hiller F (1949) Die Bedeutung des mesodermalen Gewebes bei der Nervenregeneration. Experimentelle Untersuchungen an Nervenverletzungen und Transplantaten. Dtsch Z Nervenheilk 160:176–195
3. Schröder JM (1972) Zur Feinstruktur der Degeneration und Regeneration im peripheren Nerven. Med Mitteilungen 46, B. Braun-Melsungen, S 37–57
4. Weiss P, Taylor C (1946) The viability of isolated nerve fragments and its modification by methylene blue. J Cell Comp Physiol 27:87–103

Vascularization of the Peripheral Nerve After Epineural Suture

M. Lehmann, M. A. Konerding, and M. Blank, Essen/FRG

Introduction

A sufficient revascularization is the basis for repair of a nerve after trauma. The complexity of the peripheral nerve's vascular system has been pointed out by several authors. Lundborg and Branemark (1968) distinguished two integral but independent systems, the "extrinsic" one consisting of nutritive epi- and perineural vessels and the "intrinsic" one consisting of an intrafascicular endoneural plexus (Fig. 1). If one of these systems breaks down, the other is

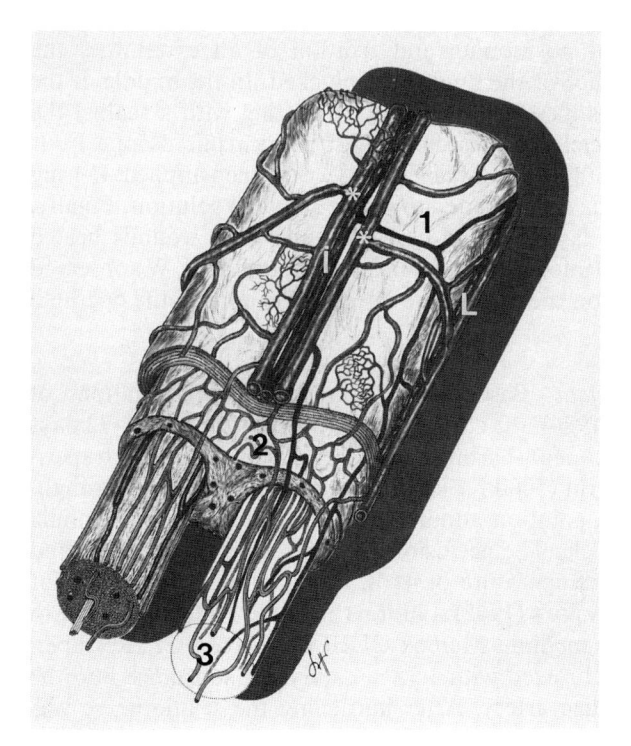

Fig. 1. Schematic drawing of the vascularization of the sciatic nerve based on Lundborg and Branemark (1968), Hiramatsu (1982), and on our own studies. *1*, Epineurium with lateral (*L*) and intrafascicular (*i*) vascular bundles; *2*, perineurium with perineural plexus; *3*, endoneural plexus; *, vascular sphincters

able to undertake the whole blood supply of the nerve so that damage cannot occur (Bateman 1962; Lundborg and Branemark 1968). This is not possible after complete cutting of the nerve. A revascularization becomes necessary instead of a compensatory change in the circulation rate.

The aim of this work is to document the revascularization of the sciatic nerve in domestic chickens after complete cutting and epineural suture by means of the corrosion cast technique.

Material and Methods

Our laboratory animals were 24 homozygote, female, immature, 18-week-old chickens (*Gallus domesticus*) of the HNL breed, weighing 735–1135 g. These animals have the advantage of a high temperature, ranging from 40.5 to 43.5 °C (average 41 °C; Wittke 1972). This indicates that they have a high metabolic rate as well as rapid clinical and morphological regeneration processes (Glees and White 1961; Glees 1961).

Operation Procedure. The chickens were anaesthetized with mepivacaine (Scandicain). After lateral positioning and fixation of all extremities the feathers of the lateral surface of the thigh were plucked. In the middle of the thigh the sciatic nerve was dissected. After sharp cutting with a scalpel the protruding tissue of the fascicles was resected using a surgical microscope. Four or five epineural sutures (Ethicon 10×0, metric 0.2) were then applied. During the operation the nerve was moistened with a 0.75% NaCl solution. Finally, the wound was closed in layers. In all cases the operative wounds healed without complications. No infections or damages could be found. We observed a small decubital necrosis on the dorsal side of the ankle joint of the operated leg in only two cases.

Corrosion Cast Technique. Based mainly on the recommendations of Lametschwandtner et al. (1984), the chickens were thoracotomized 3–22 days after the operation in deep pentobarbital anaesthesia 30 min after intraperitoneal application of heparin (5000 IU/kg body weight). They were exsanguinated with a 0.7% NaCl solution administered through a button cannula inserted into the left ventricle. The perfusion pressure varied between 80 and 110 mm Hg at a solution temperature of 41 °C. The animals were fixed for maximally 5 min in Karnovsky's (1965) solution (pH 7.40, 1660 mosmol) with up to 450 ml. The casting medium Mercox CL2B or Mercox CL2R (Japan Vilene, Japan) was injected mixed with 1.75% catalyzing substance into the descending aorta or the iliac artery. After hardening the sciatic nerve was dissected and macerated with Soluene 350 (Packard), a quarternary ammonium base, over 12–18 h. After drying and mounting on holders the specimen were sputtered with gold in an argon atmosphere and examined with a Stereoscan 180 (Cambridge) at 1013 kV.

Results

When the sciatic nerve is cut, its vessels – the endo- and perineural plexus and the lateral and interfascicular main vessels – are also damaged. It could be confirmed histologically that from the 3rd postoperative day small branches of the epineural vessels began to spread out. These were tortuous and varied in diameter (15–35 μm; Fig. 2). Their luminal surface was irregular and differed from that of normal epineural vessels. After the 6th day we saw the first complete vascular bridging of the neuromas. The vessels of the peri- and epineural plexus grew out at random and had netlike connections to one another. Besides the tortuous and coiled vessels there were rather straight

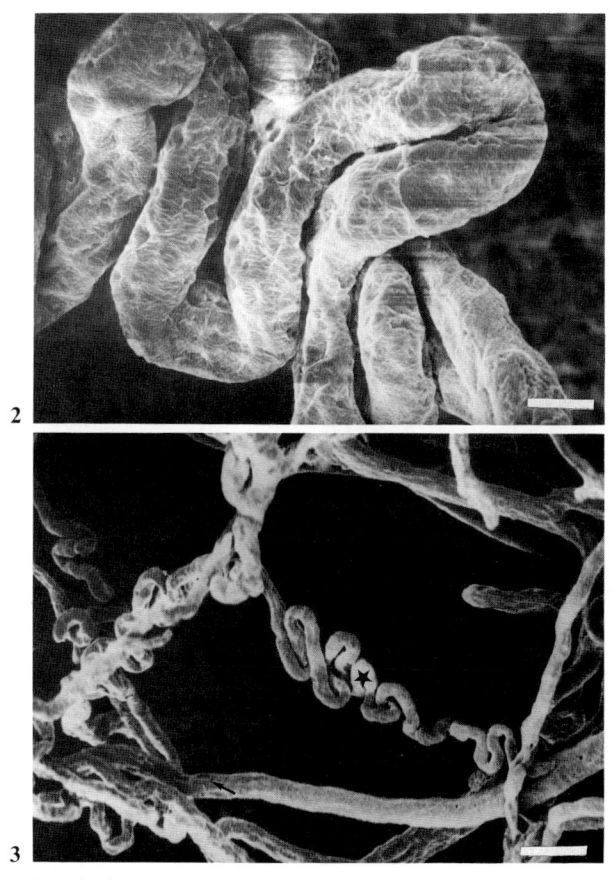

Fig. 2. Corrosion cast of newly developed epineural vessels 4 days after nerve suture. Sciatic nerve, chicken. *Bar*, 20 μm

Fig. 3. Epi- and perineural vessels of the sciatic nerve in the suture region 11 days after operation. *, Tortuous capillaries anastomosing with one another; *arrow*, impressions of endothelial cell nuclei; *bar*, 50 μm

vessels with a regular surface profile (Fig. 3). Here one could see impressions of endothelial cell nuclei. With the corrosion cast technique and histological methods we could rarely find vessels in the endoneural region. The epi- and perineural vessels surrounding the neuroma spread into the tissue. The main epineural axial vessels were dilated (Fig. 4), but a reanastomosis of them could not be confirmed until the 18th day. After 22 postoperative days the main epineural vessels bridged the suture (Fig. 5). The interfascicular vessels still had an irregular shape. The epi- and perineural plexuses reached nearly normal density although they had an irregular arrangement. In the endoneural region vessels could always be depicted in this stage. Later the diameter of the neuroma in the region of the suture decreased.

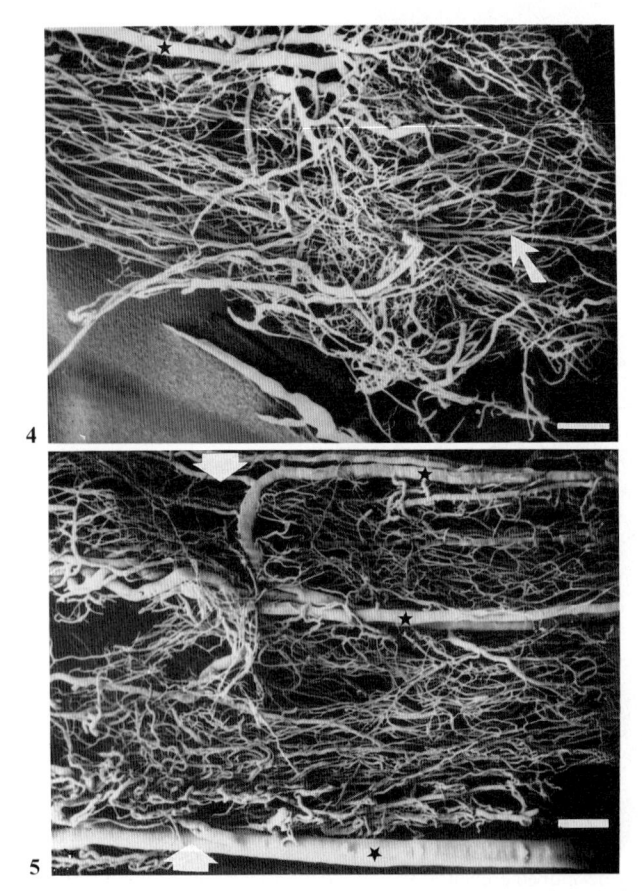

Fig. 4. Vessels in suture region 18 days after operation. *, interfascicular, main epineural vessels; *arrow*, endoneural vessels; *bar*, 500 μm

Fig. 5. Vessel topography of the sciatic nerve 22 days after suture. *Arrow*, Direction of cut; *, main epineural vessels; *bar*, 500 μm

Discussion

The epineural nerve suture has become the most common suture technique (Kleinert and Griffin 1973; Daniel and Terzis 1977). Employing this technique, we regularly found neuroma of varying sizes. We consider this due to the damage to the perineurium that normally holds the intrafascicular structures close together. The traumatization of the nerve causes a protrusion of intrafascicular tissue. In spite of resection and immediate suture the function of the perineurium is destroyed, which is the preliminary condition for an appropriate intrafascicular milieu (Lundborg 1979). This may explain why Orgel and Terzis (1977) favoured the perineural suture to the epineural one based on electron microscopic and electrophysiological studies.

The timing of vascularization is determined by the size of the neuroma. We saw the first complete bridging on the 8th day. This correlates with the angiographic results of Hassler (1969) who found the first vessels after 5 days. Their arrangement and luminal structure differed considerably from normal vascular anatomy. Further investigations should establish whether the perineural suture with development of smaller neuroma or improved quality of axonal repair by suppression of all mechanical stresses (De Medinacelli and Freed 1983) induces a more rapid revascularization and better healing of the nerve.

References

Bateman JE (1962) Trauma to nerves in limbs. Saunders, Philadelphia/PA
Daniel RK, Terzis JK (1977) Reconstructive microsurgery. Little Brown, Boston/MA
De Medinacelli L, Freed WJ (1983) Peripheral nerve reconnection: immediate histologic consequences of mechanical support. Exp Neurol 81:459–468
Glees P (1961) Experimentelle Markscheidendegeneration durch Triorthokresylphosphat und ihre Verhütung durch Cortisonacetat. Dtsch Med Wochenschr 86:1175–1178
Glees P, White WG (1961) The absorption of tri-ortho-cresylphosphate through the skin of hens and its neurotoxic effects. J Neurol Neurosurg Psychiatry 24:271–274
Hassler O (1969) Vascular reactions after experimental nerve section, suture and transplantation. Acta Neurol Scand 45:335–341
Hiramatsu Y (1982) Stereoscopic observation of the microvasculature of peripheral nerves. Acta Med Okayama 36 (4):263–275
Karnovsky MJ (1965) A formaldehyde-glutaraldehyde fixative of high osmolality for use in electron microscopy. J. Cell Biol 27:137A–138A
Kleinert HE, Griffin JM (1973) Technique of nerve anastomosis. Orthop Clin North Am 4:907–915
Lametschwandtner A, Lametschwandtner U, Weiger T (1984) Scanning electron microscopy of vascular corrosion cast technique and applications. Scanning Electron Microsc II:663–695
Lundborg G (1979) The intrinsic vascularization of human peripheral nerves: structural and functional aspects. J Hand Surg 4:34–41
Lundborg G, Branemark PI (1968) Microvascular structure and function of peripheral nerves. Vital microscopic studies of the tibial nerve in the rabbit. Adv Microcir 1:66–88
Orgel MG, Terzis JK (1977) Epineural vs perineural repair: an ultrastructural and electrophysiological study of nerve regeneration. Plast Reconstr Surg 60:80–91
Wittke G (1972) Physiologie der Haustiere. Parey, Berlin Hamburg

Vascularization of the Peripheral Nerve in Laboratory Animals

M. A. KONERDING, M. LEHMANN, and M. BLANK, Essen/FRG

Introduction

Fetterman and Spitler (1940), among others, have concluded that vascular diseases lead to ischemic neuropathies. Basing his conclusions on the first systematic studies, Adams (1942) distinguished three kinds of vessels: nutritive vessels, epineural vessels, and an intrafascicular plexus. Blunt (1959), Waksman (1961), and Lang (1962) confirmed these results.

A very important contribution came from Lundborg and Branemark (1968). They discovered that the microcirculation consisted of two integral systems independent of one another, the "extrinsic" consisting of nutritive epineural vessels and a perineural plexus, and the "intrinsic" consisting of an intrafascicular plexus. According to these authors the intrinsic system is able to undertake the nutrition of the whole nerve if the extrinsic system breaks down, for example, through a surgical mobilization of a larger part of the nerve. Hiramatsu (1982), who has carried out the only work on the microvasculature of peripheral nerves using corrosion casting techniques, partially agreed with these findings.

The aim of this study was to demonstrate the vascularization of the peripheral nerve by means of microcorrosion casting and freeze-broken nerves in order to provide an improved three-dimensional illustration and to extend basic knowledge for further experimental studies.

Material and Methods

Our studies used 14 female, 18-week-old chickens of the HNL breed weighing 735–1135 g. Additionally, the sciatic nerves of 11 12-week-old Wistar rats of both sexes weighing 160–240 g were studied.

Corrosion Casting Technique. Following recommendations of Lametschwandtner et al. (1984) and Hodde et al. (1980), we have chosen the following procedure. In deep pentobarbital anesthesia (Nembutal, 80 mg/kg body weight intraperitoneally) the animals were thoracotomized 30 min after intraperitoneal application of heparin (Liquemin, 5000 IU/kg body weight). The rats were exsanguinated with up to 250 ml 0.9% NaCl solution, the chickens with up to 450 ml 0.7% NaCl solution. The solution was applied by means of an olive-tipped cannula inserted into the left ventricle. The perfusion pressures were 80–110 mmHg and the solution temperatures 41 °C for chickens and 37°–39 °C for rats. The animals were fixed for a maximum of 5 min in Karnovsky's (1965) solution (pH 7.40, 1660 mosmol) to a total of 450 ml. In the region of the lower thoracic vertebral bodies, the thoracic aorta was dissected, the button cannula inserted and advanced into the right and left common iliac arteries or the external iliac arteries. In these vessels 20 ml (rats) or 50 ml (chickens) of the casting medium Mercox CL-28 B or Mercox CL-2 R (Japan Vilene, Japan) mixed with 1.75% catalyzing substance was injected. After 4 h in a waterbath at 40 °C the specimens were completely hardened. The sciatic nerve was dissected and macerated 12–18 h with a quarternary ammonium base (Soluene 350, Packard). After drying and mounting on holders the specimens were sputtered with gold in an argon atmosphere and examined with a Stereoscan 180 scanning electron microscope (Cambridge) at 10–13 kV acceleration voltage.

Freeze-Broken Specimens. After perfusion with saline and fixation as described above, parts of the nerves of approximately 10 mm in length were dissected free and postfixed for 4 h in Karnovsky's solution (1965) at 4 °C. The specimens were washed in cacodylate buffer and contrasted in osmic acid solution (Dalton 1955). They were dehydrated in ascending grades of alcohol and amyl acetate. From the pure amyl acetate the specimens were transferred to fluid propane gas in a liquid nitrogen environment. After complete freezing they were broken with a scalpel. Then the specimens were retransferred to amyl acetate, dried in liquid CO_2 by the critical-point method, mounted on specimen holders, and sputtered in an argon atmosphere. They were examined with a Stereoscan 180 scanning electron microscope (Cambridge) at an acceleration voltage of 15–20 kV.

Results

The sciatic nerve of the rat and that of the chicken receives major arterial branches not only from the external sciatic artery but also from the smaller arteries of the neighboring tissues such as muscles. These nutritive vessels have a connective tissue of their own, the mesoneurium (see Smith 1966; Nobel and Black 1974). These flow into the epineural vessels.

The main epineural vessels form a lateral vascular bundle on both sides of the sciatic nerve and an interfascicular vascular bundle along the axial direction of the nerve (Fig. 1). The main arterial and venous epineural vessels are connected by transverse (Fig. 1) or diagonal anastomoses (Fig. 2). A plexuslike vascular network is formed on some main epineural vessels and several small vessels and capillaries. One artery is usually accompanied by one or two parallel veins (Fig. 2). This arrangement is discontinued when the larger muscular branches of the nerve ramify. These do not further have the arrangement of the epineural vessels as typical in the sciatic nerve (Fig. 3).

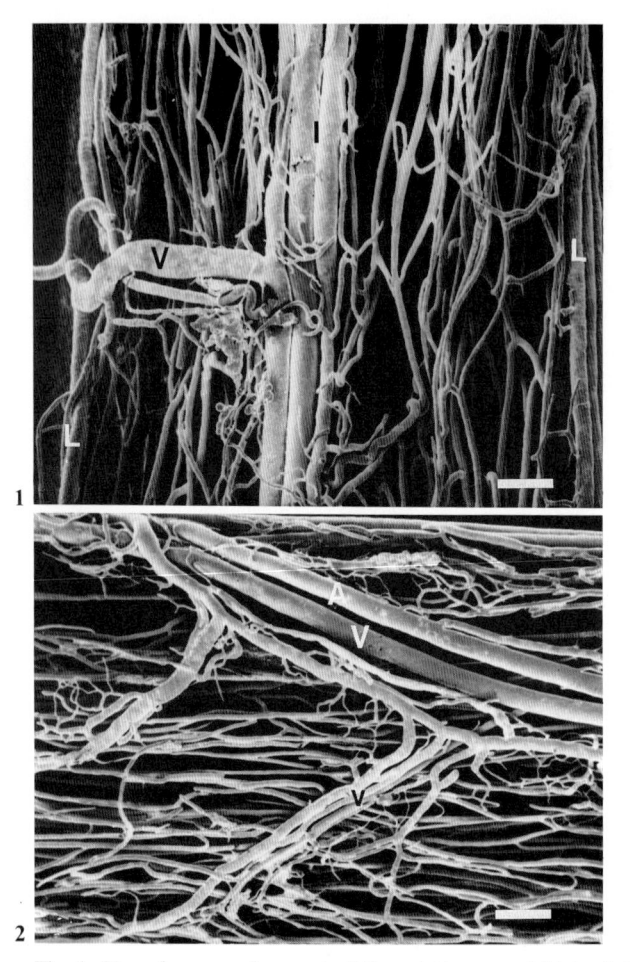

Fig. 1. Vascular corrosion cast of the sciatic nerve (chicken). Demonstration of epineural vessels. *I*, Interfascicular; *L*, main lateral epineural vessels; *V*, venous anastomoses between main vessels; *bar*, 300 μm

Fig. 2. Vascular corrosion cast of the sciatic nerve (chicken). *v*, Venous anastomosis of epineural main vessels; *A*, artery; *V*, vein; *bar*, 300 μm

Arteries and veins show a circular contractive profile probably having a regulative function (Fig. 4). The endothelia of the main arteries have an ovoid shape and are orientated in a longitudinal direction (Fig. 4, inset). The endothelia of the main veins are not ovoid but irregular.

The perineural as well as the epineural vessels are characterized by their longitudinal arrangement. However, the partly wavelike vessels have several cross-connections to one another (Fig. 5). The vascular density of this plexus seems to be more intense in the chicken than in the rat. In the border region of the peri- and epineural plexuses numerous anastomoses can be seen which are

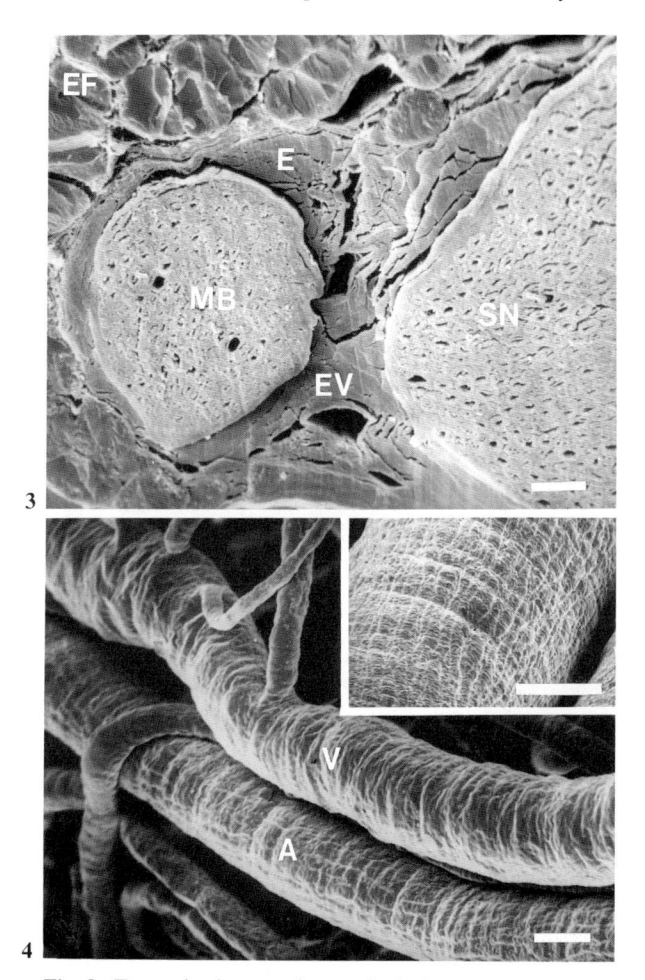

Fig. 3. Freeze-broken specimen of sciatic nerve (rat) in the region of branching muscular ramus. *E*, Epineurium; *EV*, epineural vessels; *EF*, epineural fat; *SN*, sciatic nerve; *MB*, muscular branch; *bar*, 30 μm

Fig. 4. Corrosion cast of chicken sciatic nerve. Surface structure of epineural arteries (*A*) and veins (*V*). Note the circular contraction profiles. *Bar*, 20 μm. *Inset*, longitudinally orientated endothelial cell-borders of an artery; *Bar*, 10 μm

characterized by sphincterlike constrictions (Fig. 6). In vessels running inwards and outwards from the peri- to the endoneural vessels, we detected a considerable amount of constrictions and dilatations (Fig. 7). We have observed such changes in the diameters both in arteries and in veins. Of course it was not always possible to define the border between peri- and endoneural vessels in the corrosion casts with certainty. This pertained mainly to the veins.

The vessels of the endoneural region of the fascicles also have a mainly axial arrangement. They depict a wavelike form, as do the perineural vessels (Fig. 8). There are not as many circular constrictions as in the peri- or epineural vessels.

Fig. 5. Survey of perineural vessels of the sciatic nerve (chicken). Note the side to side anastomosis (★) and the dichotomous branching (➡). *Bar*, 100 µm

Fig. 6. Shunt connection (*S*) of two arterioles between peri- and endoneural plexus with sphincterlike impressions (corrosion cast, rat). *Bar*, 30 µm

Fig. 7a, b. Long constrictions of venous vessels (➡) in the border region of peri- and endoneural plexus corrosion cast, chicken). *Bar*, 100 µm

Fig. 8. Corrosion cast of chicken sciatic nerve. Endoneural capillaries with sphincterlike constriction of lumen (➡). *Bar*, 50 µm

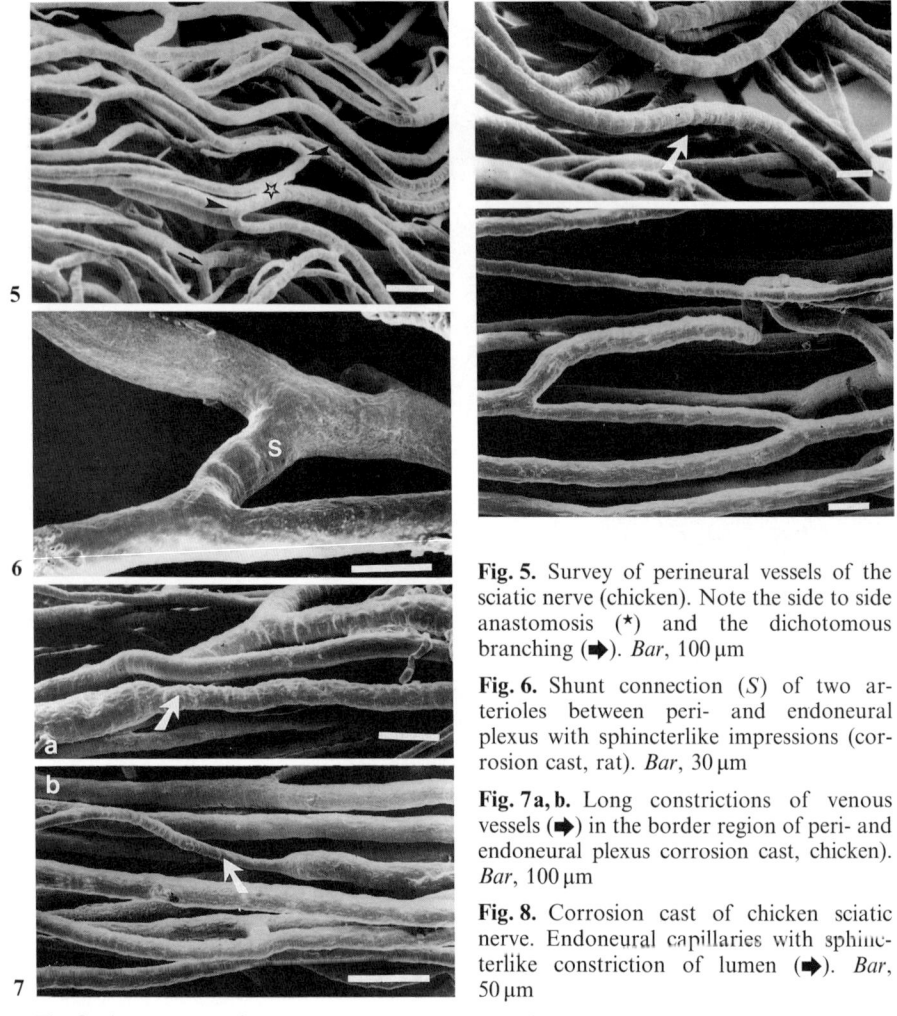

Fig. 9. Anastomoses between endoneural vessels of chicken sciatic nerve. Vascular corrosion cast. *Bar*, 50 µm

Between the vessels there are several diagonally and longitudinally orientated anastomoses (Fig. 9). In freeze-broken specimens and corrosion casts we could not find any significant differences between the densities of endoneural vessels of the rat and those of the chicken.

Discussion

There have already been a number of detailed studies on the vascularization of the peripheral nerve of animals (e.g., rabbits; Lundborg and Branemark 1968)

as well as of human beings (e.g., Lundborg 1979). These studies still provide an important model for the microcirculation of peripheral nerve. However, it is not yet possible to give a correct view of the vascularization with intravital microscopic or microangiographic methods.

Stöhr (1980), Carter et al. (1972), Eames and Lange (1967), and Raff and Asbury (1968) regarded a disturbed microcirculation as the cause for development of many neuropathies. In order to verify damaging influences such as trauma, pressure, vibration, or metabolic imbalance to the nerve or its vessels with a model it was necessary to have an in toto demonstration of the vascularization. This is possible by corrosion casting. Hiramatsu (1982) demonstrated the microvasculature of peripheral nerves in dog and human samples with this technique. In agreement with him, we substantially confirm the circulatory model established by Lundborg and Branemark (1968) and subsequently improved by Lundborg (1975).

In addition, we discovered the presence of sphincterlike structures by scanning electron microscopy in the vessels of all plexuses, although less frequently in the endoneural plexus. The circular constriction profiles are probably caused by smooth-muscle constrictions of the vascular wall probably leading to intravital changes in the diameter and blood flow. Although these constrictions are also visible in some micrographs, Hiramatsu (1982) did not comment on them. The great number of cross-communications between epi-, peri-, and endoneural vessels might explain why a short breakdown of one of these systems (e.g., as a consequence of a mobilization of a nerve) does not lead to a generalized ischemia of the whole nerve. The high vascular density might confirm Lundborg's findings (1975) that only a part of the whole endoneural plexus is perfused, and that there are vessels in reserve which are brought into play when required. It is also possible that the intense proximity of the vessels in the epineural plexus supports the stabilization of the nerve in its surroundings.

The meandering of the endoneural capillaries is probably responsible for the fact that the nerve can be distended to 115% of its length without any nutritive harm (Lundborg and Rydevik 1973). Waksman (1961) and Lang (1962) stated that mainly capillaries are to be found in the endoneural space. Together with Hiramatsu (1982), we cannot confirm this finding.

Altogether, our studies of the vascularization of the sciatic nerve showed that there are no significant differences between rats and chickens, so that experimental results in these species can be compared with one another.

References

Adams WE (1942) The blood supply of nerves. I. Historical review. J Anat 76:323–341
Blunt MJ (1959) The vascular anatomy of the median nerve in the forearm and hand. J Anat 93:15–22
Carter DC, Lee PW, Gill W, Johnston RJ (1972) The effect of cryosurgery on peripheral nerve function. J R Coll Surg (Edinb) 17:25–31
Dalton AJ (1955) A chrome-osmium fixative for electron microscopy. Anat Rec 121:281

Eames RA, Lange LS (1967) Clinical and pathological study of ischemic neuropathy. J Neurol Neurosurg Psychiat 30:215–226

Fetterman JL, Spitler DK (1940) Vascular disorders of peripheral nerves. J Am Med Assoc 114:2275–2279

Hiramatsu Y (1982) Stereoscopic observation of the microvasculature of peripheral nerves. Acta med. Okayama 36(4):263–275

Hodde KC, Nowell JA (1980) SEM of microcorrosion casts. Scanning Electron Microsc. II: 88–106

Karnovsky MJ (1965) A formaldehyde-glutaraldehyde fixative of high osmolality for use in electron microscopy. J Cell Biol 27:137a–138a

Lametschwandtner A, Lametschwandtner U, Weiger T (1984) Scanning electron microscopy of vascular corrosion casts – technique and applications. Scanning Electron Microsc II:663–695

Lang J (1962) Über das Bindegewebe und die Gefäße der Nerven. Z Anat Entw Gesch 123:61–79

Lundborg G (1975) Structure and function of the intraneural microvessels as related to trauma, edema formation, and nerve function. J Bone Joint Surg 57(A):938–948

Lundborg G (1979) The intrinsic vascularization of human peripheral nerves: structural and functional aspects. J Hand Surg 4:34–41

Lundborg G, Branemark PI (1968) Microvascular structure and function of peripheral nerves. Vital microscopic studies of the tibial nerve in the rabbit. Adv Microcir 1:66–88

Lundborg G, Rydevik B (1973) Effects of stretching the tibial nerve of the rabbit: a preliminary study of the intraneural circulation and the barrier function of the perineurium. J Bone Joint Surg 55(B):390–401

Nobel W, Black D (1974) The microcirculation of peripheral nerves: techniques for perfusion and microangiographic, macrophotographic, and photomicrographic recordings in animals. J Neurosurg 41:83–91

Raff MC, Asbury AK (1968) Ischemic mononeuropathy and mononeuropathy multiplex associated with diabetes mellitus. New Eng J Med 279:17–22

Smith JW (1966) Factors influencing nerve repair. I. Blood supply of peripheral nerves. Arch Surg 93:335–341

Stöhr M (1980) Iatrogene Nervenläsionen (iatrogenic nerve lesions). Thieme, Stuttgart New York, S 26–65

Waksman BH (1961) Experimental study of diphtheritic polyneuritis in the rabbit and guinea pig. III. The blood-nerve barrier in the rabbit. J Neuropathol Exp Neurol 20:35–77

Primate Peripheral Nerve Anastomosis with CO_3 Laser

J. E. Bailes[1], D. G. Kline[2], I. Ciric[1], A. R. Hudson[3], and J. W. Cozzens[1], Evanston[1] and New Orleans[2]/USA, Toronto[3]/Canada

Introduction

The CO_2 laser has become widely used for its ability to vaporize neoplasms of the central nervous system and in neuroablative procedures. New research in laser engineering and laboratory experimentation has led to our ability to bond tissues using CO_2 laser energy in the milliwatt range with a small and accurate delivery system. These technological improvements have been utilized in an attempt to develop a better method of anastomosing blood vessels, nerves, fallopian tubes, and vas deferens and in closing dura. We investigated the use of the milliwatt CO_2 laser for peripheral nerve repair in a higher animal model for inference of the possibility of human application of this technique.

Method and Results

Fourteen adult monkeys of mixed sexes (12 *Macaca* rhesus, 2 African green) underwent general anesthesia with ketamine and halothane. Standard exposure of the sciatic nerve complex was performed bilaterally. The peroneal nerve was isolated and a 2-cm segment was removed. The sural nerve was harvested for use as interposition grafts for interfascular placement using CO_2 laser at 70–100 mW, continuous mode, and spot size of 150 µm (Bioquantum Microsurgical Laser, Model 7600, Bioquantum Technologies, Houston, Texas, USA). The opposite limb underwent a conventional nerve repair with 9–0 nylon suture. The animals were allowed to recover without dietary or activity restraints and were sacrificed at 5, 7, 10, and 13 months postoperatively. Nerve conduction velocities and nerve action potentials were recorded preoperatively and before killing of the animals.

All animals survived the operative procedure without obvious complications. By observation, there was no apparent discrepancy in functional motor recovery in limbs with laser as compared to suture repairs. At the time of killing, there was no gross discernable morphological difference between laser-assisted and suture anastomosed nerves, nor was there any instance of dehiscence. Preliminary nerve conduction velocities and nerve action potentials appear comparable for the two methods of repair. Detailed morphometric analysis is underway, with final results pending.

Discussion

Initial work with "tissue welding" involved the performance of laser-assisted vascular anastomoses (LAVA). Both end-to-end [1] and end-to-side [2, 3] anastomoses were possible with virtually a 100% patency rate [4, 5], adequate anastomotic strength [6], and lack of significant endothelial injury [7]. LAVA could be performed in roughly one-third of the time required for suture anastomoses, leading to a shortened clamp time and, theoretically, less end-organ ischemia. However, as more experience was gained, it was noted that there was a significant rate of aneurysm formation with both CO_2 [8] and argon sources [9], believed to be secondary to thermal damage to elastic elements in the tunica medica. Until this phenomenon is resolved, the clinical use of LAVA is not recommended [10].

It followed the attempt to repair peripheral nerves with the CO_2 laser. Fischer et al. demonstrated the feasibility of such technique in rat sciatic nerves with 5-W pulsed CO_2 laser energy with a 0.6-mm spot size directed tangentically. Microscopic analysis suggested that nerves repaired with laser had less scarring and constriction at the repair sites due to a lack of a suture-induced foreign body response [11]. Almquist has reported the successful use of argon laser for primate nerve anastomoses. A qualitative assessment showed a large amount of axonal regeneration into the distal stump, minimal outgrowth of axons at the repair site, no deleterious effect of laser on underlying axonal microtubules, and minimal connective tissue proliferation [12].

Preliminary work in our laboratory involved sutureless laser-assisted nerve anastomosis (LANA) in rat sciatic nerves with both end-to-end and interposition graft repairs. Electrophysiological assessment showed no statistically significant difference in nerve conduction velocities between LANA specimens and control suture anastomoses. Morphologically, more small non-myelinated fibers, fibers with intact myelin sheaths and viable Schwann's cells were seen in distal segments of LANA as compared to sutured nerves. In this early work, tensile strength was suboptimal, as 25% of end-to-end and 12% of grafted nerves showed dehiscence [13]. It was felt that with more experience and less tension on the repair site, this limitation could be overcome. Indeed, in the present primate experiment, no instance of dehiscence was seen.

Thus, it seemed that laser irradiation of rat sciatic nerves did not present subsequent regrowth of axons across the anastomotic site, nor was electrophysiological conduction significantly altered. Previous investigators have shown, with the ruby laser, that cranial and peripheral nerves were more resistent to laser energy than the brain or spinal cord [14, 15]. Others demonstrated no detrimental effects to underlying neural structures or subsequent axonal regrowth following CO_2 laser application to rat peripheral nerves [16]. Laser beam transection of neurites in single-cell cultures has not prevented regeneration [17, 18]. Due to the superlative regenerative capacity of the rat, an analogous study in a primate model was necessary before extrapolation to the human was possible. The purpose of the work reported herein was to provide laser repair data in such a model.

The utilization of laser to bond nerves is an attractive idea for several reasons. First and foremost is the possibility of an improved healing response based on two theories. First, laser repair obviates the need for suture material with its attendant foreign body response. This intrinsic cellular reaction is also associated with an ingrowth of fibrous tissue from the surrounding area into the repair site. Secondly, it is plausible that as the laser creates a "water-tight" seal at the repair site, a locally biochemically favorable environment may be created. The ability to achieve such a seal has been shown with the use of laser for dural closure [19]. Another advantage of laser repair is that it may provide the ability to join nerves which otherwise could not be reapproximated, due either to small fascicular size or to a location of limited access or exposure. Least important is the fact that laser anastomosis can be performed in roughly one-third of the time required for suture anastomosis.

Laser nerve anastomosis has been shown to be technically feasible in rats and primates with both CO_2 and argon sources while preliminary studies have shown no detrimental effects and favorable healing. The ultimate prediction of human applicability of LANA rests on detailed morphometric analysis of nerve segments including axon fiber counts, which we expect to be forthcoming soon.

References

1. Quigley MR, Bailes JE, Kwaan HC et al. (1985) Microvascular anastomosis using the milliwatt CO_2 laser. Lasers Surg Med 5:357–365
2. Quigley MR, Bailes JE, Kwaan HC et al. (1987) Laser-assisted end-to-side anastomosis. J Reconst Microsurg 3:277–279
3. Sartorius CJ, Shapiro A, Campbell RL et al. (1986) Experimental laser-assisted end-to-side microvascular anastomoses. Microsurgery 7:79–83
4. Quigley MR, Bailes JE, Kwaan HC et al. (1985) Histologic comparison of suture versus laser-assisted vascular anastomosis. Surg Forum 36:508–510
5. Serure A, Withers EH, Thompsen S et al. (1983) Comparison of carbon dioxide laser-assisted microvascular anastomosis and conventional microvascular sutured anastomosis. Surg Forum 34:634–636
6. Quigley MR, Bailes JE, Kwaan HC et al. (1985) Comparison of bursting strength suture and laser-anastomosed vessels. Microsurgery 6:229–232
7. Bailes JE, Quigley MR, Kwaan HC et al. (1985) Fibrinolytic activity following laser-assisted vascular anastomosis. Microsurgery 6:163–168
8. Quigley MR, Bailes JE, Kwaan HC et al. (1986) Aneurysm formation after low-power carbon dioxide laser-assisted vascular anastomosis. Neurosurgery 18:292–299
9. Pribil S, Powers SK (1985) Carotid artery end-to-end anastomosis in the rat using the argon laser. J Neurosurg 63:771–775
10. Quigley MR, Bailes JE, Kwaan HC et al. (1985) Laser-assisted vascular anastomosis. Lancet 1:334
11. Fischer DW, Beggs JL, Kenshalo DL et al. (1985) Comparative study of microepineurial anastomoses with the use of CO_2 laser and suture techniques in rat sciatic nerves. Neurosurgery 17:300–308
12. Almquist EE, Nachemson A, Auth D et al. (1984) Evaluation of the use of the argon laser in repairing rat and primate nerves. J Hand Surg 9(A):792–799
13. Bailes JE, Quigley MR, Cerullo LJ et al. (1986) Sutureless CO_2 laser nerve anastomosis: histology and electrophysiologic analysis. Lasers Surg Med 6:248

14. Brown TE, True C, McLaurin RL et al. (1967) Laser irradiation. II. Long-term effects of laser radiation on certain intracranial structures. Neurology 17:789–796
15. Stellar S, Polanyi TB, Bredemeier HC (1974) Lasers in surgery. In: Wolbarsht ML (ed) Laser applications in medicine and biology, vol 12. Plenum Press, New York, pp 241–293
16. Fischer DW, Beggs JL, Shetter AG et al. (1983) Comparative study of neuroma formation in the rat sciatic nerve after CO_2 laser and scalpel neurectomy. Neurosurgery 13:287–294
17. Rieske E, Kreutzberg GW (1978) Neurite regeneration after cell surgery with laser microbeam irradiation. Brain Res 148:478–483
18. Gross GW, Lucas JH, Higgins ML (1983) Laser microbeam surgery: ultrastructural changes associated with neurite transection in culture. J Neurosci 3:1979–1983
19. Heiferman KS, Quigley MR, Cerullo LJ et al. (1986) Dural welding with CO_2 laser. Lasers Surg Med 6:248

Laser-Assisted Sciatic Nerve Anastomoses and Transplants

F. Ulrich, K. H. Reiners, and T. Sander, Düsseldorf/FRG

Introduction

In an initial study on laser-assisted microanastomoses with the 1.32-µm Nd:YAG laser, the fusion effect could be attributed to structural alterations of collagen fibers (Schober et al. 1986). Alterations of the nerve coats and subsequent tissue reactions in this region accompanying this effect also suggested a certain leader function for sprouting fibers in terms of a neuromatous neurotization. To obtain further functional information supplementary electrophysiological investigations of nerve anastomoses produced with laser assistance were performed.

Material and Methods

By means of the modified Nd:YAG laser (1.318 µm; 200 µm light conductor; MBB-Medizintechnik, Munich, FRG) end-to-end ($n = 53$) nerve anastomoses and ($n = 16$) transplants of the sciatic nerve of adult rats were performed. In order to be able to carry out the microsurgical operations with extreme precision, a micromanipulator (OPMILAS YAG, Carl Zeiss, Oberkochen, FRG) fixed on the surgical microscope was used. Whereas additional holding sutures were not necessary in the 1-cm-long nerve transplants, two additional holding threads were applied in the nerve anastomoses. Electromyographic investigations were performed 3–4 weeks after the laser-assisted anastomoses and transplants. Anastomoses and transplants carried out with conventional microsurgical suture technique were used as control groups.

Results

Two microscopically visible dehiscences could be detected in the 69 laser-assisted nerve fusions performed. The time course of regeneration of the sciatic nerve was investigated neurographically in the group which had received a nerve anastomosis by suture and a group treated with the laser-assisted anastomosis technique with regard to the following parameters: (a) time of the first occurrence of a reinnervation potential in the small muscles of the foot determined by stimulation of the sciatic nerve proximal to the anastomosis site;

(b) time course and quality of regeneration determined on the basis of the time interval from anastomosis until occurrence of a reinnervation potential of 50 µV or 700 µV as well as the latency to the target muscles on day 70 after the operation.

A typical regeneration course is shown in Fig. 1 for an animal of the group of laser-assisted anastomoses. It is seen that the potential amplitude gradually increases again after the first occurrence of a very low and polyphasic reinnervation potential on day 35, and that the latency to the target muscle is simultaneously shortened in accordance with the progress of myelination. The

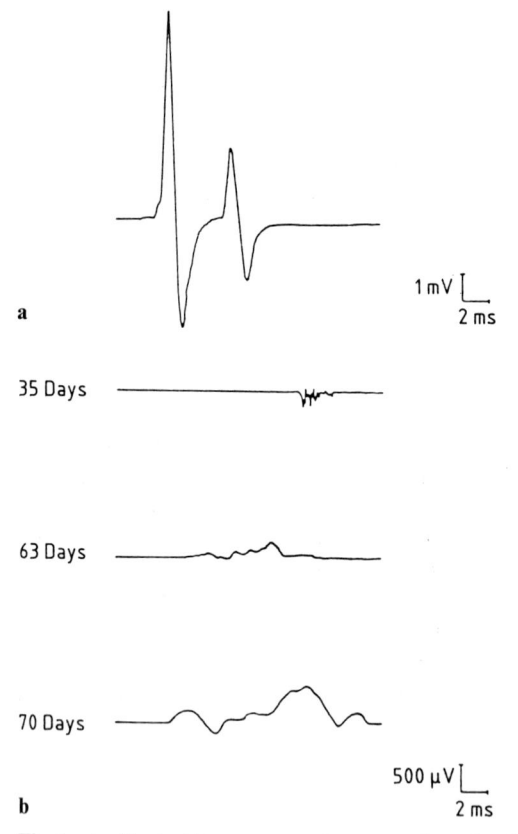

Fig. 1 a, b. Typical time course of regeneration after laser-assisted anastomosis of the sciatic nerve of the rat. The compound muscle action potential of the small foot muscles after proximal stimulation of the nerve is shown. **a** The potential before severance and reanastomosis of the nerve. Besides the M response, the F wave is also typically obtainable. **b** The reinnervation potentials are shown after the respective time interval given after the operation. The first reinnervation potential was obtained after 35 days in this case. It has a very low amplitude and has an appreciably prolonged latency in accordance with the still small degree of myelination. In the further course, the potential amplitude increases, and the latency is shortened at the same time in the course of progress of myelination. On day 70 after the operation, the amplitude of the potential is only about one-tenth of the original value, but the latency is only about twice as long as before the nerve division

results of the interval comparison up to attainment of the above amplitudes are shown in Figs. 2 and 3 with a comparison between the suture and laser anastomosis groups. The differences in the course of regeneration are not significant between the two groups, but a trend to earlier attainment of a higher potential (700 µV) was shown in the group with laser-assisted anastomosis with a rather earlier occurrence on average of a reinnervation potential of 50 µV amplitude in the sutured group.

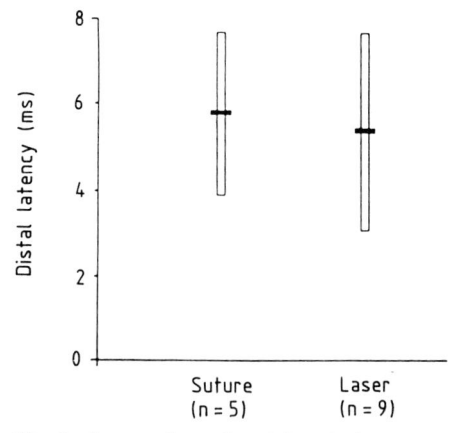

Fig. 2. Average latencies of the sciatic nerve to the small foot muscles ($\pm$ standard deviation) of the groups with sutured or laser-assisted anastomosis on day 70 after the operation. There is no difference between the two groups with regard to the shortening of the latencies

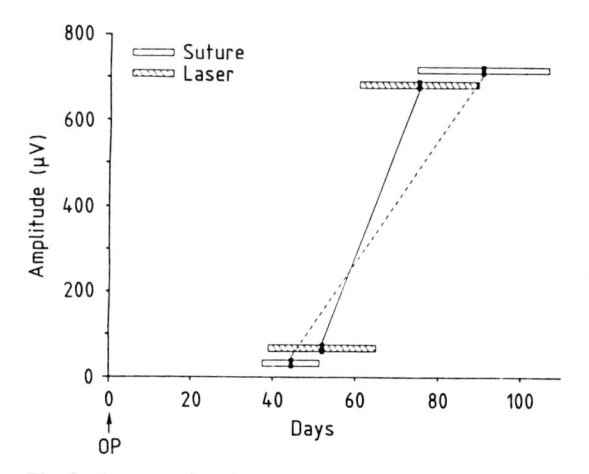

Fig. 3. Average time interval in days ($\pm$ standard deviation) (*abscissa*) until attainment of potential amplitudes of a reinnervation potential of 50 µV or 700 µV for the groups with suture and laser-assisted anastomosis. The time differences are not significant for the two potential amplitudes. In the group with laser-assisted anastomosis, however, there is a trend to slight delay (on average 8 days) up to attaining an amplitude of 50 µV, but the further regeneration course tends to be accelerated, so that the higher amplitude of 700 µV is reached on average 15 days earlier than in the group with suture

The evaluation of the corresponding findings in the animals with nerve transplants has not yet been completed. Therefore histological results including a synoptic discussion will be presented separately.

References

1. Beggs JL, Fischer DW, Shetter AG (1986) Comparative study of rat sciatic nerve microepineurial anastomoses made with carbon dioxide laser and suture techniques. II. A morphometric analysis of myelinated nerve fibers. Neurosurgery 18:266–269
2. Schober R, Ulrich F, Sander T, Dürselen H, Hessel S (1986) Laser-induced alteration of collagen substructure allows microsurgical tissue welding. Science 232:1421–1422
3. Ulrich F, Bock WJ (1986) Laser assisted repair of small blood vessels with the 1.3 µm Nd:YAG laser. In: Waidelich W, Kiefhaber P (eds) Laser/Optoelektronik in der Medizin. Springer, Berlin Heidelberg New York Tokyo, pp 418–423

Some Ultrastructural Aspects of Regeneration in 1.32 µm Nd:YAG Laser-Assisted Peripheral Nerve Transplantation*

R. Schober, F. Ulrich, and T. Sander, Düsseldorf/FRG

Introduction

Various types of lasers have already been tested as a substitute for sutures in microsurgical peripheral nerve anastomoses (Almquist et al. 1984; Fischer et al. 1985; Ulrich et al. 1986). In a histological evaluation of experiments using this technique, the 1.32 µm Nd:YAG laser has been found to be suitable but not appreciably superior to epineurial suture alone (Schober et al. 1988). It was advocated to use the 1.32 µm Nd:YAG laser with its inherent property of precise coagulation in peripheral nerve transplantation, a procedure where so far laser application has been restricted to the milliwatt CO_2 laser (Richmond 1986). In this report we give an account of some ultrastructural features pertinent to the outcome of regeneration in such an experimental design. A final evaluation must await the conclusion of a larger experimental series, technical details of which are described in another contribution to this volume (Ulrich et al.).

Material and Methods

This study was based on four autologous rat sciatic nerve transplants using the 1.32 µm Nd:YAG laser with or without two additional stay sutures at each intersection. After epineurial adaptation, several welding points were applied with a laser adjustment of 12.5 W power output, 0.2 mm spot diameter, and 0.1 s duration of exposure, corresponding to an energy density of 3400 J/cm^2. One animal was killed immediately, the others after 1, 2, or 3 weeks. The nerves were carefully dissected by aid of an operating microscope and fixed by immersion in 2.5% glutaraldehyde buffered to pH 7.4 with 0.1 M sodium cacodylate. The tissue was processed according to standard procedures, including postfixation with 1% osmium tetroxide and embedding in Spurr's epoxy resin. Each nerve was divided into five blocks, securing transverse sections of the proximal and distal stumps and the graft, and longitudinal sections of the proximal and distal anastomosis. Sections 1 µm thick for light

---

* This research was supported by the Ministerium für Wissenschaft und Forschung des Landes Nordrhein-Westfalen, FRG.

microscopy were stained with toluidine blue. Thin sections were stained with uranyl acetate and Reynold's lead citrate and examined in a Zeiss 1a electron microscope.

Results

The effects of laser application at the proximal and distal site of anastomosis were well marked by strong bulging of the coagulated epineurial collagen and by a slight superficial brownish discoloration (Fig. 1). The contours of chronic preparations were generally smooth except for some lateral adhesions and for an occasional focal narrowing due to a slight dehiscence of endoneural contents (Fig. 2).

Microscopic examination revealed the changes of Wallerian degeneration and of vigorous regeneration. Axon sprouts with incipient myelination were present in well-formed bands of Büngner in the transplant and in the distal segment by weeks 2 and 3. They were also present in the coagulated epineurial collagen overlying and connecting the nerve stumps (Fig. 3). This was first invaded both by cells showing fine structural characteristics of fibroblasts and by cells with larger, more lightly stained nuclei often in mitosis and with copious amounts of cytoplasm. Capillary sprouting then preceded or was concomitant with the ingrowth of nerve fibers. The old perineurium progressively dissolved, and cells derived from the granulation tissue in the periphery of the nerve flattened up to form a layer resembling a new nerve sheath. The interposed coagulated epineurial collagen, in places as broad as the endoneurium, was subdivided by mesenchymal cells with elongated processes lying roughly parallel to each other and concentric to the nerve (Fig. 4). Sprouting nerve fibers, on the other hand, were mostly oriented longitudinally and parallel to the nerve. The formation of miniature fascicles was well visualized in the homogeneous and at first largely acellular coagulated collagen. In electron micrographs of week 2, isolated axons or axonal growth cones were not detected. Instead, they were in close contact with or were invested by large cell processes most likely representing Schwann cells, although a basal lamina was not clearly present (Fig. 5). Other cells or cell processes without basal lamina surrounded these axon – Schwann cell complexes in a manner suggestive of immature perineurium. By week 3, the differentiation was advanced enough for a clear recognition of miniature fascicles. Axon–Schwann cell complexes showed incipient myelination and were surrounded by a continuous basal lamina. The sheath of Henle consisted of one or several flattened cell layers with points of contact, clearly identifiable as perineurial in nature although a continuous basal lamina or pinocytotic vesicles were not present (Fig. 6). In areas close to the proximal anastomosis where the perineurium was largely dissolved, the old confinements of the fascicle could be barely recognized due to the merging of a dense population of miniature fascicles with the regeneration groups separated in endoneural compartments.

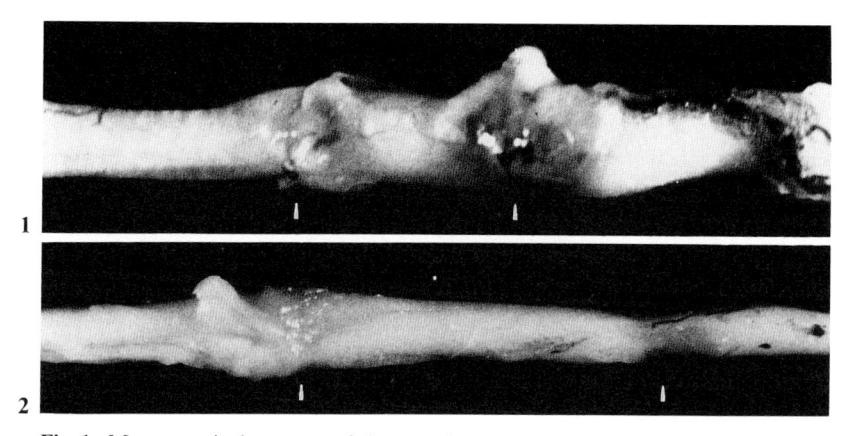

Some Ultrastructural Aspects of Regeneration 171

Fig. 1. Macroscopical aspect of laser-assisted rat sciatic nerve transplantation, acute preparation. *Arrows*, sites of anastomosis

Fig. 2. Similar preparation to that in Fig. 1, 7 days survival; slightly smaller magnification

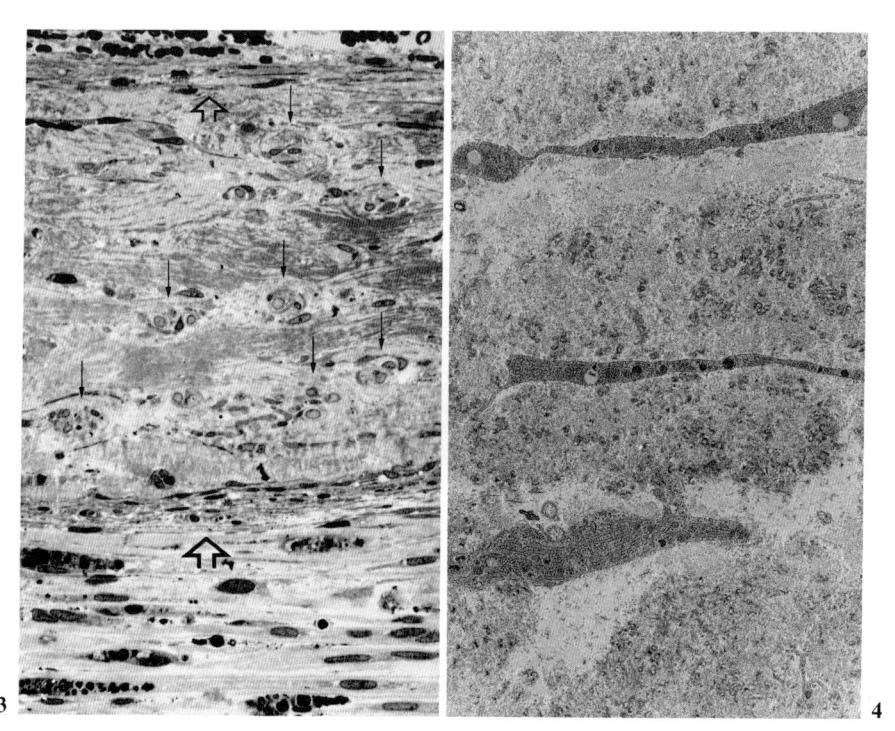

Fig. 3. Distal end of the graft, 2 weeks survival. The broadly widened epineurium is demarcated by the perineurium (*large open arrow*) and at the outer circumference by a newly formed lamellar sheath (*small open arrow*). The coagulated collagen is pierced by aberrant nerve fibers with early fasciculation (*arrows*). (Oblique section, toluidine blue; ×340)

Fig. 4. Lamellar arrangement of cell processes in a transverse section of the coagulated epineurium of the graft; 2 weeks survival. (×3500)

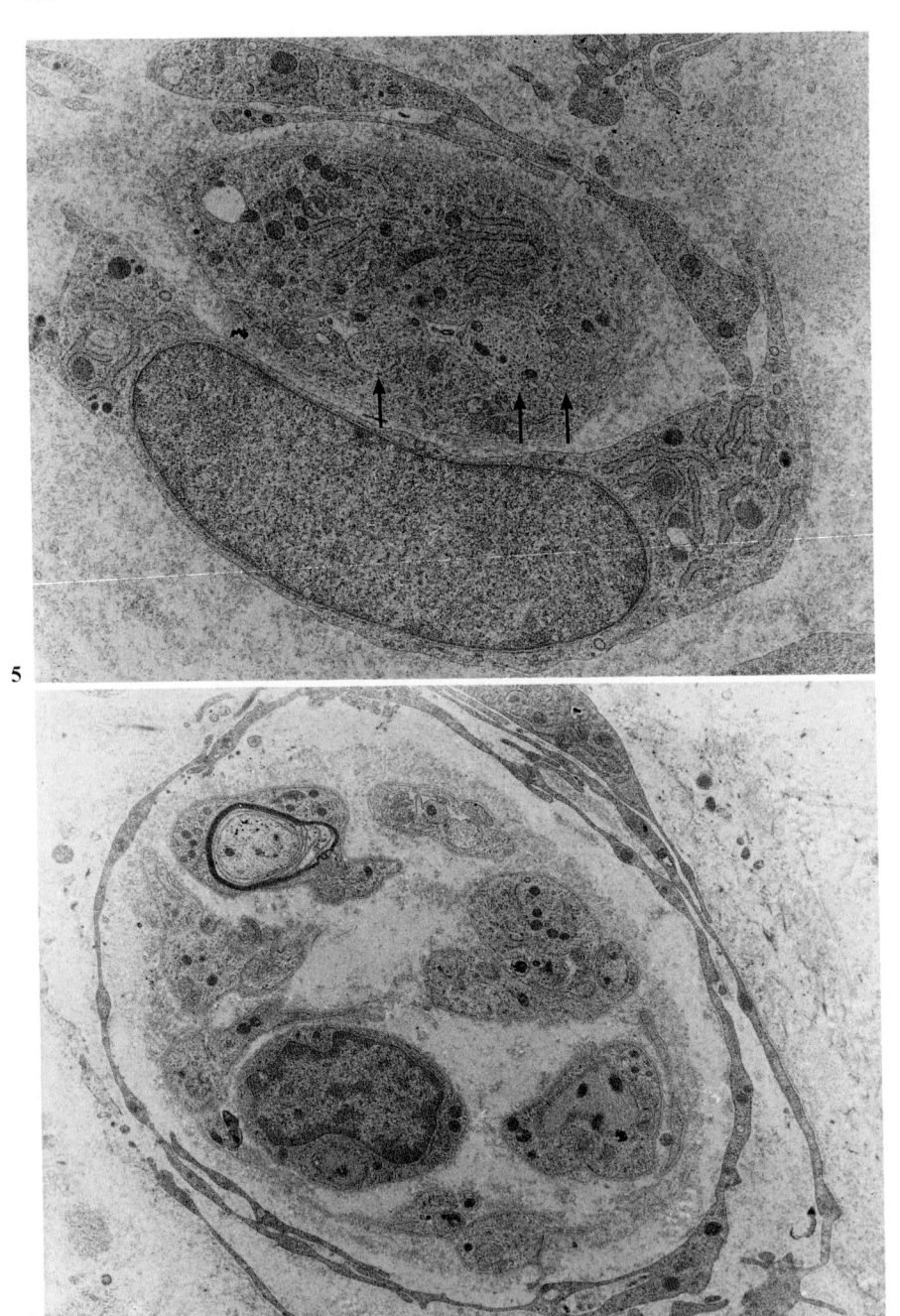

Fig. 5. Incipient fasciculation of immature cells and cell processes including axons (*arrows*) within the coagulated graft epineurium; 2 weeks survival. (×9300)

Fig. 6. Later stage showing a clearly outlined miniature fascicle; 3 weeks survival. (×7500)

Discussion

The interest in these experiments does not lie in the evaluation of laser-assisted nerve transplantation but rather in the advantages that this model offers for the study of peripheral nerve regeneration. The eventual outcome of nerve repair after laser application will have to be assessed in a controlled long-term study using physiological and quantitative histological methods such as has already been done in laser-assisted nerve anastomoses (Beggs et al. 1986). It will be strongly dependent on details of microsurgical manipulation, and even under identical conditions a large variation in the degree of regeneration can be expected (Hudson et al. 1979). Potential benefits of the use of the 1.32 µm Nd:YAG laser, consisting of a reduction of suture granulomas and possibly of an additional "neuromatous neurotization" of the graft, have already been documented (Schober et al. 1986).

The exposure to Nd:YAG laser irradiation at the energy densities applied appears not to be detrimental to axonal regeneration or myelination and afflicts principally the sheath structures of the nerve. It is the usual course of Wallerian degeneration and regeneration that the latter undergo an extensive remodeling with "compartmentation", and in the early stages of this process it is impossible on fine structural grounds to discriminate between endoneural fibroblasts, perineurial cells, and possibly also Schwann cells (Thomas and Jones 1967; Morris et al. 1972). Corresponding changes, even in the absence of outgrowing axons, have also been described in nerve grafts (Ahmed and Weller 1979; Jenq and Coggeshall 1986), and the associated problems of histogenetic derivation are also apparent from the results of the present study. Their solution certainly requires more sophisticated methods, an example of which is found in the recent immunohistochemical detection of Schwann cells preceding the ingrowth of axons during muscle development (Noakes and Bennett 1987).

In posttraumatic peripheral nerve regeneration, a growth-supporting influence of Schwann cells has long been suggested from observations of their initial swarming out and their progressive transformation with neurotization. At the same time, the experimental advantages of an acellular matrix, as realized, for example, with an agar-filled tube, have been pointed out (Edinger 1918). Since the coagulated collagen in Nd:YAG laser-assisted transplantation provides a largely acellular natural matrix at the sites of anastomosis without introduction of other artificial devices, this model appears to be particularly suitable for such investigations.

References

1. Ahmed AM, Weller RO (1979) The blood-nerve barrier and reconstitution of the perineurium following nerve grafting. Neuropathol Appl Neurobiol 5:469–483
2. Almquist EE, Nachemson A, Auth D, Almquist B, Hall S (1984) Evaluation of the use of the argon laser in repairing rat and primate nerves. J Hand Surg (Am) 9:792–799
3. Beggs JL, Fischer DW, Shetter AG (1986) Comparative study of rat sciatic nerve microepineurial anastomoses made with carbon dioxide laser and suture techniques. II. A morphometric analysis of myelinated nerve fibers. Neurosurgery 18:266–269
4. Edinger L (1918) Untersuchungen über die Neubildung des durchtrennten Nerven. Dtsch Zeitschr Nervenheilk 58:1–32
5. Fischer DW, Beggs JL, Kenshalo DL Jr, Shetter AG (1985) Comparative study of microepineurial anastomoses with the use of CO_2 laser and suture techniques in rat sciatic nerves. I. Surgical technique, nerve action potentials, and morphologic studies. Neurosurgery 17:300–308
6. Hudson AR, Hunter D, Kline DG, Bratton BR (1979) Histological studies of experimental interfascicular graft repairs. J Neurosurg 51:333–340
7. Jenq CB, Coggeshall RE (1986) The effects of an autologous transplant on patterns of regeneration in rat sciatic nerve. Brain Research 364:45–56
8. Morris JH, Hudson AR, Weddell G (1972) A study of degeneration and regeneration in the divided rat sciatic nerve based on electron microscopy. IV. Changes in fascicular microtopography, perineurium and endoneural fibroblasts. Z Zellforsch 124:165–203
9. Noakes PG, Bennett MR (1987) Growth of axons into developing muscles of chick forelimb is preceded by cells that stain with Schwann cell antibodies. J Comp Neurol 259:330–347
10. Richmond IL (1986) The use of lasers in nerve repair. In: Fasano AV (ed) Advanced intraoperative technologies in neurosurgery. Springer, Wien New York, pp 175–183
11. Schober R, Ulrich F, Sander T, Dürselen H, Hessel S (1986) Laser-induced alteration of collagen substructure allows microsurgical tissue welding. Science 232:1421–1422
12. Schober R, Ulrich F, Sander Th (1988) A histological evaluation of experimental nerve anastomoses with the 1.32 µm Nd:YAG-laser. Adv Neurosurg 16:31–35
13. Thomas PK, Jones DG (1967) The cellular response to nerve injury. II. Regeneration of the perineurium after nerve section. J Anat 101:45–55
14. Ulrich F, Sander T, Bock WJ (1986) Anastomosis of the sciatic nerve of the rat with the modified Nd:YAG laser. A preliminary report. In: Waidelich W, Kiefhaber P (eds) Laser/Optoelektronik in der Medizin. Springer, Berlin Heidelberg New York Tokyo, pp 414–417

Experimental Peripheral Nerve Crush Lesion
I. Posttraumatic Metabolic Responses of Spinal Motoneurons Over Time

A. C. NACIMIENTO and C. MARX, Homburg (Saar)/FRG

Introduction

The present study is part of a systematic examination of changes ensuing in spinal motor unit components (motoneuron, axon, muscle fibers) following peripheral nerve lesions requiring repair. Our main objective is to set up an experimental base-line for a quantitative evaluation of therapeutic strategies aimed at mobilizing and enhancing the potential for regeneration of the injured motor unit, such as investigating the effectiveness of neurotrophic factors or assessing various approaches to microreconstruction of injured nerves [4, 9, 11, 12, 14, 23, 24, 27, 29, 30, 31, 33, 35, 45].

Assessment of the responses of the cell body to axonal lesions [2, 3, 15, 16, 47, 50, 51] is of paramount importance in estimating and predicting the potential for regeneration following peripheral nerve injury [8, 9, 10, 14, 24, 42]. Various therapeutic strategies, including the timing of microsurgical nerve repair, have been discussed in terms of patterns of metabolic changes in the affected motoneurons [8, 9, 10, 14, 24, 33, 38, 43, 45]. Metabolic responses to axonal injury have been studied in a variety of neurons [2, 3, 6, 19, 20, 36, 40, 46, 47]. However, there is a wide range of variability in the reported results, probably because of the broad spectrum of experimental designs used. This must be taken into account when evaluating results [6].

In the present work we evaluated the metabolic responses of single spinal motoneurons after crushing and partial excision of the sciatic nerve in rats. This experimental design was chosen because (a) these lesions represent the experimental counterpart of those focal traumatic nerve injuries showing the highest (crushing injuries) and the lowest (cutting injuries) degrees of clinical recovery [37, 38, 41, 42, 43], (b) the sharp clinical and histopathological distinctions between them are widely used in the classification of nerve injuries [37, 38, 41, 43], and (c) attempts at explaining the differences observed in the spinal motoneuron after these two types of lesion may help in the recognition of the factors underlying some of the poor clinical results observed following posttraumatic nerve reconstruction.

Applying histochemical and computer-assisted cytophotometric methods, we measured posttraumatic changes in activity of four enzymes used as metabolic markers: glucose 6-phosphate dehydrogenase (G6PDH) and 6-phosphogluconate dehydrogenase (6PGDH), key enzymes in the pentose phosphate pathway, a metabolic system located in the cytosol which generates

NADPH and pentoses needed for the biosynthesis of nucleotides [5, 13, 17, 20, 22], cytochrome oxidase (CO) [53, 54, 55, 56, 57] as indicator of levels of oxidative capacity, and acetylcholinesterase (AChE) to monitor neurotransmitter metabolism [2, 3, 36, 40, 46, 47]. A preliminary report has been published [28].

Material and Methods

Animal Preparation. The experiments were performed in 50 adult Sprague-Dawley male rats with 250–300 g body weight. Sciatic nerve lesions made on the right side under pentobarbital anesthesia (i.p. 65 mg/k) were standardized as follows. In 22 animals, the nerve was crushed at a point 1 cm distal to its emergence from the gluteal musculature. With appropriate tweezers and under operation microscope control, a nerve stretch 2 mm long was crushed for 60 s. Histological sections confirmed completeness of the crush lesion. For transec-

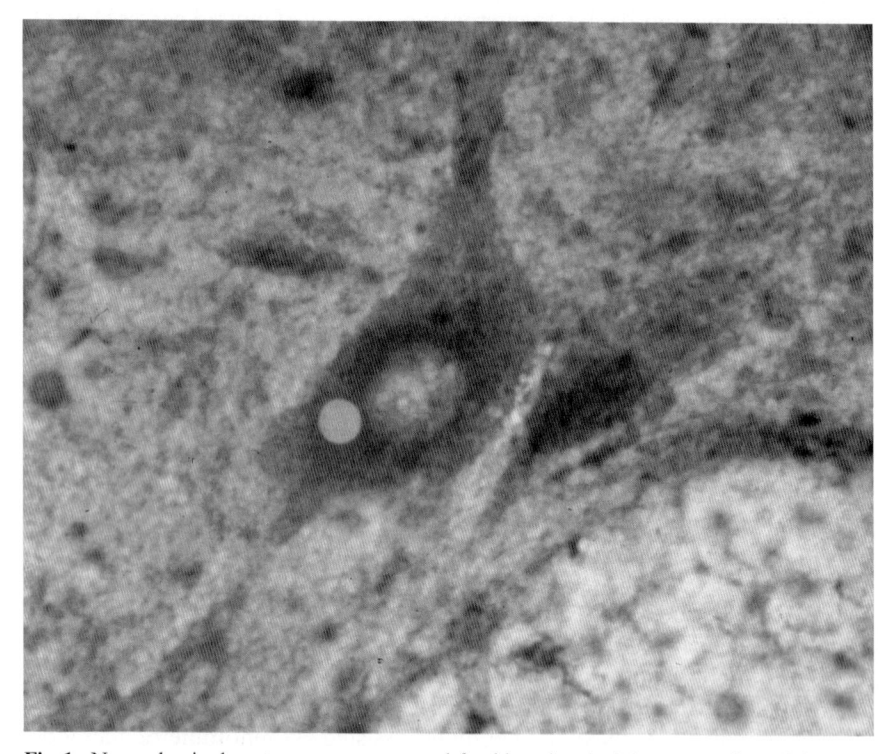

Fig. 1. Normal spinal motoneuron, processed for histochemical demonstration of G6PDH activity and measurement of its intensity by quantitative cytophotometry. Extinction reactions of the reaction product were made at cytoplasma spots such as the one illustrated here, with a measuring aperture diameter of 2.5 µm. Only motoneurons with an exactly delineated nucleus were measured

tion, in 23 animals a nerve segment about 3 cm long was exposed and transected at the same point chosen for crushing. The proximal stump was ligated, and a length of nerve about 2 cm long distal to the cut was excised. Sham operations were carried out on the contralateral side. In five intact animals control measurements were performed under identical experimental conditions except for injury. At 3 days, and 1, 2, 4, 6, and 8 weeks following injury the animals were reanesthetized as before, the spinal cord exposed, and a length quickly excised between segments T10 and S2 and immediately frozen in hexane at $-65\,°C$.

Histochemistry and Cytophotometry. Sections from spinal cord segments L3 and L4 were cut serially at 20 μm with a cryostat and processed for histochemical demonstration in the cytoplasm of single motoneurons in Rexed's lamina IX of the reaction products of G6PDH 6PGDH [20], CO [53], and AChE [25]. In pilot experiments incubation times were optimized for each enzyme. Cytophotometry was carried out with a Leitz MPV microphotometric unit coupled to a computer system. At least 20 spinal motoneurons were investigated at random on each side, in sections 80–100 μm apart. Measurements were made only in motoneurons showing sharply and exactly delineated nuclei. Cytophotometric extinction readings were taken at five randomized cytoplasm spots with a measuring aperture diameter of 2.5 μm (Fig. 1). Extinction measurements were fed into the computer system for conversion into absorbance values, calculation of mean values for each side, and statistical analysis. Results are expressed as ratios of mean absorbance values of operated to control sides.

Changes in absorbance ratios over time following both types of injury were analyzed statistically by means of the Wilcoxon non-parametric ranking test.

Results

Pentose Phosphate Pathway Enzymes. Absorbance ratios in intact animals had a range of 0.98–1.04 for G6PDH (Fig. 2) and 0.95–1.05 for 6PGDH (Fig. 3). Following both crush and transection injuries, there was an acute and significant increase in activity of both enzymes already measurable 3 days postinjury. Afterwards there were differences between time patterns. After crush, increases showed a biphasic trend until the 4th (G6PDH) and the 6th (6PGDH) week, with a transient stabilization at 2 weeks. Following transection, elevation in enzyme activity peaked at the 2nd week, whereas a differential tendency set in after the 4th week, when G6PDH reactivity was already markedly reduced, and that of 6PGDH reactivity was still significantly high. In the crush group, there was a gradual return to control levels between the 6th and 8th week, while in the transection group significant decreases were found at 6 and very low levels at 8 weeks postinjury. In general, there was a tendency for 6PGDH reactivity to be more stimulated by crush than by transection

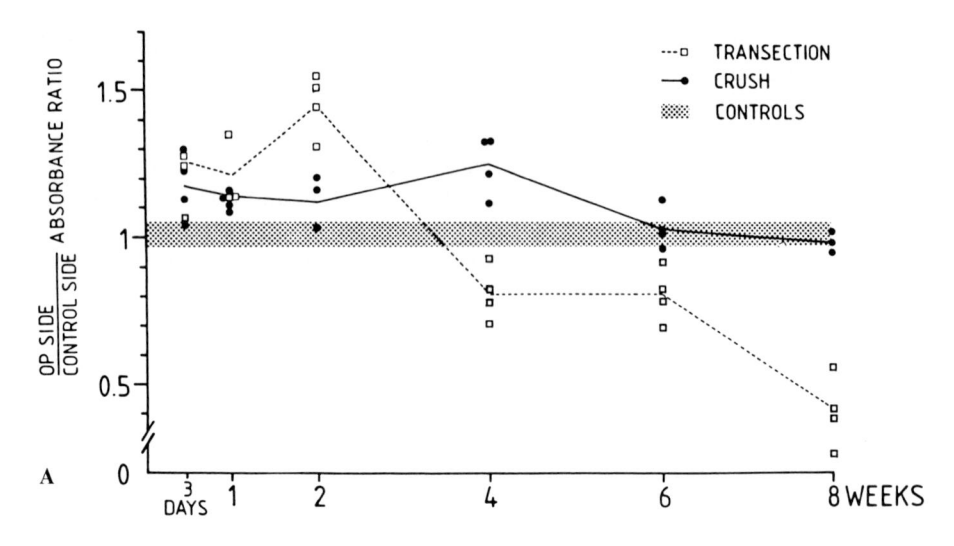

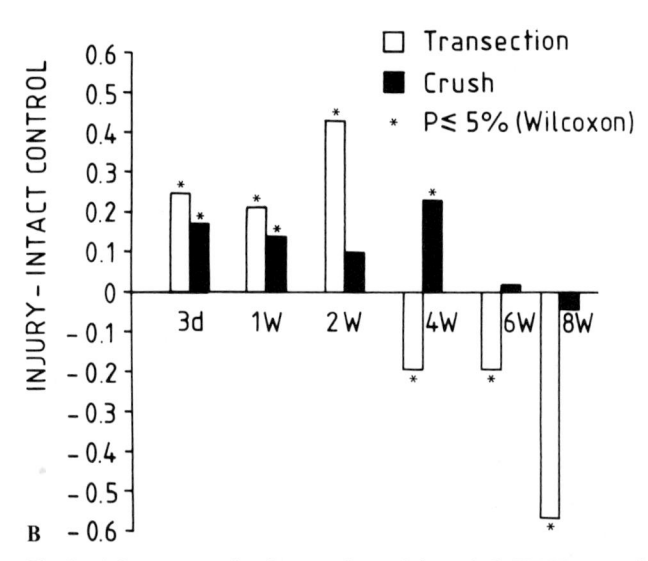

Fig. 2. A Posttraumatic changes in activity of G6PDH over time after either crush or transection injury. In this, and in the following similar subsequent curves, each data point represents the ratio of mean absorbances of enzyme reaction product in the operated side to mean absorbance in the control side in one animal, measured cytophotometrically, as shown in Fig. 1, at five cytoplasm spots in each of at least 20 single spinal motoneurons on each side. *Shaded belt*, range of absorbance ratios obtained in this manner in five intact control animals **B** Mean changes in G6PDH reactivity relative to those measured in intact control animals. In this, and in similar subsequent graphs, the height of each column represents the mean value of all data points for each posttraumatic time. Relative changes where obtained by subtracting each of these means from the mean absorbance ratio in intact control animals, taken as 1. Increases in reactivity result in positive, decreases in negative values. Statistical differences between data points in injured and in intact control animals were evaluated by the Wilcoxon non-parametric ranking test

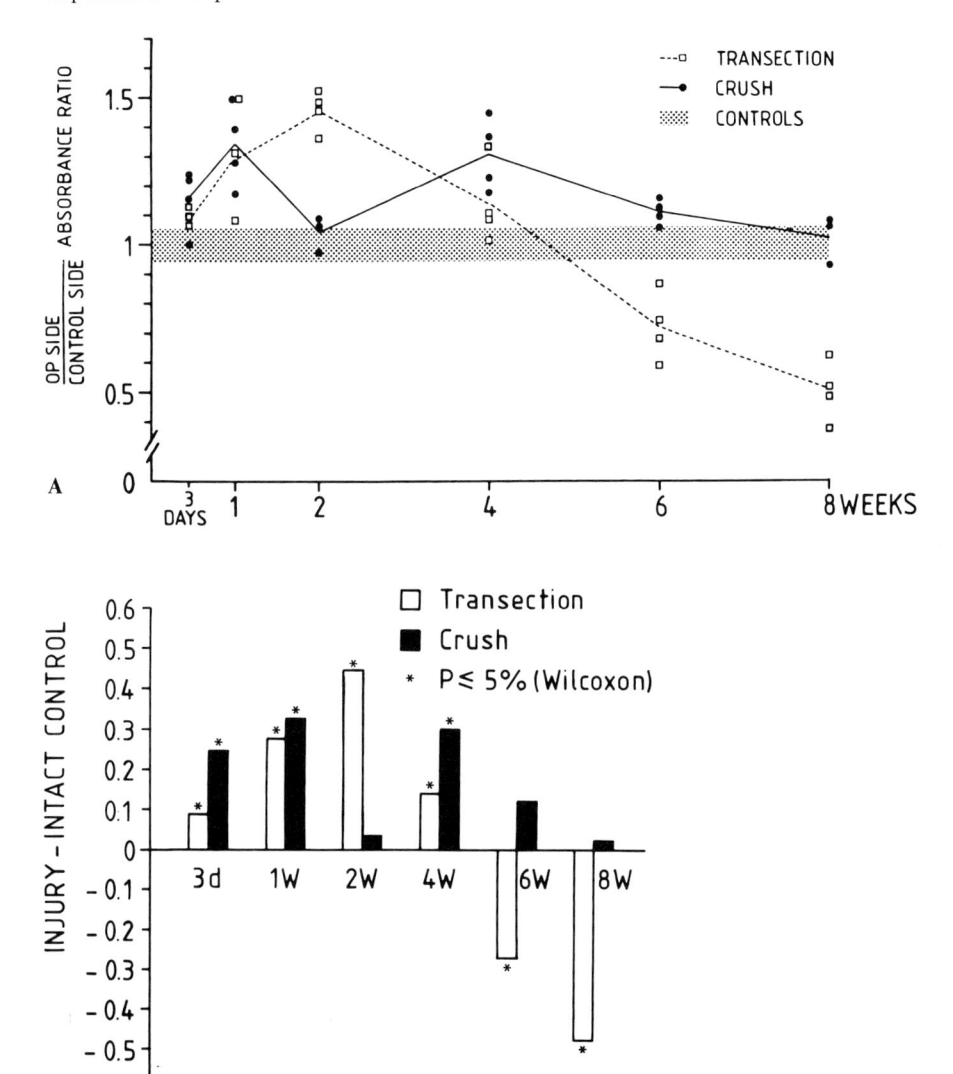

Fig. 3. A Posttraumatic changes in activity of 6PGDH as a function of time after crush or transection injury. Details as in Fig. 2A. **B** Mean changes in 6PGDH reactivity relative to those measured in intact control animals. Detail as in Fig. 2B

injury. Net mean magnitude, temporal course, and statistical significance of these changes relative to those obtained in intact control animals are presented in Figs. 2B and 3B.

Cytochrome Oxidase. Ratios in unoperated animals varied between 0.98 and 1.08 (Fig. 4). In the early phase, activity of this enzyme underwent a significant reduction at 3 days postinjury after both kinds of lesions. There followed an activity overshoot at the 1st week which was shared by both injury types but reached significant levels only after transection. Following a common return to control values at the 2nd week a progressive decrement began at the 4th week after both lesions. Following crush it settled at moderate but significantly subnormal levels at the 6th and 8th week. After transection, reduction was already much stronger at the 4th week, reaching its lowest levels at the 8th week. Final balance of these changes is shown in Fig. 4B.

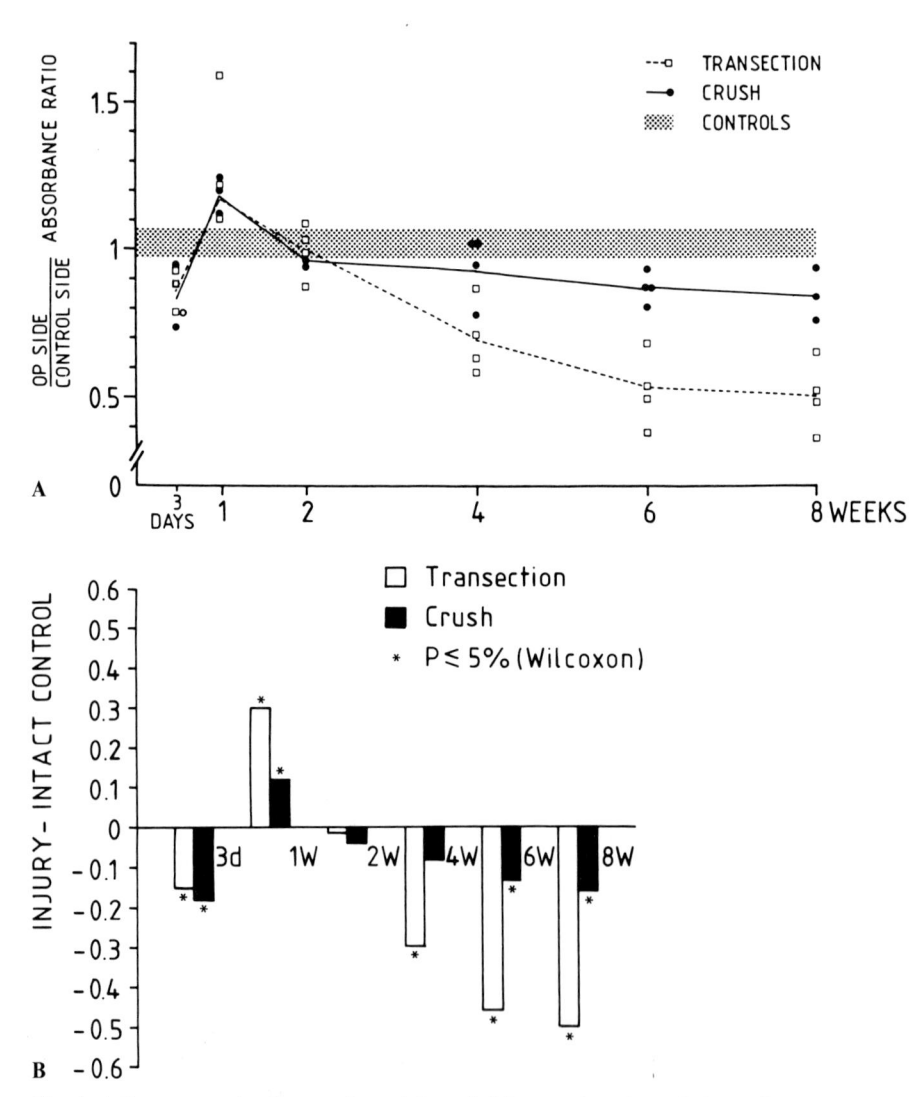

Fig. 4. A Posttraumatic changes in activity of CO as a function of time after crush or transection injury. Details as in Fig. 2A. **B** Mean changes in CO reactivity relative to those measured in intact control animals. Details as in Fig. 2B

Acetylcholinesterase. In the control groups ratios ranged from 0.93 to 1.09 (Fig. 5). Following both crush and transection, enzyme activity decreased non-significantly in the acute, 3 days to 1 week postinjury phase. There was a return to the base line at the 2nd week. Thereafter, enzyme activity decreased again after both lesions but at different rates and levels. Following crush decrease was moderate and not significant, whereas after transection activity reduction became progressively stronger, reaching significantly low levels at the 8th week. The corresponding net changes are shown in Fig. 5B.

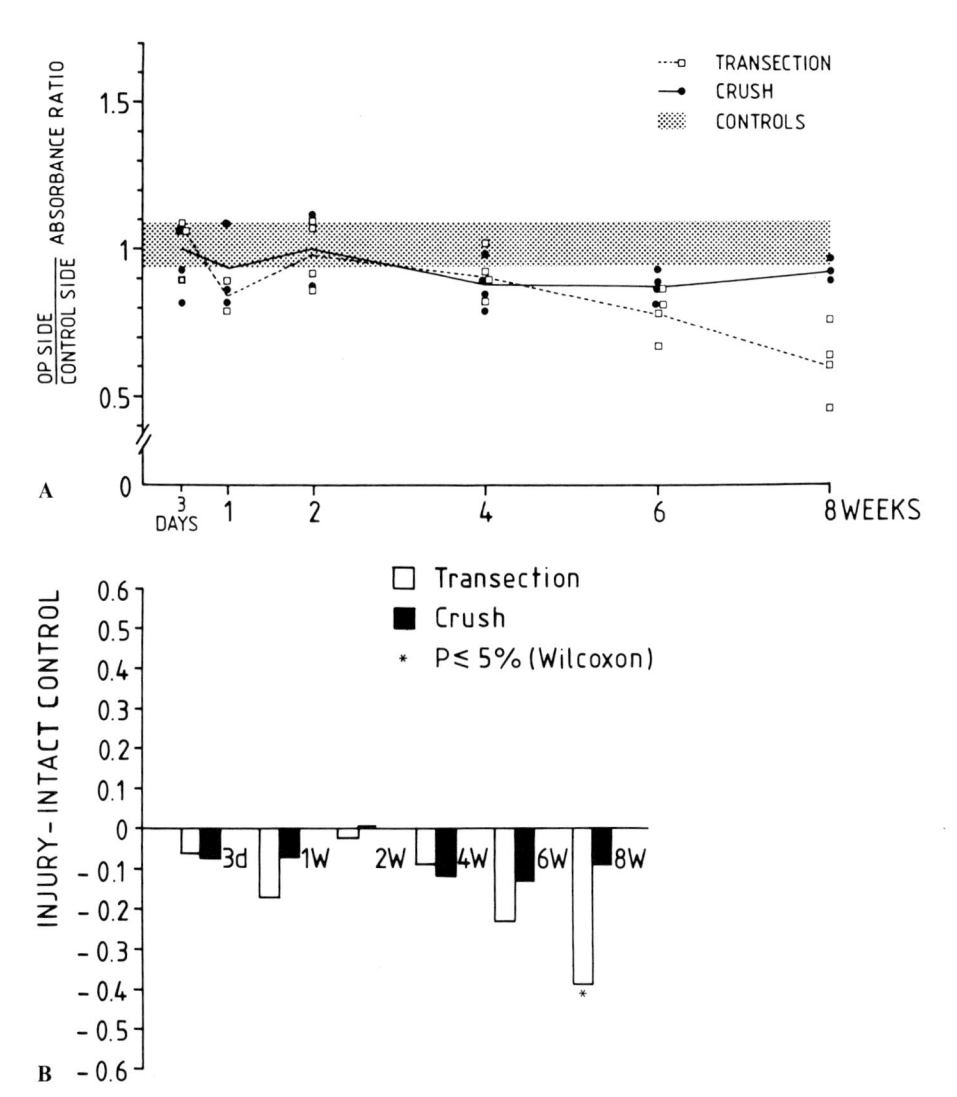

Fig. 5. A Posttraumatic changes in activity of AChE as a function of time after crush or transection injury. Details as in Fig. 2A. **B** Mean changes in AChE reactivity relative to those measured in intact control animals. Details as in Fig. 2B

Discussion

Pentose Phosphate Pathway Enzymes. The posttraumatic increase in G6PDH and 6PGDH activities reported here is in agreement with many previous observations [2, 3, 20, 26, 39, 40, 46]. However, direct quantitative comparison in spinal motoneurons of magnitude and time course of this metabolic response to standardized types of injury, has not been reported before. This analysis demonstrates clear differences between lesions. At 2 weeks reactivity was peaking for both enzymes, while following crush there was a tendency to return to the base-line. At 4 weeks, however, reactivity after crush increased again, whereas following transection a reduction set in which was particularly marked for G6PDH. Thereafter, in contrast to a fluctuation within control levels after crush, the deleterious effects of transection progressed steadily until the end of the observations.

Under normal conditions, only a very small proportion of glucose metabolism in the adult mammalian brain is processed through the pentose phosphate pathway or hexose monophosphate shunt [22], a multifunctional system the main function of which is to synthetize NADPH to convert hexoses into pentoses, particularly ribose 5-phosphate. The contribution of the shunt is larger following short-term electrical stimulation [13], in the inmature brain [17], and in predominantly myelinated tracts [5] where there is a need for lipid synthesis, which depends on the NADHP produced by this pathway. The activation of the shunt produced by axonal injury probably subserves mainly the biosynthesis of nucleotides [51].

Our results suggest that this metabolic shift may contribute to sustaining axonal regeneration during the initial 4 weeks after both types of injury. At this time, however, crucial differences appear. The downward trend after transection probably reflects the experimentally programmed failure of axons to establish functional contact with muscle. In contrast, the second increase in reactivity following crush may be associated with functional reconnection. In fact, in experiments reported in a companion paper (Adler and Nacimiento, this volume) we observed good recovery of size of extensor digitorum longus muscle fibers following crush lesion of the peroneal nerve at 4 weeks postinjury, while after transection reduction in fiber size made further significant progress.

Cytochrome Oxidase. While G6PDH and 6PGDH are located in the cytosol, CO is a mitochondrial enzyme which reacts and adjusts rapidly to changing oxidative demands in a variety of nerve cells, including spinal motoneurons [57]. These demands are posed mainly by the processes of ion transport maintaining resting and synaptic potentials. Pure conductile activity does not require energy in comparable amounts, with the result that CO activity in the white matter is generally low [7]. Systematic studies of CO reactivity in neurons in the somatosensory, visual, and auditory systems have shown a clearly positive correlation with levels of spontaneous and excitatory synaptic activity [53, 54, 55, 56]. In the present experiments, the significant increase in CO reactivity 3 days after both types of injury may reflect an acute effect of trauma upon the oxidative steady state capacity of the affected motoneurons. The following high reactivity at 1 week indicates a sharp, short-term increase in oxidative demands, especially after transection injury. Particularly noteworthy is the subsequent reduction in reactivity at the 2nd week after crush, signaling a slowly progressing decrease of oxidative capacity. This suggests a posttraumatic lability in the capacity of spinal motoneurons to adjust to the new demands placed upon the cell body by regeneration processes, in remarkable contrast to the vigorous stimulation of biosynthetic metabolism denoted by the increase in G6PDH and 6PGDH activities. The pronounced and progressive reactivity decrease after transection is an indication of the profound posttraumatic depression of oxidative metabolism expected from this kind of lesion. In terms of quality of functional recovery, this feature seems to indicate, at least within our observation time of 8 weeks, that crush injury may produce a long-lasting reduction in the oxidative capacity of spinal motoneurons, which in turn may hamper recovery and/or increase the vulnerability of the cell body to additional lesions.

Acetylcholinesterase. The reduction in AChE reactivity at all times after both injuries did not reach statistical significance until the 8th week. This fact does not negate the existence of a consistent pattern. Thus, the initial reactivity decrement may be reversible, as shown by the transient recovery at the 2nd week. Further, reduction after transection proceeds at a slow but clearly progressive rate. In contrast, changes after crush remained at discretely subnormal but stable levels. As in the case with CO reactivity, there were indications of incomplete recovery after crush injury, at least until the 8th week, in spite of the clear signals of reconnection that we could observe in extensor digitorum longus fibers 4 weeks after peroneal nerve crush in the study mentioned above (Adler and Nacimiento, this volume). The observed decrease in AChE reactivity is in agreement with previous results obtained in spinal motoneurons following axonal lesions [36, 40], a finding which can be generalized to various types of neurons and species [2, 3, 46, 47].

The Nature of Late Activity Changes After Transection. It is not possible from the present results to offer an unambiguous explanation for the low activity level of all enzymes at the 8th week. Longer observation times are needed to define final outcome in our experimental conditions. Nevertheless, this finding reflects the close association between the metabolic state of the cell body after axon injury and the ability of axonal endings to accomplish effective target-organ reconnection [14, 16, 52]. Lack of reconnection switches the metabolic state of the cell body to an inactivity mode, which may lead in some neurons to atrophy and death and in others to a low but potentially reversible steady-state level [50, 51, 52]. This quiescent stage may be switched back to the active mode by reconnection, even many months after injury, as shown, for example, by functionally effective repair by grafting [14, 30, 31, 45]. Recognition of the factors underlying this plasticity is of crucial clinical interest.

Metabolic Responses of the Cell Body to Axonal Injury and Timing of Nerve Repair. Increases in the reactivity of some intracellular enzymes, particularly those of the pentose phosphate pathway, demonstrated in various types of neurons 2–3 weeks following injury to their axons [8, 9, 10, 19, 20, 39] gave rise to the proposition that the timing of nerve repair might be optimized by making it coincide with this neuronal state [8, 9, 14]. This view led to the proposal of early secondary repair as an effective strategy for improving the potential for regeneration in reconstructed nerves [8, 9, 14]. An analysis of this concept in the light of our own results leads to the following considerations. (a) There is no proof that posttraumatic stimulation of G6PDH and 6PGDH lasts beyond the critical turning point between the 2nd and 3rd week postinjury, to support axonal growth with biosynthetic activities at a time in which chances for successful reconnection by repair cannot be safely established. (b) CO reactivity was found to be significantly low at the 4th week, pointing to a decreased oxidation capacity which may enhance the vulnerability of motoneurons to the additional injury necessarily involved in preparation of the nerve for repair. (c) AChE reactivity is consistently lowered after injury, and there are no indications that early secondary repair may at this time reverse this trend and activate neurotransmitter metabolism at the rate required for functional reconnection.

The metabolic effects of a second lesion have been studied on facial motoneurons in the rat following either crush or transection injury of the facial nerve [46]. The nerve was lesioned once on one side and twice, with an interval of 2 weeks, on the other. Changes in G6PDH, 6PDGH, AChE, and 5' nucleotidase (a marker for glia proliferative activity) were measured at various times up to 4 weeks postinjury and compared. It was found that the posttraumatic burst of biosynthetic activity after the second lesion was, except for a brief phase 1–3 days postinjury, consistently weaker than that following the single lesion, reaching similar levels at the 3rd and 4th week. AChE activity which was already weaker after the single lesion, was further lowered by the second. 5' Nucleotidase activity was higher after the second lesion for only 1–3 days postinjury; thereafter both single- and second-lesion sides did not differ. These results suggest that a second lesion may partially impair posttraumatic biosynthetic regenerative activity and severely depress neurotransmitter metabolism in the cell body.

These considerations do not lend experimental support to the notion of an optimum time for early repair based on metabolic reactions of neurons to single or repeated axonal injuries. As a result, we agree with Sunderland [43, 44], that the concepts underlying early secondary repair do not have an adequate experimental basis.

The discovery of nerve growth factor [48, 49] and a growing family of neurotrophic agents, including motoneuron growth factors [1, 18, 21, 32], led to the concept that trophic homeostasis is an essential requirement for adequate neuronal function. The metabolic state of the cell body is a basic factor in maintaining this equilibrium, which is lost after nerve injury. Therefore it is of great clinical interest to find ways of stimulating the metabolic function of motoneurons in connection with repair of their injured axons. Magnitude and time course of changes in enzyme activity obtained in this study followed consistent, highly reproducible and predictable patterns. As a result, these changes may function as sensitive indicators and reliable predictors of well-defined metabolic reactions of spinal motoneurons to peripheral nerve lesions. It is concluded that the present experimental paradigms are suitable for testing the effectiveness of pharmacological and/or microreconstruction means of influencing neuronal metabolism in a clinically relevant context.

Summary

Metabolic reactions over time of single motoneurons in spinal cord segments L 3 and L 4 in the rat to standardized crush or unrepaired transection lesions of the sciatic nerve were studied in terms of changes in activity of the enzymes G6PDH and 6PGDH, two key enzymes of the pentose phosphate pathway which generate NADPH and pentoses for biosynthesis of nucleotides: CO, an indicator of oxidative capacity, and AChE, which reflects neurotransmitter metabolism. Enzyme activity was demonstrated histochemically and its changes measured by computer-assisted cytophotometry at 3 days, and 1, 2, 4, 6, and 8 weeks following injury.

In an early phase up to the 4th week, there was, following both crush and transection lesions, a marked increase in activity of G6PDH and 6PGDH of various degrees. The activity elevation following crush outlasted that measured after transection. CO activity decreased at 3 days postinjury, increased at 1 week, and returned to control levels at 2 weeks. In a late phase activity of the pentose phosphate pathway enzymes stabilized to control conditions after crush injury but declined progressively to subnormal levels following transection, while CO activity decreased after both lesions, moderately following crush and strongly after transection. AChE activity was lower at all post-traumatic times.

The metabolic state of the cell seems to switch between the active and inactive modes depending on the ability of axon terminals to reestablish neuromuscular connections. The higher potential for regeneration following crush lesion may depend on its high safety factor for functional reconnection.

The present experiments did not provide evidence supporting the arguments underlying the concept of early secondary repair.

Magnitude and time course of the observed changes were consistent, highly reproducible and predictable. They are considered to be suitable for quantitative evaluation of pharmacological and/or microreconstruction approaches aimed at influencing the metabolic state of motoneurons in connection with nerve repair.

References

1. Anderson KJ, Dam D, Lee S, Cotman CW (1988) Basic fibroblast growth factor prevents death of lesioned cholinergic neurons in vivo. Nature 332:360–361
2. Barron KD, Dentinger MP, Rodichok LD. The axon reaction of central and peripheral mammalian neurons: a comparison. In: Ref. 14., pp 17–26
3. Barron KD (1983) Comparative observations on the cytologic reactions of central and peripheral nerve cells to axotomy. In: Kao CC, Bunge RP, Reier PJ (eds) Spinal cord reconstruction. Raven Press, New York, pp 7–40
4. Brushart TM, Mesulam MM (1980) Alteration in connections between muscle and anterior horn motoneurons after peripheral nerve repair. Science 208:603–605
5. Buell MV, Lowry OH, Roberts NR, Chang MW, Kapphahn J (1958) The quantitative histochemistry of the brain. V. Enzymes of glucose metabolism. J Biol Chem 232:976–993
6. Cammermeyer J (1969) Species differences in acute retrograde neuronal reaction of the facial and hypoglossal nuclei. Journal für Hirnforschung 11:13–29
7. Creutzfeldt OD (1975) Neurophysiological correlates of different functional states of the brain. In: Ingvar DH, Lassen NA (eds) Brain work. Alfred Benzon Symposium VIII. Academic Press, New York, pp 21–46
8. Ducker TB, Kempe LG, Hayes GJ (1969) The metabolic background for peripheral nerve surgery. J Neurosurg 30:270–280
9. Ducker TB, Kauffman FC (1977) Metabolic factors in surgery of peripheral nerves. Clin Neurosurg 24:406–424
10. Engh CA, Schofield BH (1972) A review of the central response to peripheral nerve injury and its significance in nerve regeneration. J Neurosurg 37:195–203
11. Fischer DW, Beggs JL, Kenshalo DL, Shetter AG (1985) Comparative study of microepineurial anastomoses with the use of CO_2 laser and suture techniques in rat sciatic nerves: part 1. J Neurosurg 17:300–308
12. Fawcett JW, Keynes RJ (1986) Muscle basal lamina: a graft material for peripheral nerve repair. J Neurosurg 65:354–363
13. Giacobini E, Jongkind JF (1968) Pentose shunt enzymes in the crustacean stretch receptor neuron after impulse activity. Acta Physiol Scand 73:255–256
14. Gorio A, Millesi H, Mingrino S (eds) (1981) Posttraumatic peripheral nerve regeneration. Raven Press, New York
15. Grafstein B, McQuarrie IG (1978) Role of nerve cell body in axonal regeneration. In: Cotman CW (ed) Neuronal plasticity. Raven Press, New York, pp 155–195
16. Grinnell AD, Herrera AA (1981) Specificity and plasticity of neuromuscular connections. Long-term regulation of motoneuron function. Prog Neurobiol 17:203–282
17. Guerra RM, Melgar E, Villavicencio M (1967) Alternative pathways of glucose metabolism in fetal rat brain. Acta Biochim Biophys 148:356
18. Gurney ME, Heinrich SP, Lee MR, Shu Yin H (1986) Molecular cloning and expression of neuroleukin, a neurothrophic factor for spinal and sensory neurons. Science 234:566–574
19. Härkönen MHA, Kauffman FC (1974) Metabolic alterations in the axotomized superior cervical ganglion of the rat. I. Energy metabolism. Brain Res 65:127–139
20. Härkönen MHA, Kauffman FC (1974) Metabolic alterations in the axotomized superior cervical ganglion of the rat. II. The pentose phosphate pathway. Brain Res 65:141–157
21. Hofer MM, Barde Y-A (1988) Brain-derived neurotrophic factor prevents neuronal death in vivo. Nature 331:261–262
22. Hostetler KY, Landau BR (1967) Estimation of the pentose cycle contribution to glucose metabolism in brain tissue in vivo. Biochem 6:2961–2964
23. Kline DG, Hudson AR, Bratton BR (1981) Experimental study of fascicular nerve repair with and without epineurial closure. J Neurosurg 54:513–520
24. Kline DG, Hudson AR (1985) Selected recent advances in peripheral nerve injury research. Surg Neurol 24:371–376

25. Koelle GB, Friedewald JS (1949) A histochemical method for localizing cholinesterase activity. Proc Soc Exp Biol Med 70:617–622
26. Kreutzberg GW (1963) Changes of coenzyme (TPN) diaphorase and TPN-linked dehydrogenase during axonal reaction of the nerve cell. Nature 199:393–394
27. Lundborg G, Dahlin LB, Danielson N, Hansson H, Johannesson A, Longo F, Varon S (1982) Nerve regeneration across an extended gap: a neurobiological view of nerve repair and possible neuronotropic factors. J Hand Surg 7:580–587
28. Marx C, Nacimiento AC (1987) Quantitative histochemistry of enzyme changes over time in rat spinal motoneurons following axotomy. Abstr Soc for Neurosc 13:182, 8
29. Medinaceli L de, Wyatt R, Freed W (1983) Peripheral nerve reconnection: mechanical, thermal, and ionic conditions that promote the return of function. Exp Neurol 81:469–487
30. Millesi H (1981) Reappraisal of nerve repair. Surg Clin North Am 61:321–340
31. Millesi HN (1987) Nerve grafting. In: Terzis JK (ed) Microreconstruction of nerve injuries. Saunders, Philadelphia, pp 232–237
32. Oppenheim RW, Haverkamp LJ, Prevette D, McManaman JL, Appel SH (1988) Reduction of naturally occurring motoneuron death in vivo by a target-derived neurotrophic factor. Science 240:919–922
33. Orgel MG (1984) Epineurial versus perineurial repair of peripheral nerves. Clin Plast Surg 11:101–104
34. Rexed B (1952) The cytoarchitectonic organization of the spinal cord in the cat. J Comp Neurol 96:415–466
35. Samii M, Scheinpflug W (1974) Klinische, elektromyographische und quantitativ histologische Untersuchungen nach Nerventransplantation. Acta Neurochir 30:1–29
36. Schwarzacher H (1958) Der Cholinesterasegehalt motorischer Nervenzellen während der axonalen Reaktion. Acta Anat 32:51–65
37. Seddon HJ (1943) Three types of nerve injury. Brain 66:237–288
38. Seddon HJ (1972) Surgical disorders of the peripheral nerves. Churchill Livingstone, Edinburgh London
39. Sinicropi DV, Kauffman FC, Burt DR (1979) Axotomy in rat sympathetic ganglia: reciprocal effects on muscarinic receptor binding and 6-phosphogluconate dehydrogenase activity. Brain Research 161:560–565
40. Söderholm U (1965) Histochemical localization of esterases, phosphatases and tetrazolium reductases in the motor neurones of the spinal cord of the rat and the effect of nerve division. Acta Physiol Scand (Suppl 256) 65:1–60
41. Sunderland S (1951) Classification of peripheral nerve injuries producing loss of function. Brain 74:491–516
42. Sunderland S (1952) Factors influencing the course of the regeneration and the quality of recovery after nerve suture. Brain 75:19–54
43. Sunderland S (1978) Nerve and nerve injuries, 2nd ed. Churchill Livingstone, Edinburgh
44. Sunderland S (1980) Clinical and experimental approaches to nerve repair in perspective. In: Jewett DL, McCarroll HR (eds) Nerve repair and regeneration. Mosby, St. Louis Toronto London, pp 337–355
45. Terzis JK (ed) (1987) Microreconstruction of nerve injuries. Saunders, Philadelphia London Toronto
46. Tetzlaff W, Kreutzberg G (1984) Enzyme changes in the rat facial nucleus following a conditioning lesion. Exp Neurol 85:547–564
47. Tetzlaff W, Graeber MB, Kreutzberg GW (1986) Reaction on motoneurons and their microenvironment to axotomy. Exp Brain Res (Suppl) 13:3–8
48. Thoenen H, Barde Y-A (1980) Physiology of nerve growth factor. Physiol Rev 60:1284–1335
49. Thoenen H, Korsching S, Heumann R, Acheson A (1985) Nerve growth factor. Ciba Found Symp 116:113–128
50. Watson WE (1970) Some metabolic responses of axotomized neurones to contact between their axons and denervated muscle. J Physiol (Lond) 210:312–343

51. Watson WE (1974) Cellular responses to axotomy and to related procedures. Br Med Bull 30:112–114
52. Watson WE (1976) Cell biology of brain. Chapman & Hall, London
53. Wong-Riley M (1979) Changes in the visual system of molecularly sutured or enucleated cats demonstrable with cytochrome oxidase histochemistry. Brain Res 171:11–28
54. Wong-Riley M, Welt C (1980) Histochemical changes in cytochrome oxidase of cortical barrels following vibrissal removal in neonatal and adult mice. Proc Natl Acad Sci USA 77:2333–2337
55. Wong-Riley M, Walsh SM, Leake-Jones PA, Merzenich MM (1981) Maintenance of neuronal activity by electrical stimulation of unilaterally deafened cats demonstrable with the cytochrome oxidase technique. Ann Otol Rhinol Laryngol (Suppl 82) 90:30–32
56. Wong-Riley M, Carroll EW (1984) Effect of impulse blockage on cytochrome oxidase activity in monkey visual system. Nature 307:262–264
57. Wong-Riley M, Kageyama GH (1986) Localization of cytochrome oxidase in the mammalian spinal cord and dorsal root ganglia, with quantitative analysis of ventral horn cells in monkeys. J Comp Neurol 245:41–61

Experimental Peripheral Nerve Crush Lesion
II. Short-Term Reinnervation Changes in Fast Muscle Fibers

G. ADLER and A. C. NACIMIENTO, Homburg (Saar)/FRG

Introduction

From the clinical point of view, quality of muscle reinnervation following peripheral nerve injury constitutes a crucial element in the assessment of effectiveness of nerve repair. We analyzed this problem in a standardized experimental paradigm in the rat. By means of morphometrical, histochemical, and ultrastructural methods we studied acute posttraumatic changes in selected parameters indicating reinnervation of single fibers in extensor digitorum longus (EDL) and extensor hallucis longus (EHL) muscles following a standardized crush injury of the peroneal nerve. We quantified these changes 2 and 4 weeks postinjury against the background provided by those developing in a parallel experimental group in which muscle reinnervation was prevented by peroneal nerve unrepaired excision. These muscles represent predominantly the fast type and are identical in histochemical profile, ultrastructure, and the time course of reinnervation. A preliminary report has been published [1].

Material and Methods

Nerve Lesions. The investigation was carried out in 12 Sprague-Dawley rats which underwent either resection ($n = 6$) or crush ($n = 6$) of the peroneal nerve on the right side under intraperitoneal pentobarbital anesthesia (7 mg/100 g body weight). In the resection group, a 1-cm stretch of peroneal nerve was removed and the proximal stump ligated. The crush lesion was made with appropriate tweezers. A 1-cm-long nerve segment remained between the distal end of the resection or the crush lesion and the EDL and EHL muscles.

Muscle preparation. Muscles were excised on the operated side 2 ($n = 3$) and 4 ($n = 3$) weeks after each type of lesion. At this time body weight ranged between 360 and 400 g. Control observations were made on both sides in each of three intact animals. Excised EDL muscles were frozen in n-hexane at $-70\,°C$ and stored at this temperature. The animals were subsequently perfused through the heart with a solution of 1% formaldehyde and 2% glutaraldehyde in phosphate buffer. The EHL muscles were removed, and immersion fixation was performed for 2 days in the same solution. From the midportion of the EDL muscles 8-µm transverse sections were cut in a cryostat and air-dried. They were stained for myofibrillar ATPase activity following either alkaline or acid preincubation [2] and for succinic dehydrogenase (SDH) activity [10]. By inspection of ATPase- and SDH-stained serial sections the fibers were classified into slow oxidative (SO), fast oxidative glycogenolytic (FOG), and fast glycogenolytic (FG) [11]. The entire cross-section of the muscle was drawn by means of a side-tube projection of the microscopical image. From these drawings, number and cross-sectional area of the muscle fibers for each fiber type were measured using a digitizing graphic tablet.

The EHL muscles were postfixed in 1 % osmium tetroxide and embedded in epoxy resin. Transverse and longitudinal semithin sections of 1 μm thickness were performed and stained with methylene blue. Capillaries and muscle fiber nuclei were counted. Mitochondrial fraction was measured in 100-nm ultrathin sections cut in a longitudinal plane, mounted on formvar-filmed grids, and contrasted with lead citrate and uranyl acetate. At an original magnification of 9600, a strip of one sarcomere width was photographed entirely through five fibers of each muscle. The mitochondrial fraction was evaluated in this strip. The fiber area was normalized to a uniform sarcomere length of 2.25 μm, and a 2-μm-wide field at each side was excluded to avoid distortion of the results from subsarcolemmal mitochondria accumulations [5]. Statistical significance was calculated by means of Student's t test.

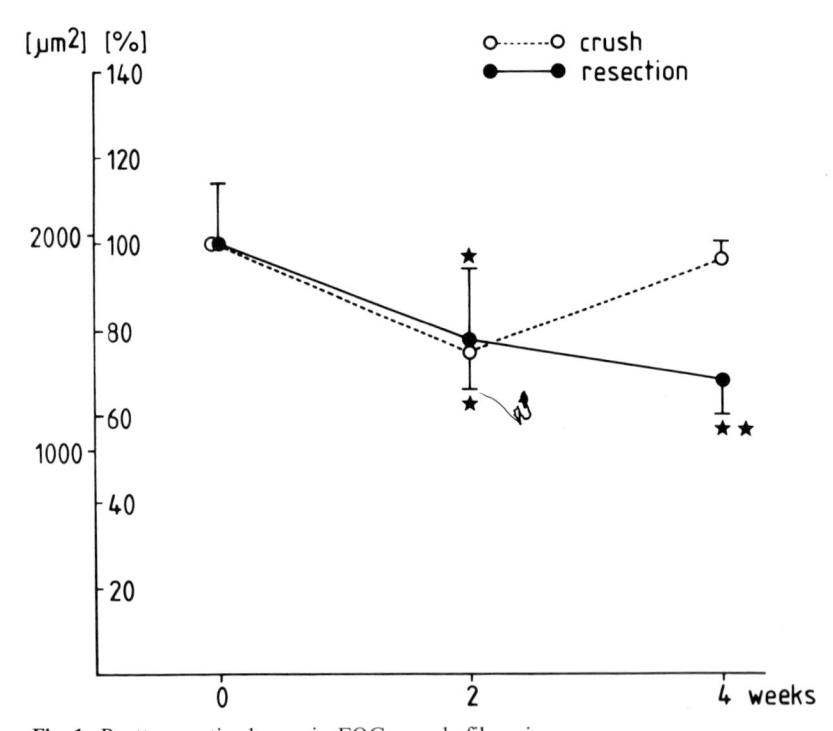

Fig. 1. Posttraumatic change in FOG muscle fiber size

Results

Two weeks following both types of lesions there was a marked decrease in the size of FOG (Fig. 1) and FG (Fig. 2) fibers. Four weeks after resection this decrease further progressed at a slower rate, whereas following crush injury fiber size recovered to normal values. After 4 weeks size decrease in FG fibers due to resection was larger than that in FOG fibers ($p < 0.01$). SO fibers did not change significantly.

Four weeks following crush lesion of the peroneal nerve fiber type composition changed significantly (Fig. 3). The number of FOG fibers was increased by 30%, and that of FOG fibers was reduced by about the same amount. The total number of muscle fibers in control animals was 1999 ± 787. It did not change significantly in the operated ones.

Two weeks after nerve resection or crush, the number of capillaries per muscle fiber was reduced to 80% of control value (Fig. 4). Here again differences between lesion types were apparent at 4 weeks posttrauma. After resection capillary number decreased further to 70%, while following crush injury there was complete recovery. Since in both experimental groups mean fiber size decreased, as described above, there was an overall increase in capillary density.

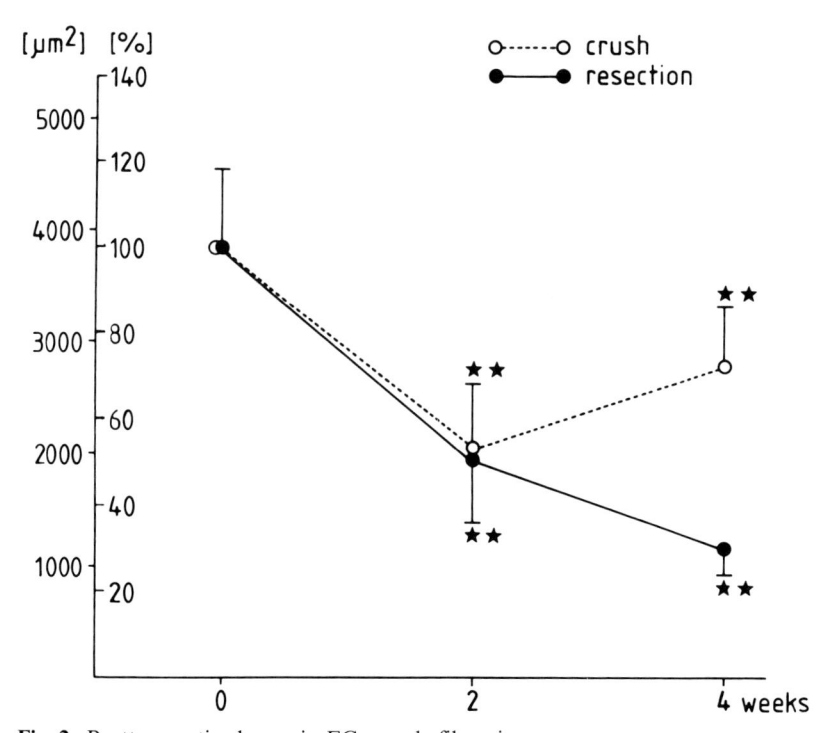

Fig. 2. Posttraumatic change in FG muscle fiber size

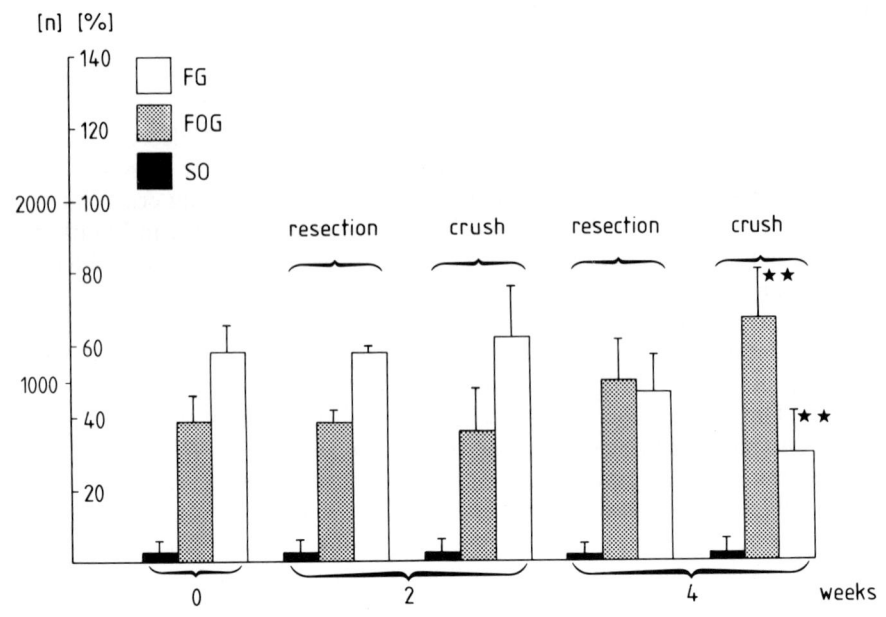

Fig. 3. Posttraumatic changes in histochemical profile of EDL muscle fibers. ** $p < 0.01$, compared to preinjury values

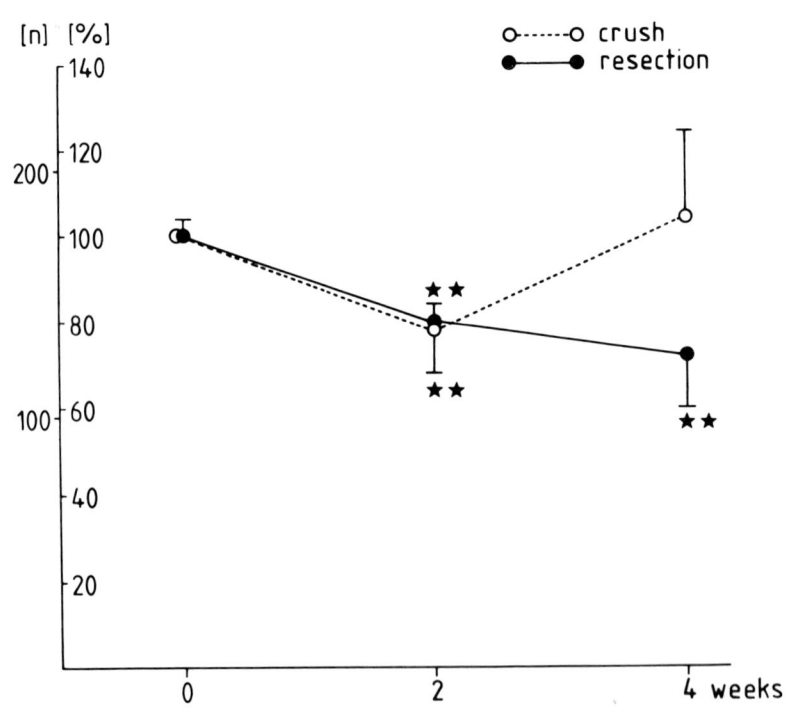

Fig. 4. Posttraumatic changes in capillary number in EHL muscle fibers. ** $p < 0.01$, compared to preinjury values

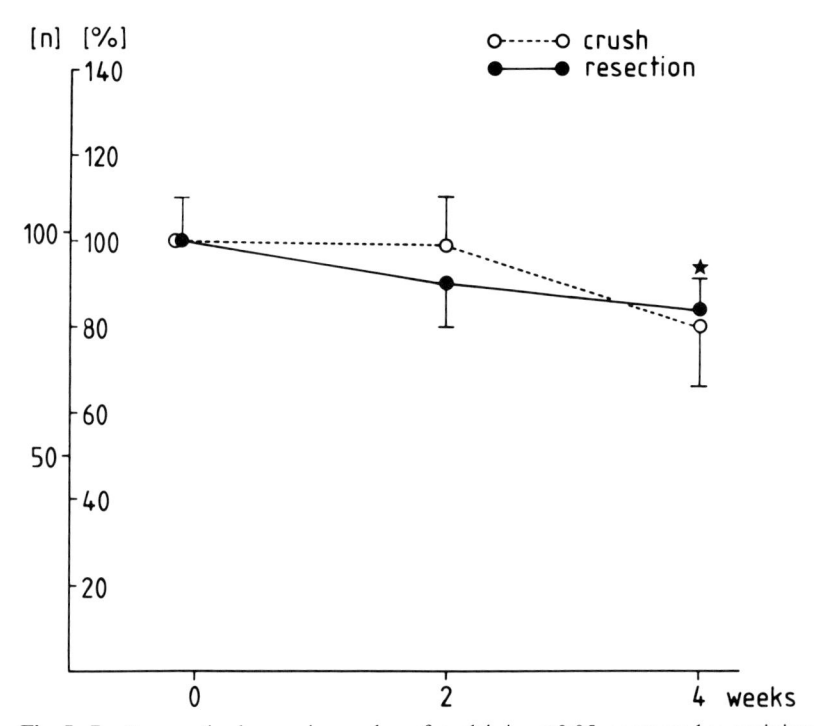

Fig. 5. Posttraumatic changes in number of nuclei. * $p < 0.05$, compared to preinjury values

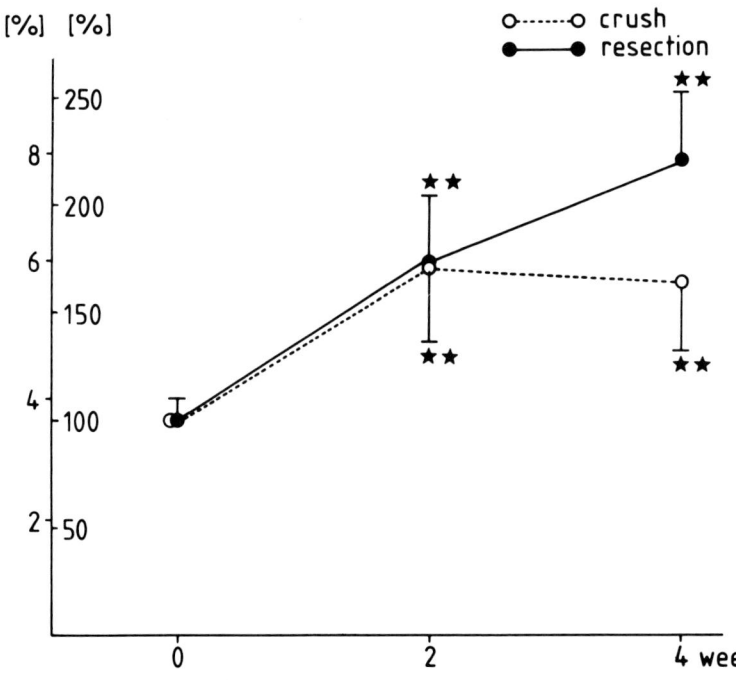

Fig. 6. Posttraumatic change in mitochondrial fraction. ** $p < 0.01$, compared to preinjury values

The number of nuclei per muscle fiber tended to decrease slightly after nerve resection (Fig. 5). Following crush lesion, no significant changes could be observed.

Number, size, and shape of mitochondria changed markedly in the operated animals (Fig. 6). In longitudinal sections, the number of mitochondria was reduced, size was increased and their shape became elongated, with the long axis parallel to the longitudinal axis of the muscle fibers. These changes probably reflect a change of the mitochondria in spatial orientation with their long axis shifting from the transverse to the longitudinal axis of the muscle fibers. Following nerve resection, the mitochondrial fraction increased to 180% of the control value after 2 weeks and to 220% after 4 weeks. As this increase is inversely about proportional to mean fiber size, the absolute mitochondrial volume seemed to be unchanged. After nerve crush, the mitochondrial fraction was increased to 170% after both the 2nd and 4th week. An augmentation in mitochondrial volume suggested by changes in fiber size from 60% to 70% of control values between the 2nd and the 4th postinjury week did not reach statistical significance.

Discussion

Results of measurements of the expected decrease in fiber size following peripheral nerve transection carried out in anterior tibial muscle after sciatic nerve injury [9] are in agreement with those reported here. There is a similar agreement with size measurements made 2–3 weeks following crush lesion of the sciatic nerve in soleus and plantaris muscles [7]. However, the quantitative changes over time in fiber composition described in the present work have not been previously reported.

In this context, it seems better suited to the purpose of this investigation to relate histochemical profiles to a physiological variable such as resistance to fatigue rather than to twitch time [3]. This physiological–histochemical correlation defines the following three groups: fast, fatiguable (FG type); fast, fatigue-resistant (FOG type); and slow, fatigue-resistant (SO type). On this basis, our finding of a significant increase in the amount of FOG fibers 4 weeks after crush injury discloses a functional rearrangement directly related to the ongoing reinnervation events in the acute postinjury phase. Inasmuch as preinjury distribution is restored in the chronic state (2 months postinjury; Adler and Nacimiento, unpublished results), this phenomenon seems to be a transitional one. Nevertheless, this reorganization points to a postinjury plasticity in the affected motor units attributable, for example, to a phase of polyneuronal reinnervation, which in turn may be influenced by factors affecting postinjury reinnervation.

In a recent study, capillary distribution in rat fast muscles following nerve crush was found to be closely related to muscle fiber type [8]. The conclusion was drawn that capillary supply seems to match changes in metabolic demand of the muscle. Our observations concerning time course, magnitude, and direction of changes in capillary number following both types of lesion are in agreement with and clearly support this notion.

Measurements of mitochondrial mass in the initial phase of denervation showed no significant changes [6]. Our results confirm this finding, thus casting doubts as to the usefulness of this type of ultrastructural analysis as a postinjury evaluation parameter.

This study was aimed at defining the suitability of various regeneration parameters as predictors in the quantitative assessment of (a) the potential for regeneration of motor units following peripheral nerve injury and (b) therapeutic approaches to mobilize this potential. We found that serial measurements of changes in fiber size of functionally defined histochemical profiles and capillary number proved to be reproducible and predictable parameters. Accordingly, we are applying these criteria to the studies of the pharmacological actions of putative neurotrophic factors currently under way in our laboratory.

Summary

Size and histochemical profile of EDL muscle fibers changed with a characteristic and reproducible time-dependent pattern within the first 4 postinjury weeks following either crush or resection of the peroneal nerve. At the 4th week there was in particular a large increase in the number of fast, fatigue-resistant fibers.

Capillary number in EHL muscle fibers changed with a time course consistent with this posttraumatic rearrangement of fiber type composition. In contrast, neither number of nuclei nor mitochondrial fractional volume were useful indicators of ongoing reinnervation processes.

Fiber size, functionally defined histochemical profiles, and capillary distribution showed high levels of short-term posttraumatic plasticity. This quality allows them to function as reliable predictors for quantitative assessment of reinnervation events in the acute postinjury phase following peripheral nerve lesions.

References

1. Adler G, Mautes A, Hübschen U, Nacimiento AC (1987) Time dependent changes in histochemical profile of a fast muscle following nerve transection or crush in the rat. Pflügers Archiv 408 (Suppl. 1): R 81
2. Brooke MH, Kaiser KK (1969) Some comments on the histochemical characterization of muscle adenosine triphosphatase. J Histochem Cytochem 17: 431–432
3. Burke RE, Levine DN, Zajac FE III, Tsairis P, Engel WK (1971) Mammalian motor units. Physiological-histochemical correlations in three types in cat gastrocnemius. Science 174: 709–712
4. Coster W de, Reuck J de, Eecken H vander (1985) Early changes in experimental denervated rat gastrocnemius muscle. Acta Neuropathol (Berl) 67: 114–120

5. Eisenberg BR (1983) Quantitative ultrastructure of mammalian skeletal muscle. In: Peachy LD (ed) Handbook of Physiology. Vol. 10. American Physiological Society, Bethesda/MD, pp 73–112
6. Engel AG, Stonnington HH (1974) Morphological effects of denervation of muscle. A quantitative ultrastructural study. Ann NY Acad Sci 228:68–88
7. Jaweed MM, Herbison GJ, Ditunno JF (1975) Denervation and reinnervation of fast and slow muscles. A histochemical study in rats. J Histochem Cytochem 23:808–827
8. Large J, Tyler KR (1985) Changes in capillary distribution in rat fast muscles following nerve crush and reinnervation. J Physiol (Lond) 362:13–23
9. Lindboe CF, Presthus J (1985) Effects of denervation, immobilization and cachexia on fibre size in the anterior tibial muscle of the rat. Acta Neuropathol (Berl) 66:42–51
10. Nachlas MM, Tsou K-C, de Souza E, Cheng C, Seligman AM (1957) Cytochemical demonstration of succinic dehydrogenase by the use of a p-nitrophenyl substituted ditetrazole. J Histochem Cytochem 5:420–436
11. Peter JB, Barnard RJ, Edgerton VR, Gillespie CA, Stempel KE (1972) Metabolic profiles of three fiber types of skeletal muscle in guinea pigs and rabbits. Biochemistry 11:2627–2633

Structural Changes of the Peripheral Nerve After Pressure Lesions in the Domestic Fowl

M. Blank, M. A. Konerding, H.-E. Nau, and P. Wenzel, Essen/FRG

This paper deals with the histological alterations found in the ischiadic nerve of the domestic fowl after compression with aneurysm clips. The corresponding clinical and electrophysiological findings are described elsewhere in this volume (Nau et al.).

Methods

After exsanguination, perfusion fixation was performed with Karnovsky's solution. The prepared ischiadic nerves of the experimental and healthy sides were photographed and measured. One part of the preparations was studied by light microscopy and morphometry and another part by scanning electron microscopy (Stereoscan 180, Cambridge, UK). By light microscopy the injured and the intact nerves were cut in serial sections in steps of 15 mm. The modified Kodoussek silver-stain technique described by Blank et al. (1978) was used for morphometric examination. For scanning electron microscopical examinations a postfixation in 1% osmium tetroxide solution was performed. These were dried by the critical point method by carbon dioxide sputtered by gold in argon atmosphere.

Results

In the ischiadic nerve of the killed animal we found a bloody imbibition and circular compression at the site of the clip directly after the end of clipping. In this acute stage there were no differences in the diameter of the nerve. Light microscopy also revealed a normal diameter of the nerve at the site of the compression, but the degree of silver staining was reduced. This was due to a spotty discoloration of the myelin structures. Also, the axons and the axolemma of the axons showed various impregnations. Thirty minutes after the end of compression there was almost no silver impregnation, but a marked edema, especially in the center of compression. One hour after the compression the edema had spread in both directions from the lesion.

When killing the animal about 80 days after the compression, we found a marked swelling distal to the site of lesion. There were no differences in the

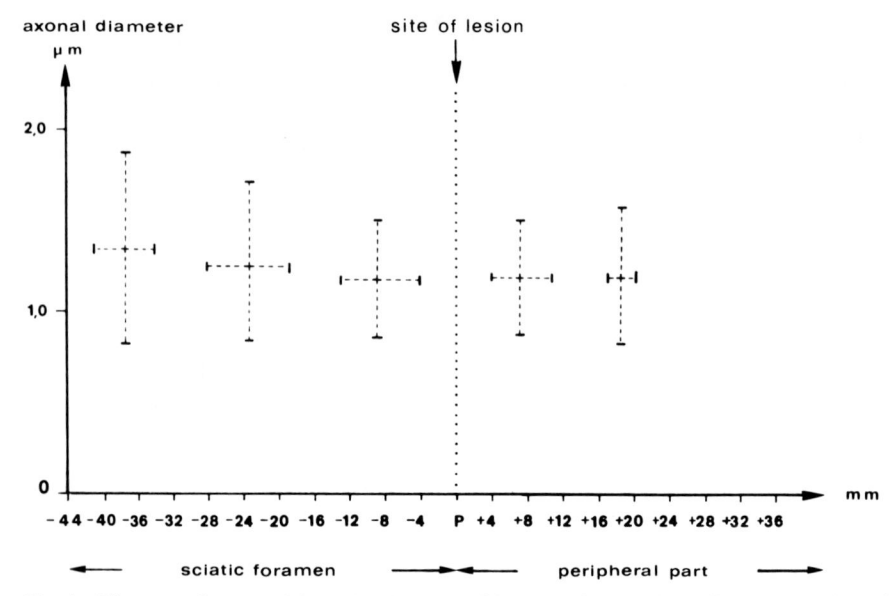

Fig. 1. Diameter of axons of the ischiadic nerve of domestic fowl 80 days after compression of a duration of 2–24 h. Measurements were done in 200 axons at each position in the different parts of the nerve in ten animals. No significant differences were seen along the nerve

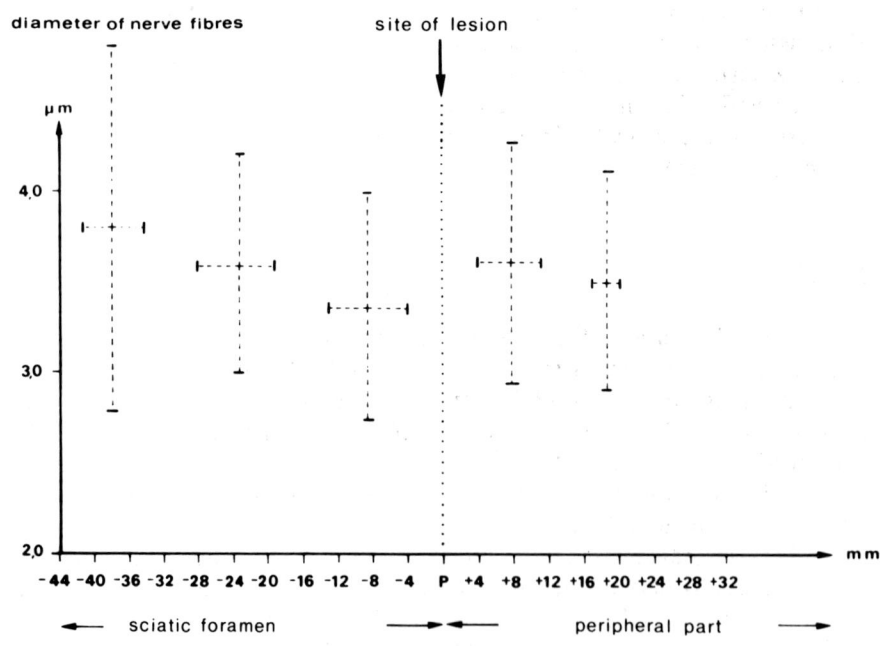

Fig. 2. Diameter of the nerve shows no statistically significant changes before and after the site of the lesion. Measurements as in Fig. 1

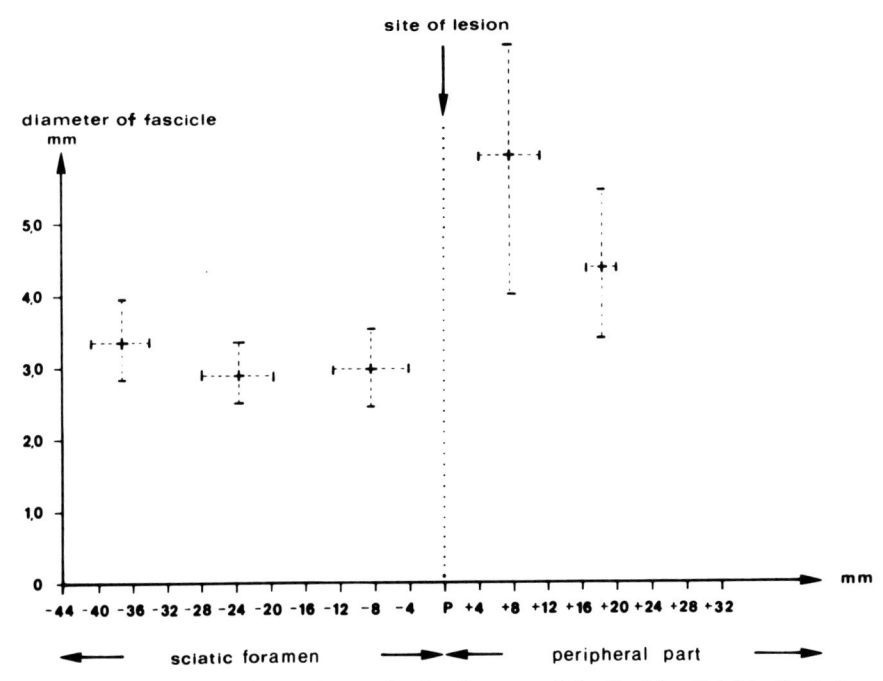

Fig. 3. Statistically significant changes in the diameter of the fascicles distal to the lesion. Measurements as in Fig. 1

degree of swelling between the nerves with varying durations of compression. This swelling could be verified as an edematous one. There seemed to be differences in the morphological pictures of the nerves depending on the duration of compression, although in these animals there were no differences in the clinical and electrophysiological findings. The increase in the nerve diameter could be due to an increase of the substance between the nerve fibers.

Morphometry of the normal ischiadic nerve of the domestic fowl showed an increase in the diameter of the nerve in the proximodistal direction, but a constant diameter of the myelin sheaths and the axons. Eighty days after the compression we found no differences in the diameter of the myelin sheaths or the axons (Figs. 1, 2) but a marked increase in the diameter of the fascicle distal to the lesion (Fig. 3).

Upon scanning electron microscopy we could demonstrate the increase in connective tissue. Between the different layers of the perineurium there were clefts filled with amorphous material. The surface of the perineural membrane was markedly rough, and substantial granula were observed. This sometimes seemed to be broken. Amorphous substances and fibrocytic elements were also found in the endoneural space. The cytoorganelles in the axons were also changed.

Conclusions

These experiments have shown that the quick disappearance of the nerve conduction may be due to the rapid structural changes of the peripheral nerve. In the acute stage an edema spreads along the nerve, proximally and distally from the site of the compression. The circular constriction is seen in this acute stage but cannot be found in later stages. The swelling distal to the site of the lesion may be due to chronic changes following the acute edema. In this stage the diameter of the nerve is increased, which is due to an increase in the interfascicular connective tissue. Although the diameter of the myelin sheaths and axons is not markedly changed upon light microscopy, there are remarkable alterations to be found upon scanning electron microscopy. These might be responsible for the fact that the nerve conduction velocity before the lesion is not reached in the follow-up and recovery. The key to all these alterations seems to lie in the structural changes of the vessels (see Konerding et al., this volume).

Reference

Blank M, Lehmann M, El-Hifnawi ES (1978) Eine Modifikation der Kodoussekschen Silberimprägnationsmethode, die für elektronenmikroskopische Vergleichsuntersuchungen geeignet ist. Beitr Elektronenmikroskop Direktabb Oberfl 11:263–268

Computed Tomography in Peripheral Nerve Pathology

A. ALEXANDRE, F. DI PAOLA, F. DI TOMA, P. CISOTTO, D. BILLECI, and A. CARTERI, Treviso/Italy

Computed tomography (CT) is a universally employed diagnostic tool of proven utility. While it is routinely used in central nervous system pathology, it has rarely been employed in the study of peripheral nervous system lesions, particularly if the involved specialist is not a neurosurgeon. We present here our experience in a preoperative study of patients in whom anatomical and pathological data have been sought by means of CT scans.

Patients and Methods

Between 1 January 1985 and 1 June 1987, 262 patients affected by peripheral nerve lesions of varying etiology underwent clinical study and surgical treatment in the Division of Neurosurgery at Padua University in Treviso, Italy. These included 186 cases of carpal tunnel syndrome, 15 ulnar nerve entrapments at the elbow, 15 traumatic lesions of the upper extremity with involvement of one, two, or of all three major nerve trunks, 20 traumatic or tumoral lesions of the brachial plexus, 10 traumatic lesions of the sciatic or anterior tibial nerve, 8 lipomas located in the forearm or the leg, and 6 cases of Morton's metatarsalgia.

All patients underwent careful anamnestic and clinical study and complete electrophysiological investigation of the nervous and muscular functions of the involved anatomical area. Moreover, a careful radiological study was performed by means of CT scan and enhanced CT. Measurements of tissue absorption are given in Hounsfield units (HU). On this scale, neurogenic tumors, lipomas, and scar tissue have a specific value, allowing distinction from muscles, vessels, parenchymatous tissues and bony structures. The association of radiological data with electrical evaluation has proved to be very helpful in assessing the anatomical site of the lesion.

Results and Discussion

Since the ultimate purpose of surgery is complete removal of the lesion with preservation of nervous functions, the most refined and presice definition of the anatomical features of an area affected by pathological processes which displace and distort nervous and muscular structures is desirable. The features of CT are spatial resolution and density measurement. The element which allows the identification of a single anatomical structure inside an area is the specific density of adipose tissue interposed in thin hypodense layers between muscles, expanding lesions, and vessels. CT allows the collection of three-dimensional data about the shape and anatomical relationships of masses with peripheral nerves and vessels. Of invaluable help to the surgeon is knowledge of the exact diameter of pathological processes. Comparing the pathological area with the corresponding contralateral normal anatomy is of help here.

Neurogenic tumors are classically masses of solid density, above 30 HU, because of the presence of dense bundles of collagen. Some authors have reported lower density values [1, 2, 4], in some instances even lower than -40 HU. Kumar et al. [3] have presented five pathological factors which may explain this variability: the percentage of Schwann's cells rich in lipids, the presence of adipocytes for transformation of fibroblasts in neurofibromas, the adhering of perineural adipose tissue in plexiform neurofibromas, the coalescence of cystic space in type B schwannomas, and the cystic degeneration secondary to necrosis in neurofibromas and neurofibrosarcomas. In our opinion, no pathological indication for differentiating among these tumors is presently obtainable from CT scans. Lipoma is another tumor which is classically diagnosed by CT scan; it is clearly delimited and has a homogeneous density from -70 to -130 HU [1].

Venous administration of contrast media allows definition of the entity of tumor vascularity and clarifies the exact location of vessels in the operative field. Also, the apparent density of nerves is reinforced by contrast media, and they are thereby more easily identified even if displaced and compressed.

The CT examination may contribute to distinguishing malignant from benign lesions. The latter have a well-defined contour and a homogeneous density while malignant lesions have shaded contours and inner areas of varying density. Neurogenic tumors, such as neurofibromas and schwannomas, are often clearly delimited lesions. Their density, slightly less than that of muscles, is homogeneous, and their shape is fusiform. All these features and their location in neurovascular bundles may strongly suggest the correct diagnosis.

In cases of traumatic peripheral nerve lesions CT is less helpful. Since the density of scar tissue does not differ from that of nerves, and both are enhanced by contrast media, nervous structures are not clearly recognized when surrounded by fibrotic processes which eliminate the hypodense adipose tissue and extend irregularly in all torn tissues. The extension of fibrosis is visualized, and its relationships to neighboring vessels and muscles are clarified.

CT data, together with electrophysiological information and clinical evaluation, give the surgeon the possibility of better understanding the problems that he will have to face during surgery, with a clear anticipation of anatomical distortions and of the consequent dangers.

References

1. Lemaitre L, Rèmy J, Saint-Michel J (1986) Masses et pseudo-masses mèdiastidales. In: Vasile N (ed) Tomodensitometrie corps entièr. Vigot, Paris, pp 91–143
2. Lemaitre L, Gosselin B, Smith M, Ramon P, Lafitte JJ, Servais B, Remy J (1982) Localisation abdominales des thymomes invasifs. J Radiol 63:485–494
3. Kumar AJ, Kuhajda P, Martinez CR, Fishmane K, Jezic DV, Siegelman SS (1983) Computed tomography of extracranial nerve sheath tumors with pathological correlation. J Comput Assist Tomogr 7:857–865
4. Naidich DP, Zerhouni EA, Siegelman SS (1984) Mediastinum: computed tomography of the thorax. Raven Press, New York

Initial Experiences with MRI in the Diagnosis of Peripheral Nerve Lesions

W. E. Braunsdorf, H. D. Kuhlendahl, F. Koschorek, and H.-P. Jensen, Kiel/FRG

Following our successful experiences with MRI in the diagnosis of soft-tissue alterations of the spine [1], we have attempted to determine whether MRI may be helpful in the preoperative diagnosis of peripheral nerve lesions.

Material and Method

Seven patients with peripheral nerve lesions were investigated by a 1.5 Tesla superconducting magnet. The following parameters were used: BO 1.5 Tesla, matrix 256×256, slice thickness 2.5–5 mm, SE technique with TR 500 ms, TE 30 ms. Two patients had a traumatic injury of the brachial plexus, three a traumatic peripheral nerve injury, and two peripheral nerve tumors. Four of the seven patients were later operated on, and MRI and surgical results were compared. A careful follow-up was carried out with postoperative clinical and electrophysiological investigations performed as preoperatively, so that the reliability of MRI diagnosis could be determined.

Results

One patient had a posttraumatic lesion of the axillar and suprascapular nerves before surgical exploration. By MRI a substantial brachial plexus lesion could not be verified. A continuous improvement was seen without operation. The second patient developed a brachial plexus lesion after resection of a cervical rib. By MRI a compressive scar could be excluded. This patient also improved without operation. Three patients with peripheral nerve injuries were investigated to confirm whether an interruption in continuity could be observed, or stump neuromas could be visualized. MRI in one of these patients verified a neurotmesis together with stump neuromas. In another, MRI confirmed the preservation of continuity of the avulsed peroneal nerve. The third of these patients had a cut median nerve; movement artifacts did not allow determination of the severity of the injured nerve. Neurinomas in two patients of the median and ulnar nerve could be visualized by MRI, including the differential diagnosis to ganglia (Figs. 1, 2). These findings were confirmed by the operation.

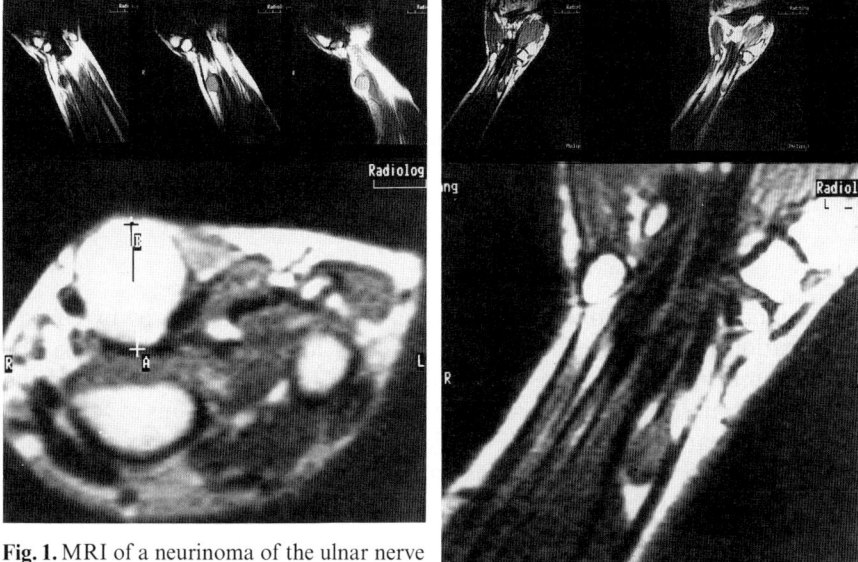

Fig. 1. MRI of a neurinoma of the ulnar nerve
Fig. 2. MRI of a neurinoma of the median nerve

Conclusion

Summarizing our initial experiences, we believe that MRI may be helpful in the preoperative diagnosis of peripheral nerve lesions, especially concerning the interruption of continuity and formation of stump neuromas and neurinomas. Further investigations must be performed to obtain better information as to the reliability of this method.

Electroneurography and electromyography are helpful in brachial plexus lesions to estimate the extension of the lesion. The decision for a surgical exploration is nevertheless problematic. In both of our patients, EMG/ENG only confirmed the results of clinical investigation. The morphological exclusion or confirmation of interruption of continuity or compressive scar formation by means of MRI is essential for planning the surgical procedure. In peripheral nerve injuries and tumors of peripheral nerves EMG and ENG are inexact for localizing the lesion and its extension and also for distinguishing between interruption and compression of the nerve. MRI by high resolution technique enables a safe distinction preoperatively.

Since the preparing of this paper we now examined further 37 patients with peripheral nerve lesions and found the above mentioned criteria.

Reference

1. Braunsdorf WE, Koschorek F, Jensen H-P (1987) MRI in complications of neurosurgical spine surgery. In: Walter W, Brandt M, Brock M, Klinger M (eds) Advances in Neurosurgery 16. Springer, Berlin Heidelberg New York Tokyo, pp 222–226

Modern Imaging Procedures in Peripheral Nerve Lesions

D. Stolke, U. Kunz, and V. Seifert, Hanover/FRG

The diagnosis of a peripheral nerve lesion should, even today, be by clinical examination means alone. However, neurophysiological procedures may be used to confirm the diagnosis and especially to reveal the precise site of the lesion. As modern imaging procedures are able to visualize lesions of very small size, and no part of the body is excluded from this new type of examination, we tried to find even small lesions causing peripheral nerve palsies. Upon palpating a space-occupying lesion or provoking pain by applying pressure to the nerve or the tissue in its immediate neighborhood, we asked our radiologist for a CT scan, MRI, ultrasound examination, or digital substraction angiography. And indeed, in these cases we could confirm a lesion interrupting or compressing the course of the peripheral nerve.

Case 1. A 26-year-old man (Fig. 1) complained of a progressive weakness in his foot. Upon examination there was tenderness in the immediate neighborhood of the head of the fibula and a weakness of the peroneal and tibialis anterior muscles. Neurophysiological examinations localized the lesion at the knee joint region. CT scan revealed a small hypodense lesion that appeared under microsurgical operation as a neurofibroma.

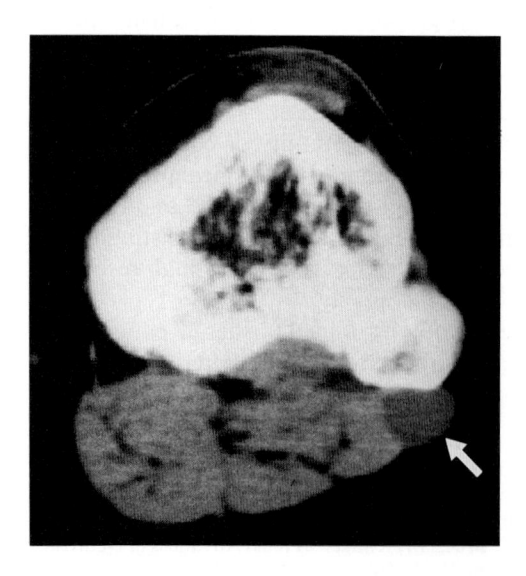

Fig. 1. Neurofibroma (*arrow*) at the head of the fibula

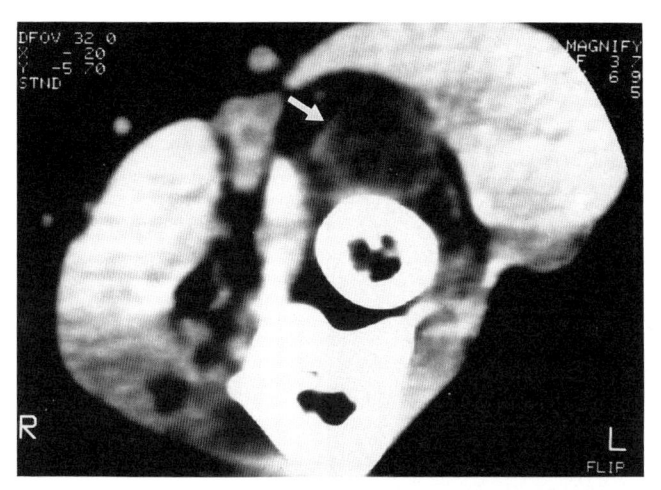

Fig. 2. Cystic space-occupying lesion (ganglion; *arrow*) causing a wristdrop syndrome

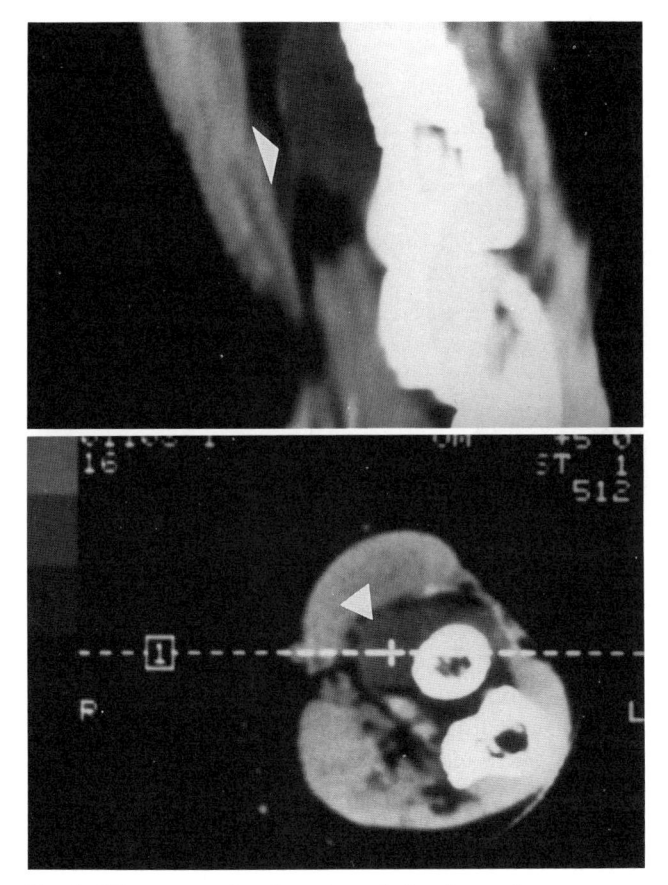

Fig. 3. CT scan reveals a hypodense lesion (*arrows*)

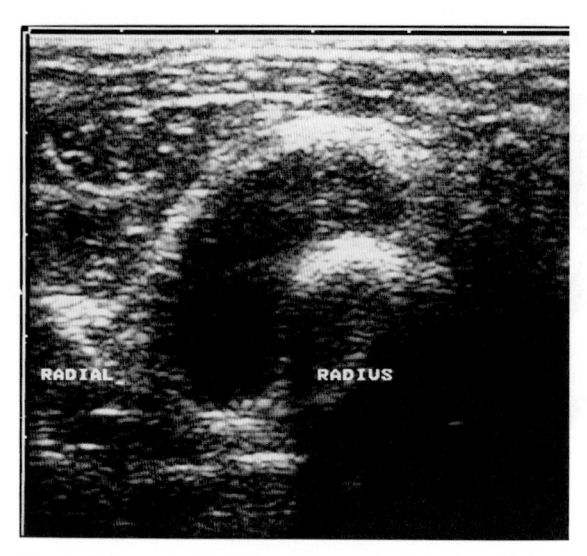

Fig. 4. Ultrasound indicates a hypoechoic lesion. (Same case as Fig. 3)

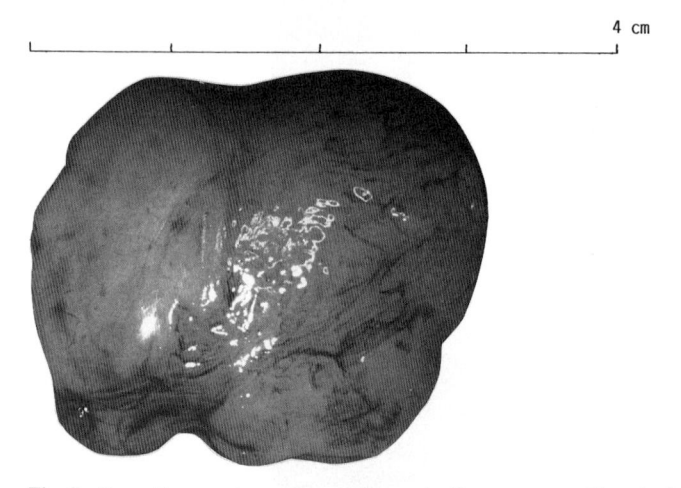

Fig. 5. Operative specimen (neurofibroma). (Same case as Figs. 3, 4)

Case 2. A 53-year-old woman (Fig. 2) complained of progressive extensor weakness of the wrist and fingers (wristdrop). On examination the radial nerve palsy could be interpreted as a supinator channel syndrome. However, as there seemed to be a certain swelling and a tenderness, we asked for a CT scan; this revealed a hypodense lesion that was confirmed by the ultrasound examination. On surgery this turned out to be a ganglion of the elbow joint.

Case 3. A 73-year-old woman (Figs. 3–5) complained of a progressive wristdrop. Once again, the patient was admitted because of a supinator channel

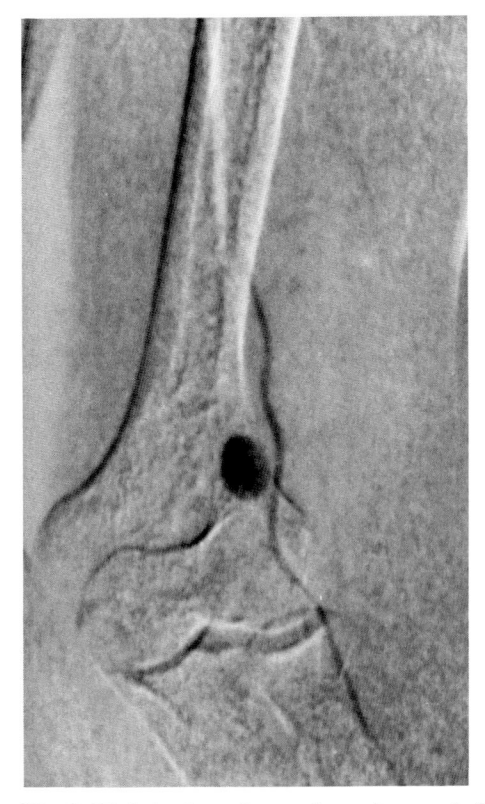

Fig. 6. Digital subtraction angiography reveals false aneurysm after brachial arteriography causing median nerve palsy

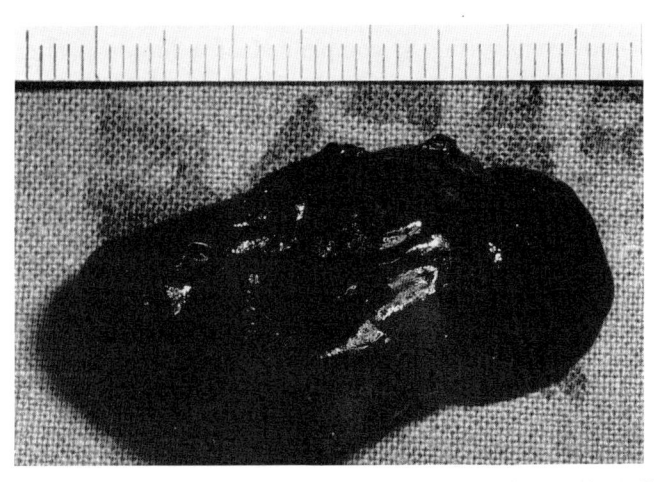

Fig. 7. Specimen of the extirpated false aneurysm. (Same case as Fig. 6)

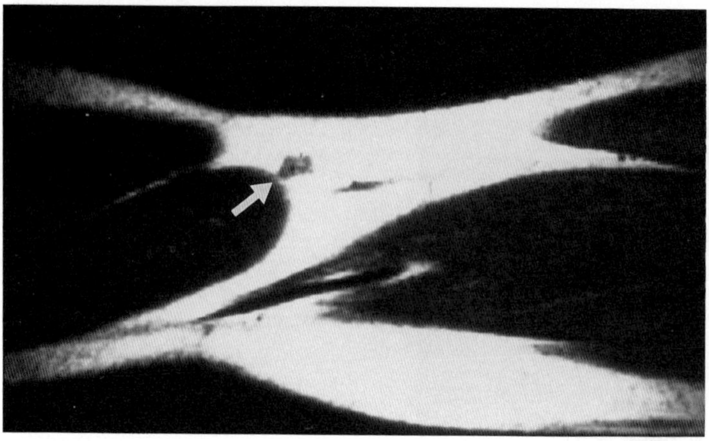

Fig. 8. MRI reveals calcified tendon of the lateral gastrocnemius muscle causing footdrop symptoms

syndrome. CT scan revealed a hypodense lesion that turned out to be a neurofibroma of the radial nerve. Under microsurgical procedure it was extirpated totally.

Case 4. A 61-year-old man (Figs. 6, 7) suffering from a coronary heart disease underwent a brachial catheterization for coronary angiography. Two days later a progressive median nerve palsy developed which was nearly complete when he arrived at our department. A digital substraction angiography revealed a false aneurysm of the brachial artery compressing the median nerve. On exploration the false aneurysm was excised, the artery wall defect sutured, and the nerve decompressed.

Case 5. A 25-year-old woman (Fig. 8) complained of a footdrop after a short walk. There was tenderness proximal to the head of the fibula. Electrophysiological examinations showed slowing of the conduction velocity in this area; MRI revealed a lesion in the tendon of the lateral gastrocnemius muscle which could be a bony lesion. On exploration the ossified part of the gastrocnemius tendon which compressed the common peroneal nerve could be excised.

We have pointed out that the diagnosis of a peripheral nerve lesion should be accomplished by clinical and neurophysiological means. Nevertheless the peripheral nerve lesion should also be diagnosed by modern imaging procedures. These procedures may provide a deeper understanding of pathophysiological problems, as they have in other fields of neurosurgery and medicine.

Acknowledgements. We thank all coworkers of the Center for Radiology for performing all imaging procedures that we needed.

References

1. Haagle JR, Altidi RJ (1983) Computed tomography of the whole body. Mosby St. Louis Toronto
2. Lissner J, Seiderer M (1987) Klinische Kernspintomographie. Enke, Stuttgart
3. Mumenthaler M, Schliack H (1977) Läsion peripherer Nerven. Thieme, Stuttgart
4. Nadimi M (1986) Digitale Subtraktionsangiographie in der Neuroradiologie. Thieme, Stuttgart New York
5. Sunderland S (1978) Nerves and nerve injuries. Churchill Livingstone, Edinburgh London New York
6. Stuhler T (1987) Ultraschalldiagnostik des Bewegungsapparates. Springer, Berlin Heidelberg New York Tokyo

Success of Sensory Evoked Potentials in Patients with Median Compression Syndrome and Additional Neuropathy

M. Conzen, R. Kramer, and F. Oppel, Bielefeld/FRG

Introduction

Conventional EMG and peripheral nerve conduction studies are common in detection of peripheral nerve lesions. In severe traumatic lesions of peripheral nerves sensory nerve action potentials may not be recordable for many weeks. In some patients additional neuropathies, such as toxic polyneuropathy, influence the interpretation of electrophysiological measurements. Sensory evoked potentials (SEP) may be used to document sensory nerve continuity when sensory nerve action potentials are unrecordable because they are too small or too desynchronized. The ability to monitor SEP in the absence of a sensory nerve action potential implies that incoming peripheral signals have been amplified within the CNS [2, 5].

Material and Methods

In our study SEP were monitored in 30 patients with carpal canal syndrome and additional neuropathy. There were 21 women and 9 men; ages ranged from 30 to 75 years with an average age of 55.3. The cause of neuropathy was uremia in 12 cases and severe diabetes mellitus in 18. Motor conduction time was first measured with a conventional EMG examination using bipolar needle electrodes. SEP were then monitored.

The median nerve was stimulated at the level of the wrist and second finger via 9 mm disc electrodes. Resistance was reduced to less than 5000 Ω by filling them with electrocardiographic solution. The anode was placed directly over or adjacent to the nerve, with the cathode placed 2–3 cm from the anode. The stimulus intensity used was equal to or greater than the sum of the sensory and motor thresholds. (We used a Schwarzer stimulator and averager.) The duration of the stimulus was 0.3 ms at a repetition rate of 4–5/s. Between 225 and 2000 stimuli were obtained for each average. The responses were stored on flexible discs and plotted on paper for review. Cortical potentials were obtained via disc electrodes located at the vertex (C_z) and referred to the linked ear electrodes and midfrontal region (F_z) [8].

In all cases we measured both nerves, the compressed and the contralateral median nerve. Two normal persons and two patients with only median compression syndrome served as controls.

Results

Our 30 patients showed all the neurological signs of carpal canal syndrome, with characteristic motor and sensory deficit and paresthesia nocturna. The additional polyneuropathy complicated the clinical and neurological symptoms. The carpal canal syndrome is diagnosed in most cases by EMG and electroneurography. A prolonged distal latency in the median nerve and a decreased sensory conduction value between the second finger and wrist, the findings proximal thereto remaining normal, are regarded as typical electroneurographic findings. In patients with polyneuropathy there are reduced motor and sensory conduction velocities (Fig. 1) [2, 6, 7].

Table 1 shows our electroneurographic findings. The motor and sensory distal latencies are characteristically prolonged, but the motor and sensory conduction velocities at the forearm are decreased. In carpal canal syndrome examination of the sensory conduction velocity is generally regarded as the more reliable method [2]. We could measure the sensory distal latency in only six cases, with a mean value of 4.1 ms. Ludin and Tackmann pointed out that the absence of an antidromic nerve action potential may not be assessed as definitely pathological [7].

SEP findings are shown in Table 2. In 26 patients the orthodromic nerve action potential could be determined. The mean value of 18 was 24.2. The four missing values are regarded as pathological.

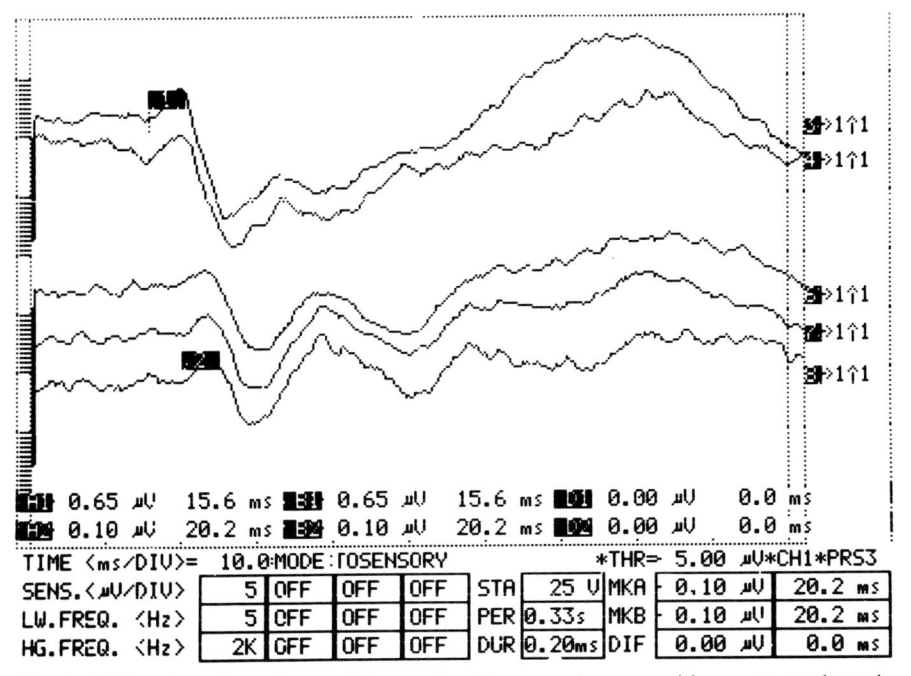

Fig. 1. SEP at the wrist and second finger of median nerve in a case with severe carpal canal syndrome and polyneuropathy

Table 1. Electroneurographic findings

	n	Mean
Motor distal latency	30	5.4 ms
Motor conduction velocity (wrist–elbow)	30	36.8 m/s
Sensory distal latency	6	4.1 ms
Sensory conduction velocity (wrist–elbow)	10	40.9 m/s

Table 2. SEP Findings

	n	Mean
Distal latency finger II	26	24.2
Wrist	30	17.6
Normal finger II	2	17.6
Normal wrist	2	16.0

Discussion

The method of SEP offers a view of physiologic anatomy to examine the peripheral nervous system and the large fiber sensory tracts in the CNS. Conventional EMG and peripheral nerve conduction studies are common in detection of peripheral compression nerve syndrome and neuropathies. In severe lesions of peripheral nerves sensory nerve action potentials may not be recordable with the conventional technique, for example, in patients with median nerve compression syndrome and severe additional neuropathy. SEP may be used in these cases to document sensory nerve function and to determine whether the sensory loss of median nerve is caused by diabetic neuropathy or by median compression syndrome at the wrist. The ability to elicit on SEP in the absence of a sensory nerve action potential, or when the potential is too small or too desynchronized, implies that incoming peripheral inputs have been amplified within the CNS [1–4]. Stimulation of the sensory median nerve at the second finger and at the wrist allows the estimation of conduction velocity by subtracting the latencies of the N 19 peaks. The values of conduction velocity are measured at the contralateral upper limb and show delays of sensory conduction in the very portion of the carpal ligament. In all cases with renal disease and diabetes mellitus we found an abnormal conduction time between wrist and brachial plexus; some patients showed an abnormal conduction time between lower medulla and cortex [9].

Neuropathies that disrupt the myelin, as in our cases, slow the conduction velocity and may reduce amplitude. Additional EMG testing is needed to determine the function of the motor units. In one case with a severe polyneuropathy we measured a motor conduction velocity at the forearm with 23 m/s and at the wrist with 12 m/s caused by additional carpal canal syndrome. The operative findings confirmed the diagnosis. On the other hand we know the distal accentuated polyneuropathy with extreme latency delay. SEP change correlates with decompression of the nerve. These findings are important when sensory nerve action potentials cannot be recorded preoperatively to secure the surgical decompression. Patients with severe polyneuropathy have a reduced capacity for nerve recovery. Therefore the postoperative results are not comparable with those of single carpal canal syndrome.

References

1. Ball GJ, Saunders MG, Schnabl J (1971) Determination of peripheral sensory nerve conduction velocities in man from stimulus response delays of the cortical evoked potentials. Electroenceph Clin Neurophysiol 30:409
2. Chiappa KH (1983) Evoked potentials in clinical medicine. Raven Press, New York
3. Cracco J, Castells S, Mark E (1980) Conduction velocity in peripheral nerve and spinal afferent pathways in juvenile diabetics. Neurology 30:370–371
4. Eisen A, Elleker G (1980) Sensory nerve stimulation and evoked cerebral potentials. Neurology 30:1097–1105
5. Greenberg RP, Ducker TB (1982) Evoked potentials in the clinical neurosciences. J Neurosurg 56:1–18
6. Ludin HP (1980) Electromyography in practice. Thieme, Stuttgart New York
7. Ludin HP, Tackmann W (1984) Polyneuropathien. Thieme, Stuttgart New York
8. Nuwer MR (1986) Evoked potential monitoring in the operating room. Raven Press, New York
9. Vaziri D, Pratt H, Saiki JK, Starr A (1981) Evaluation of somatosensory pathways by short latency evoked potentials in patients with end-stage renal disease maintained on hemodialysis. Int Y Artif Organs 4:17–22

Intraoperative Analysis of the Function of Peripheral Nerves with Sensory Evoked Potentials

R. STOBER, St. Gallen/Switzerland

Introduction

In contrast to microsurgical vascular anastomosis, in which the functional capacity of the stumps can be checked directly, nerve adaptation takes place to structures which do not allow a primary appraisal of their functional capacity. The morphological appearance of the cross-section of the nerve allows detection of fascicular structures even at low magnification, but is does not allow determination of whether axons capable of regeneration are present on the cut surface. Only electrical stimulation allows the function of the central nerve stump to be checked. It was formerly necessary that the patient reports pain, and the operation therefore had to be carried out under local anesthesia; however, today the report of pain can be replaced by the monitoring of evoked potentials, thus allowing surgery under general anesthesia. What information can be obtained intraoperatively from the nerve cross-section with this technique?

Position of the Regeneration Capacity

In principle, the intactness of the sensory conduction from the nerve cross-section to the cerebral cortex is checked with the monitoring of sensory evoked potentials. Especially in nervous reconstructions in injuries that have occurred some time in the past, the point of stimulation for the monitoring of sensory evoked potentials is often situated surprisingly far proximal to the injury site. In 14 such reconstructions of old nerve injuries (older than 1 year), the site of monitoring was more than 2 cm proximal to the cut surface of the nerve with its intact macroscopic appearance. We have retained the position of stimulability with the insertion of the sural interponates because we suspect that an optimal regeneration stimulus is applied only with trimming at this site. In almost all cases, early peripheral progress of the Hoffmann-Tinel sign is an indication that nervous regeneration has indeed commenced. The degree of return of function differs, but a complete absence of nerve regeneration was observed in only one case.

Sensorimotor Differentiation

For sensorimotor reconstruction appropriate to function, the monitoring of evoked potentials provides in principle the possibility of detecting a motor fascicle at the proximal end of the nerve by absence of the stimulus response. However, this applies only to the case in which a normal sensory evoked potential can be recorded on stimulation of the overall nerve. A second precondition is an adequate specialization of one or several fascicles, which contain mainly motor fiber components. This is the case in the median nerve especially at the level of the wrist (motor thenar branch) and in the region of the forearm before the emergence of the muscular branches for the flexor muscles.

In the ulnar nerve sensory motor fascicle differentiation is also possible in the region of the wrist, and in the radial nerve such a possibility of distinction exists at the level of the elbow, where sensory parts of the superficial radial nerve branch off from the mainly motor components. Such a differentiation requires that the nerve stump be split into several fascicles over 4–5 mm, so that single stimulation is possible without jumping over to the entire cross-section. The stimulus intensity is to be reduced accordingly. In the single-blind trial, the fascicles which do not reveal a sensory response in the evoked potentials can be isolated with a relatively high certainty with a double sequential measurement (separate operation of the stimulus electrode and the registration instrument). Anatomical orientations can help to simplify the process of measurement. Thus, for example, the radial parts of the nerve are analyzed more carefully in the median nerve at the level of the wrist than the ulnar components, since the motor fascicle for the thenar is to be expected with high probability in the radial half.

Analysis of Root Function

In brachial plexus damage, the function of the anterior root can be confirmed with intraoperative monitoring of sensory evoked potentials. Besides the decision as to the possibility of reconstruction, which depends on the given proximal connections, the decision as to whether replantation is to be carried out in tear-amputations of the upper arm also depends on the intactness of the sensory plexus root. In our opinion, the large-scale replantation of an upper arm is admissible only when there are prospects of nervous regeneration.

The monitoring of evoked potentials in the peripheral nerve reconstruction has been used 103 times at my former department, the Clinic for accident surgery, hand, plastic and reconstructive surgery of Ulm University since 1981. A sensorimotor fascicle differentiation was carried out 30 times. In these cases, there was a complete absence of return of motor function in two cases in a period of follow-up observation of 1–3 years (both cases in the ulnar nerve). Evoked potentials have been used to determine the limit of resection in old peripheral nerve injuries in 53 cases. There was complete absence of nerve regeneration in only one case postoperatively. In this case, we decided not to sacrifice a further 3 cm of nervous tissue up to the site of the stimulability of the nerve because of the length of the nerve defect to be bridged over. In 20 cases, evoked potentials have been used in reconstruction of plexus injuries. In two cases, no functional root components could be found at all, which is why we switched to an intercostal transfer. The remaining 18 plexus reconstructions all had a functional gain from the operation over a period of follow-up observation of 3–5 years.

Intraoperative monitoring of sensory evoked potentials is a measurement technique which provides intraoperative information on the functional capacity of the proximal nerve stump. With adequate consideration of this information, indications can be established more strictly, and reconstructions can be carried out with greater prospects of success.

Functional Changes of Single Motor Units After Nerve Suture*

R. Dengler, Bonn/FRG and R. B. Stein, Edmonton/Canada

It is well known that the alpha-motoneuron controls the functional properties of its motor unit (MU). A particular role is played by the motoneuron size, which is closely correlated with MU parameters such as voluntary recruitment threshold, axonal conduction velocity (CV), twitch force, and contraction speed, and muscle fiber fatigability ("size-principle" of Henneman et al. [5]). Some of these parameters can be determined in humans to be used for MU characterization [2, 6, 7].

We have studied MU recruitment thresholds, axonal CVs, and twitch forces in normal subjects and in either one patient with a resuture of a completely severed ulnar and median nerve. We were interested in the changes of these parameters in reinnervated MUs and, in particular, in whether the sprouting motoneurons were able to reestablish the above size relationships in the newly formed MUs.

Methods

The muscles studied were the first dorsal interosseus (FDI) and the abductor pollicis brevis (APB). The action potentials of single MUs were recorded by tungsten electrodes of the type used for microneurography [9]. The contraction force was measured by a virtually isometric strain gauge positioned between thumb and index finger (FDI) or at the radial aspect of the thumb (APB). The recruitment threshold for a single MU was determined as the force required to activate it and to keep it firing repetitively. Spike-triggered averaging [6] was used to assess the MU twitch forces. The associated axonal CVs were measured using a method described very recently [1, 7].

Results

Normal Subjects. Figure 1 illustrates a record obtained from a MU in the FDI. The action potential of the MU is shown in trace A during voluntary activation and in C and D in response to stimulation at the wrist and the elbow,

---

* This research was supported by the Deutsche Forschungsgemeinschaft.

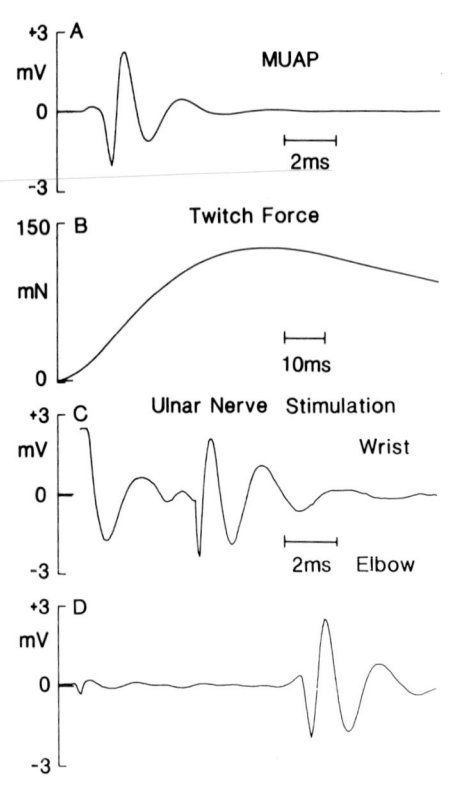

Fig. 1. A Action potential of a MU (*MUAP*) in the FDI of a normal subject during voluntary innervation. **B** Associated twitch force. **C, D** Action potential of the same MU in response to wrist (**C**) and elbow (**D**) stimulation. Note the latency difference used to calculate the axonal CV

respectively. The twitch force (B) was fairly high and corresponded well with the fast axonal CV (62 m/s) as well as with the high voluntary recruitment threshold of the MU. The CV was calculated from the distance of the stimulation sites and the latency difference of the responses in C and D. Recruitment threshold, twitch force, and axonal CV are size-related and therefore also interrelated. Figure 2 shows the relations for 11 MUs recorded in the FDI of a normal subject. Both the axonal CV and the twitch force were positively correlated with the threshold, i.e., they increased with increasing threshold in line with the "size principle" of Henneman [5].

Median Nerve Lesion. The data in Fig. 3 were obtained from a 17-year-old woman with a distal median nerve lesion at the transition from wrist to palm. The nerve was completely severed and resutured more than 2 years prior to the investigation. The result was excellent, and there was no atrophy or weakness of the thenar muscles. Eight MUs were analyzed in detail. As in normals, axonal CVs and recruitment thresholds were positively correlated although the

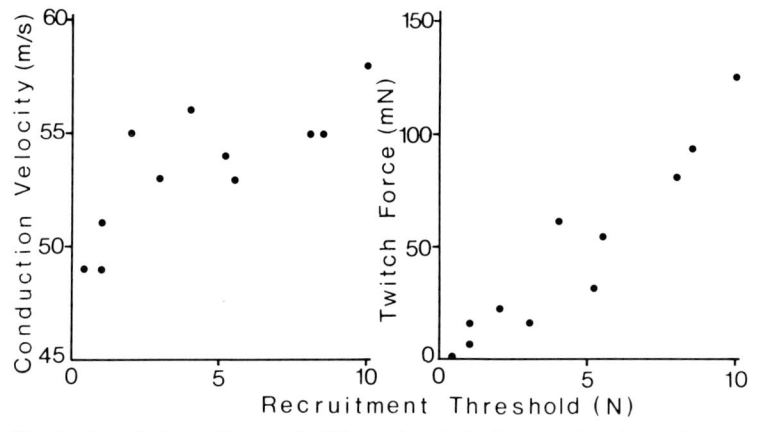

Fig. 2. Correlation of axonal CVs and twitch forces with the voluntary recruitment thresholds of 11 MUs in the FDI of a normal subject. There is a strong positive correlation in both cases

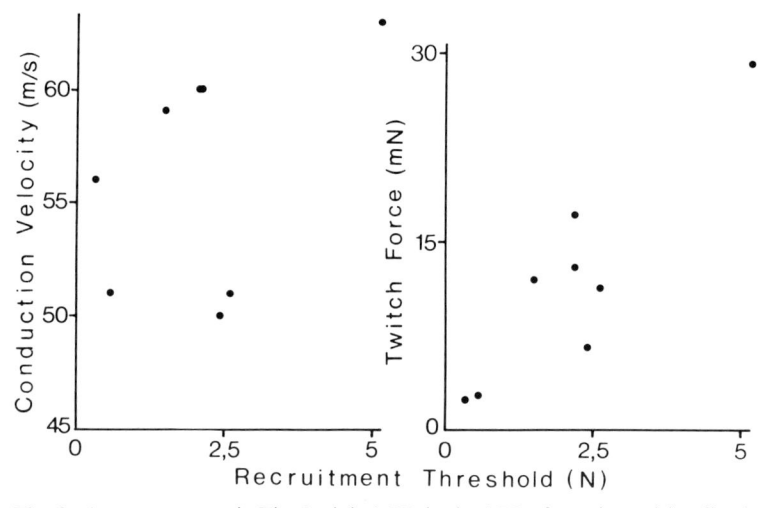

Fig. 3. Arrangement as in Fig. 2; eight MUs in the APB of a patient with a distal median nerve suture. The normal positive correlations are reestablished

values may have been somewhat more scattered. The range of the axonal CVs (50–64 m/s) was normal, as expected, because the suture was distal to the studied nerve segment. The relationship between twitch force and recruitment threshold resembled that of normal subjects. It can be concluded that the motoneurons were able to reestablish the normal size relationships in the newly formed MUs.

Ulnar Nerve Lesion. Figure 4 illustrates data from the FDI of a 52-year-old man with an ulnar nerve lesion in the elbow region. The nerve was resutured

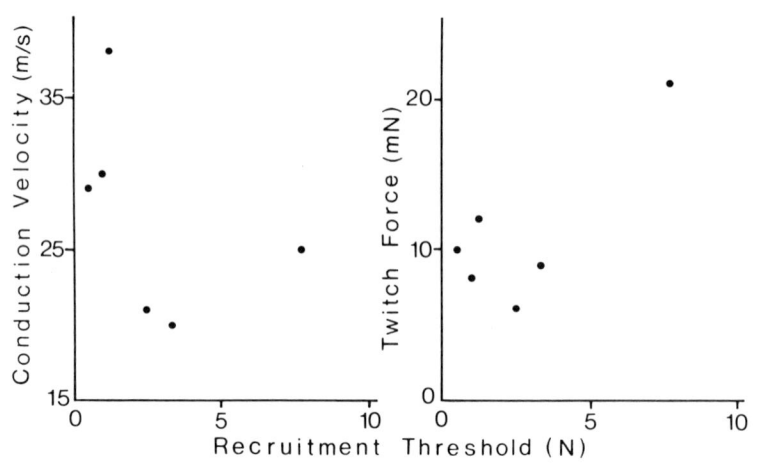

Fig. 4. Arrangement as in Fig. 2; six MUs in the FDI of a patient with an ulnar nerve suture at the elbow. Axonal CVs and twitch forces are reduced, and the normal interrelations between the MU parameters are lost

about 3 years prior to the investigation. The clinical outcome was moderate, and there was some atrophy and weakness (MRC 4) of the ulnar nerve-supplied hand muscles. Six MUs were studied in detail. The axonal CVs were greatly reduced (20–38 m/s). Recruitment thresholds and axonal CVs did not show any relationship, and the correlation between thresholds and twitch forces was only weakly positive. The twitch forces appeared to be reduced, with the highest measured value at 22 mN. Obviously, this patient with a proximal ulnar nerve lesion had a worse regeneration than the patient with the distal median nerve lesion, and the size relations of the MU parameters were not reestablished.

Discussion

The function of newly formed MUs after nerve severance and suture may be fairly normal, as observed in the case with the distal median nerve lesion. The young age of the patient and the short distance between suture and target muscles probably favored this outcome. The normal axonal CVs proximal to the suture indicate that the axons either preserved their diameters and myelin sheaths or regained them if there was any retrograde degeneration. This case also shows that motoneurons under favorable circumstances are able to reinnervate and to modify muscle fibers in such a way that the newly formed MUs develop the normal size relationships [4] necessary for well-coordinated movements.

The case with the proximal ulnar nerve lesion illustrates the obstacles to such a favorable outcome. The longer distance between the lesion site and the target muscles and perhaps the older age of the patient may have played a role. The slowed axonal CVs probably indicate reduced axonal diameters and/or poor remyelination. The reduced twitch forces cannot be accounted for only by a bias in selection but are likely to point to a diminished number of muscle fibers per MU. As a consequence of the above changes, the normal interrelations between the MU parameters were not reestablished, and their value as measures of motoneuron size was restricted. The size relationship may have been further obscured by misdirection of the growing axons which could reinnervate their original as well as other ulnar nerve supplied muscles, as known from animal studies [3]. The impact of axonal misdirection has been investigated and discussed very recently in great detail by Thomas et al. [8]. This explains why patients with ulnar nerve lesion frequently do not regain sufficient control of their hand muscles even if they had good reinnervation.

In conclusion, modern surgical techniques have greatly improved the chances for nerve regeneration and muscle reinnervation. A problem that remains unresolved, however, is axonal misdirection. Intensive research in this area is necessary if nerve regeneration is to result in satisfying movement control also in more proximal lesions.

Acknowledgement. The study was carried out at the Department of Physiology of the University of Alberta, Edmonton, Canada.

References

1. Dengler R, Stein RB, Thomas CK (1988) Axonal conduction velocity and force of single human motor units. Muscle & Nerve 11:136–145
2. Freund HJ, Büdingen HJ, Dietz V (1975) Activity of single motor units from human forearm muscles during voluntary isometric contractions. J Neurophysiol 38:933–946
3. Gillespie MJ, Gordon T, Murphy PR (1986) Reinnervation of the lateral gastrocnemius and soleus muscles in the rat by their common nerve. J Physiol (Lond) 372:485–500
4. Gordon T, Stein RB (1982) Reorganization of motor-unit properties in reinnervated muscles of the cat. J Neurophysiol 48:1175–1190
5. Henneman E, Somjen G, Carpenter DO (1965) Functional significance of cell size in spinal motoneurons. J Neurophysiol 28:560–580
6. Milner-Brown HS, Stein RB, Yemm R (1973) The contractile properties of human motor units during voluntary isometric contraction. J Physiol (Lond) 228:280–306
7. Stein RB, Dengler R (1986) A method to measure motor axon conduction velocity in man. J Neurosci Meth 17:229–230
8. Thomas CK, Stein RB, Gordon T, Lee RG, Elleker MG (1987) Patterns of reinnervation and motor unit recruitment in human hand muscles after complete ulnar and median nerve section and resuture. J Neurol Neurosurg Psychiat 50:259–268
9. Vallbo AB, Hagbarth KE, Torebjörk HE, Wallin BG (1979) Somatosensory, proprioceptive and sympathetic activity in human peripheral nerves. Physiol Rev 59:919–957

Outcome of Clinical Function in Relation to Motor, Sensory Nerve Conduction, Somatosensory Evoked Potentials and EMG After Suture of Median and Ulnar Nerves

W. Tackmann, Höxter/FRG

Introduction

The relationship between results of electrophysiological examinations on human nerves during the course of regeneration after a traumatic transection and suture or grafting have shown disappointing results. In the majority of papers concerning this subject only results of parameters of motor nerve fibres were given, since sensory nerve action potentials generally could not be recorded. This was due mainly to the inappropriate recording techniques used in these studies. Therefore no correlations between clinical and electrophysiological results were found. Only Buchthal and Kühl (1979) were able to show a correlation between the recovery of tactile sensibility and the increase in cumulative amplitude of the sensory nerve action potential over a period of 40 months after suture. They examined three patients, two children and one young adult. Two patients had a primary suture, and the third was grafted.

In the present study 46 nerves from 42 patients were examined clinically and electrophysiologically 4–59 months after nerve repair. All the patients had a transection of median or ulnar nerves or both near the level of the wrist. Of the 46 nerves, 24 were primarily sutured, 8 had a secondary suture, and 14 were grafted.

The following electroneurographical parameters were studied: distal motor latency, amplitude of evoked muscle action potentials, sensory nerve conduction velocity, maximum amplitude, and cumulative amplitude.

In addition, somatosensory evoked potentials (SSEP) were studied. The results from these examinations were compared with data obtained from examinations of the healthy side. By means of needle electromyography spontaneous activity, mean duration of motor unit action potentials, incidence of polyphasic potentials, and pattern during full effort were studied. Sensory recovery was scaled using the schedule of Nicholson and Seddon (1957); furthermore, two-point discrimination was tested. Methods have been described elsewhere in detail (Tackmann et al. 1983, 1985). An example of electrophysiological results is presented in Fig. 1.

Results

Distal motor latencies could not be recorded in two nerves; they were normal in three nerves. In the other 41 nerves there was a prolongation up to more than

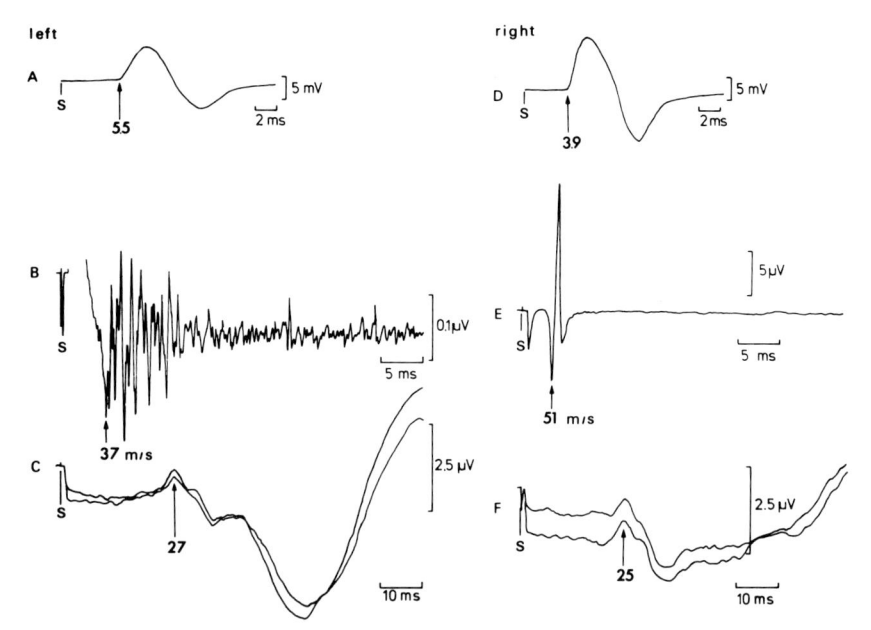

Fig. 1 A–F. Electrophysiological results in a 23-year-old patient 24 months after primary suture of the left median nerve. **A, D** Distal motor latencies. **B, E** Sensory conduction. **C, F** SSEP. **A–C** left. **D–F** Right

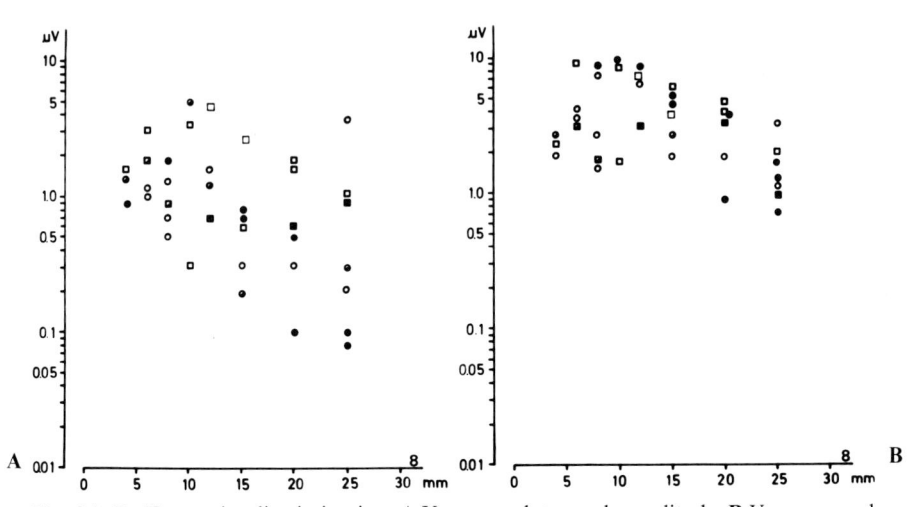

Fig. 2 A, B. Two-point discrimination. **A** Versus peak-to-peak amplitude. **B** Versus cumulative amplitude

300% compared with the healthy side. Amplitudes of evoked muscle action potentials ranged from 50 µV to 19 mV, which was 1%–109% of that of the control side. Maximum sensory nerve conduction velocities were 21–50 m/s, 38%–100% of the healthy side. Maximum amplitudes of sensory nerve action potentials ranged from 0.08 µV to 5 µV – 0.8%–28% of the control side. These values increased significantly with time after operation. This relationship was more pronounced for the cumulative amplitude, which ranged from 0.74 to 9.5 µV – the equivalent of 4.4%–90.5% of the control side. Needle electromyography showed spontaneous activity in 36 of 46 muscles. A complete loss of voluntary muscle activity was seen in two muscles, 8 and 27 months, respectively, after grafting. Motor unit potentials were normal in only three extremities.

Comparing electrophysiological data with clinical results, there was a significant relationship between two-point discrimination grade in the sensibility score of Nicholson and Seddon (1957) and maximum amplitude of sensory nerve action potentials. This relation was more pronounced when comparing clinical data with results obtained for the cumulative amplitude of sensory nerve action potentials as seen in Fig. 2.

Despite a statistically significant correlation this relationship was not very strong. Therefore, we consider electrophysiological results to be inappropriate predictors for the degree of clinical recovery.

SSEP may be helpful in demonstrating regeneration when neither sensory nor evoked muscle action potentials can be recorded. However, care must be taken not to confuse early components with activity from other nerves.

References

Buchthal F, Kühl V (1979) Nerve conduction, tactile sensibility, and the electromyogram after suture or compression of peripheral nerve. A longitudinal study in man. J Neurol Neurosurg Psychiat 42:436–451
Nicholson OR, Seddon HJ (1957) Nerve repair in civil practice. Br Med J 2:1065–1071
Tackmann W, Brennwald J, Nigst H (1983) Sensory electroneurographic parameters and clinical recovery of sensibility in sutured human nerves. J Neurol 229:195–206
Tackmann W, Kaeser HE, Nigst H, Pfeiffer P, Brennwald J, Gloor D (1985) Motorische, sensible elektroneurographische und elektromyographische Resultate sowie somatosensorisch evozierte Potentiale im Vergleich mit klinischen Befunden nach Nervennaht. Fortschr Neurol Psychiat 53:123–133

Intraoperative Somatosensory Evoked Potential Diagnoses in Brachial Plexus Lesions

P. MAILÄNDER, E. SCHALLER, M. MÖCKEL, A. BERGER, and G. F. WALTER, Hannover/FRG

The evaluation of the brachial plexus by the aid of somatosensory evoked potential (SSEP) monitoring was first described by Zalis et al. in 1970 and Zverina and Kredba as well as Rosen et al. in 1977. In 1984 Sugioka reported on the importance of SSEP monitoring in distinguishing between traction lesions distal and proximal to the dorsal root ganglia in the operating room.

We compared the SSEP of a root or nerve fascicle with the histological picture of the central nerve stump, as a morphological correlate to the electrophysiological findings. Since 1985 we have examined 37 patients with brachial plexus lesions by intraoperative SSEP recording. We used 0.1 ms rectangular stimulation with 0.5–13 mA stimulus and 3–5 Hz frequency by a signal processor DISA 2000 N. To exclude distant field potentials we used an analysis time of only 10–50 ms and tried to isolate the bipolar electrode against the situs by India rubber. High- and low-pass filters were set 2 kHz and 20 Hz. Reactions were averaged over 50–200 stimuli. The SSEPs were recorded by locating the active electrode in the skin of the contralateral somatosensory evoked point (CP_3 or CP_4) and the reference electrode at the midfrontal area (Fz). For monitoring the effect of anesthesia on SSEP and checking the system we used the stimulation of the intact contralateral median or ulnar nerve. The principles involved here are illustrated by two clinical examples.

The first case is that of a 23-year-old who experienced complete paralysis of his right arm after a motorcycle accident with rupture of the subclavian artery and the AC joint. Four months after the trauma the brachial plexus was dissected, and we found an infraclavicular lesion with a rupture of all three fascicles (Fig. 1). After the dissection we stimulated the axillary nerve and

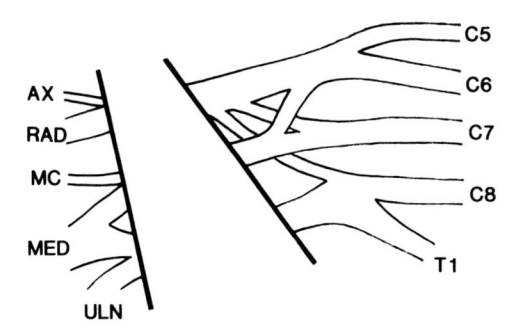

Fig. 1. Situs of case 1

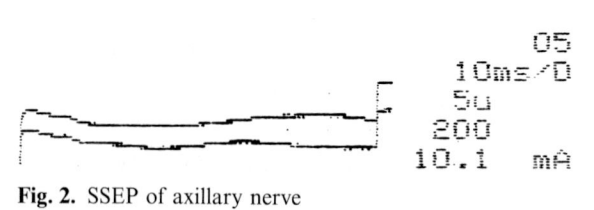

Fig. 2. SSEP of axillary nerve

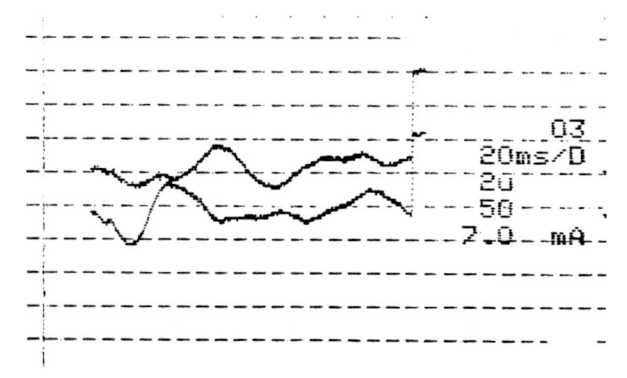

Fig. 3. SSEP of a neuroma in the dorsal fascicle

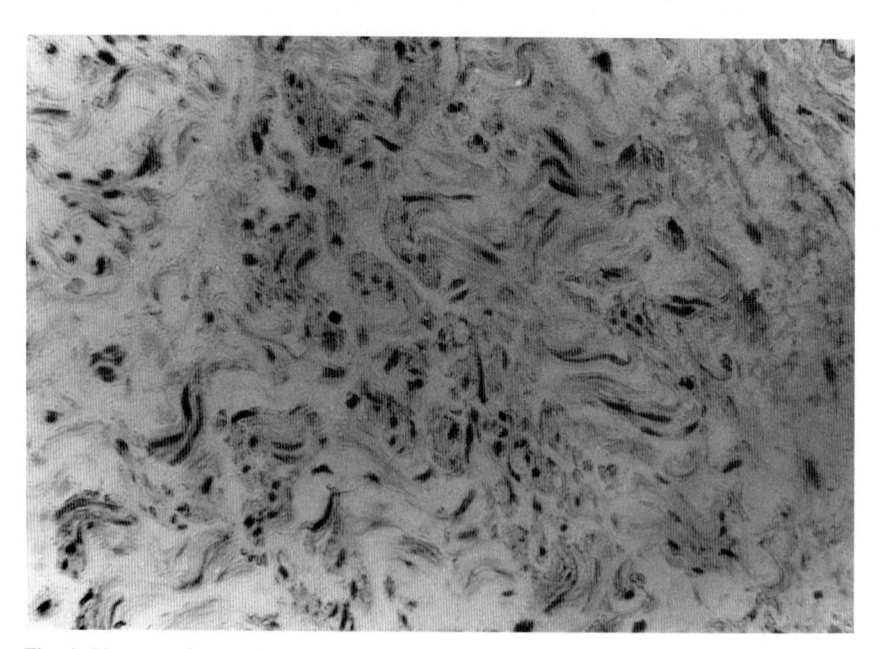

Fig. 4. Neuroma in the dorsal fascicle. (Trichrome; ×400)

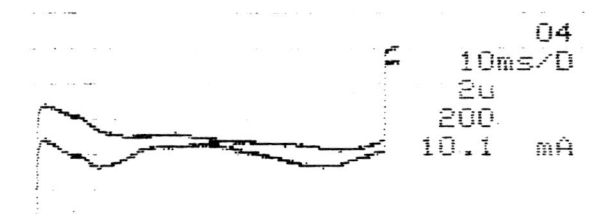

Fig. 5. SSEP of the proximal stump of dorsal fascicle after the resection of the neuroma

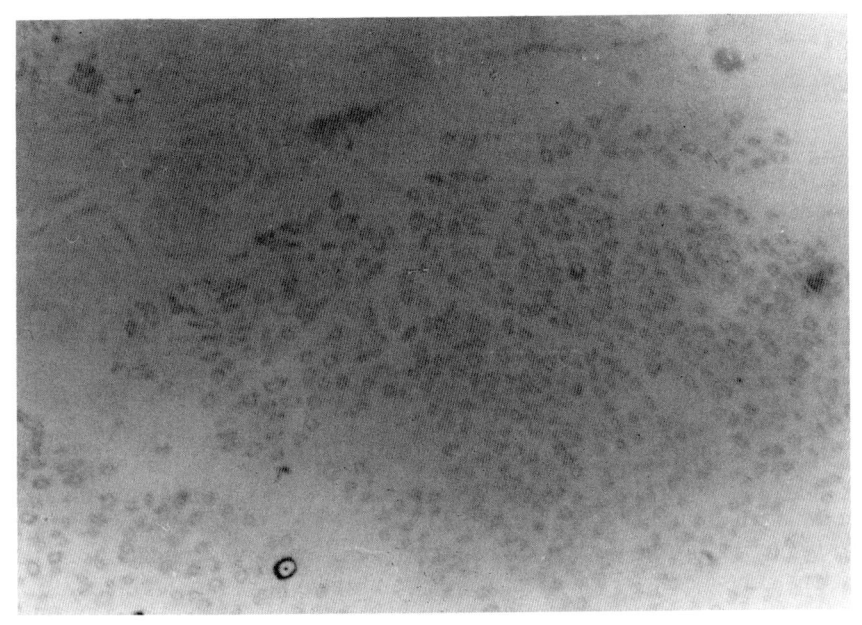

Fig. 6. Sufficient density of neurons in the proximal stump of the dorsal fascicle. (Semithin; ×800)

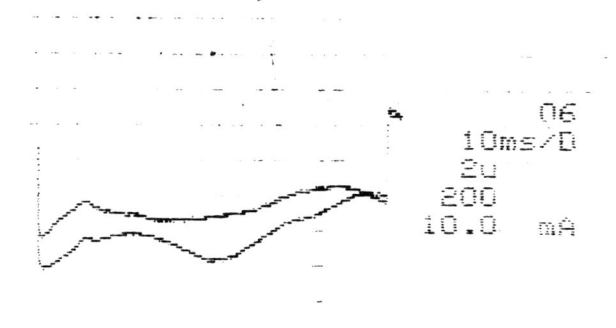

Fig. 7. SSEP of the medial fascicle

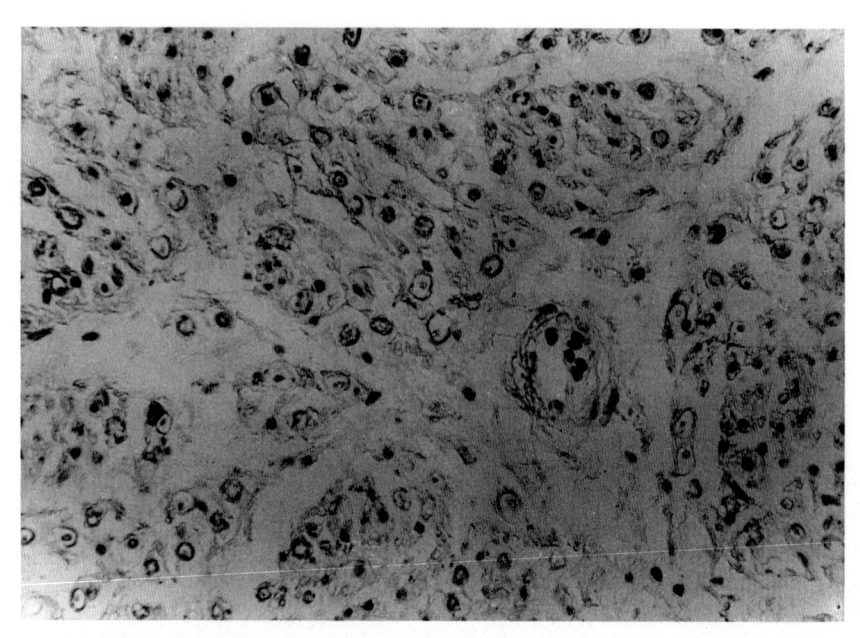

Fig. 8. Nearly normal structure in the medial fascicle. (Trichrome; ×800)

obtained no reproducible SSEP (Fig. 2). We then stimulated the proximal stump of the dorsal fascicle, again without reproducible potential (Fig. 3). By histology we found a neuroma (Fig. 4) which was resected. Then, 2 cm more proximal we found a reproducible SSEP (Fig. 5) in the dorsal fascicle. The corresponding histological picture showed a fascicle with particularly intact neurons (Fig. 6). In the medial fascicle we also found a reproducible SSEP (Fig. 7) and a nerve stump with particularly intact neurons (Fig. 8). The reconstruction was done by nerve grafts to the median and musculocutaneous nerve and by a vascularized ulnar nerve graft to the radial nerve.

The second case is that of a 22-year-old who suffered rupture of the AC joint and a complete paralysis of the brachial plexus as the result of a

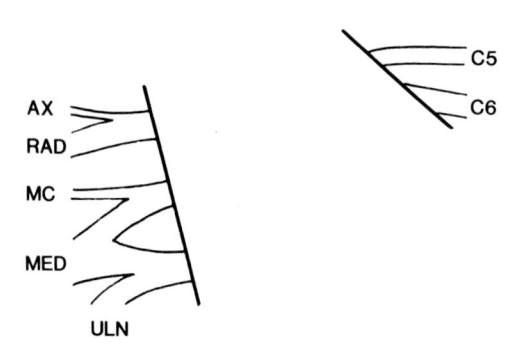

Fig. 9. Situs of case 2

Fig. 10. SSEP of C 5

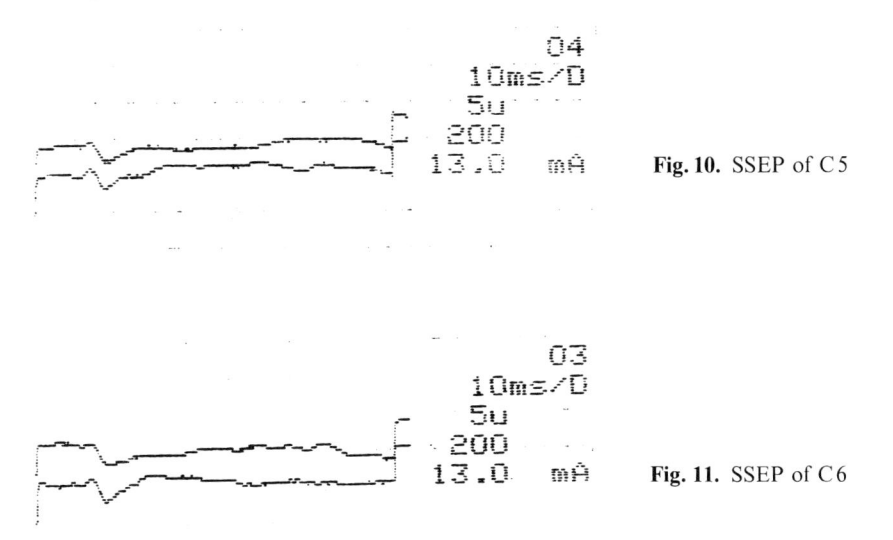

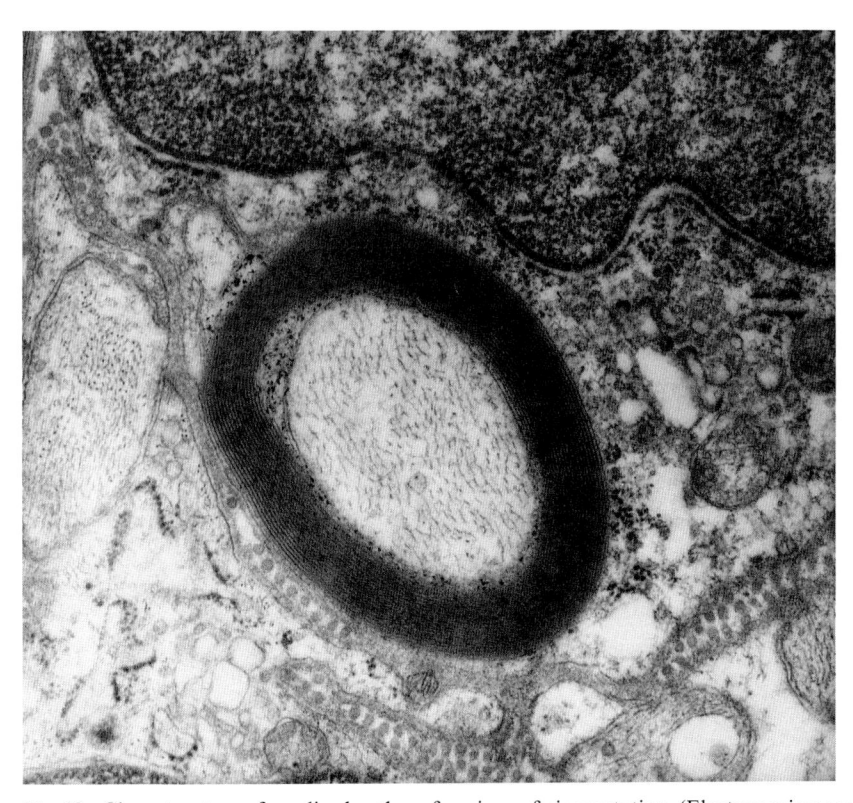

Fig. 11. SSEP of C 6

Fig. 12. Clear structure of myelin sheaths, a few signs of pigmentation. (Electron microscopy; ×31 500)

motor cycle accident. Five months after the trauma the brachial plexus was dissected, and we found a rupture of the roots C 5 and C 6 and an avulsion of C 7, C 8, and T 1 (Fig. 9). The SSEPs in the roots C 5 and C 6 were reproducible (Figs. 10, 11). Electron microscopy of the proximal nerve stumps in C 5 and C 6 showed myelinated fibers of intact neurons (Fig. 12).

In our opinion, intraoperative SSEP monitoring can help provide objective information about the quality of a proximal nerve stump in addition to the subjective judgement of the surgeon under the operating microscope. By histology a morphological control of the SSEP is possible.

References

Berger A, Zaunbauer W, Ganglberger J, Meissl G (1976) Die Computersensometrie als eine objektive Untersuchung der Sensibilität im Fingerbereich. Handchirurgie 8:3–5

Rosen I, Sörnäs R, Elmqvist D (1977) Cervical root avulsion – electrophysiological analysis with electrospinogram. Scand J Plast Reconstr Surg 11:247–250

Schröder JM (1983) Degeneration und Regeneration nach Plexus brachialis-Verletzungen. In: Hase U, Reulen HJ (eds) Läsionen des Plexus brachialis. De Gruyter, Berlin New York, p 65

Sugioka H, Tsuyama N, Hara T, Nagana A, Tachibana S, Ochiai N (1982) Investigation of brachial plexus injuries by intraoperative cortical somatosensory evoked potentials. Arch Orthop Traumat Surg 99:143–151

Sugioka H (1984) Evoked potentials in the investigation of traumatic lesions of the peripheral nerve and the brachial plexus. Clin Orthop Rel Res 184:85–92

Sugioka H (1986) Electrodiagnosis in evaluation of traction lesions of brachial plexus. Peripheral Nerve Repair and Regeneration 1:53–58

Zalis AW, Oester YT, Rodriquez AA (1970) Electrophysiologic diagnosis of cervical nerve root avulsion. Arch Phys Med Rehabil 51:708–710

Zverina E, Kredba J (1977) Somatosensory cerebral evoked potentials in diagnosing brachial plexus injuries. Scand J Rehabil Med 9:47–54

Postoperative Changes in Nerve Conduction Times After Neurolysis of the Distal Median Nerve

S. A. Rath, H. J. Klein, A. Kühn, and V. Wippermann, Günzburg/FRG

Introduction

The median nerve conduction velocity and particularly the delayed distal latency of the muscular response potential (DML, distal motor latency) constitute – in addition to the clinical symptoms – the electrophysiological confirmation of carpal tunnel syndrome [2, 3, 6]. Since, however, a clinically relevant carpal tunnel syndrome in need of surgical therapy may also be found with normal nerve conduction times, DML is only an additional diagnostic measure secondary to the clinical signs [1, 4]. Furthermore, neurophysiological methods do not permit the differentiation of patients by those suited for conservative treatment and those who must be operated on. It is also not possible to derive any prognostic statements from the preoperative measurements [4].

Concerning the postoperative measurements, Sunderland reported that abnormal distal latencies persist long after motor and sensory functions have recovered completely [5]. Nevertheless, there is no differentiated analysis of changes in latency and their correlation to clinical findings pre- and postoperatively. This study was therefore performed with the objective of comparing the early postoperative measurements of DML and the amplitude of the muscular response potential with the preoperative values and the pre- and postoperative findings, because this permitted an intra-individual correlation.

Material and Methods

From 1 January 1987 to 30 August 1987, 60 patients undergoing surgical decompression for carpal tunnel syndrome were examined immediately prior to the procedure as well as 14 days postoperatively. The DML and the amplitude of the muscular response potential (MRP) were measured both times. The patients were 17 men and 43 women, aged 25–81 years; the average age of the women was 53 years and that of the men was 52. The operation was performed 39 times on the right and 21 times on the left side.

Results

All patients were free of pain after surgery. With regard to DML, a complete conduction block was found in five cases postoperatively. Four of these had

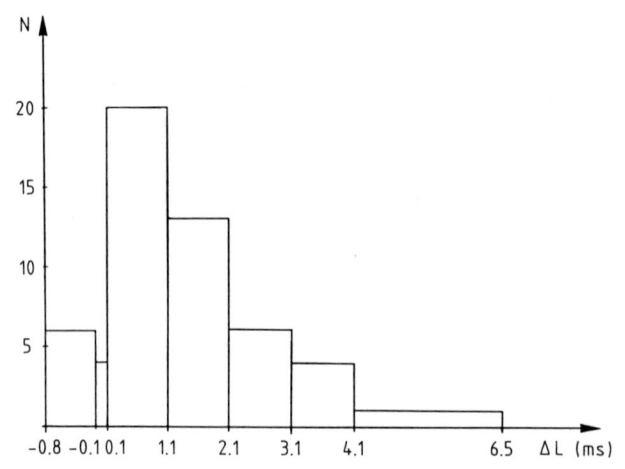

Fig. 1. Changes in DML of the median nerve 2 weeks after surgical decompression of carpal tunnel syndrome ($n = 54$)

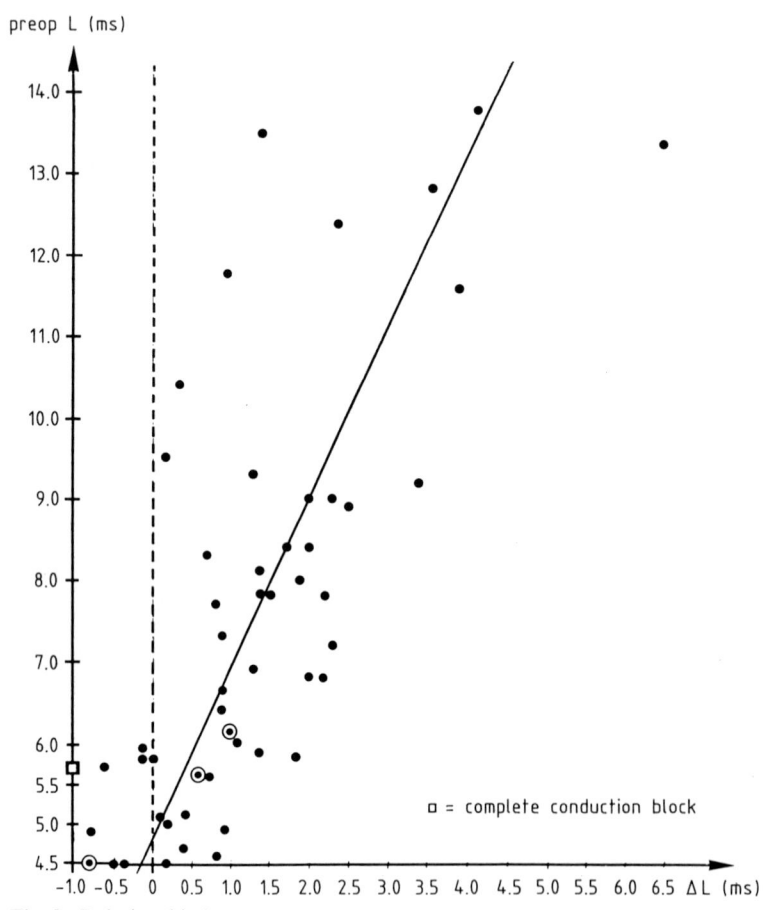

Fig. 2. Relationship between preoperative prolongation of DML and changes in conduction velocity 2 weeks after surgical decompression

existed preoperatively, and one was new. In one patient with a complete conduction block before the operation, a muscular action potential (7.8 ms) was again elicited postoperatively.

Thus there were 54 pre- and postoperative nerve conduction times available for comparison (Fig. 1). Concerning the reproducible accuracy of measurement, Hopf et al. [2] assumed a range of 0.2 ms, so that a difference in the pre- versus postoperative latency between -0.1 and $+0.1$ was considered an unchanged finding ($n = 4$). Four further patients were also unchanged, because they had a conduction block both pre- and postoperatively. An improvement in DML of 0.2–1.1 ms was observed in 20 patients and a reduction of 1.2–2.1 ms in 13 patients. Six cases showed an improvement of 2.2–3.1 ms, four cases of 3.2–4.1 ms, and one case of 6.5 ms. In six patients there was a delay of the postoperative DML (from -0.2 to -0.8 ms), and one patient with a preoperative latency of 5.7 ms had a complete nerve conduction block after surgery. It should be noted that a postoperative deterioration occurred only

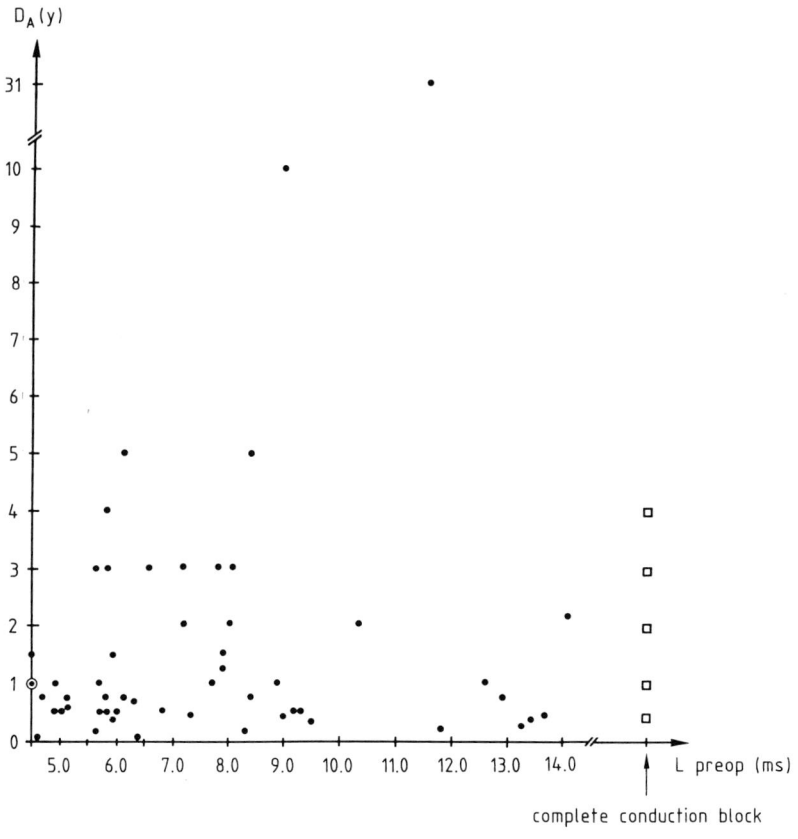

Fig. 3. Relationship between preoperative duration of disturbances (D_A) in years and preoperative DML

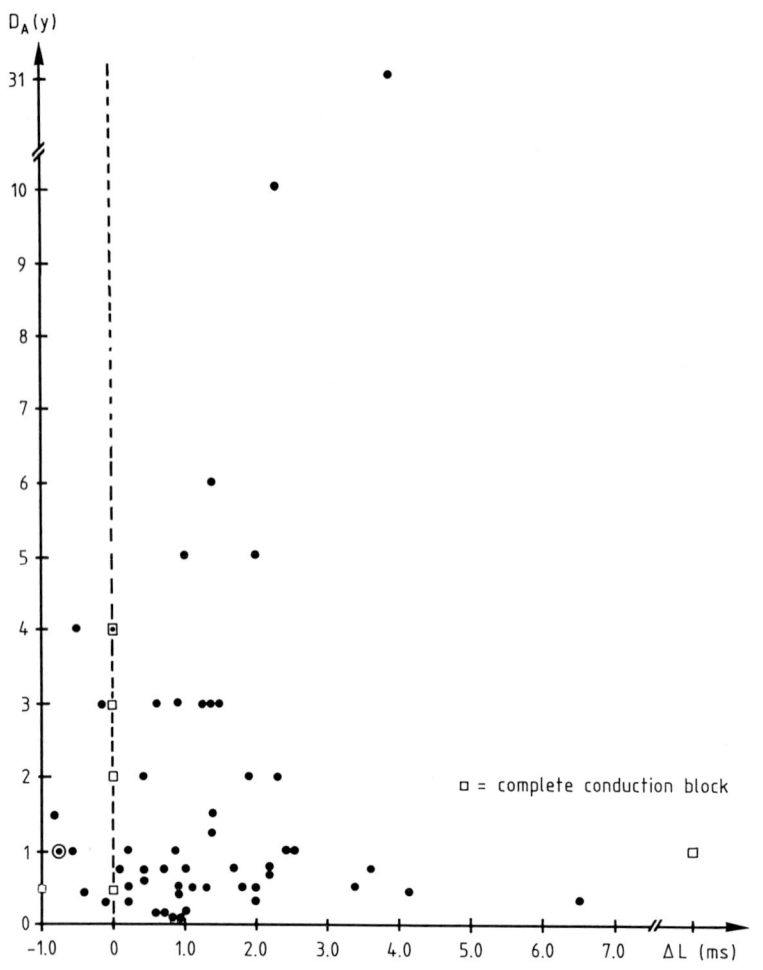

Fig. 4. Relationship between duration of disturbances (D_A) in years to changes in DML 2 weeks after surgical decompression, with regard to precondition conduction velocity

with preoperative values below 5.9 ms. The longer the preoperative latency, the better was the postoperative improvement of latency on average (Fig. 2).

There was no correlation between the history of disease duration and preoperative latency (Fig. 3), nor between history of disease duration and postoperative changes in latency (Fig. 4). The correlation between postoperative improvement of latency and preoperative clinical findings shows the least average improvement of latency (0.9 ms) in those patients who complained only of pain (SD 0.78; $n = 10$). With additional sensory impairment, the average improvement of latency was 1.25 ms (SD 1.25; $n = 21$), and with both motor and sensory impairment the improvement was rather distinct with 1.35 ms (SD 1.64; $n = 21$). Patients with medium to severe motor impairment

($n = 17$) had an average improvement of latency of 1.45 ms (SD 1.8). The average improvement of latency in all patients was 1.23 ms (SD 1.35).

In contrast to the report by Sunderland [5], a correlation was found with regard to the tendency for the regression of neurological impairment and the postoperative changes in latency. Thus, patients who showed no further impairments postoperatively had an average improvement in latency of 1.0 ms (SD 0.92). If the impairment was distinctly improved, the latency was 1.85 ms (SD 1.87) on average and 0.67 ms (SD 0.66) if the condition was unchanged (Table 1).

Table 1. Preoperative DML and DML improvement in relation to change in preexisting neurological deficits after 2 weeks

Neurological deficits	n	Preoperative DML (mean)	DML improvement (mean)
Complete recovery	19	6.5	1.02
Marked improvement	18	9.0	1.85
Unchanged	7	7.5	0.67

The behavior of the postoperative amplitude of the muscular response potential can be characterized as follows, relative to the changes in latency. If the postoperative amplitude was lower by more than half the preoperative amplitude, the average improvement in latency was 0.6 ms ($n = 16$). If the postoperative amplitude was 0.5 – 2 times the initial value ($n = 19$), the improvement in latency was 1.1 ms, and if the postoperative amplitude was more than twice as great, the average improvement in latency was 2.7 ms ($n = 13$).

Conclusion

DML in its intra-individual pre- and postoperative follow-up generally permits the observation of an improvement synchronous with the favorable clinical outcome. In those cases with preoperatively only slight augmentation of DML this electrophysiological improvement may be lacking in the early postoperative phase. This fact accords with the findings of some authors that clinically impressive pictures of carpal tunnel syndrome may have normal range latency values. Sunderland assumes an intra-individual prolongation of DML from primarily extraordinary low values in those just above normal value range [5]. In this sense in patients with preoperatively only moderate increased latency the decompression effect is less accentuated than the intermediate worsening caused by soft-tissue swelling and surgical manipulation. The more prolonged the preoperative distal latency, the more pronounced the early postoperative latency improvement became and with it the immediate net effect of the surgical decompression itself.

References

1. Goodgold J, Eberstein A (1977) Electrodiagnosis of neuromuscular diseases. Williams & Wilkins, Baltimore, pp 114–118
2. Hopf HC (1974) Elektromyographie. Thieme, Stuttgart, pp 119–127
3. Hudson A, Berry H, Mayfield F (1982) Chronic injuries of peripheral nerves by entrapment. In: Youmans JR (ed) Neurological surgery, vol. 4. Saunders, Philadelphia, London, Toronto, Mexico City, Sydney, Tokyo, pp 2430–2474
4. Leblhuber F, Reisecker F, Witzmann A (1985) Zur Frage elektrodiagnostischer Veränderungen in bezug auf die Schwere morphologischer Veränderungen beim Karpaltunnelsyndrom. In: Hohmann D (ed) Neuroorthopädie III. Springer, Berlin Heidelberg New York Tokyo, pp 332–336
5. Sunderland S (1978) Nerves and nerve injuries. Churchill Livingstone, Edinburgh London New York, pp 718–721
6. Thomas JE, Lambert EH, Csenz KA (1967) Electrodiagnostic aspects of the carpal tunnel syndrome. Archs Neurol (Chicago) 16:635–641

Outcome of Traumatic Peripheral Neuromas After Microsurgical Procedure

S. BEL and B. L. BAUER, Marburg/FRG

The successful treatment of symptomatic neuroma belongs to one of the most difficult and controversial chapters in the neurosurgical therapy of peripheral nerve injuries. Since the early nineteenth century when neuromas were described for the first time by Oldier their pathophysiology and therapy have been intensively investigated. Therapeutic viewpoints and possibilities of treatment have changed and developed in recent decades, but as yet there exists no reliable, generally applicable method for the elimination of symptomatic neuromas.

To date, more than 100 different physical and chemical methods have been tried. One can subdivide these methods into six groups according to localization:

1. Local operations: (a) simple resection of neuroma [3, 7, 8, 13, 24]; (b) exposition and transfer into healthy tissue [1, 21], for instance, into bones, as practiced by Gluck in 1880 [17]; (c) local injections into the neuroma with alcohol [8, 12], formaldehyde [1, 7, 20, 35, 36], gentian violet [7, 36], or corticosteroids [6, 32, 34, 35]; (d) treatment of the nerve endings with tantalum [1, 36, 40] or plastic caps [6, 13, 16, 31]; (e) renewed amputation of the stump [31].
2. Plexus resection; for example, Livingstone's plexus brachial resection in the case of amputation neuroma in the upper arm [25].
3. Tract operations and operations on the spinal cord: for example, rhizotomy [15, 33, 40] and chordotomy or commissural myelotomy [18, 26, 39, 40].
4. Brain operations: by stereotactic operations the pain tracks can be interrupted at various levels, for instance, at the Thalamus and postcentral gyrus [39, 40].
5. Operations on the vegetative system: Sympathetic blockade or sympathicectomy [18, 40].
6. Peripheral electrostimulation: based on the principle of the "gate-control therapy" by Melzack and Wall [28].

Although these alternative therapeutic methods exist, there is no one method at the present time which can be generally recommended.

In the Neurosurgical Clinic at the University of Marburg seven posttraumatic neuromas have been treated (Table 1). Two of these were neuromas of the median nerve of the hand after splinter and cut injuries; two were

Table 1. Seven cases of posttraumatic neuroma

Patient no.	Age (years)	Cause	Location	Operation	Outcome
1	25	Cut injury to the wrist	Median nerve	Neurolysis, scar excision	Unchanged
2	33	Cut injury to the wrist	Ulnar nerve	1. Neurolysis, scar excision, alcohol injection; resection	Unchanged
3	46	Traumatic amputation of the thigh	Ischiadic nerve	Neurolysis, scar excision, alcohol injection	Unchanged
4	31	Splinter injury to the wrist	Radial nerve	Neurolysis, scar excision, electrocoagulation; resection 2×	Unchanged
5	18	Cut injury to the wrist	Radial nerve	Resection, implantation in the bone, alcohol injection, scar excision	Unchanged
6	30	Splinter injury to the wrist	Median nerve	Neurolysis, scar excision, alcohol injection	Excellent
7	57	Knee contusion	Peroneal nerve	Resection, scar excision	Improvement

neuromas of the radial nerve, also in the hand after a cut injury. The amputation neuromas were those of the ischiadic nerve after a traumatic leg amputation; one was a neuroma of the common peroneal nerve in the area of the head of the fibula which had been crushed in an automobile injury. In all these cases, the neuromas were exposed, and the surrounding scar tissue resected. Four were injected with 70% alcohol. In three cases the neuroma was primarily surgically removed. In patient 4 (Table 1) the neuroma resection led to a renewed neuroma formation at the site of removal for the nerve implant, the stump of the sural nerve. Renewed resection and transplantation of the nerve were not successful. In patient 5 the neuroma of the radial nerve was primarily resected and implanted in the radius. Because of continuing pain, the revision was followed by injection of 70% alcohol.

The difficulties of neuroma treatment (which often begin at diagnosis) can be demonstrated by the case of a 67-year-old patient (patient 1, Table 2), who was referred to us with the diagnosis "amputation neuroma after thigh amputation." He had been treated several times in other clinics without success. In spite of the presence of a palpable amputation neuroma, the thorough neurological examination did not yield a certain diagnosis. There was neither evidence for the typical neuroma pain upon tapping nor the burning

Table 2. Two cases of uncertain diagnosis

Patient no.	Age (years)	Cause	Location	Operation	Outcome
1	67	Traumatic amputation of the thigh	Ischiadic nerve	Laminectomy L5	Excellent
2	67	Traumatic amputation of the calf	Ischiadic nerve	Laminectomy L5	Excellent

pain of causalgia. Phantom limb pain was also absent. The diagnosis of sciatica, however, could not be confirmed in the shortened thigh despite EMG tests. We therefore decided to carry out a myelography, which to our surprise showed evidence of an extensive osteochondrotic and spondyloarthritic lumbar canal stenosis. Laminectomy of the 5th lumbar vertebra finally led to freedom from pain in the patient. A similar case was also observed in another 67-year-old patient (patient 2, Table 2), who was also subjected to laminectomy L5 and was also free from pain after the operation.

References

1. Battista A, Cravioto HM, Budzilovich GN (1981) Painful neuroma: changes produced in periphal nerve after fascicle ligation. Neurosurgery 9(5):589–600
2. Bernstein JJ, Pagnanelli D (1982) Long-term axonal apposition in rat sciatic nerve neuroma. J Neurosurg 57:682–684
3. Biddulph SL (1972) The preventional treatment of painful amputation neuroma. J Bone Joint Surg 54(B) 2:379
4. Braun RM (1982) Epineural nerve suture. Clin Orthop Rel Res 163:50–56
5. Brown HA (1944) Internal neurolysis in the treatment of peripheral nerve injuries. Clin Neurosurg VII:99–110
6. Burke B (1978) A preliminary report on the use of silastic nerve caps in conjunction with neuroma surgery. Foot Surg 17(2):52–57
7. De Carvalho Pinto VA (1954) A comparative study of the methods for the prevention of amputation neuroma. Surg Gyn Obst 99:492–496
8. Defalque RJ (1982) Painful trigger points in surgical scars. Anesth Analg 61:518–520
9. Dick W (1982) Der Morton'sche Vorfußschmerz. Orthopäde 11:235–244
10. Dobyns JH, Linscheid RL (1972) Bowler's thumb – diagnosis and treatment. J Bone Joint Surg 54(A)4:751–755
11. Dogliotti AM, Teneff S, Micheli E (1948) Amputationi e disarticolationi. In: Dogliotti AM, Technica operativa, vol. 1. Edit. Torinese, Torino
12. Dogliotti AM (1931) Traitement des syndromes douloureux de la peripherie par l alcoolisation sub-arachnoidienne des racines posterieures a Leur emergence de la moelle epiniere. Press Med 39:1249–1252
13. Eaton RG (1980) Painful neuromas. Management of Peripheral Nerve Problems. Pain: 194–202
14. Farley HH (1965) Painful stump neuroma. Minnesota Medicine: 347–350
15. Foerster O, Gagel O (1932) Die Vorderseitenstrangdurchtrennung bei Menschen. Z Ges Neurol Psychiat 138:1–98

16. Frackelton WH, Teasley JL, Tauras A (1972) Neuromas in the hand treated by nerve transposition and silicone capping. J Bone Joint Surg 54(A)2:813
17. Gluck T (1880) Über Neuroplastik auf dem Wege der Transplantation. Arch Klin Chir 25:606–616
18. Goldhahn WE (1977) Operationen bei therapieresistenten Schmerzen nach peripheren Nervenverletzungen. Psychiat Neurol Med Psychol (Leipz) 29(2):64–76
19. Gonzalez-Darder J, Barbera J, Abellan J, Mora A (1985) Centrocentral anastomosis in the prevention and treatment of painful terminal neuroma. An experimental study in the rat. J Neurosurg 63:754–758
20. Huber GC, Lewis D (1920) Amputation neuromas, their development and prevention. Arch Surg (Chicago) 1:85–113
21. Kline DG (1980) Evaluation of the neuroma in continuity. Management of Peripheral Nerve Problems. Pain: 450–461
22. König HJ, Themann H, Hiller U, Gullotta F (1987) Prevention of neuroma formation by neodym yag laser-experimental observations. Acta Neurochir (Wien) 87(1–2):63–69
23. Laborde KJ, Kalisman M, Tsai TM (1982) Results of surgical treatment of painful neuromas of the hand. Hand Surg 7(2):190–193
24. Lagarrigue J, Chavoin JP, Belahouari L, Scavazza R (1982) Traitement des neuromes douloureux par anastomose nerveuse en anse "piege a neurome". Neurochirurgie 28:91–92
25. Livingstone WK (1943) Pain mechanism: a physiological interpretation of causalgia and its related states. Mac Millan, New York, p 83–113
26. Long DM (1976) Cutaneous afferent stimulation for the relief of pain. Prog Neurol Surg (Basel) 7:35–51
27. Melzack R, Bromage PR (1973) Experimental phantom limbs. Exp Neurol 39:261–269
28. Melzack R, Wall P (1965) Pain mechanism: a new theory. Science 150:971–979
29. Milgram JE (1980) Morton's neuritis and management of post-neurectomy pain. Management of Peripheral Nerve Problems. Pain:202–215
30. Powers KS, Norman D, Edwards MSB (1983) Computerized tomography of peripheral nerve lesions. J Neurosurg 59:131–136
31. Riddoch G (1941) Phantom limbs and body shape. Brain 64:197–222
32. Robbins TH (1977) The response of tender neuromas and scars to triamcinolone injection. Brit J Plast Surg 30:68–69
33. Sindow M, Fischer G, Goutelle A, Mansuy L (1974) La radicelolotomie, posterieure selective. Neuro.-Chir. 20:391–408
34. Smith DC (1962) Treatment of digital stump neuromata. J Bone Joint Surg 44(B)1:227
35. Smith JR, Gomez NH (1970) Local injection therapy of neuromata of the hand with triamcinolone acetonide. J Bone Joint Surg 52(A)1:71–83
36. Snyder CC, Knowles RP (1965) Traumatic neuromas. J Bone Joint Surg 47(A)3:641
37. Wall PD, Gutnick M (1974) Properties of afferent nerve impulses originating from a neuroma. Nature 248:740–743
38. Wall PD, Seet WH (1967) Temporary abolition of pain in man. Science 155:108–109
39. White JC (1946) Painful injuries of nerves and their surgical treatment. Am J Surg 72(3):468–488
40. White JC, Hamlin H (1945) New uses of tantalum in nerve suture; control of neuroma formation. J Neurosurg 2:402

Femoral Nerve Lesion in Surgery of the Hip

G. BINDL, Stuttgart/FRG

Reports about complications in surgery of the hip generally involve infection and loosening of the prosthesis. Neurologic complications are rare (Table 1), but these complications increase in difficult or repeated revisions (Table 2). In most cases the sciatic nerve is concerned (Griss et al. 1982; Karpf et al. 1976; Lambiris et al. 1981; Rubovszky 1977; Weber et al. 1976). The femoral nerve is endangered by pressure from Hohmann retractors (Fig. 1). While interference with the femoral nerve is not expected using an anterolateral approach to the hip because the nerve is protected by iliopsoas muscle, anatomic conditions may have changed in revision of the arthroplasty. A case of this is described in the present report.

A 62-year-old woman had a first hip replacement on the left side in July 1981 and one on the right side in September 1981 (Fig. 2). The left side remained strongly anchored, but on the right side the hip prosthesis was changed twice due to loosening. In September 1983 the right side became infected, and the

Table 1. Nerve lesions in hip replacement – first implantation: review of literature

Author	Year	n	Femoral nerve	Sciatic nerve	Peroneal nerve	Percentage
Boitzy	1973	309	3	–	–	1.0
Buchholz and Noack	1973	3205	–	60	–	1.5
Coventry et al.	1974	2012	5	12	–	0.85
Karpf et al.	1976	1000	–	22	–	2.2
Weber et al.	1976	2012	–	14	–	0.7
Rubovszky	1977	1536	11	3	–	0.9
Dietschi	1978	1136	11	–	6	1.5
Lambiris et al.	1981	880	–	4	–	0.45
Griss et al.	1982	4043	–	18	–	0.45

Table 2. Nerve lesions in hip replacement – revisions: review of literature

Author	Year	n	Femoral nerve	Sciatic nerve	Peroneal nerve	Percentage
Amstutz et al.	1982	66	–	–	5	7.5
Griss et al.	1982	461	–	5	–	1.1
Schuster	1984	152	7	–	2	5.9

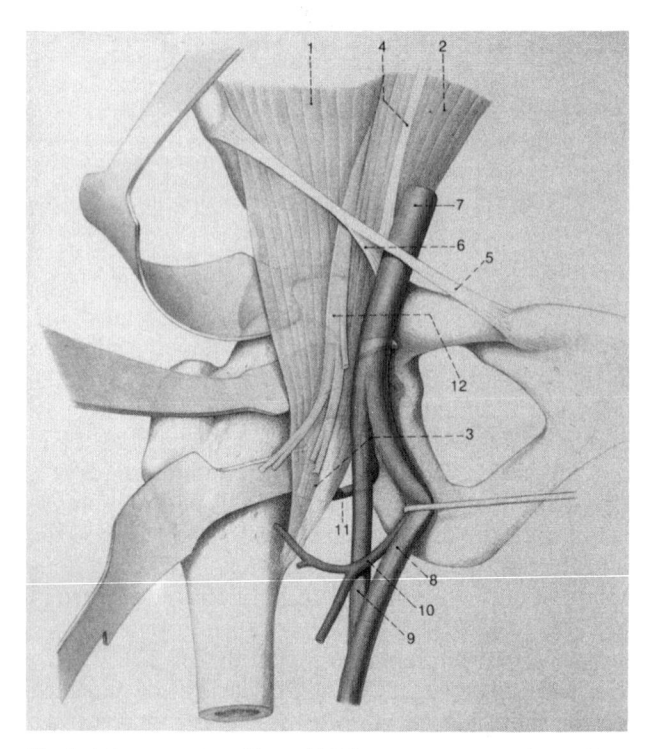

Fig. 1. The correct position of Hohmann retractors (according to Bauer)

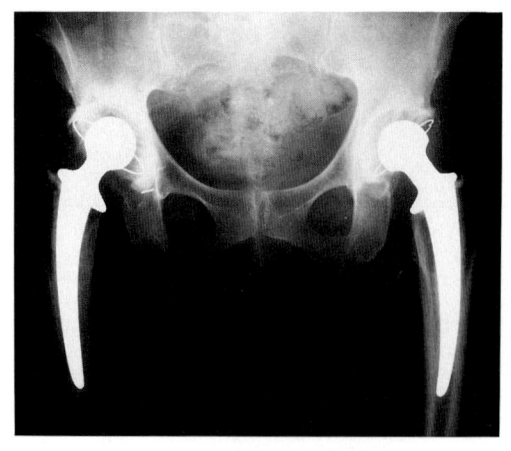

Fig. 2. Total hip replacement on both sides

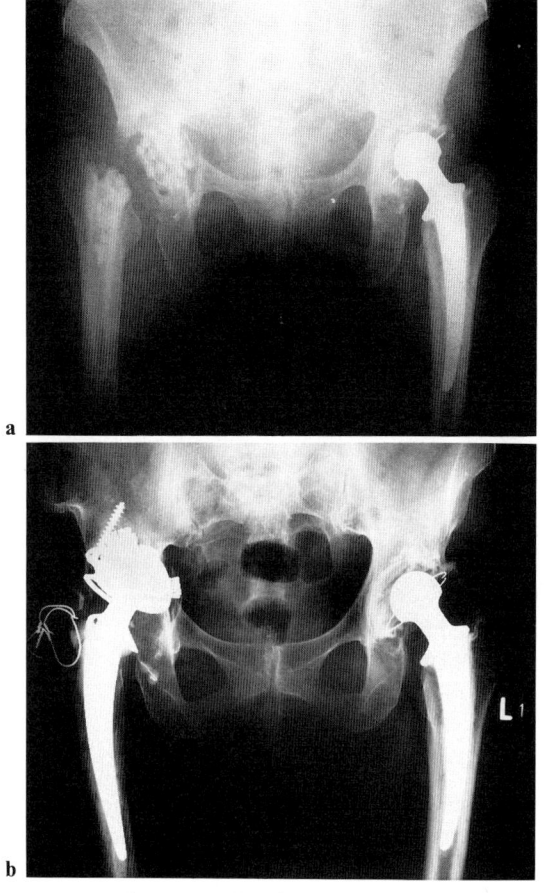

Fig. 3. a The huge cavity after removing the prosthesis on the right side. **b** The position of the new implanted prosthesis

implant was removed completely (Fig. 3). In the pelvis a huge cavity remained, and the acetabular floor was perforated. The infection soon came to an end. Because of severe shortening, pain, and instability of the hip a cementless acetabular component and a cemented shaft component were implanted in November 1985. Because of the four previous operations the anatomical situation was irregular. The scar went deep into the pelvis and changed the position of the femoral vessels and femoral nerve. While removing this scar from the cavity of the former acetabulum the femoral nerve was cut. The identification of the nerve during the operation occurred by chance. At the end of the revision of the arthroplasty the femoral vessels and the femoral nerve were prepared by a separate iliofemoral approach. The veins were intact. The defect of the femoral nerve was 5 cm long. It was bridged by four cables. The coordination of the cables to the fascicles was optional. After 1.5 years the

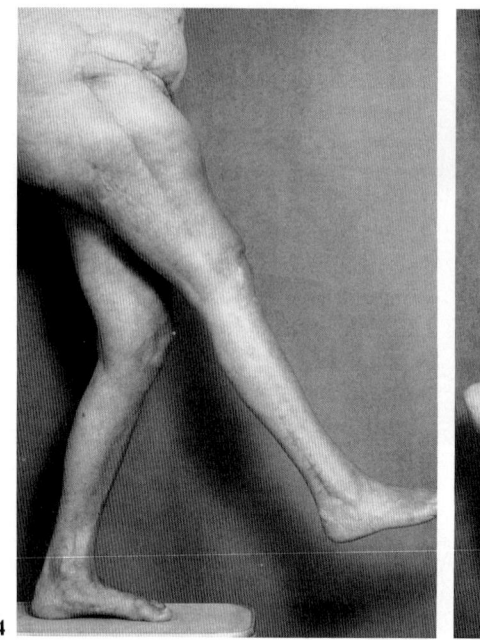

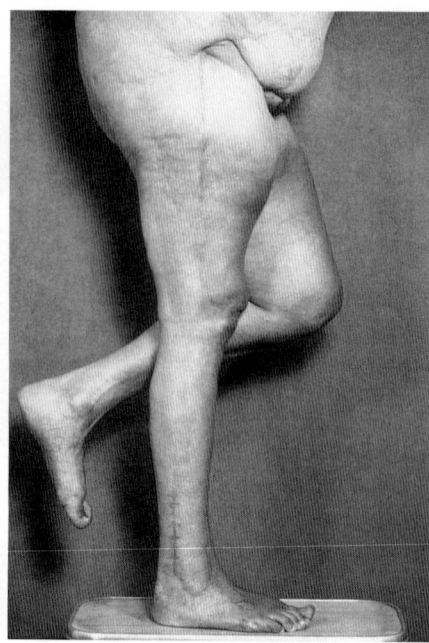

Fig. 4. The patient is able to extend the right leg
Fig. 5. The patient is able to stabilize the leg by quadriceps muscle

vastus lateralis and rectus femoris muscles showed signs of reinnervation. The vastus intermedius is still without any innervation. The patient is able to extend the leg fully and to lift it (Fig. 4). Furthermore, the patient is able to stand and stabilize the right leg completely. The artificial joint is without signs of loosening or infection (Fig. 5).

References

Amstutz HC, Steven MD, Riyaz H Jinnah, Larry Mai (1982) Revision of aspectic loose total hip arthroplasties. Clin Orthop 170:21–33
Boitzy A (1973) Allgemeine operative Komplikationen bei Totalendoprothesen der Hüfte. In: Cotta H, Schulitz H-P (Hrsg) Der totale Hüftersatz. Thieme, Stuttgart
Buchholz HW, Noack G (1973) Results of the total hip prothesis "St. George". Clin Orthop 95:201–210
Coventry MB, Beckenbaugh RD, Nolan DR, Jlstry (1974) 2012 Total hip arthroplasties: a study of postoperative course and early complications. J Bone Joint Surg 56(A):273–284
Dietschi C (1978) Zur Problematik des künstlichen Hüftgelenks Schriftreihe der med.-orth. Technik, Bd 3. Gentner, Stuttgart
Griss P, Hackenbroch M, Jäger M, Preussner B, Schäfert T (1982) Findings on total hip replacement for ten years. Aktuelle Probleme in Chirurgie und Orthopädie, Bd 21
Karpf PM, Ludwig U, Beck W (1976) Periphere Nervenläsionen beim prothetischen Hüftgelenksersatz. Orthop Praxis 12:675–677

Lambiris E, Stoboy W, Bortz W (1981) Aseptische Komplikationen bei der Totalarthroplastik am Hüftgelenk. Unfallchir 7:242–248

Rubovszky S (1977) Neurologische Komplikationen nach Hüfttotalendoprothesen. Akt Traumatol 7:303–310

Schuster G (1984) Komplikationen nach Reoperationen von Hüfttotalendoprothesen. Dissertation, Universität Freiburg

Weber ER, Daube JR, Coventry MB (1976) Peripheral neuropathies associated with total arthroplasty. J Bone Joint Surg 58(A):66–69

Isolated Traumatic Nerve Lesions of the Extensor Pollicis Longus and Brevis Muscles

C. TIZIAN and L. DÖBLER, Hofheim (Taunus)/FRG

Introduction

Isolated peripheral lesions of the muscular branches of the radial nerve on the forearm are rare injuries. They are mostly caused by a pointed instrument, only a small skin lesion is seen on the extensor side of the forearm. In comparison to sensible nerve lesions, peripheral muscular nerve injuries are in most cases neither diagnosed nor treated at the first examination. Due to the lack of sufficient diagnosis of the nerve injury most of the patients need secondary reconstruction.

After passing the upper arm, the radial nerve (C 5 – C 8) crosses the elbow joint on the flexor side and divides at the level of the head of the radius into its two terminal branches, the superficial and the deep branch. The deep branch perforates the superinator muscle obliquely and separates into numerous muscular branches, such as those to the extensor pollicis brevis and longus muscles [1]. Isolated damage to the peripheral muscular branches leads to paralysis of the extensor pollicis longus and brevis muscles, resulting in an extension insufficiency of the MP and IP joints of the thumb, while the first metacarpal joint shows regular function [2]. Due to a thick soft-tissue coverage consisting of skin, subcutaneous tissue, and muscle the Tinel sign is not seen in the majority of the cases.

Case Report

A 20-year-old patient was injured with a pointed knife. Primary treatment consisting of wound débridement and skin closure was carried out elsewhere. Six weeks later the patient was admitted to our clinic showing paralysis of the extensor pollicis brevis and longus muscles. No Tinel-Hoffmann sign was present. Until surgery 2 weeks later physical therapy and electric stimulation of the aforementioned muscles were initiated.

The surgical procedure started with exposure of the deep branch of the radial nerve from proximal to distal. Before entering the muscle bellies of the extensor pollicis longus and extensor pollicis brevis, the two nerve branches were completely divided, showing two neuromas (Fig. 1). After resection of the neuromas and the nerve endings back to the healthy tissue, a defect of 4.5 cm each was bridged using a vascularized cutaneous antebrachii nerve graft. After immobilization for ten days physical therapy and selective electric stimulation

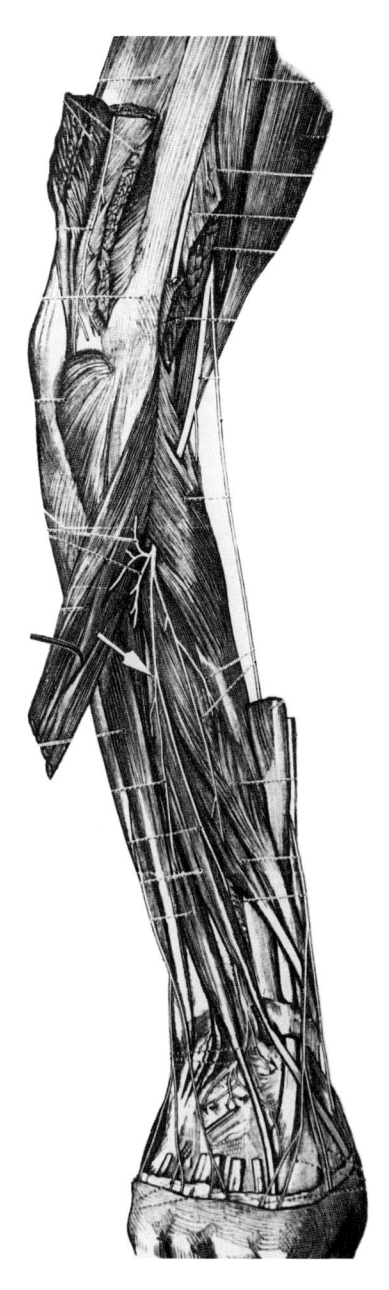

Fig. 1. Division of nerve branches (*arrow*)

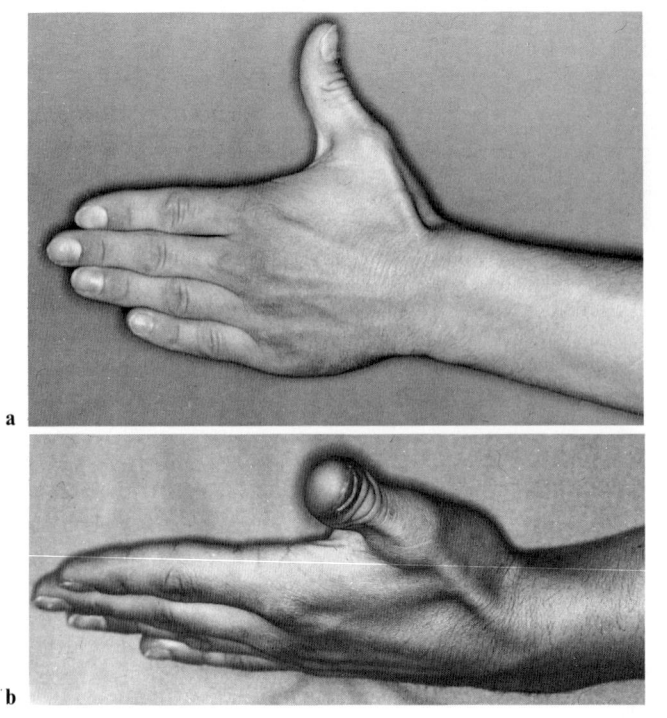

Fig. 2a, b. Achievement of full function of the extensor pollicis longus and brevis muscles

were continued. Six months after surgery full function of the two muscles was observed (Fig. 2).

Discussion

In isolated lesions of peripheral muscular branches of the radial nerve the primary reconstruction is, if possible, the most sufficient treatment. As most of such lesions are recognized later, secondary reconstruction using nerve grafts is indicated. Physical therapy and selective electric stimulation of the paralyzed muscles are necessary for ultimate achievement of full function. As shown by our case, nerve reconstruction using vascularized nerve grafts can result in complete functional rehabilitation. Therefore, even in this type of injury where the transposition of the extensor indices proprius–tendon represents an acceptable procedure, the reconstruction using nerve grafts is indicated as first choice.

References

1. Kahle W, Lenhardt H, Platzer W (1976) Color atlas and textbook of human anatomy. Georg Thieme, Stuttgart
2. Millesi H (1977b) Interfascicular grafts for repair of peripheral nerves of the upper extremity. Orth Clin North Am 8:387

Peripheral Nerve Involvement in Recklinghausen's Disease

M. TATAGIBA, A. KLEIDER, W. BINI, A. SEPEHRNIA, J. BRENNECKE, G. PENKERT, and M. SAMII, Hannover/FRG

Introduction

Neurofibromatosis is a relatively common inherited disease of the nervous system with a frequency of about 1 in 3000 births and affecting about 20000 people in the Federal Republic of Germany. It consists of at least two distinct genetic diseases: neurofibromatosis 1, as described by Friedrich von Recklinghausen and characterized by café-au-lait spots and subcutaneous neurofibromas, and neurofibromatosis 2, recently established as a separate entity and characterized by bilateral acoustic neuromas [1–3, 21, 26].

Involvement of peripheral nerves by tumors is one of the usual features of Recklinghausen's disease. They include neurofibromas that may occur in deeper peripheral nerves and result in functional compromise of limbs and in pain and cause cosmetic disfigurements [2, 9, 11, 12, 22–25]. The tumors may be either schwannomas or neurofibromas, both arising from the nerve sheath. In some plexiform neurofibromas malignant transformation into malignant neurilemmomas may take place [4–8, 13–16].

Clinical Material

From January 1978 to September 1987, 53 patients with neurofibromatosis were operated on in our clinic. Of these, 36 had bilateral acoustic neuromas, and 8 had peripheral nerve tumors. In these 8 patients a total of 15 operations were performed. Complete excision was the procedure for 12 tumors, and a partial removal was performed in 3. In 4 of the 12 tumors nerve excision was necessary to achieve complete removal. A microsurgical reconstruction with a sural nerve graft was performed in one case (Table 1). Pain and motor

Table 1. Surgical procedures (number of operations)

	Complete removal	Incomplete removal
Neurolysis	3	1
Resection of cutaneous nerve	5	1
Resection of nerve trunk with grafting	1	0
Resection of nerve trunk without grafting	3	1
	12	3

Table 2. Indications and histology (number of tumors)

	Operations	Neurofibroma (plexif. NF)	Schwannoma	Malignant schwannoma
Pain	7	2	3	2
Motoric impairment	3	3(1)	–	–
Diagnostics	5	2(1)	–	3
Cosmetic	–	–	–	–
	15	7(2)	3	5

Table 3. Sites of tumors

	Tumors
Head and neck	1
Supraclavicular	1
Upper extremity	8
Retroperitoneum	1
Lower extremity	4
	15

Table 4. Involved nerves

	Tumors
Supraclavicular nerve	1
Brachial plexus	3
Radial nerve	3
Median nerve	1
Antebrachial cutaneous nerve	1
Femoral nerve	1
Superficial peroneal nerve	1
Skin nerves	4

impairment were the most frequent symptoms observed preoperatively (Table 2). The sites of the lesions and the involved nerves are presented in Tables 3 and 4.

Case Reports

Case 1. A 20-year-old woman operated on in our clinic for bilateral acoustic neuroma was readmitted 2 years later suffering from pain and swelling in the left forearm and in the supraclavicular fossa as well as from progressive hand movement impairment for several months. A surgical exploration was performed. Two schwannomas were found and completely removed from the median antebrachial cutaneous nerve (Fig. 1) and from a C8 fascicle in the

Fig. 1. Schwannoma Antoni A-type of the antebrachial cutaneous nerve

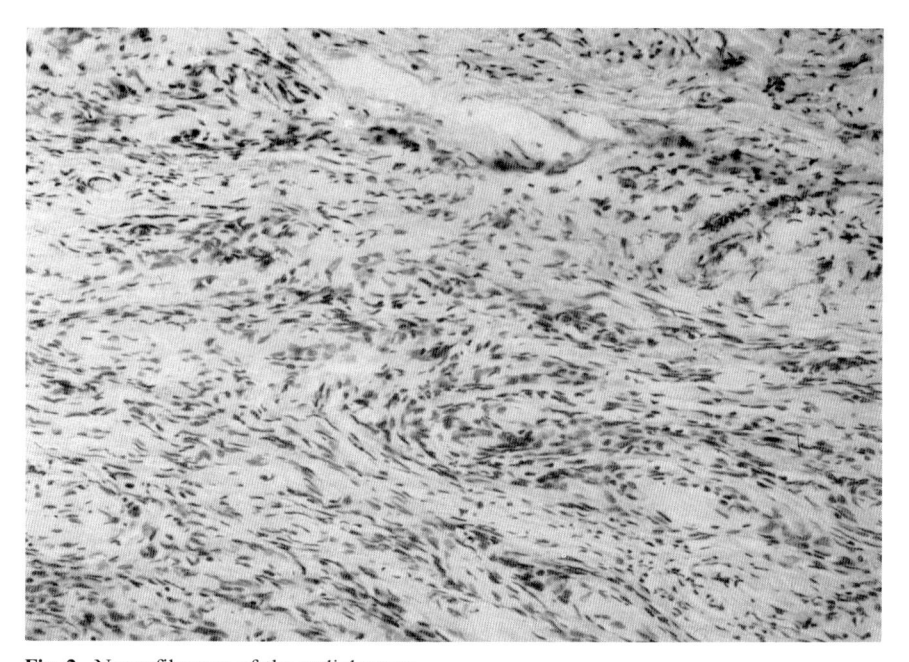

Fig. 2. Neurofibroma of the radial nerve

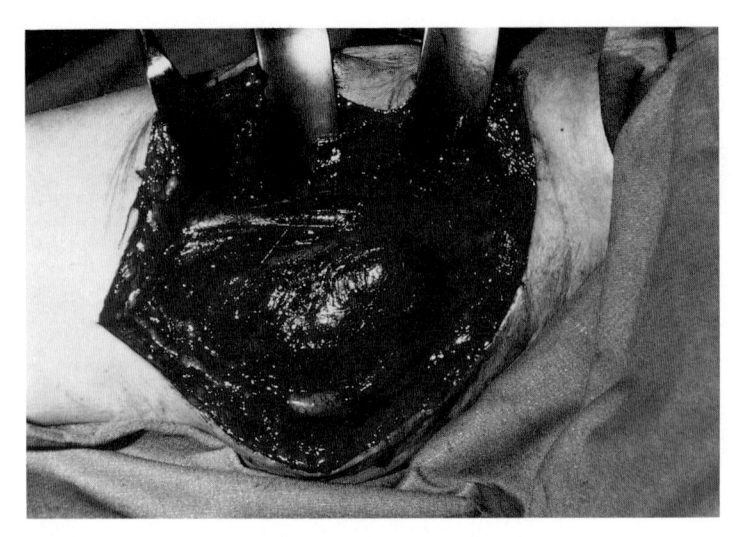

Fig. 3. Malignant schwannoma arising from the upper arm

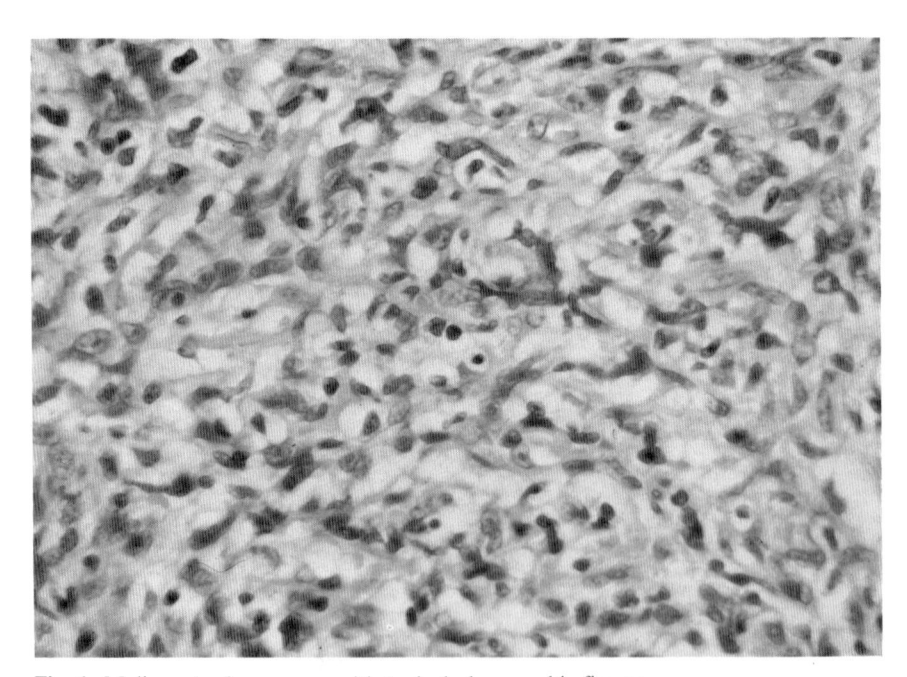

Fig. 4. Malignant schwannoma with typical pleomorphic figures

supraclavicular fossa. The patient achieved pain relief after the operation. A follow-up of 10 months showed no tumor recurrence and an improvement in hand movements.

Case 2. An 18-year-old man was operated on in our clinic for bilateral acoustic neuroma and spinal cord meningioma. He was newly admitted due to a mass in the right forearm causing progressive radial palsy. We performed a surgical exploration and removed completely a neurofibroma of the right radial nerve (Fig. 2). Sural grafting (8 cm) was performed in this case. After 3 years there was no redurrence of tumor.

Case 3. A 50-year-old man suffering from the peripheral form of neurofibromatosis had already been operated on for a malignant schwannoma in the region of the groin 10 years before his last admission in our clinic. Because of painful swelling masses multiple surgical explorations were made in this patient with excision of malignant schwannomas in the region of the groin and subaxilla (Figs. 3, 4). The prognosis in this case was poor. Amputation of the right arm was indicated.

Discussion

As peripheral nerve involvement is common in Recklinghausen's disease, patients with the classical form of generalized Recklinghausen's disease should be kept under observation to note excessive growth of certain tumors or other complicating features that may be amenable to surgical treatment.

Based on our experience, and in accordance with the literature [10, 17–19, 22–25], we believe that an operative treatment is indicated in the case of: (a) increased size of tumor that causes pain or interferes with activity, (b) rapid progression in size with the danger of malignancy, and (c) cosmetic disfigurements. Furthermore, surgical removal of small tumors for microscopic study or for cosmetic effect has not been followed by increased growth phenomena and is not contraindicated. Plexiform neurofibromas within the subcutaneous tissue may be treated by extirpation, and no nerve repair is necessary. Neurofibromas with involvement of major nerve trunks should not imply sacrifice of the nerve unless accurate diagnosis of a malignant degeneration is obtained. In this case sacrifice of nerves and repair by nerve graft may be performed.

The sural nerve itself may be affected, or neurofibromas can appear in the graft at a later stage [20]. This should be kept in mind when planning the surgical therapy.

References

1. Canale DJ, Bebin J (1972) Von Recklinghausen's disease of the nervous system. In: Virhn PJ, Bruyn GW (eds) Handbook of clinical neurology, vol 14. North Holland Publ, Amsterdam New York, pp 132–162
2. Riccardi VM, Eichner JE (1986) Neurofibromatosis. Phenotype, natural history and pathogenesis. Johns Hopkins Univ Press, Baltimore
3. Kanter WR, Eldrige R, Fabricant R, Allen JR, Koerber T (1980) Central neurofibromatosis with bilateral acoustic neuroma: genetic, clinical and biochemical distinctions from peripheral neurofibromatosis. Neurology 30:851–859
4. Kramer W (1970) Tumors of nerves. In: Virhn PJ, Bryun GW (eds) Handbook of clinical neurology, vol 8. North Holland Publ, Amsterdam, pp 412–512
5. Russel DS, Rubinstein LJ (1977) Pathology of tumors of the nervous system, 4th edn. Edword Arnold Ltd, London [Williams & Wilkins, Baltimore]
6. Seddon HJ (1972) Surgical disorders of the peripheral nerves. Churchill Livingstone, Edinburgh
7. Harkin JC, Reed RJ (1969) Tumors of the peripheral nervous system. In: Atlas of tumor pathology, 2nd series, fascicle 3. Armed Forces Institute of Pathology, Washington DC
8. Harkin JC, Reed RJ (1982) Tumors of the peripheral nerval system. In: Atlas of tumor pathology, 2nd series, fascicle 3 (Suppl). Armed Forces Institute of Pathology, Washington DC
9. Harkin JC (1980) Differential diagnosis of peripheral nerve tumors. In: Omer GE Jr, Spinner M (eds) Management of peripheral nerve problems. Saunders, Philadelphia London Toronto, pp 657–668
10. Ariel I (1980) Current concepts in the management of peripheral nerve tumors. In: Omer GE Jr, Spinner M (eds) Management of peripheral nerve problems. Saunders, Philadelphia London Toronto, pp 669–693
11. Urich H (1983) Pathology of tumors of cranial nerves, spinal nerve roots and peripheral nerves. In: Dick PJ, Thomas PK, Lambert EH (eds) Peripheral neuropathy, vol 2. Saunders, Philadelphia, pp 2253–2299
12. Brooks D (1983) Clinical presentation and treatment of peripheral nerve tumors. In: Dick PJ, Thomas PK, Lambert EH (eds) Peripheral neuropathy, vol 2. Saunders, Philadelphia, pp 2236–2251
13. Storm FK, Eiber FR, Mirra J, Morton DL (1980) Neurofibrosarcoma. Cancer 45:126–129
14. Ducatman BS, Scheithauer BW, Piepgras DG, Reiman HM, Ilstrup DM (1986) Malignant peripheral nerve sheath tumors. Cancer 57:2006–2021
15. Arpornchayanon O, Hirota T, Itabashi M, Nakajima T, Fukuma H, Beppu Y, Nishikawa K (1984) Malignant peripheral nerve tumors: a clinicopathological and electron microscopic study. Jpn J Clin Oncol 14(1):57–74
16. Sorensen SA, Mulvihill JJ, Nielsen A (1986) Long-term follow-up of von Recklinghausen neurofibromatosis. Survival and malignant neoplasms. N Engl J Med 314(16):1010–1015
17. Barfred T, Zachariae L (1975) Neurofibroma in the median nerve treated with resection and free nerve transplantation. Scand J Plast Reconstr Surg 9:391–396
18. Corradi M, Guardoli A (1984) Neurofibromatosi multipla dell'arto superiore. Arch Putti Chir Organi Mov 34:391–396
19. Tognetti F, Poppi Martinelli P, Pozzati E (1983) Recovery of nerve function following operation for solitary neurofibroma in the elderly. Neurochirurgia 26:149–151
20. Samii M (1986) Surgery of facial nerve paralysis. No Shinkei Geka 14(8):943–955
21. Seizinger BR, Roleau GA, Ozelius LJ, Lane AH, Faryniarz AG, Chao MV, Huson S et al. (1987) Genetic linkage of von Recklinghausen neurofibromatosis to the nerve growth factor receptor gene. Cell 49:589–594
22. Roback HB, Kirshner H, Roback E (1981/82) Physical self-concept changes in a mildly, facially disfigured neurofibromatosis patient following communication skill training. Int J Psychiatry in Med 11(2):137–143

23. Adkins JC, Ravitch MM (1977) The operative management of von Recklinghausen's neurofibromatosis in children, with special reference to lesions of the head and neck. Surgery 82(3):342–348
24. Rothenstein M, Beitbart EW (1981) Korrektive operative Therapie beim Morbus Recklinghausen. Z Hautkr 56(24):1578–1583
25. Griffith BH, Lewis VL, McKinney P (1985) Neurofibromas of the head and neck. Surg Gynecol Obstet 60:534–538
26. Seizinger BR, Martuza RL, Gusella JF (1986) Loss of genes on chromosome 22 in tumorigenesis of human acoustic neuroma. Nature 322:644–647

Clinical Aspects of Entrapment Neuropathies of Peripheral Nerves

M. Mumenthaler, Bern/Switzerland

Introduction

The terminology regarding neuropathy has become more and more vague. Too often the entity of neuropathy, due to an entrapment in a physiological narrow path, has been extended to the compression syndromes due to external pressure and to those due to additional pathological factors in the critical anatomical zone. This presentation is limited to the original concept of entrapment neuropathy: a peripheral nerve lesion presenting without evident external cause and localized in one of those anatomical zones where the nerve passes through a narrow path.

General Clinical Characteristics and Diagnostic Criteria

The beginning of symptoms and signs is in general insidious and slowly progressive. Depending on which nerve is involved, the symptoms may be localized pain, sensory loss, and/or motor weakness. Either of these three elements may be prominent. Among the clinical signs the exact determination of a sensory loss and/or an analysis of the motor weakness permits determination of which peripheral nerve is involved and localization more or less exactly of the site of lesion. Some specific clinical tests give additional information about the site of entrapment and the mechanism of the lesion, for example, pressure or tapping at the site of compression frequently evokes local or irradiating pain or paresthesias; maneuvers stretching the nerve at the site of entrapment may also increase the symptoms, e.g., the cross-body action in the incisura scapulae syndrome (see below). This may also be achieved by maneuvers which in some way enhance the pressure at the entrapment site, such as the Phalen test in carpal tunnel syndrome by diminishing the width of the carpal canal. Additional ancillary methods may make important contributions to the clinical diagnosis. In particular, electromyographic and electroneurographic tests (motor and sensory conduction) add to the precise localization of the site of lesion. Local anesthetic blocks may confirm the diagnosis by relieving pain.

Frequency

Fifteen years ago we analyzed the outpatients with peripheral nerve lesions in the Department of Neurology and Neurosurgery at the University Hospital of Bern over a 9-year period [56]. The 3465 cases represented 17.3% of the total of 20000 outpatients seen; 1574 had non-traumatic lesions of peripheral nerves, which represented approximately 45% of the peripheral nerve cases. Among these 1574, not all were entrapment neuropathies as defined above. However, in approximately two-thirds of them no external or additional cause for the peripheral nerve lesion could be found. Therefore, at that time 922 outpatients suffered from, or 4.6% of all entrapment neuropathies. Most of these – 709 – had carpal tunnel syndrome.

We have now updated these numbers and have analyzed the 11-year period 1975–1985, considering the peripheral nerve lesions not primarily due to a traumatic cause. These 5938 cases represent 9.3% of the 63808 outpatients seen in this period (Table 1). Among the 5938 non-primarily traumatic cases, however, only 4590 were actual entrapment neuropathies without external

Table 1. Patients with non-traumatic lesions of the peripheral nerves seen in an 11-year period (1975–1985)

	n
Radial nerve at the upper arm (callus)	5
Radial nerve at the upper arm, external pressure	91
Radial nerve, R. profundus[a]	71
Median nerve, processus supracondylaris[a]	2
Median nerve, compression at the upper arm	57
Carpal tunnel syndrome[a]	4051
Ulnar nerve, processus supracondylaris[a]	3
Ulnar nerve, pathology at elbow	69
Ulnar nerve, external pressure at elbow	544
Ulnar nerve, at elbow with luxation[a]	48
Ulnar nerve at wrist, non-traumatic	87
Long thoracic nerve, Rucksack paralysis	1
Brachial plexus, thoracic outlet[a]	106
Brachial plexus, radiotherapy	32
Cheiralgia paresthetica	5
Peroneal nerve, external pressure	226
Lumbar plexus, pressure	69
Saphenous nerve, non-traumatic[a]	30
Tibial nerve, tarsal tunnel syndrome, posttraumatic	101
Tarsal tunnel syndrome, spontaneous[a]	15
Sensory nerve of the foot, compression	23
Meralgia paresthetica[a]	229
Ilioinguinal nerve (after surgery and other causes)	38
Ilioinguinal nerve, spontaneous[a]	5
Morton's toe[a]	30
Total	5938

[a] Entrapment neuropathies ($n = 4590$).

causes; they represented 77.3% of the non-primarily traumatic peripheral nerve lesions and 7.2% of all patients seen as outpatients over this period. A large majority, 4051 cases, had carpal tunnel syndrome. This very high number is due partly to the presence of a very active Department of Hand Surgery in our hospital, which sends us a large number of its patients for electrophysiological evaluation. The high percentage of entrapment neuropathies and their gratifying surgical treatment fully justify the interest that physicians devote to this diagnostic group.

Signs and Symptoms of Entrapment Neuropathies of Individual Peripheral Nerves

In this review there is no space for an exhaustive description of the entrapment syndromes of the individual peripheral nerves. We therefore limit ourselves to those aspects which are either of particular diagnostic importance or, on the basis of our experience, not well enough known. We have given a more exhaustive description of this type of peripheral nerve lesion in a monograph which provides more details and numerous references [57]. In addition, there are also other monographs on this subject [42, 71, 76].

Entrapment of Brachial Plexus in the Thoracic Outlet

The anatomical sites of entrapment are the scalenus passage and the costoclavicular passage. Clinically a diffuse brachial pain is frequently present, but this is by no means sufficient to make the diagnosis. A strong argument in favor of a scalenus syndrome is the presence of a cervical rib [1], and the likelihood of an entrapment of the brachial plexus in the scalenus passage becomes very high when in addition signs indicating a lower plexus lesion are present, e.g., pain radiating to the ulnar digits and atrophy of small hand muscles including the thenar eminence. A sensory loss of the $C8/D1$ segment may confirm this etiology, but this is frequently absent when the chronic entrapment is due to a cervical rib or a tight band [21] between the lateral process of $C7$ and the first rib. The classical maneuvers aimed at showing a compression of the subclavian artery in the scalenus or costoclavicular passage are positive in a large number of normal individuals and are therefore not as helpful as often supposed. Electrophysiological tests measuring orthodromic sensory conduction can add arguments to the clinical elements [82] as can arteriography showing vascular compression in certain arm positions [12].

Entrapment of the Suprascapular Nerve in the Scapular Notch (Incisura Scapulae Syndrome)

Anatomically the notch is bridged by a ligament under which the nerve runs. Here it can be mechanically irritated by repetitive movements [3, 35] or compressed by a ganglion [57]. In spite of the lack of cutaneous sensory fibers in the suprascapular nerve, a dull pain in the shoulder is a prominent symptom, due to the fibers for deep sensation from the shoulder joint. The isolated atrophy and paresis of the supra- and infraspinatus muscles is typical. Additional pain can be provoked as follows: the patient puts the hand of his affected side on his opposite shoulder and elevates his elbow to a horizontal plane. The examiner pulls the patient's elbow towards the opposite side. This "cross-body action" causes pain in the affected shoulder.

Entrapment of Axillary Nerve in the Quadrilateral Space

The axillary nerve is a branch of the posterior fascicle of the brachial plexus. It runs together with the posterior humeral circumflex artery through the quadrilateral space. This is bounded laterally by the collum chirurgicum of the humerus, cranially by the subscapular and teres minor muscles, medially by the long head of the triceps, and caudally by the teres major muscle. In this space the nerve is very rarely entrapped in the absence of exogenous causes, mainly in active young people [11, 48]. This may cause upper arm pain, reproduced by forced abduction and external rotation of the upper arm. There is tenderness posteriorly over the quadrilateral space, and arteriography shows a segmental interruption of flow in the posterior humeral circumflex artery during abduction and external rotation [48]. There is in general no motor weakness of the deltoid muscle or sensory loss at the external aspect of upper arm.

Entrapment of the Deep Branch of Radial Nerve in the Supinator Canal

The deep branch of the radial nerve is purely motor. This branch goes from the cubital fossa in a spiral course around the proximal radius dorsally. Here it is embedded in the supinator muscle which has its origin at the lateral epicondylus of the humerus, at the capsule of the elbow joint, and at the dorsal edge of the ulna. The thin muscle plate lies directly on the radius, and the spiral course of its fibers crosses at right angle the deep branch of the radial nerve. The nerve penetrates and leaves the muscle through a slit with fibrotic edges. The deep branch contains nerve fibers for the extensor carpi ulnaris, extensor digiti minimi and extensor digitorum, extensor pollicis longus and brevis and abductor pollicis longus muscles. The fibers for the brachioradial muscle, for the extensor carpi radialis longus and brevis as well as those for the supinator itself, however, leave the main nerve before the deep branch enters the canal in the supinator muscle. This supinator syndrome [6, 22, 29, 45, 80] is therefore characterized clinically by a purely motor paralysis. Unusual efforts of the forearm may precede the clinical symptoms. In general, the first sign is a weakness of the extensor digiti minimi, and then progressively the other muscles innervated by the deep branch become successively paralyzed. The extension of the radial part of the hand is still possible due to the normally functioning extensores carpi radiales muscles. Pain is absent or at least never prominent. Some local tenderness over the supinator muscle may, however, be present. The syndrome may also be bilateral [65].

Entrapment Syndromes of the Ulnar Nerve

The ulnar nerve at the elbow goes through the narrow canal in the groove dorsally from the medial epicondylus. This groove is bridged by the epicondylo-olecranic ligament. In addition, every flection movement of the elbow joint narrows the diameter of this canal due to several factors. The ligament tightens, the medial head of the triceps muscle is pulled down into the groove, and the nerve itself is stretched and pulled against the medial border of the canal [15, 55, 57]. These physiological elements per se may be sufficient to produce symptoms and signs when the arm is used intensively or kept in a flexed position. There is a nearly constant slowing of the conduction velocity in the cubital canal [30]. Intraneural pressure measurements in the canal in corps have demonstrated that in the straight position the pressure is 7 mmHg, while in right angle flexion the pressure increases to 11–14 mmHg. In maximal flexion with extended wrist it may be as high as 46 mmHg [64]. Additional factors may also intervene, e.g., arthritic deformations, posttraumatic sclerotic tissue changes, or ganglions. Pain is always a presenting symptom, a local dull pain at the elbow with irradiations to the ulnar edge of the hand and to the little finger. Paresthesias and sensory loss may be present, and eventually a weakness of interossei may appear. The nerve in the groove at the elbow is tender to local pressure. Electroneurography is very useful in localizing the site of lesion.

At the hand the terminal stem of the ulnar nerve formed by both the motor deep and the mixed superficial branches passes through the so-called canal of Gujon [23, 26, 54, 73, 77]. This is formed by fiber bands which from the pisiform bone go to the retinaculum flexorum. A truly spontaneous entrapment at this site, however, is rare, and in most cases additional factors – such as chronic pressure, e.g., by working tools or a ganglion – are present. The symptoms are those of a dull local pain at the wrist and paresthesias at the volar aspect of the ulnar 1 1/2 fingers, and the motor deficit of the hypothenar and interosseus muscles can be demonstrated. The sensation on the dorsal aspect of the ulnar territory at the hand is normal, and there is no motor weakness of the ulnar flexors of the forearm and deep flexors of the fourth and fifth fingers.

Entrapment Neuropathies of the Median Nerve

The median nerve crosses at least four narrow passages. At the distal upper arm it perforates the medial septum intermuscularis brachii from dorsal to volar. In 1% of cases a supracondylar process [55], as a phylogenetic residual, is present, and the so-called Struthers ligament connects the tip with the medial epicondylus. The trunk of the median nerve passes beneath the ligament, which may also be present in the absence of a bony supracondylar process. Rarely, this spur [17, 24, 55] or the ligament [75, 78] may cause a compression of the median nerve, characterized by pain and paresthesias in the radial fingers and a preacher's hand type of motor paralysis.

In the proximal forearm the nerve penetrates between the two heads of the pronator teres [4]. Here it may be compressed and irritated, for example, by repetitive movements of the forearm [38, 72, 79]. Cramps, pain, and paresthesias in the radial fingers are the most prominent symptoms, and local pressure over the pronator muscle is painful. Weakness of forearm muscles has been observed, and writer's cramp has been attributed to this mechanism [37, 46].

The anterior interosseus nerve is a motor terminal branch of the median nerve. It leaves the main nerve stem under the flexor digitorum superficialis muscle midway at the forearm and innervates the flexor pollicis longus and flexor digitorum profundus muscles for the index and the middle finger as well as the pronator quadratus. A lesion of this distal motor branch is seen not only after a forearm fracture but also spontaneously (Kiloh-Nevin syndrome) [14, 18, 28, 34, 59, 61, 74]. There is no pain but an atrophy of the flexor muscles just mentioned and the incapacity to flex the distal phalanx of the thumb and index finger. The patient is no longer able to put these two fingers together in order to form the letter O.

The most frequent entrapment neuropathy is due to a compression of the median nerve at the wrist in the carpal tunnel. The canal is formed by the carpal bones and covered by the retinaculum flexorum. This ligament connects the tubercula of the scaphoid and trapezoid bone with the pisiform bone and the hamulus ossis hamati. The nerve passes through the canal together with the tendons of the long flexor of the thumb and the deep and superficial flexors of the fingers with the tendon sheaths, the nerve being the most superficial structure running just beneath the retinaculum flexorum. The most narrow point in the canal lies 2.5 cm distal to its entrance. The width of the canal in symptom-free individuals is $2.53 \text{ cm}^2 \pm 0.15$, while in laborers with symptoms or signs of a carpal tunnel syndrome the canal has a width of $1.75 \pm 0.21 \text{ cm}^2$ [8]. The pressure inside the canal is increased threefold when the wrist is flexed by 90°, as is done in the Phalen test and even more in 90° extension [2, 19]. The typical symptoms of carpal tunnel syndrome are by now well known [5, 57]. In the beginning nocturnal paresthesias and diffuse pain in the hand and quite frequently in the whole arm up to the shoulder or even the neck are present. Shaking the arm and rubbing the hands releaves the pain. Upon waking in the morning, the hand feels numb and looks swollen, but in the initial phase all disturbances disappear during the day. Only after many months a numbness and sensory loss at the radial finger tips in daytime is observed. A paralysis of the short abductor of the thumb becomes evident, and the width of grip between thumb and index is reduced. The patient is therefore no longer able, for example, to grip a bottle (bottle sign). Pain can be produced by local pressure at the retinaculum flexorum and paresthesias by a 1-min hyperflexion (Phalen test) or hyperextension of the wrist. EMG is only extremely rarely normal, if motor and orthodromic as well as antidromic sensory conduction are measured.

Entrapment Neuropathies of the Thoracic Spinal Nerves

The terminal branches of these nerves can be entrapped as their dorsal fibers pass through clefts in the fascia covering the superficial back muscles. In the dorsal region this may cause the notalgia paresthetica [66]. This is characterized by a localized pain in the back between scapula and the spine. This spot is tender, and one finds a dollar-sized local sensory loss. The pain can be temporarily eliminated by a local nerve block. A similar local pain is attributed to the analogous mechanism in the lumbar region [31, 69]. Subcutaneous fat tissue may cause a compression of the nerve branches in the fascial clefts.

The medial cutaneous branches of the caudal thoracic nerves may be entrapped at their passage through the rectus abdominis muscle or the fascia covering these muscles. This rectus abdominis syndrome [36, 70] causes a local pain, particularly in active contraction of the muscles. Local tenderness and even sensory loss can be demonstrated and sometimes even denervation in EMG.

Entrapment Neuropathy of the Ilioinguinal Nerve

The terminal sensory branch of this nerve, the anterior cutaneus branch, passes through the external oblique, a few inches medial from the anterior superior iliac spine. A spontaneous entrapment of the nerve at this passage [41, 53] causes local pain in the groin. The patient keeps the hip slightly flexed in walking and lying. A sensory loss at the groin as well as at the labium majus or at the scrotum and at the proximal medial aspect of the thigh may be present. Local tenderness near the anterior superior iliac spine and augmentation of pain by hyperextension of hip must be looked for.

Entrapment of the Lateral Femoral Cutaneous Nerve in the Inguinal Ligament

This syndrome, the meralgia paresthetica, is due to an entrapment of the purely sensory nerve at its passage through the inguinal ligament [9, 33, 58, 67]. At this passage the nerve also makes a change of its course of nearly 90°. A pull on the inguinal ligament by a protruding abdominal wall in obesity, a long-lasting extension of the hip, or strenuous physical activity including abdominal muscle activity may trigger the clinical symptoms. They are characterized by a burning pain at the anterolateral aspect of the thigh, the site of cutaneous distribution of this sensory nerve. Hyperextension of the hip increases, flexion lessens the pain. There is also local tenderness at the lateral aspect of the inguinal ligament.

Entrapment of the Obturator Nerve in the Canalis Obturatorius

This rare condition is in general due either to a herniation in the obturator canal, a tumor, or inflammatory or posttraumatic changes in this region. The symptoms, the so-called Howship-Romberg syndrome [27, 39], are characterized by pain at the inner side of the knee and sometimes a spasm or contraction [16] of adductor muscles. One may find a sensory loss at the distal and medial part of the thigh, a motor weakness of adductor muscles, and loss of the adductor reflex.

Entrapment Syndrome of Femoral Nerve

Only the longest sensory terminal branch of the femoral nerve, the saphenus nerve, may show spontaneous entrapment. The saphenus nerve runs distally in the adductor canal (Hunter) together with the femoral artery. Where it leaves the canal through the vastoadductorial membrane, it may be chronically compressed [52]. Pain and sensory loss at the medial side of the lower leg follows.

A few inches proximal to the medial condylus the infrapatellar branch separates from the saphenous nerve. This branch pierces the fascia and may be entrapped at this site by the edges of the fascial slit [39, 40, 42, 47, 49]. Pain and sensory loss, the neuropathia patellae (gonalgia paresthetica) [81] are then present at the medial side and distal to the patella.

Entrapment Neuropathies of the Tibial Nerve

This nerve can be entrapped spontaneously at two sites. At the tarsal tunnel [13, 32, 44, 51, 62, 63, 68] the nerve together with the artery and veins travels behind the internal malleolus in one of the compartments formed by septal subdivisions of the retinaculum flexorum ligament. The tendons of the flexor digitorum and flexor hallucis longus run through separate compartments. In most cases a sprain of the ankle precedes the symptoms, but sometimes no triggering cause can be found, and one must consider these spontaneous cases as entrapment syndrome. Local pain at the medial aspect of the ankle or pain in the sole of the foot enhanced by walking is a presenting symptom. One finds a local tenderness behind the internal malleolus, the sole is dry, and sometimes a sensory loss is present here. The patient is no longer able to spread apart his toes (always compare with the opposite side).

The digitales plantares communis nerves are terminal branches of the tibial nerve. They are located between the metatarsal bones, and at the level of the heads of these bones they give rise to the terminal digitales plantares proprii nerves. Here they may be subjected to chronic compression by the neighboring heads of the metatarsal bones. This entrapment syndrome, Morton's toe, [7, 25, 50, 60] is most frequent in the third or fourth interdigital space and is much more frequent in women. It is characterized by a local pain in the forefoot, in the beginning only in walking, later even spontaneously. A transverse compression of the anterior part of the foot or a local displacement of the neighboring heads of the metatarsal bones evokes an acute pain. This is temporarily eliminated by a conduction block of the common interdigital nerve from the dorsal interdigital space.

Entrapment of the Terminal Branch of the Deep Peroneal Nerve at the Dorsum of the Foot

This rare entrapment site lies under the pars cruciformis vaginae fibrosae (also called ligamentum cruciatum or retinaculum extensorum) at the dorsum of the foot. The terminal branch of the deep peroneal nerve travels under this ligament. An entrapment at this site is sometimes called anterior tarsal tunnel syndrome [10, 20, 43]. It is characterized mainly by pain and a sensory loss dorsally over the first interdigital space. One can also demonstrate a motor weakness of the short extensors at the dorsum of the foot.

Acknowledgement. We gratefully acknowledge the help of Nicole Kühl for assembling the data for Table 1 from our patient files.

References

1. Adson AW, Coffey JR (1927) Cervical rib. A method of anterior approach for relief of symptoms by divison of the scalenus anticus. Ann Surg 85:839–857
2. Aminoff MJ (1979) Involvement of peripheral vasomotor fibres in carpal tunnel syndrome. J Neurol Neurosurg Psychiat 42:649–655
3. Augustin P, Verdure L, Samson M (1976) Le syndrome du nerf sus-scapulaire à l'étroit. Une neuropathie canalaire souvent méconnue. Rev Neurol 132:219–222
4. Beaton LE, Anson BJ (1939) Relation of median nerve to pronator teres muscle. Anat Rec 75:23–26
5. Benini A, (1975) Das Karpaltunnelsyndrom und die übrigen Kompressionssyndrome des Nervus medianus. Thieme, Stuttgart
6. Benini A, Di Martino E (1976) Die Schädigung des Ramus profundus nervi radialis (Supinatorsyndrom). Die dissoziierte Radialislähmung vom proximalen Unterarmtyp. Schweiz Med Wochenschr 106:639–643
7. Betts LO (1940) Morton's metatarsalgia. Neuritis of fourth digital nerve. Med J Aust 1:514–515
8. Bleecker ML, Bohlmann M, Moreland R et al. (1985) Carpal tunnel syndrome: role of carpal canal size. Neurology (Minneap) 35:1599–1604
9. Bollinger A, (1961) Die Meralgia paraesthetica. Klinisches Bild und Pathogenese anhand von 158 eigenen Fällen. Schweiz. Arch Neurol Neurochir Psychiat 87:58–102
10. Borges LF, Hallett M, Selkoe DJ, Welch K (1981) The anterior tarsal tunnel syndrome. Report of two cases. J Neurosurg 54:89–92
11. Cahill BR, Palmer RE (1983) Quadrilateral space syndrome. J Hand Surg 8:65–69
12. Castaigne P, Laplane D et al. (1969) Etude de neuf cas de côte cervicale et d'un cas d'apophysomégalie avec complications neurologiques, tous opérés, dont huit comportent une artériographie sous-clavière. Rev Neurol 120:210–214
13. De Sèze S, Dreyfus P, Denis A et al. (1970) The tarsal tunnel syndrome. Clinical and electromyographic study. Ann Phys Med 13:133–149
14. d'A. Fearn CB, Goodfellow JW (1965) Anterior interosseous nerve palsy. J Bone Joint Surg 47(B):91–93
15. Feindel W, Stratford J (1958) The role of the cubital tunnel in tardy ulnar palsy. Canad J Surg 1:287–300
16. Fettweis E (1966) Kniegelenks- und Hüftgelenkskontrakturen bei narbiger Irritation des sensiblen Astes des Nervus obturatorius. Dtsch Med Wochenschr 91:313–314
17. Gantert F, Alzheimer C (1956) Der Processus supracondylicus humeri als Ursache von Medianusschädigungen (Ein Beitrag zur Differentialdiagnose der Schmerzzustände im Bereich des Armes). Nervenarzt 27:349–353
18. Gardner-Thorpe C (1974) Anterior interosseous nerve palsy: spontaneous recovery in two patients. J Neurol Neurosurg Psychiat, 37:1146–1150
19. Gelberman R, Hergenroeder P, Hargens A et al. (1981) The carpal tunnel syndrome. A study of carpal tunnel pressures. J Bone Joint Surg 63(A):380–383
20. Gessini L, Jandolo B, Pietrangeli A (1984) The anterior tarsal syndrome. Report of four cases. J Bone Joint Surg 66(A):786–787
21. Gilliatt RW, Willison RG, Dietz V, Williams IR (1978) Peripheral nerve conduction in patients with a cervical rib and band. Ann Neurol 4:124–129

22. Goldman S, Honet JC et al. (1969) Posterior interosseous nerve palsy in the absence of traume. Arch Neurol (Chic) 21:435–441
23. Gosset J, Apoil A (1972) Les paralysis tronculaires par compression nerveuse à l'avant-bras. (Nerfs médian, cubital et radial). Ann Chir 26:119–130
24. Goulon M, Lord G, Bedoiseau (1963) L'atteinte du médian et du cubital par apophyse sus-épitrochléenne. A propos de deux observations. Presse Méd 71:2355–2357
25. Greenfield J, Rea J, Ilfeld F (1984) Morton's interdigital neuroma. Indications for treatment by local injections versus surgery. Clin Orthop 185:142–144
26. Guyon F (1861) Note sur une disposition anatomique propre à la face antérieure de la région du poignet et non encore décrite. Bull Soc Anat (Paris) 36:184–186
27. Heckl RW (1976) Die Obturatoriusneuralgie. Akt Neurol 3:199–202
28. Huffmann G, Leven B (1976) N.-interosseus-anterior-Syndrom. Bericht über 4 eigene und 49 Fälle aus der Literatur. J Neurol 213:317–326
29. Hustead AP, Mulder DW, MacCarthy CS (1958) Nontraumatic, progressive paralysis of the deep radial (posterior interosseous) nerve. Arch Neurol (Chic) 79:269–274
30. Kaeser HE (1963) Diagnostische Probleme beim Karpaltunnelsyndrom. Dtsch Z Nervenheilk 185:453–470
31. Kaeser HE, Hochstätter A von (1973) Neurologische Schmerzursachen. Gynäkologe 6:138–144
32. Keck C (1962) The tarsal-tunnel syndrome. J Bone Joint Surg 44(A):180–182
33. Kilburn P (1957) Meralgia paraesthetica. Lancet II:952
34. Kiloh L, Nevin S (1952) Isolated neuritis of the anterior interosseous nerve. Brit Med J I:850–851
35. Komar J (1976) Eine wichtige Ursache des Schulterschmerzes: Incisura scapulae-Syndrom. Fortschr Neurol Psychiat 44:644–648
36. Komar J, Varga B (1975) Syndrome of the rectus abdominis muscle. A peripheral neurological condition causing abdominal diagnostic problems. J Neurol 210:121–125
37. Komar J, Szegavari M (1983) Der peripher-neurologische Hintergrund des Schreibkrampfes: mittlere N. medianus-Läsion. Nervenarzt 54:322–325
38. Kopell HP, Thompson WAL (1958) Pronator syndrome. Confirmed case and its diagnosis. New Engl J Med 259:713–715
39. Kopell HP, Thompson WAL (1960) Peripheral entrapment neuropathies of the lower extremity. New Engl J Med 262:56–60
40. Kopell HP, Thompson WAL (1960) Knee pain due to saphenous nerve entrapment. New Engl J Med 263:351–353
41. Kopell HP, Thompson WAL, Postel AH (1962) Entrapment neuropathy of the ilioinguinal nerve. New Engl J Med 266:16–19
42. Kopell HP, Thompson WAL (1963) Peripheral entrapment neuropathies. Williams & Wilkins, Baltimore
43. Krause K-H, Witt T, Ross A (1977) The anterior tarsal tunnel syndrome. J Neurol 217:67–74
44. Lam SJS (1967) Tarsal tunnel syndrome. J Bone Joint Surg 46(B):87–92
45. Löser R, Prill A et al. (1972) Das nichttraumatische Supinatorlogensyndrom des N. radialis und seine Abgrenzung zum zervikalen Wurzelreizsyndrom. Z Neurol 201:337–347
46. Marchetti N, Bachechi P, Barbieri E, Guido G (1978) Sindromi nervose canalicolari degli arti ad eziologia non traumatica. Liviana, Padova
47. Martinelli P, Montagna P, Coccagna G (1982) Neuropathy of the infrapatellar branch of the saphenous nerve in the differential dignosis of knee pain. Ital J Neurol Sci 2:153–154
48. McKowen HC, Voorhies RM (1987) Axillary nerve entrapment in the quadrilateral space. J Neurosurg 66:932–934
49. Moller BN, Helmig O (1984) Patellar pain treated by neurotomy. Arch Orthop Traum Surg 103:137–139
50. Morton TG (1876) A peculiar and painful affection about the fourth metatarsophalangeal articulation. Am J Med Sci 71:37–45

51. Mosimann W, Mumenthaler M (1969) Das posttraumatische Tarsaltunnelsyndrom. Mitteilung von 35 eigenen Beobachtungen. Helv Chir Acta 36:547–560
52. Mozes M, Quaknine GE, Nathan H (1975) La névralgie du nerf saphène interne. Une forme inhabituelle d'atteinte du nerf crural. Nouv. Presse Méd 4:2099–2101
53. Mumenthaler A, Mumenthaler M et al. (1965) Das Ilioinguinalis-Syndrom. Beschreibung von 7 eigenen Beobachtungen. Dtsch Med Wochenschr 90:1073–1078
54. Mumenthaler M (1958) Die Ulnarislähmung an der Handwurzel. Klinik und Therapie anhand von 30 eigenen Fällen. Schweiz Arch Neurol Psychiat 82:229–272
55. Mumenthaler M (1961) Die Ulnarisparesen. Thieme, Stuttgart
56. Mumenthaler M (1973) Some clinical aspects of nontraumatic mechanical lesions of peripheral nerves. Analysis of 3465 personal cases. Schweiz Arch Neurol Neurosurg Psychiat 112:229–237
57. Mumenthaler M, Schliack H (1987) Läsionen peripherer Nerven, 5. Aufl. Thieme, Stuttgart
58. Nathan H (1960) Gangliform enlargement on the lateral cutaneous nerve of the thigh. Its significance in the understanding of the aetiology of meralgia paraesthetica. J Neurosurg 17:843–850
59. Neundörfer B, Kröger M (1976) The anterior interosseous nerve syndrome. J Neurol 213:347–352
60. Nissen KI (1948) Plantar digital neuritis. J Bone Joint Surg 30(B):84–94
61. O'Brien D, Upton ARM (1972) Anterior interosseous nerve-syndrome. J Neurol Neurosurg Psychiat 35:531–536
62. Oh SJ, Sarala PK, Kuba T et al. (1979) Tarsal tunnel syndrome: electrophysiological study. Ann Neurol 5:327–330
63. O'Malley GM, Lambdin CS, McCleary GS (1985) Tarsal tunnel syndrome. Orthopedics 8:758–760
64. Pechan J, Julis I (1975) The pressure measurement in the ulnar nerve. A contribution to the pathophysiology of the cubital tunnel syndrome. J Biomech 8:75–79
65. Penkert G, Schwandt D (1979) Beidseitige, nicht traumatische Radialis-profundus-Läsion. Nervenarzt 50:783–787
66. Pleet AB, Massey EW (1978) Notalgia paresthetica. Neurology (Minneap) 28:1310–1313
67. Privat JM, Claustre J, Simon L, Gros C (1980) La méralgie paresthésique: Syndrome canalaire méconnu. Neurochirurgie 26:239–242
68. Radin EL (1983) Tarsal tunnel syndrome. Clin Orthop 181:167–170
69. Richter HR (1971) Discushernien und Einklemmungssyndrome der Rami dorsales der lumbalen und sakralen Spinalnerven. Schweiz. Arch Neurol Neurochir Psychiat 101:75–86
70. Rutgers MJ (1986) The rectus abdominis syndrome: a case report. J Neurol 233:180–181
71. Schaumburg HH, Spencer PS, Thomas PK (1983) Disorders of peripheral nerves. Davis, Philadelphia
72. Seyffarth H (1951) Primary myoses in the M. pronator teres as cause of lesion of the N. medianus (the pronator-syndrome). Acta Psychiat Scand (Suppl) 74:251–254
73. Shea DJ, McClain EJ (1969) Ulnar-nerve compression syndromes at and below the wrist. J Bone Joint Surg 51(A):1095–1102
74. Smith BH, Herbst BA (1974) Anterior interosseous nerve palsy. Arch Neurol (Chic) 30:330–331
75. Smith RV, Fisher RG (1973) Struthers ligament: a source of median nerve compression above the elbow. Case report. J Neurosurg 38:778–779
76. Stewart JDK, Aguayp AJ (1983) Compression and entrapment neuropathy. In: Dyck PJ, Thomas PK, Lambert EH, Bunge R (eds) Peripheral neuropathy, 2nd ed. Saunders, Philadelphia, pp 1435–1457
77. Stolke D, Seidel BU, Schliack H (1980) Das Syndrom der Loge de Guyon oder die Ulnarisparese am Handgelenk unter Bevorzugung des Ramus profundus. Akt Neurol 7:161–165

78. Suranyi Leslie (1983) Median nerve compression by Struthers ligament. J Neurol Neurosurg Psychiat 46:1047–1049
79. Thompson WAL, Kopell HP (1959) Peripheral entrapment neuropathies of upper extremity. New Engl J Med 260:1261–1265
80. Vichare NA (1968) Spontaneous paralysis of the anterior interosseous nerve. J Bone Joint Surg 50(B):806–808
81. Weigert M, Friedebold G, Klems H (1971) Fehler und Gefahren beim totalen Hüftgelenkersatz. Z Orthop 104:659–676
82. Wulff CH, Gilliatt RW (1979) F waves in patients with hand wasting caused by a cervical rib and band. Muscle and Nerve 2:452–457

Evaluation of the Various Routine Neurophysiological Parameters in Diagnosis of Carpal Tunnel Syndrome

L. Rabow and H. Holmgren, Umeå and Linköping/Sweden

Introduction

Since operation for carpal tunnel syndrome (CTS) is a comparatively easy procedure, it is often carried out without any neurophysiological investigation in patients with a typical clinical picture. There are even those who claim that there is no neurophysiological pathology during the day as long as the patients have symptoms only during the night, which is not unusual in the early stage of the disease. Our own experience, however, is that all patients with a neurophysiologically confirmed diagnosis of CTS improve after operation, while patients with more or less identical symptoms but with normal neurophysiological findings do not.

Against this background we have evaluated the specificity and sensitivity of the various routine neurophysiological parameters as regards clinical symptoms of CTS and their improvement after surgery.

Material and Methods

Our 48 patients, 33 women and 15 men, aged 21–80 years (mean, 50 ± 14), had clinical CTS as defined elsewhere [1] and had at least one pathological neurophysiological sign of CTS. Each patient was examined before and 6 months after a successful operation, i.e., when the patient reported a complete restitution or a significant improvement.

The following neurophysiological parameters were studied: sensory conduction velocity (SCV) with distal latency (SDL), motor conduction velocity (MCV) with distal latency (MDL), and EMG and perception thresholds for touch and vibration. The threshold for touch was determined according to a method described by Lindblom [2]. For measuring the vibratory sense a vibrameter (Biothesiometer, Biomed, Ohio, Mass) was used. The other techniques and normal values are described in our previous paper [1]. The patients were operated on with a simple sectioning of the flexor retinaculum, with and without an epineurolysis. As reported earlier [1] the epineurolysis did not affect the results. The clinical examination was carried out after 6 months and followed up with a questionnaire after 3 years.

Results

Of the patients with CTS 91% had a pathological SCV before operation, and this was still abnormal after clinical restitution in 72%, in spite of a significant increase in mean SCV for the group as a whole. A prolonged SDL characterized 77%; this normalized after clinical restitution in all but 25%. Regarding MDL, the sensitivity was somewhat lower than for SCV and SDL: 67% of the patients with CTS were abnormal. This parameter showed, however, the highest specificity, since only 17% of the patients were abnormal after clinical restitution.

Table 1. Results of investigations

Neurophysiological parameters	Abnormal findings	
	Before operation	After operation
Sensory conduction velocity	91%	72%
Sensory distal latency	77%	23%
Motor conduction velocity	40%	32%
Motor distal latency	67%	17%
EMG, denervation	55%	26%
Tactile perception threshold	54%	24%
Biothesiometry	57%	24%

EMG, Denervation, Vibration Threshold, and Biothesiometry. The sensitivity was fairly low, about 50% for all these parameters, and the specificity was also less good than for SDL and MDL (Table 1). Decline in amplitude of the M response can also be seen in CTS, although this is not a very sensitive parameter.

Discussion

The most interesting finding is perhaps that most patients in this series had a pathologically prolonged sensory conduction velocity even after a complete clinical restitution. It must be pointed out, however, that the mean SCV was significantly increased for the group as a whole.

It is certainly true that SCV will remain slow depending on impaired function in the remyelinated fibers, which are only as functional as the most severely affected internodes [3], but the fact remains that a prolonged SCV does not necessarily cause clinical symptoms and may therefore very well precede a manifest CTS. Prolongation of the distal motor latency is the motor counterpart of delayed sensory conduction. The incidence of abnormality is high, although the test is not as sensitive as sensory conduction. This has been confirmed by many authors [4–6].

Comparing the median distal motor latency to that of the ulnar gives a slight increase in sensitivity. EMG is less useful than nerve conduction studies in the evaluation of CTS. It is said that abnormalities occur only in more advanced cases, indicating axonotmesis.

In conclusion, one must be careful to diagnose CTS if the sensory conduction velocity is normal. Prolonged motor distal latency 6 months after operation for CTS should throw some doubt on the adequacy of the procedure.

References

1. Holmgren-Larsson H, Leszniewski M, Lindén U, Rabow L, Thorling J (1985) Internal neurolysis or ligament division only in carpal tunnel syndrome – results of a randomized study. Acta Neurochir 74:118–121
2. Lindblom U (1974) Touch perception threshold in human glabrous skin in terms of displacement amplitude on stimulation with single mechanical pulses. Brain Res 82:205–210
3. Rasminsky M (1973) The effects of temperature on conduction in demyelinated single nerve fibres. Arch Neurol 28:287–295
4. Loong SC (1977) The carpal tunnel syndrome: a clinical and electrophysiological study of 250 patients. Proc Aust Assoc Neurol 14:51–62
5. Thomas PK (1960) Motor nerve conduction in the carpal tunnel syndrome. Neurology 10:1045–1050
6. Thomas JE, Lambert EH, Cseuz KA (1967) Electrodiagnostic aspects of the carpal tunnel syndrome. Arch Neurol 16:635–641

Relationships Between Preoperative Symptoms, Electrophysiological and Intraoperative Findings, and the Outcome in Patients with Carpal Tunnel Syndrome

H.-E. Nau and B. Lange, Essen/FRG

Introduction

The shorter the duration of symptoms and the less their severity, the better seems the prognosis for improvement in complaints and disorders of a disease. One can suppose that the clinical symptoms correlate with objective findings. In carpal tunnel syndrome, preoperative findings and outcome seem to be connected with weakness or atrophy of abductor pollicis brevis muscle and failure of long-term benefit [9]. Electrophysiological tests have proved their value in early [1, 7, 24] and differential diagnosis [12, 19, 22]. But it is not certain that there is a significant correlation between the degree of electrophysiological alterations and the degree of nerve compression [10]. In spite of different opinions about the preoperative value of electrophysiological examinations, the improvement or normalization of nerve conduction velocity after operation is generally supposed to correspond to the relief of symptoms [3–6, 14, 17, 20].

Our investigation sought to determine the relationships between pre- and intraoperative conditions including the clinical symptoms and electrophysiological tests before operative procedures.

Patients and Methods

Our investigation included 55 hands of 44 patients (33 women, 11 men; average age of the women 54, of the men 51 years). All underwent decompression of the median nerve in the carpal tunnel. In our clinic pre- and postoperative clinical and electrophysiological investigations were done in all patients. One patient was left-handed. Eleven patients (eight women, three men) suffered from bilateral carpal tunnel syndrome. The time of postoperative examination ranged from 2 months to 8 years (average 37 months).

Pareses and sensory disturbances were classified according to Röttgen and Wüllenweber [18] and Seddon [21], the electromyographic alterations according to Liesegang [13] and Simpson [22]. The electromyo-neurographic investigations were done with Schwarzer electromyograph 2000/2 and concentric steel needle electrodes (DISA) from the short abductor pollicis muscle. The motor nerve conduction velocity was separately derived along the carpal tunnel and the forearm.

The results were classified as excellent (no neurological deficit, no electromyo-neurographic alterations), good (clinical symptoms, electromyo-neurographic alterations markedly improved), satisfactory (clinical symptoms better, electromyo-neurographic alterations unchanged), or not satisfactory (clinical symptoms, electromyo-neurographic alterations unchanged or worse).

Results

The typical brachialgia paresthetica nocturna depended on the duration of symptoms and was found especially in a short duration of symptoms. Concomitant motor deficits improved excellently in those patients with nocturnal brachialgia. Positive signs in the provocation tests (Hoffmann-Tinel sign, flexion/extension tests) were seen in patients with shorter duration of symptoms. The motor deficits of patients with preoperative sensory deficit and without postoperative sensory improvement did not improve at all. The severity of paresis and atrophy depended on the preoperative duration of symptoms. In nearly all these cases (longer histories and atrophy) the operation revealed gross alterations of the median nerve. A statistically significant recovery was found in patients with motor deficits but without atrophies. Electromyographic alterations reflected paresis and muscle atrophy very early and well.

There was no connection between the degree of the alterations of the ligament and the duration of symptoms. The alterations of intention patterns improved depending on the severity and the duration of the alterations in the preoperative course with the exception of alterations in patients with a history longer than 1 year and with thenar atrophy. In accordance with complaints and severity of symptoms the nerve conduction velocity was decreased in the carpal tunnel. Postoperatively there was quick improvement. Nerve conduction velocity measuring was more useful for therapy control than for prognostic hints. The favorable and unfavorable signs in regard to the outcome are summarized in Table 1.

Table 1. Pre- and intraoperative findings in regard to the outcome

Favorable signs	Unfavorable signs
Short history	Atrophy
Brachialgia paresthetica nocturna	Marked gross morphological alterations
Positive provocation tests	
Absence of atrophy	
EMG: (spontaneous activity) good intention pattern	

Discussion

Brachialgia paresthetica nocturna was found in cases with short histories. This may point to an earlier lesion of the thinner pain-conducting nerve fibers, which may be supported by the findings of early reduced sensory conduction velocities [8]. It was a good sign for the outcome.

Motor deficits of patients with postoperatively persisting sensory deficit did not improve. In half of these patients we found a preoperative atrophy of thenar muscles so that – if not the median nerve – the reacting organ (muscle) was irreversibly impaired before the operation. Similar findings were reported by Mühlau et al. [15]. Thus muscle atrophy and the corresponding electromyographic alterations were signs of an unfavorable outcome. Positive provocation tests in short histories were described also by Rickenbacher [17]. In these cases there were no atrophies, but some already showed intraoperative alterations when decompression was performed. These might be due to the different etiologies and pathogenesis. The positive tests may be an early sign of primary morphological alterations around the nerve.

Intraoperatively, alterations of the nerve (augmentation of connective tissue, signs of compression) were more frequent than alterations of the ligament (thickening). This may also point to the different causes in pathogenesis. There was no connection between the degree of alterations of the ligament and the duration of symptoms. In contrast to these results, the intraoperative finding of augmented connective tissue could be seen in patients with symptoms lasting longer than half a year.

Electromyography seems useful to objectify motor deficits, the acuteness of the lesion and the differential diagnosis. Signs of denervation were found in cases with shorter and longer histories when the process was still going on. Postoperatively there was no spontaneous activity. This means that the surgical treatment could stop the process. The alterations of intention patterns improved depending on the severity and the duration of the alterations in the preoperative course. No relief was seen in hands with a history longer than 1 year and with thenar atrophy, which is understandable because the processes of the muscular transformation are reversible only in functional and not organic lesions, such as muscle atrophy.

The electroneurographic alterations proximal to the lesion [23, 25] may be secondary to circulation alterations. Circulation seems to be involved because shunts of the extrinsic epineural system proximal to a compressing ligament could be seen in some patients during operation. The role of circulatory disorders has been discussed in the literature [2] and seems to be important in our own histological investigations [16] (see Gerhard et al., this volume). Corresponding to the complaints and the severity of symptoms the nerve conduction velocity was decreased in the carpal tunnel. Postoperatively, it improved quickly, which was also found by Le Quesne and Casey [11]. These quickly reversible alterations also point to the role of the circulation.

Conclusions

The results indicate that pain as the first symptom is due to metabolic alterations evoked by circulatory alterations, a fact which manifests itself primarily in special provocation conditions such as extreme flexion or extension of the hand with reducing venous and perhaps later arterial circulation. The nocturnal pain might be produced by a venous stasis caused by the lack of muscle pump. This is why the presence of positive provocation tests are a good sign for the prognosis. If the circulatory disorders are prolonged, morphological changes can become manifest, such as edema and thereafter thickening of nerve connective tissue and alterations of myelin sheath. The venous stasis can enlarge proximally – evoking pain – and leads to morphological alterations with marked electrophysiological disturbances. These are reflected in reduced nerve conduction velocity proximal to the lesion. At this stage the operation can stop the process, and restoration can begin. At the stage of morphological alterations, clinically considered as muscle atrophy, an operation cannot improve deficits whereas it should be possible at the earlier stages of repetitive circulatory disturbances. The degree of the morphological alterations and the operative outcome can be estimated by electromyography.

References

1. Buchtthal F, Rosenfalck A (1971) Sensory conduction from digit to palm and from palm to wrist in the carpal tunnel syndrome. J Neurol Neurosurg Psychiat 34:243–252
2. Fullerton PM (1963) The effect of ischemia on nerve conduction in the carpal tunnel syndrome. J Neurol Neurosurg Psychiat 26:385–397
3. Gassman N, Segmüller G (1976) Das Karpaltunnelsyndrom: Indikation und Technik der epineuralen und der interfaszikulären Neurolyse. Hel Chir Acta 63:699–702
4. Glidden A, Bauer RB (1968) Carpal tunnel syndrome: a comparison of nerve conduction studies before and after treatment. Harper Hosp Bull 26:221–230
5. Godman HV, Gilliatt RW (1961) The effect of treatment on median nerve conduction in patients with the carpal tunnel syndrome. Ann Phys Med 6:137–155
6. Hongell A, Mattsson HS (1971) Neurographic studies before, after and during operation for median nerve compression in the carpal tunnel. Scand J Plast Reconstr Surg 5:103–109
7. Jacobson S (1976) The carpal tunnel syndrome. Electroenceph. Clin Neurophysiol 22:392
8. Kaeser HE (1963) 3. Elektromyographische Untersuchungen bei Diskushernien und bei Kompressionssyndromen peripherer Nerven. Schweiz Arch Neurol Neurochir Psychiat 92:64–73
9. Kulick MI, Gordillo G, Javidi T, Kilgore ES, Newmeyer III WL (1986) Long-term analysis of patients having surgical treatment for carpal tunnel syndrome. J Hand Surg 11(A):59–66
10. Leblhuber F, Reisecker F, Witzmann A (1986) Carpal tunnel syndrome: neurographical parameters in different stages of median nerve compression. Acta Neurochir 81:125–127
11. Le Quesne PM, Casey EB (1974) Recovery of conduction velocity distal to a compressive lesion. J Neurol Neurosurg Psychiat 37:1346–1351
12. Lichtman DM, Florio RL, Mack GR (1979) Carpal tunnel release under local anesthesia: evaluation of the outpatient procedure. J Hand Surg 4:544–546

13. Liesegang J (1975) Neurophysiologische Untersuchungen bei zervikalen Kompressionssyndromen. Thesis, Essen
14. Maxion H, Wessinghage D, Leng E (1972) Untersuchungsbefunde nach konservativer und operativer Behandlung des Karpaltunnelsyndroms. Med. Welt 14:714–726
15. Mühlau G, Both R, Kunath H (1984) Carpal tunnel syndrome – course and prognosis. J Neurol 231:83–86
16. Nau H-E (1982) Klinische und tierexperimentelle Untersuchungen zu Druckläsionen peripherer Nerven. Thesis, Essen
17. Rickenbacher M (1971) Karpaltunnelsyndrom. Spätergebnisse nach operativer Behandlung des Karpaltunnelsyndroms. Klinische und elektromyographische Nachkontrolle von 24 Fällen. Hel Chir Acta 38:359–366
18. Röttgen P, Wüllenweber R (1974) Die Chirurgie der peripheren Nerven. In: Olivecrona H, Tönnis W, Krenkel W (Hrsg) Handbuch der Neurochirurgie, Bd 7/3. Springer, Wien New York S 269–497
19. Rogoff JB (1978) Electrical study in carpal tunnel syndrome. Arthritis and Rheumatism (Atlanta) 21:865
20. Schoenhuber R, Bortolotti P, Malavasi P, Landi A (1984) Elektromyographie und Elektroneurographie in der Nachuntersuchung von Karpaltunnelsyndrom-Patienten. Neurochirurgia 27:144–145
21. Seddon HJ (1942) Classification of nerve injuries. Brit Med J II:237–239
22. Simpson JA (1975) Terminology of electromyography. In: Remond A (ed) Handbook of electroencephalography and clinical neurophysiology, Vol. 13. Elsevier, Amsterdam, pp 16-B-132–136
23. Stöhr M, Petruch F, Scheglman K, Schilling K (1978) Retrograde changes of nerve fibres with the carpal tunnel syndrome. An electroneurographic investigation. J Neurol 218:287–292
24. Thomas JE, Lambert EH, Cseuz KA (1967) Electrodiagnostic aspects of the carpal tunnel syndrome. Arch Neurol 16:635–641
25. Thomas PK (1960) Motor nerve conduction in the carpal tunnel syndrome. J Neurol Neurosurg Psychiat 26:520–527

Morphological and Pathogenetic Considerations in Entrapment Syndromes

L. GERHARD, V. REINHARDT, E. KOOB, and H.-E. NAU, Essen/FRG

Introduction

The damage to peripheral nerves by entrapment is due to compressive mechanisms that occur where the nerves are normally confined to narrow anatomic passage pathways and are therefore susceptible to compression. This definition does not include any details about the pathogenetic mechanisms in entrapment syndromes. It is also known that the peripheral nerves are more susceptible to mechanical injury in special metabolic conditions such as alcoholism, diabetes mellitus, malnutrition syndromes, and endocrine disturbances. The best known entrapment neuropathy is the carpal tunnel syndrome (CTS) of the median nerve. Other syndromes of the ulnar and radial nerves as well as of the peroneal nerve are less frequent and therefore less well investigated. Only little attention has been paid to the "painful hand" (interosseous ramus of radial nerve syndrome, IRS).

Material and Methods

We investigated patients with CTS and with IRS. In order to investigate normal morphological conditions in the carpal tunnel studies were done in autopsy cases.

The control group consisted of 17 hands in 9 patients (four men and five women, aged 17–81 years) who died because of various cerebral diseases (brain injuries, SAH) and without clinical signs of median nerve entrapment in the carpal tunnel. The contents of the carpal tunnel was removed in toto. After formalin fixation the tissue was embedded in paraffin. Division of the blocks in longitudinal and transverse diameters followed. From each block serial sections were performed. Staining was done with the methods described for biopsies.

In 24 patients (aged 23–60 years) with clinically and electrophysiologically established CTS the removed parts of the ligament were investigated. Staining was with hemalaun-eosin, PAS, Gomori, Sudan black B nuclear fast red, elastica van Gieson, and Ladewig methods. The syndrome of IRS was investigated in 55 patients with operative resection of the interosseous ramus of the deep radial nerve (Fig. 1) which include now 100 investigated cases.

Inflammatory 54.5%
f:m = 25:5

30

Miscellaneous 3.6%
f:m = 2:0

Posttraumatic 7.3%
f:m = 3:1

2

4

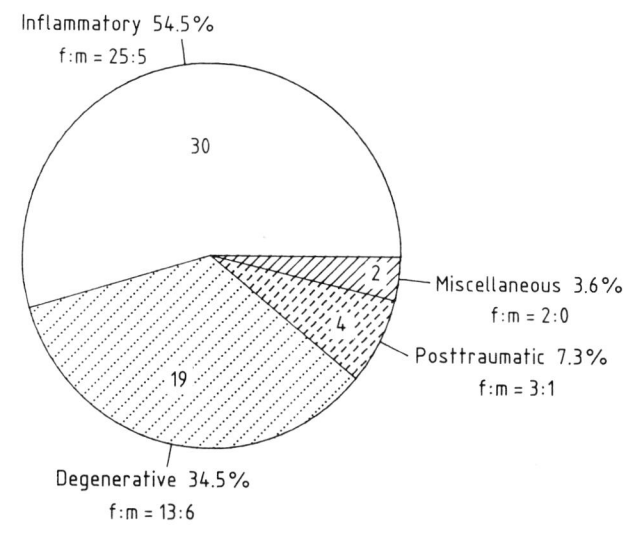

19

Degenerative 34.5%
f:m = 13:6

Fig. 1. Disease groups in patients with resection of interosseous ramus of the radial nerve

Results

Autopsy Cases (*CTS*). In all specimen portions of the muscles were found on the ulnar or radial side of the carpal tunnel ligament. The muscles of the hypothenar had an origin with a large angle, in contrast to the thenar muscles which originated in a sharp one. The diameter of the muscle fibers varied substantially. The variation in muscle fiber diameter was independent of age. In one old patient there were many ring fibers (type I) in the thenar muscles. In a young patient we found a high percentage of fatty tissue in the muscles as well as significant fibrosis. The ligament consisted of collagenous tissue and elastic parts. As a rule, its thickness was 2–3 mm. In two cases we found small nerve fascicles penetrating the ligament. Above the ligament there were Vater-Paccini bodies, at least one in each case but as a rule more than one. Their distribution was variable between ulnar and radial position.

The median nerve had the typical morphology of a peripheral nerve. In some older patients we found a marked intrafascicular augmentation of collagen and arteriosclerotic changes of epi- and intraneural vessels. The fascicles varied in size and were septated. In one case there was a proliferation of fibrocytes between perineurium and myelin sheath. A thickening of perineurium was seen in one patient only. There was a marked vascularization of endo- and epineurium. Certain changes in groups and chains of fibrocytes – Renaut's bodies – with production of much intracytoplasmatic fibrous material were found in the close neighborhood of the perineurium. In two cases we found these bodies in a great number and in each fascicle. Their distribution was documented in comparison with the normal one (Fig. 2).

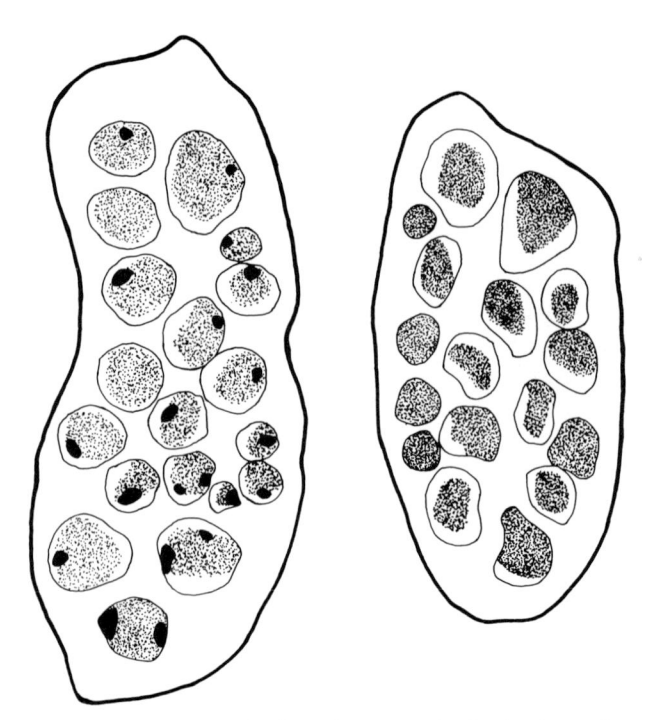

Fig. 2. Schematic distribution of Renaut's bodies in the median nerve in the carpal tunnel at the left compared to normal findings at the right

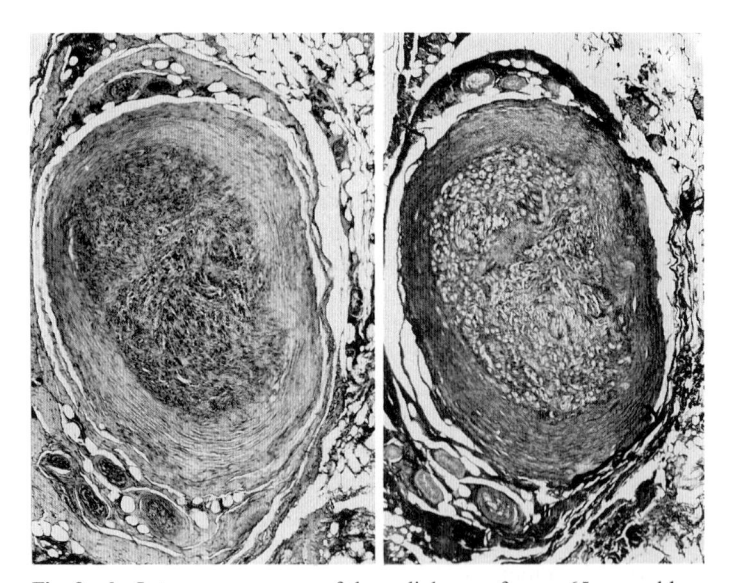

Fig. 3a, b. Interosseous ramus of the radial nerve from a 65-year-old woman suffering from primary chronic polyarthritis, thickening of perineural sheath, demyelination (**a**) and intrafascicular fibrosis (**b**). (**a** Sudan black B nuclear fast red, ×54; **b** Elastica van Gieson, ×54)

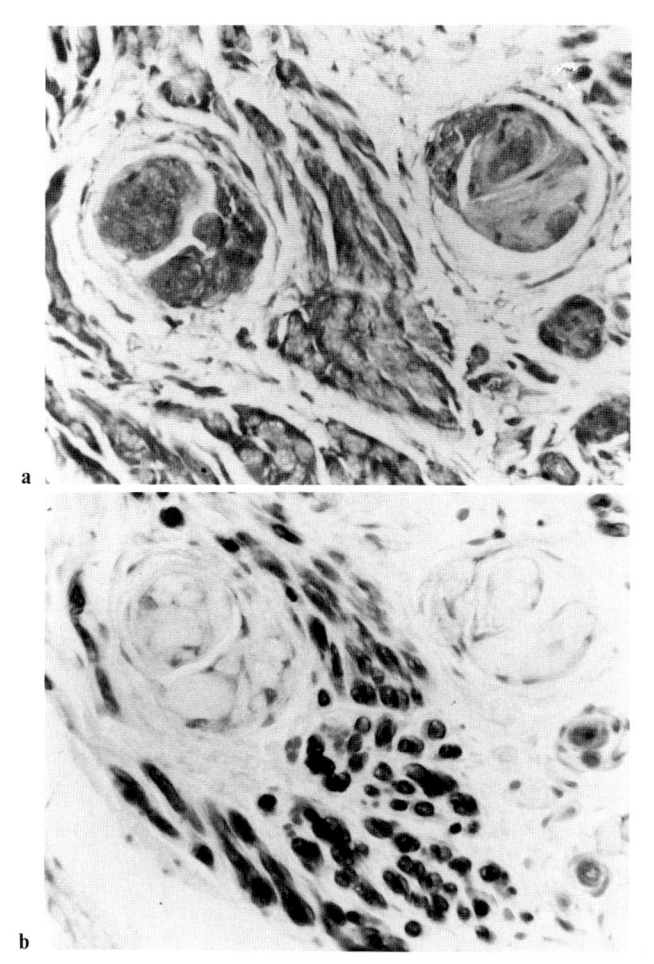

Fig. 4a, b. Small bundle of myelin sheaths pushed asunder by Renaut's bodies and fibrotic areas. (**a** Elastica van Gieson, ×320; **b** Sudan black B nuclear fast red, ×320)

The tendons showed no remarkable alterations in different ages. The vessels demonstrated alterations in a variable degree independent of age. We found sclerosis of the vessel wall and hyalinosis. Near the ligament smaller vessels had a large endothelial layer. A marked meandering of nearly all vessels could be seen inside of and close to the carpal tunnel.

Bioptic Material of Patients with CTS. All alterations described for the carpal tunnel ligament in the control group could be found in the bioptic material as well. In some bioptic cases we recognized marked alterations of small nerve fascicles penetrating the ligament: thickened perineural sheath with increased collagen, liquid and connective tissue cells in the space between the perineural sheath and the nerve fiber, some Renaut's bodies with tendency to hyalinosis, and the vessels still more serpentiform.

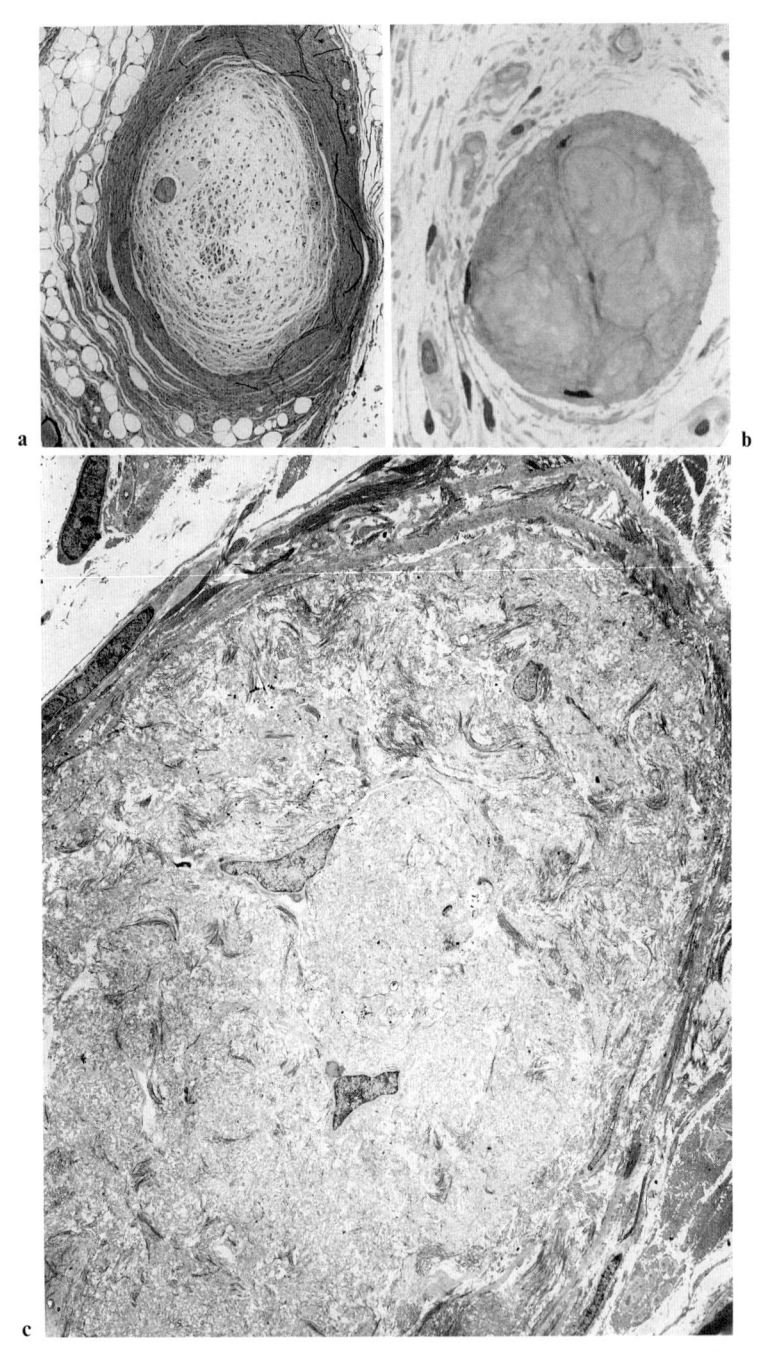

Fig. 5a–c. Ramus interosseus nervi radialis. **a** Much thickened perineural sheath, few myelinated axons and a large Renaut's body. **b** Higher magnification of the Renaut's body. **c** Ultrastructure of Renaut's body with fibrillated and granular matrix. (**a, b** Semithin section; **a** ×54; **b** ×563; **c** ×2550)

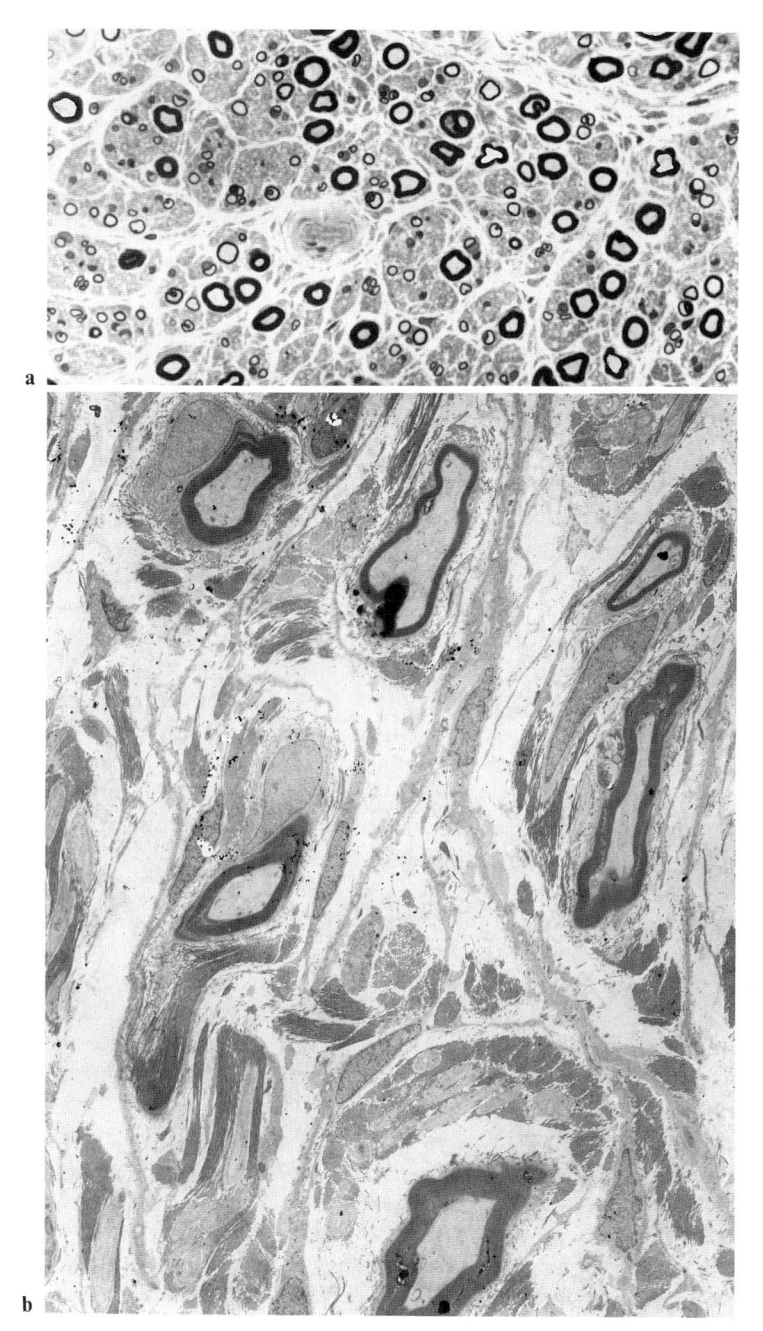

Fig. 6a. Interosseous ramus of the radial nerve with very different thickness of myelin sheath in the semithin section in spite of equal callibers of the axons. **b** Ultrastructure of myelinated axons, demonstrating the different diameter of myelin sheath and fibrosis. (**a** Semithin section; ×563; **b** ×2550)

Biopsies of Patients with IRS. The advantage of the studies of the interosseous nerve (IRS) compared with those in CTS was that the morphological changes of the resected nerve could be investigated. We found the following histological changes: (a) increased thickness of the perineural sheaths either generalized or in distinct parts (Fig. 3) and cytoplasmic changes in cells of the perineural sheath (Fig. 4); (b) demyelination and remyelination of axons (Figs. 3, 6); (c) loss of axons; (d) fibrosis and proliferation of Schwann's cells; (e) formation of Renaut's bodies (Fig. 5); and (f) mucoid changes inside the fascicle.

Discussion

It must be assumed that the pathogenesis of entrapment syndrome is similar in all compressive neuropathies. Therefore it should be possible to correlate and discuss the morphological findings in the two investigated syndromes.

Carpal Ligament. We could confirm that there were no regular alterations due to age or fibrosis in and around the ligament. Tanzer (1959) and Sunderland (1968) discussed whether the thickening of the ligament could lead to median nerve compression. Neither author saw a connection between the thickening of the ligament and the development of CTS. This was supported by our findings. Pathological changes in perforating nerve fascicles, the number and position of Meissner's bodies, and the findings in the muscles which insert in the carpal ligament are of interest in the connection with the CTS, but one may speculate that they are a link in the regulation of the tension of the carpal ligament. This may be a self-regulation system (Nau 1982).

Perineural Sheath. In only one control case of the median nerve a thickening of the perineural sheath was found. However, nothing is yet known about changes in the perineural sheath in pathological conditions in CTS. In nearly all investigated cases the interosseous ramus showed an increased thickness of perineural sheath up to four or five times the normal. Since the patients suffered from different etiologies – degenerative as well as traumatic or inflammatory – the lesion must have a pathogenetic factor common to all groups. Therefore we consider compression as the most convincing reason for this alteration. In addition, the penetrating angle of the nutritive vessels was changed, and the length of the penetrating channel was increased by the thickness of the perineural sheath. The same was found for small branches of the nerve itself. We believe that the impressive thickening of the perineural sheath is in itself a pathogenetic factor. Venous drainage may be one of the affected mechanisms. The cellular density and the obvious proliferation zone of the perineural sheath on the internal border of the perineural sheath was seen frequently in the interosseous ramus and once in the median nerve of the control group. This phenomenon leads to an obliteration between the neural fascicle and the perineural sheath. We also conclude that the growth of the thickened perineural sheath starts from the inner layers. It cannot be decided whether edema is a reason or cause of these changes. An age-related thickness as suggested by Cottrell (1940) cannot be supported by our findings, neither in the median nerve of the autopsy cases nor in the ramus interosseous.

Edema. We found edema in a large number of rami interossei, some of them staining positive for mucoid material. Even small cysts with lipoid and mucoid material have been found inside the fascicle. Therefore fibrosis may be the result of such an increased fluid content in the fascicle.

Myelin Sheath. Myelin sheath in the IRS group showed de- and remyelination at the time of investigation. This was especially recognizable by electron microscopy. The breakdown of myelin was only infrequently recognized. The number of myelin sheath is sometimes much decreased, and groups and single myelinated fibers are pushed asunder by collagen tissue and Renaut's bodies. However, the absolute loss of myelin fibers is difficult to judge in these cases, since the increase in collagen and interstitial space might simulate a loss of myelinated fibers. Our findings agree with some reports in the literature (Dellon and Seif 1978; Carr and Davis 1985). We have not seen changes in the axoplasm, but in some areas sprouting was suggested inside of single Schwann's cells.

Renaut's Bodies. Corresponding to the increase in thickness of the perineural sheath and the fibrosis inside the fascicle Renaut's bodies of all sizes were frequently recognized. These seem to be an additional sign of pathological changes although the meaning of the Renaut's bodies is still unclear. Renaut's bodies are normal structures in peripheral nerves. Their number is increased in compressed nerves (Asbury and Johnson 1978). An increased number of Renaut's bodies was found in horses and donkeys (Asbury and Johnson 1978). Perhaps there are connections to the pain of racing horses and the denervating operations in them. Hyalination of Renaut's bodies is generally considered a pathological sign. This occurred frequently in the IRS group. The ultrastructure of Renaut's bodies demonstrates inside mesenchymal cells two types of cytoplasmatic substances, one of them a fibrillar one. These changes could also be recognized in cells of different layers of the perineural sheath. Immunhistology supports the origin of Renaut's bodies from the perineural sheath.

Sometimes Renaut's bodies were interpreted as ischemic lesions (Dyck et al. 1984 b) or as fibrinoid degenerations (Carr and Davis 1985). On the basis of our findings and because of the intracytoplasmic changes of the mesenchymal cells in Renaut's bodies these interpretations are highly improbable. A connection with age of the patient could not be seen, in contrast to the reports of Asbury and Johnson (1978) and Dyck et al. (1984a). The distribution may be important. In one case with occupational trauma (a secretary) we found an increased number of Renaut's bodies. This is in accord with Krücke (1955), who believed the appearance of Renaut's bodies to be caused by a pressure mechanism. In 1978 Asbury et al. also described an increased number of Renaut's bodies in the close neighborhood of joints.

Vessels. A specific finding in epineural vessels and vessels around the ligament and the joints seemed to be their meandering. We believe that this provides additional space and width in stretching movements (protective mechanism). This may be the morphological correlate to functional adaption, especially in extreme positions of the hand. It is understandable that stasis in such a vascular system can lead to a varicose space-occupying phenomena. This relates our findings to the experimental results by Weisl and Osborne (1964) and Lundborg (1975), who discussed an edema after obliteration of vasa vasorum and intrafascicular edema as a cause for the lesion in compression. A special biological factor for venous drainage may be the oblique penetration of vessels through the perineural sheath. A similar situation was found for the vessels inside the carpal tunnel ligament. Smaller vessels with a thicker layer of endothelium regularly penetrated the carpal tunnel ligament and showed signs of stasis and edema. For the marked serpentiform vessels of the carpal tunnel an increased disposition for stasis and edema could be presumed. This was also recognizable in the IRS group, where especially the tortuous supply of the submucous tissue is remarkable. This is even exaggerated in chronic inflammatory conditions of the joints, as in PCP.

We cannot determine whether these alterations of the vessels and recurrent stasis and edema could evoke functional alterations in the myelin sheath and axon. However, it is possible that recurrent disturbances of the metabolism could lead to alterations of nerve conduction velocity. Irreversible alterations seemed to appear only after longer lasting pathological conditions. This hypothesis might explain the quick normalization of nerve conduction velocity after decompression which was seen by Buchthal and Rosenfalck (1971). This persistent stasis and edema followed by demyelination is known by other diseases of the peripheral nerve and by changes in the central nervous system.

With regard to the interosseous ramus the additional question as to a possible correlation between morphological changes and pain cannot be answered. As Dyck et al. (1984) have recently stated, there is yet no specific morphological correlate which would explain pain. In their opinion this can be extended also to the possible explanation of pain in causalgia, which was thought to be caused by isolated preservation of autonomic fibers.

References

Asbury AK, Johnson PC (1978) Pathology of peripheral nerve, vol 9. Saunders, Philadelphia London Toronto, pp 24–31
Buchthal F, Rosenfalck A (1971) Sensory conduction from digit to palm and from palm to wrist in the carpal tunnel syndrome. J Neurol Neurosurg Psychiat 34:243–252
Carr D, Davis P (1985) Distal posterior interosseous nerve syndrome. J Hand Surg 10(A):873–878
Cottrell L (1940) Histologic variations with age in apparently normal peripheral nerve trunks. Arch Neurol 43:1138–1150
Dellon AL, Seif SS (1978) Anatomic dissections relating to posterior interosseous nerve of the carpus, and the etiology of dorsal wrist ganglion pain. J Hand Surg 3(a):326–332

Dyck PJ, Thomas PK, Lambert EH, Bunge R (1984a) Peripheral neuropathy, vol 1, Saunders, Philadelphia London Toronto, pp 823–827

Dyck PJ, Thomas PK, Lambert EH, Bunge R (1984b) Peripheral neuropathy, vol 2. Saunders, Philadelphia London Toronto, pp 2031–2033

Krücke W (1955) Die Renautschen Körperchen. In: Lubarsch O, Henke F, Rössle R (Hrsg) Handbuch der speziellen pathologischen Anatomie und Histologie, Bd 13/5. Springer, Berlin Göttingen Heidelberg

Lundborg G (1975) Structure and function of the intraneural microvessels as related to trauma, edema formation, and nerve function. J Bone Joint Surg 57(A):930–947

Nau H-E (1982) Klinische und tierexperimentelle Untersuchungen bei Druckläsionen peripherer Nerven. Habilitationsschrift, Essen

Sunderland S (1968) Nerves and nerve injuries. Compression lesions of the median nerve in the carpal tunnel. E & S Livingstone, Edinburgh London, pp 800–807

Tanzer C (1959) The carpal-tunnel syndrome. J Bone Joint Surg 41(A):626–634

Weisl H, Osborne GV (1964) The pathological changes in rats' nerves subject to moderate compression. J Bone Joint Surg 46(B):297–306

Pitfalls in Surgery for Carpal Tunnel Syndrome

H.-P. RICHTER, Günzburg-Ulm/FRG and G. ANTONIADIS, Fulda/FRG

Introduction

Surgery for carpal tunnel syndrome is considered safe, simple, and highly successful. Some surgeons therefore proceed directly and cut the transverse carpal ligament in patients with pain and paresthesias in the hand and reserve preoperative electrophysiological investigations at most for those with questionable symptoms.

In larger series of operated patients, on the other hand, a 5% – 10% failure rate has been reported, with either no or only minor improvement following surgery. Impairment following surgery has been seen in 1% – 4% of cases in various series comprising more than 100 patients (Beringer 1972; Cseuz et al. 1966; Lehner and Heinz 1976; Phalen 1972). In the extensive literature concerning the carpal tunnel syndrome, only a few publications deal exclusively with failures and complications after surgical therapy (Büchler et al. 1983; Conolly 1978; Das and Brown 1976; Hudson et al. 1987; Langloh and Linscheid 1972; Louis et al. 1985; Wadström and Nigst 1986). Our own findings in 48 patients reoperated on for persisting or recurring symptoms of carpal tunnel syndrome are reported in the present paper.

Clinical Material

A total of 48 reoperations on the carpal tunnel were performed because the symptoms of median nerve compression either persisted or recurred following the first operation. In 22 cases, the transverse carpal ligament was found either to be entirely intact (9/22) or incompletely severed (13/22). In the remaining 26 cases, scarring around the median nerve had caused the clinical problems. Only the former group represents true pitfalls, whereas the cases of the latter group are considered to be recurrences.

Discussion

Carpal tunnel surgery may be unsuccessful for three reasons.

Long-Standing Neurological Deficit. Whereas there is no doubt that a severe neurological deficit does not improve postoperatively as well as a minor deficit, it is still a matter of controversy as to whether the duration of symptoms and signs is a relevant prognostic factor. Among Sakellarides' patients (1983), only 30% showed a moderate motor improvement as best achievable result when symptoms had started 2–10 years before. Likewise, sensory deficits never disappeared completely in patients with such a long history. On the other hand, Müller (1980) pointed out that motor improvement is possible even after long-standing atrophy of the thenar muscles. A poor functional outcome possibly related to a long history of neurological signs should be avoided by early diagnosis and adequate treatment of the carpal tunnel syndrome.

False-Positive Diagnosis of a Carpal Tunnel Syndrome. Half of the patients with unalleviated or recurrent symptoms and signs after carpal tunnel release reported by Hudson et al. (1987) did not have had a carpal tunnel syndrome and therefore did not profit from the operation. Patients may either have suffered from a C7 radiculopathy, or they may have been free of any peripheral nerve or spinal root involvement. The history of carpal tunnel syndrome with brachialgia paresthetica nocturna is typical and rarely misleading. However, electrophysiological examination – namely, conduction studies – is mandatory in order to substantiate the clinical diagnosis, to rule out other peripheral nerve disorders, and to avoid the false-positive diagnosis of a carpal tunnel syndrome. If the surgeon relies only on a vague history, if he does not examine the patient thoroughly, and if he does not consider electrophysiological studies necessary, a high proportion of unjustified operations may be the result. This can be avoided by exact neurological and neurophysiological examination.

Technical Problems. Problems related to the technique of median nerve decompression are probably the most important cause of unalleviated symptoms following surgery for carpal tunnel syndrome. In 22 of our 48 cases of reoperations, the transverse carpal ligament was found to be either intact (9/22) or only partially transected (13/22). Sometimes, a transverse skin incision at the wrist or a vertical incision at the distal forearm had been used, the latter then ending at the level of the wrist creases. From such incisions, the transverse carpal ligament must be severed blindly, entailing the risk not only of incomplete decompression of the median nerve but also of an inadvertent injury to the median nerve or its branches. We have compiled seven reported cases of complete median nerve transection in the course of this type of surgery (Büchler et al. 1983; Conolly 1978; Hudson 1983; Woodyard 1971).

The most important single technical factor influencing the outcome of carpal tunnel surgery is the extent of transection of the transverse carpal ligament under visual control, which is impossible from a transverse wrist incision. This transverse skin incision was initially advocated even by Phalen who later switched to a vertical incision which alone permits the exploration of tunnel pathology under visual control (Phalen 1972). The main argument in favor of such a transverse incision had been the assumption that it is less frequently followed by embarrassing keloid formation than the vertical incision (Schlesinger and Liss 1959). This was disproved by authors such as Kopell and Thompson (1976) and Semple and Cargill (1969).

To summarize, there is no acceptable argument in favor of a transverse skin incision. Such an incision is rather dangerous, even though Paine (1955) and Paine and Polyzoidis (1983) advocate their "Paine retinaculotome." Reviewing the results of these authors (1983), the high proportion of incomplete transections of the transverse carpal ligament is discouraging. The complications mentioned can be avoided by a vertical incision in the palm followed by complete transection of the ligament on its ulnar side and thus adequate decompression of the median nerve over the entire length of the tunnel. Only with this technique can the surgeon deal with the tunnel's pathology as anatomical variations, such as a transligamentous course of the motor branch of the median nerve.

Conclusion

Decompression of the median nerve in the carpal tunnel is a most advantageous operation provided that the preoperative diagnosis has been correct, and that the operation itself has been performed correctly. In order to avoid poor treatment results, preoperative evaluation and operation must be carried out as accurately and carefully as in patients with more complicated peripheral nerve disorders.

References

Beringer U (1972) Das Karpaltunnelsyndrom. Analyse von 231 Fällen mit Hinweisen auf die operativen Behandlungsergebnisse. Schweiz Med Wochenschr 102:52–58

Büchler U, Goth D, Haußmann P, Lanz U, Martini AK, Wulle C (1983) Karpaltunnelsyndrom: Bericht über 56 Nachoperationen. Handchir 15 (Suppl):3–12

Conolly WB (1978) Pitfalls in carpal tunnel decompression. Austr. New Zealand J Surg 48:421–425

Cseuz KA, Thomas JE, Lambert EH, Love JG, Lipscomb PR (1966) Long-term results of operation for carpal tunnel syndrome. Mayo Clin Proc 41:232–241

Das SK, Brown HG (1976) In search of complications in carpal tunnel decompression. Hand 8:243–249

Hudson AR (1983) Carpal tunnel syndrome in pregnancy (Letter). Canad Med Ass J 128:1348–1349

Hudson AR, Kline DG, Mackinnon SE (1987) Entrapment Neuropathies. In: Horwitz NH, Rizzoli HV (eds) Postoperative complications of extracranial neurological surgery. Williams & Wilkins, Baltimore, pp 260–282

Kopell HP, Thompson WAL (1976) Peripheral entrapment neuropathies. Krieger, Huntington New York

Langloh ND, Linscheid RL (1972) Recurrent and unrelieved carpal tunnel syndrome. Clin Orthop 83:41–47

Lehner M, Heinz C (1976) Spätresultate nach operativer Therapie des Karpaltunnelsyndroms. Eine klinische Nachuntersuchung von 60 Fällen. Schweiz Med Wochenschr 106:1673–1676

Louis DS, Greene TL, Noellert RC (1985) Complications of carpal tunnel surgery. J Neurosurg 62:352–356

Müller H (1980) Regeneration motorischer Einheiten des Nervus medianus beim veralteten Karpaltunnelsyndrom. Elektromyographische Untersuchungen. Schweiz Med Wochenschr 110:907–911

Paine KWE (1955) An instrument for dividing flexor retinaculum. Lancet 1:654

Paine KW, Polyzoidis KS (1983) Carpal tunnel syndrome. Decompression using the Paine retinaculotome. J Neurosurg 59:1031–1036

Phalen GS (1972) The carpal-tunnel syndrome. Clinical evaluation of 598 hands. Clin Orthop 83:29–40

Sakellarides HT (1983) The management of carpal tunnel compression syndrome. Follow-up of 500 cases over a 25-year period. Orthop Rev 12:77–81

Schlesinger EG, Liss HR (1959) Fundamentals, fads, and fallacies in the carpal tunnel syndrome. Am J Surg 97:466–470

Semple JC, Cargill AO (1969) Carpal tunnel syndrome. Results of surgical decompression. Lancet 1:918–919

Wadström J, Nigst H (1986) Reoperation for carpal tunnel syndrome. A retrospective analysis of forty cases. Ann Chir Main 5:54–58

Woodyard JE (1971) Decompression of the carpal tunnel. Bristol Med Chir J 86:33–36

Carpal Tunnel Syndrome: A New Surgical Approach

P. Roccella, R. Ghadirpour, A. Migliore, and G. Trapella, Ferrara/Italy

Introduction

Carpal tunnel syndrome (CTS) is an entrapment neuropathy of the median nerve at the wrist usually involving the dominant hand. It is particularly frequent in middle-aged women and is characterized by nocturnal pain in the distribution of the median nerve in the hand, paresthesias, sensory loss, weakness of the hand, and thenar muscle atrophy. In most cases treatment is surgical and consists of opening the carpal tunnel by dividing the volar ligament. After Marie and Foix in 1913 recommended the section of the flexor retinaculum in CTS, several surgical procedures have been performed (Learmonth 1933; Hunt and Luckey 1964; Eboh and Wilson 1978; Paine and Polyzoidis 1983). The typical curvilinear skin incision crossing the crease at the wrist requires, after surgical procedure, immobilization with a bulky hand dressing for several days, but it does not always avoid the developing of hypertrophic scars or dysesthesias following lesions of the palmar cutaneous branch of the median nerve. Nevertheless, the use of transverse incision, a blind procedure, is potentially dangerous for the patient because of the frequent occurrence of complications (Louis et al. 1985).

For these reasons, since January 1982 in the Department of Neurosurgery of S. Anna Hospital in Ferrara the operation has been carried out using operating microscope and the technique described below.

Methods

A slight curvilinear skin incision, about 2 cm in length, is done on the medial side of the thenar eminence to reach, but not cross, the crease at the wrist. This incision is extended through skin and subcutaneous tissue down to palmaris fascia, which is split. A partial exposure of flexor retinaculum is required, and a very small opening (2 mm in length) is made by blunt microscissors in the medial portion of the ligament. Through this opening a thin curved grooved director is introduced, distally directed, beneath the ligament as a guide the scissors, and retinaculum is cut. The same procedure is used to divide proximal portion of the ligament. The median nerve is completely exposed in the palm of the hand and neurolysis, if requested, may be carried out under high magnification. The skin is then closed with a 4–0 silk suture, and a small simple dressing is applied to the wound. A tourniquet is unnecessary because of the minimal bleeding. The operation is carried out under local anesthesia, and the patient may be discharged immediately after operation.

Between January 1982 and December 1986, 175 hands of 138 patients (37 with bilateral CTS) were operated on using this technique. Of these 138 patients, 121 were women. Ages ranged from 33 to 77 years, with a mean age of 54.5 years.

Results

In all patients nocturnal pain ceased within 72 h from surgical procedures. Paresthesias usually disappeared in 3–6 months. Only three patients required neurolysis. No complications or recurrences were observed (follow-up 8–60 months). This is not in agreement with the results of many other authors (Langloh and Linscheid 1972; MacDonald et al. 1978; Inglis 1980; May and Rosen 1981; Louis et al. 1985). All patients returned to their previous occupations in a few days.

Conclusions

Our results suggest the following observations. (a) A very short skin incision, down to but not across the wrist crease, avoids to damage the palmar cutaneous branch of the median nerve and does not require immobilization of the hand with a bulky dressing. (b) An occasional abnormal motor branch of the median nerve to the thenar eminence is preserved using a small curved grooved director during dissection of the retinaculum. (c) The use of magnification is a valuable aid during operation and it is essential whenever neurolysis is requested. (d) The short skin incision does not allow to carry out neurolysis of the median nerve beyond the wrist flexion creases; this seems to represent the only limitation of such a procedure.

References

1. Eboh N, Wilson DH (1978) Surgery of the carpal tunnel. J Neurosurg 49:316–318
2. Hunt WE, Luckey WT (1964) The carpal tunnel syndrome. Diagnosis and treatment J Neurosurg 21:178–181
3. Inglis AE (1980) Two unusual operative complications in the carpal tunnel syndrome. J Bone Joint Surg 62:1208–1209
4. Langloh ND, Linscheid RL (1972) Recurrent and unrelieved carpal-tunnel syndrome. Clin Orthop 83:41–47
5. Learmonth JR (1933) The principle of decompression in the treatment of certain diseases of peripheral nerves. Surg Clin North Am 13:905–913
6. Louis DS, Greene TL, Noellert RC (1985) Complications of carpal tunnel surgery. J Neurosurg 62:352–356

7. MacDonald RE, Lichtman DM, Hanlon JJ et al. (1978) Complications of surgical release for carpal tunnel syndrome. J Hand Surg 3:70–76
8. Marie P, Foix C (1913) Atrophie isolée de l'éminence thénar d'origine nevritique: rôle du ligament annulaire antérieur du carpe dans la pathogénie de la lésion. Rev Neurol 21:647–649
9. May JWJr, Rosen H (1981) Division of the sensory ramus communications between the ulnar and median nerves: a complication following carpal tunnel release. A case report. J Bone Joint Surg 63:836–838
10. Paine KWE, Polyzoidis KS (1983) Carpal tunnel syndrome. Decompression using the Paine retinaculotome. J Neurosurg 59:1031–1036

Anatomical Anomalies Causing Ulnar Neuropathy

H. KOLENDA, M. SCHADE, and E. MARKAKIS, Göttingen/FRG

We begin our report with the case of a 25-year-old woman with a characteristic clinical course of primary ulnar nerve compression syndrome. There had been no symptoms until she suffered a trauma to her left elbow following a sporting accident. Subsequently pain radiating from the elbow joint to the ulnar edge of the forearm and paresthesia over the supply area of the left ulnar nerve appeared. Symptoms were partially dependent on movement in the elbow joint. The neurological investigation proved hypoesthesia, hypoalgesia, and a noticeable weakness of the ulnar nerve dependent muscles. Neurophysiological investigation showed normal findings on ulnar as well as on median nerve. Plain X-rays demonstrated evidence of a processus supratrochlearis (Fig. 1). As conservative therapy had no effect, we performed an operation. The supratrochlear spur, the underlying median nerve, and the ulnar nerve up to the cubital tunnel were exposed (Fig. 2). There was no neuroma or other visible changes on either nerve. Resection of the spur led to constant remission of pain and all sensory and motor deficits.

We reviewed the case histories and plain X-rays of 143 patients with ulnar nerve irritation or compression which have been operated on over the past 10 years in our department in order to find similar abnormalities (Fig. 3). Radiograms of the elbow joint had been performed on only 22% of these patients, mainly on patients with a fracture or a trauma. Only 10% were made for diagnostic screening. No pathological findings were observed in 44% of the X-rayed sample. The rest showed mainly sequelae of former bone injuries. There was found no other processus supratrochlearis. During the review, a further seven cases of ulnar compression due to muscular anomalies were discovered, three due to an accessory anconaeus epitrochlearis muscle and four due to other muscular aberrations. In these eight cases there were no characteristic differences, such as age or succession of symptoms, compared to the other 135 cases. Volar transposition has always been successful.

The first report of an ulnar nerve compression syndrome caused by a processus supratrochlearis was presented by Panas in 1878, who found it in one of his four cases. The processus is known as a structure of the canalis supracondylicus in reptiles and mammals, the median nerve passing through it. In man it is an atavistic anomaly, present in 0.3%–2.1% of all humans. Usually it is not seen in standard radiograms, but in a special position with the elbow rotated 30° inwards it may be seen.

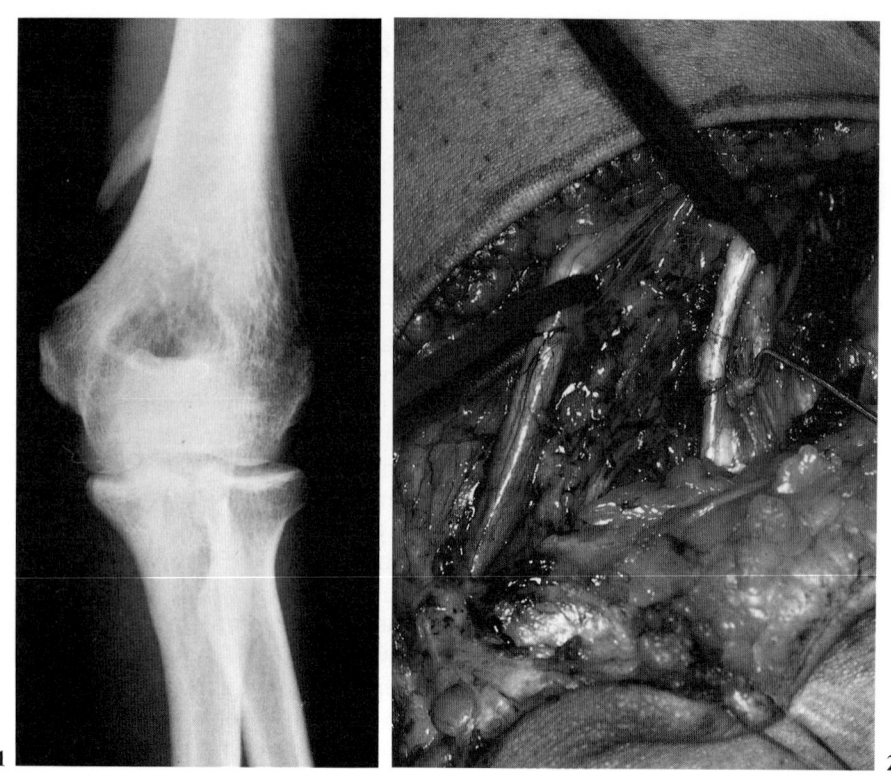

Fig. 1. Plain X-rays demonstrating a processus supratrochlearis in a special position with the elbow rotated 30° inwards

Fig. 2. Operation site exposing from *right* to *left* the processus supratrochlearis (tip of small hook), underlying median nerve and ulnar nerve up to the cubital tunnel

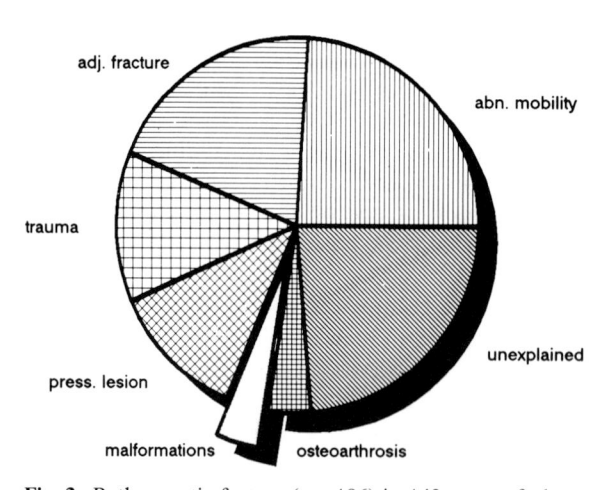

Fig. 3. Pathogenetic factors ($n = 196$) in 143 cases of ulnar nerve compression

In literature the majority of symptoms were registered on the ulnar nerve; in a few cases median nerve compression was seen. Generally it is supposed that the ulnar nerve might be stretched across the bony spur, particularly in flexion of the elbow. The topographic relation between ulnar nerve and the spur can hardly substantiate this opinion. A more reasonable explanation was given by Torres in 1971. He maintained that the processus supratrochlearis and the ligament that runs from its tip to the epicondylus medialis and the anconaeus epitrochlear muscle must be seen as unity. This muscle is found in 1% of all humans. It originates at the ligament and ends at the olecranon, crossing the ulnar nerve. Recurrent compression of the nerve by this muscle may cause the symptoms. This may explain the successful operative results either by resecting the processus or by dissecting the muscle, as we did in three of our 143 cases.

References

Panas J (1878) Sur une cause peu connue de paralysie du nerf cubital. Archives Générales de Médecine 2 (VII Serie)

Torres J (1971) Die klinische Bedeutung des Processus supratrochlearis. Handchirurgie 3:15

Neurolysis in Ulnar Nerve Entrapment Syndromes

M. Samii, Hannover/FRG

Anatomy

The ulnar nerve is the largest branch of the medial cord of the brachial plexus. Running behind the axillary vessels, it is the most posterior structure in the medial side of the arm. It generally also receives a branch from the lateral cord (C6, C7), which is the motor supply to the flexor carpi ulnaris (FCU) in the forearm. In the distal third of the arm, after having pierced the medial intermuscular septum, it is accompanied by the ulnar collateral artery and lies in front of the branch of the radial nerve to the medial head of the triceps muscle, formerly known erroneously as the ulnar collateral nerve. It leaves the arm without supplying a branch and lies in the ulnar groove of the humerus behind the medial epicondyle in direct contact with the bone. It is retained in the olecranon groove under a cover of fibrous tissue originating from the common flexor muscle.

In the forearm it barely enters the extensor compartment, disappearing between the humeral and ulnar heads of the FCU. The ulnar nerve is vulnerable at the medial epicondyle of the humerus, but it is even more easily compressed against the medial surface of the coronoid process, known as the sublime tubercle. The nerve runs down the forearm between flexor carpi ulnaris and flexor digitorum profundus, both of which it supplies. The ulnar artery accompanies it along its radial side. Emerging more superficially, just proximal to the wrist, the nerve crosses over the flexor retinaculum and passes alongside the radial border of the pisiform bone to enter the hand. Here it divides into two branches, a superficial branch supplying the palmaris brevis muscle, and then the sensibility of the ulnar 1 1/2 fingers, and a deep branch entering the palm between the origins of the flexor and abductor digiti minimi muscles and running along the concavity of the deep palmar arch. The nerve supplies several small muscles of the hand, namely the three hypothenar muscles, the ulnar lumbricals, and all the interossei, and ends with the supply to the adductor pollicis and to the flexor pollicis brevis.

Entrapment Syndromes

Cubital Tunnel Syndrome

The most common type of ulnar paralysis in clinical practice results from compression of the nerve in the olecranon groove at the elbow. The site of compression may also be distal to the medial epicondyle, between the heads of FCU and the sublime tubercle. The syndrome may arise purely from an irritation in the olecranon groove due to an increased carrying angle or to a cubitus valgus following a fracture. Another kind of olecranon defect which can cause or lead to nerve irritation is a shallow groove. The nerve constantly slips and translocates out of it causing, over a period of years, an ulnar palsy.

Chronic external compression in the region of the elbow is often occupational, but occurs as often with clerical staff as with construction workers. The fact that seems to be most uniformly documented is the long delay before the patient complains. Surgical decompression is mandatory. The principle lies in providing the nerve with an environment free of irritation. It has been conventional to translocate the nerve from the extensor to the flexor compartment of the elbow to reduce spontaneous translocations. In given cases it may be sufficient to release the cubital tunnel, but in some others medial epicondylectomy may be necessary. One should confirm that no further stretch is exerted on the nerve by the "sublime" tubercle. When the nerve is translocated, it is preferable not to make a groove in the flexor group of muscles, as this may result in a traction neuritis. Instead of transecting the entire common flexor tendon, it is preferable, burying the freed and inflamed nerve under it adjacent to the median nerve.

Guyon's Tunnel

Either one or both of the branches of the ulnar nerve in the hand may be compressed resulting in selective or complete sensory and/or motor deficits. At the wrist the superficial branch may be stretched around the pisiform bone, producing sensory impairment. The deep branch may be similarly affected in the deep palmar region. These nerves may also be injured by firmly sustained external pressure or by one or more violent blows to the palm. As with other entrapment neuropathies, this may be occupational, recreational or due to other trauma directed to the lower thenar region.

Acute lesions may be followed conservatively for several weeks, but if there are no signs of functional improvement, the nerve should be explored and, if necessary, a careful internal neurolysis is to be performed.

Summary

While in ulnar nerve luxation injuries at the level of the cubital tunnel with manifest neurological deficits, morphological changes as epineural fibrosis and

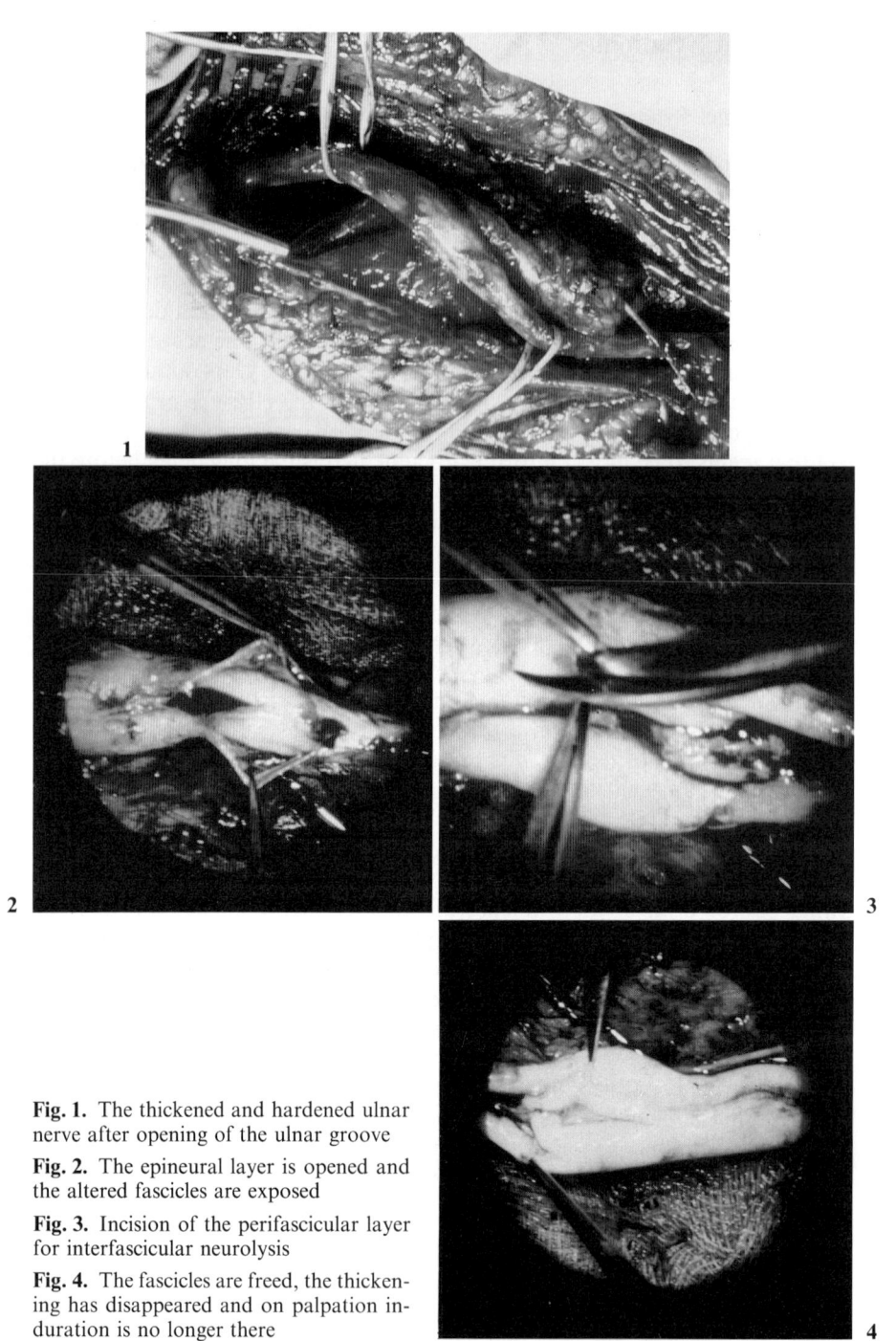

Fig. 1. The thickened and hardened ulnar nerve after opening of the ulnar groove

Fig. 2. The epineural layer is opened and the altered fascicles are exposed

Fig. 3. Incision of the perifascicular layer for interfascicular neurolysis

Fig. 4. The fascicles are freed, the thickening has disappeared and on palpation induration is no longer there

caliber changes of the affected fascicles may be slightly apparent, some years after the surgical treatment of posttraumatic compression syndromes one can observe the development of extensive fibrotic changes as well as altered fascicular calibers. These fascicles are not just enlarged, in fusiform fashion, but are also thickened and hard.

After introduction of microsurgery at the end of the 1960s, for the treatment of peripheral nerve lesions we found relatively early that the results of the surgical treatment of ulnar nerve compression syndromes were poor when such changes affecting the fascicles were present. The technique of microneurolysis we introduced in the 1970s (Samii 1977, 1980) was modified for the treatment of posttraumatic ulnar compression syndromes. The involved thickened fascicles were, after removal of the fibrotic epineurium, longitudinally and singularly slit, for this the perineurium had to be opened. As an interesting phenomenon, we observed the disappearance of the thickening and induration of the affected fascicles (Fig. 1–4). Hereby, the operative results could then be improved.

In an ulnar nerve luxation, there is seldom a fibrotic compression of the nerve fascicles, and generally a fascicular neurolysis is not necessary. The nerve fascicles are unchanged in their calibers. The results of the surgical treatment are very satisfactory and our experience has demonstrated that there is a regression of the neurological deficits within several months.

References

Kahl RJ, Samii M, Willebrand H (1972) Clinical results of perineural fascicular neurolysis. Excerpta Medica, International Congress Series No. 306:209–212

Penkert G, Moringlane JR, Samii M (1982) Beidseitig kombiniertes Karpaltunnel- und Loge de Guyon-Syndrom. Akt Neurol 9:205–207

Samii M (1977) Aspects modernes de la chirurgie des nerfs peripheriques. Editions medicales Pierre Fabre, Monography

Samii M (1980) Fascicular peripheral nerve repair. Modern Techniques in Surgery, Neurosurgery, 17, Futura Publishing Company, New York

Samii M (1980) Nerves of the head and neck. In: Management of Peripheral Nerve Problems. W. B. Saunders Company, Philadelphia: 507–547

Seddon H (1975) Surgical Disorders of the Peripheral Nerves, 2nd ed. Edinburgh, Churchill Livingstone

Thoracic-Outlet Syndrome: Limitations of the Neurophysiological Diagnosis

G. KRÄMER and A. KLEIDER, Mainz and Eltville/FRG

Introduction

The clinical diagnosis of thoracic-outlet syndrome (TOS) is often controversial. While findings are clear in classical or definite cases, they are ambiguous in the majority of patients. Because TOS surgery itself may produce severe brachial plexopathy (Wilbourn 1988), it would be of great advantage if neurophysiological methods in such cases were able to show evidence of involvement of the brachial plexus or of the lower cervical roots distal to their ganglia and thus could differentiate between TOS and other diseases.

Available Neurophysiological Methods and Their Value

Nerve Conduction Velocity Studies

As the etiology of the disease is compression of the medial parts of the brachial plexus, of the available neurophysiological methods nerve conduction studies are most likely to demonstrate the site and degree of the lesion (Smith and Trojaborg 1987).

Ulnar Nerve: Proximal. According to reports of Urschel and coworkers (Urschel et al. 1971; Urschel and Razzuk 1972) proximal ulnar nerve conduction velocity studies provided objective evidence for the diagnosis of TOS; the average normal value was described as 72 m/s, ranging from 68 to 75 (Caldwell et al. 1971) whereas the mean velocity in TOS patients was 53 m/s with a range of 32–65. The changes were clear in every case, even with mild neurological symptoms, and there was no overlap between normal controls and patients. However, other investigators found higher (76.1 m/s, Krogness 1973) as well as lower normal values (64 m/s, Sadler et al. 1975; 61.3 m/s, Jebsen 1967; 60.8 m/s, Daube 1975; 59 m/s, Cherrington 1976) or no abnormalities at all, at least in patients with the clinically diagnosed syndrome free of neurological deficits (Daube 1975).

In accordance with a comparative study of two measuring methods for the ulnar nerve conduction velocity across the thoracic outlet (London 1975) the authors of the original paper assumed that methodological aspects (use of a steel band or more flexible caliper for measuring the distances) were responsible for the differing normal values. They reemphasized their experience – based on more than 270 suspected cases studied electromyographically in a single month – with appreciable slowing of ulnar nerve conduction velocities in patients with "good criteria" for TOS and normal values in those without (Krusen and Urschel 1976). Compared to the 20 cases seen by Gilliatt and colleagues at Queen's Square in London over a 15-year period (Gilliatt 1976), a large variation in diagnostic criteria must be assumed.

Sadler and coworkers (1975) as well as Glassenberg (1981) proposed "positional" ulnar nerve conduction studies with elevated arms (limited to 90° abduction) and reported 70% pathological findings in 73 TOS patients in the neutral position and an additional 18% positive findings in the elevated position. However, their diagnostic criteria with a delay of only greater than 3 m/s compared to the normal side or neutral position does not seem to be reliable. In addition, Shahani and coworkers (1980) could not confirm their results and attributed a slowing of conduction velocity occurring in some patients to methodological errors.

Ulnar Nerve: Elbow. Ulnar nerve conduction studies across the elbow are recommended to exclude the possibility of nerve entrapment there (Swinton and Wanger 1972). In TOS they are always normal (Jerrett et al. 1984).

Ulnar Nerve: Distal. Gilliatt and coworkers described reduced or absent sensory action potentials of the ulnar nerve following stimulation of the fifth finger in five out of nine TOS patients in their first report (1970) and in 10 out of 14 other patients in a later study (1978). Normal latencies and lack of dispersion of the potentials indicated a lesion distal to the dorsal root ganglia. These results were confirmed by Morales-Blanquez and Delwaide (1982). However, in the experience of other authors only very few patients presented low-amplitude ulnar sensory nerve action potentials (e.g., 2 of 18, Jerrett et al. 1984). Maximal motor conduction velocities to the abductor digiti minimi or first interosseus muscle as well as the corresponding distal latencies were normal in all cases. These results were confirmed by other groups. Lascelles and coworkers (1977) found, for example, reduced sensory nerve action potentials from the fifth finger in 5 out of 16 patients.

Median Nerve. The distal sensory median nerve conduction velocity is an aid in the differential diagnosis between the carpal tunnel syndrome and TOS, where it is always within the normal range (Gilliatt 1976; Gilliatt et al. 1978). For the motor fibers, there may be a slight reduction in the maximal conduction velocity to the abductor pollicis brevis muscle in TOS; however, again in contradistinction to carpal tunnel syndrome the distal latency is normal (Gilliatt et al. 1970). Only few authors describe reduced amplitudes of the compound muscle action potential (Huffman 1986) or the distal sensory action potential (Morales-Blanquez and Delwaide 1982). In rare cases of prolonged distal latencies (Capistrant 1977) the hypothesis of a double-crush syndrome (Upton and McComas 1973) seems to be the most likely explanation.

F-Wave Measurement

Evoked F-wave responses are useful to measure the conduction velocity in proximal nerve segments otherwise not accessible. The usual stimulation site for determination of the ulnar nerve conduction velocity at Erb's point lies either at or below the presumed block (Eisen et al. 1977). Several authors described increased latencies on the affected side (Dorfman 1979; Jerrett et al. 1984; Kimura 1983; Wulff and Gilliatt 1979). A multiple regression analysis using arm length and ulnar forearm velocity for predicting F-wave latency in such patients was proposed by Weber and Piero (1978). However, usually normal F-wave studies were reported as well (Ryding et al. 1985; Shahani et al. 1980).

Somatosensory Evoked Potentials

The value and reliability of somatosensory evoked potentials in TOS patients is not yet clear. Median nerve evoked N9 (brachial plexus) amplitudes are always normal, whereas up to two-thirds of the patients have low amplitude ulnar N9 potentials on the affected side (Glover et al. 1981; Jerrett et al. 1984). In addition the conduction in the ulnar nerve from N9 to N13 (brachial plexus to spinal cord) was prolonged in 7 out of 18 patients. As in proximal ulnar nerve conduction studies, an increased sensitivity with dynamic arm positioning in abduction and external rotation was described (Chodoroff et al. 1985). Again, the experience of other investigators was less enthusiastic (Morales-Blanquez and Delwaide 1982; Newmark et al. 1985) or positive only in cases with already otherwise objective neurological signs such as loss of sensation, weakness, or wasting of small hand muscles (Yiannikas and Walsh 1983).

Electromyography

Electromyography of atrophic or paretic muscles can substantiate their clinical wasting and weakness (Dawson et al. 1983). However, this is seldom of additional value. Denervation in the abductor pollicis brevis and flexor pollicis brevis was described in 10 out of 16 TOS cases (Lascelles et al. 1977), all with clinical evidence of muscle weakness. Other authors (Caldwell et al. 1971; Capistrant 1977; Gilliatt et al. 1970) noted that fibrillations are rare. Findings are typical for chronic denervation with reduced number of motor units under voluntary control, which may spread to finger and wrist extensors (Caldwell et al. 1971). In cases with only very few remaining motor unit potentials, these are of high amplitude, up to 10 mV (Gilliatt et al. 1970). As noted by Dawson et al. in their book on entrapment neuropathies (1983), a careful study of the typical extent of denervation in TOS remains to be done. Surgeons tend to operate on patients whether there are electromyographic abnormalities or not (Dale and Lewis 1975).

Conclusions

The diagnosis of TOS remains primarily clinical: pain in the arm provoked by traction in combination with color changes in the hand, a radicular pattern of sensory loss, and weakness with intact tendon reflexes. A neurophysiologic examination is not always necessary. In doubtful cases it should include measurement of the ulnar sensory action potential and ulnar motor conduction at the forearm (to rule out a lesion at the elbow). Ulnar motor conduction across the thoracic outlet measured either directly or with the F-wave seems to be positive only in obvious cases. Somatosensory evoked potentials enable objective quantitative evaluation of TOS in some cases. However, as with the clinical diagnosis, the neurophysiologic findings in ambiguous cases are unfortunately not well-defined and often not of confirmative value (Dawson et al. 1983). Whether electrical or magnetic stimulation of the brachial plexus or of the spinal cord will be of any additional benefit remains to be demonstrated.

References

Caldwell JW, Crane CR, Krusen EM (1971) Nerve conduction studies: an aid in the diagnosis of the thoracic outlet syndrome. South Med J 64:210–212

Capistrant TD (1977) Thoracic outlet syndrome in whiplash injury. Ann Surg 185:175–178

Cherrington M (1976) Ulnar-conduction velocity in thoracic-outlet syndrome (letter). N Engl J Med 294:1185

Chodoroff G, Lee DW, Honet JC (1985) Dynamic approach in the diagnosis of thoracic outlet syndrome using somatosensory evoked responses. Arch Phys Med Rehabil 66:3–6

Dale WA, Lewis MR (1975) Management of thoracic outlet syndrome. Ann Surg 181:575–585

Daube JR (1975) Nerve conduction studies in thoracic outlet syndrome (abstract). Neurology 25:347

Dawson DM, Hallett M, Millender LH (1983) Entrapment neuropathies. Little, Brown & Co, Boston Toronto, pp 169–183

Dorfman LJ (1979) F-wave latency in the cervical-rib-and-band syndrome (letter). Muscle & Nerve 2:158–159

Eisen A, Schomer D, Melmed C (1977) The application of F-wave measurements in the differentiation of proximal and distal upper limb entrapments. Neurology 27:662–668

Gilliatt RW (1976) Thoracic outlet compression syndrome (letter). Br Med J 1:1274–1275

Gilliatt RW, LeQuesne PM, Logue V, Sumner AJ (1970) Wasting of the hand associated with a cervical rib or band. J Neurol Neurosurg Psychiat 33:615–624

Gilliatt RW, Willison RG, Dietz V, Williams IR (1978) Peripheral nerve conduction in patients with a cervical rib and band. Ann Neurol 4:124–129

Glassenberg M (1981) The thoracic outlet syndrome: an asessment of 20 cases with regard to new clinical and electromyographic findings. Angiology 32:180–186

Glover JL, Worth RM, Bendick PJ, Hall PV, Markland OM, (1981) Evoked responses in the diagnosis of thoracic outlet syndrome. Surgery 89:86–93

Huffman JD (1986) Electrodiagnostic techniques for and conservative treatment of thoracic outlet syndrome. Clin Orthopaed Rel Res 207:21–23

Jebsen RH (1967) Motor conduction velocity in the median and ulnar nerves. Arch Phys Med Rehabil 48:185–194

Jerrett SA, Cuzzone LJ, Pasternak BM (1984) Thoracic outlet syndrome. Electrophysiological reappraisal. Arch Neurol 41:960–963

Kimura J (1983) Electrodiagnosis in diseases of nerve and muscle: principles and practice. Davis, Philadelphia, pp 454–455

Krogness K (1973) Ulnar trunk conduction studies in the diagnosis of the thoracic outlet syndrome. Acta Clin Scand 139:597–603

Krusen EM, Urschel HC (1976) Ulnar conduction velocity in thoracic-outlet syndrome. Reply (letter). N Engl J Med 294:1185–1186

Lascelles RG, Mohr PD, Neary D, Bloor K (1977) The thoracic outlet syndrome. Brain 100:601–612

London GW (1975) Normal ulnar nerve conduction velocity across the thoracic outlet: comparison of two measuring techniques. J Neurol Neurosurg Psychiat 38:756–760

Morales-Blanquez G, Delwaide PJ (1982) The thoracic outlet syndrome: an electrophysiological study. Electromyogr Clin Neurophysiol 22:255–263

Newmark J, Levy SR, Hochberg FH (1985) Somatosensory evoked potentials in thoracic outlet syndrome (letter). Arch Neurol 42:1036

Ryding E, Ribbe E, Rosén I, Norgren L (1985) A neurophysiologic investigation of thoracic outlet syndrome. Acta Chir Scand 151:327–331

Sadler TR Jr, Rainer WG, Twombley G (1975) Thoracic outlet compression. Application of positional arteriography and nerve conduction studies. Am J Surg 130:704–706

Shahani BT, Potts F, Juguilon A, Young RR (1980) Electrophysiological studies in "thoracic outlet syndrome" (abstract). Muscle & Nerve 3:182–183

Smith T, Trojaborg W (1987) Diagnosis of thoracic outlet syndrome. Arch Neurol 44:1161–1163

Swinton NW Jr, Wanger SL (1972) Thoracic-outlet syndrome (letter). N Engl J Med 287:567

Upton ARM, McComas AJ (1973) The double crush in nerve-entrapment syndromes. Lancet 2:359–362

Urschel HC Jr, Razzuk MA (1972) Management of the thoracic outlet syndrome (current concepts). N Engl J Med 286:1140–1143

Urschel HC Jr, Razzuk MA, Wood RE, Parekh M. Paulson DL (1971) Objective diagnosis (ulnar nerve conduction velocity) and current therapy of the thoracic outlet syndrome. Ann Thorac Surg 12:608–620

Weber RJ, Piero DL (1978) F wave evaluation of thoracic outlet syndrome: a multiple regression derived F wave latency predicting technique. Arch Phys Med Rehabil 59:464–469

Wilbourn AJ (1988) Thoracic outlet syndrome surgery causing severe brachial plexopathy. Muscle & Nerve 11:66–74

Wulff CH, Gilliatt RW (1979) F waves in patients with hand wasting caused by a cervical rib and band. Muscle & Nerve 2:452–457

Yiannikas C, Walsh JC (1983) Somatosensory evoked responses in the diagnosis of thoracic outlet syndrome. J Neurol Neurosurg Psychiat 46:234–240

Diagnosis and Surgical Management of the Thoracic-Outlet Syndrome

A. Aghchi and J. Menzel, Köln/FRG

Introduction

Peripheral neuropathies of the upper extremity are too often attributed to distally located nerve compressions. By contrast, little attention is paid to proximal sites of compression characterized by the manifestation of neural and/or vascular signs (Mumenthaler und Schliack 1982; Jaeger et al. 1986; Wilhelm and Wilhelm 1985). Among these, the thoracic outlet syndrome (TOS) is of particular practical relevance (Fig. 1; Mumenthaler and Schliack, 1982). In view of the specific anatomy involved, compression of the brachial plexus and/or brachial and subclavian vessels by the scalene muscles, the first rib, or the clavicle must be considered in the differential diagnosis of this syndrome. Abnormal structures, such as the presence of cervical ribs and hypertrophic ligamentous structures, may also play an important role in the pathogenesis of TOS. In this report we describe selected cases representing examples of each of the above anatomical conditions to demonstrate the direct relationship between clinical signs and underlying morphology in TOS.

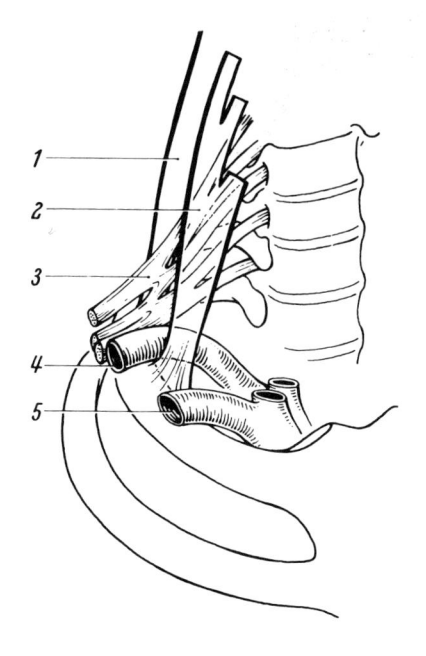

Fig. 1. Normal anatomical relationship of the crucial structures: *1*, medial scalene muscle; *2*, anterior scalene muscle; *3*, plexus brachialis; *4*, subclavian artery; *5*, subclavian vein; and the first rib. (From Mumenthaler and Schliack 1982)

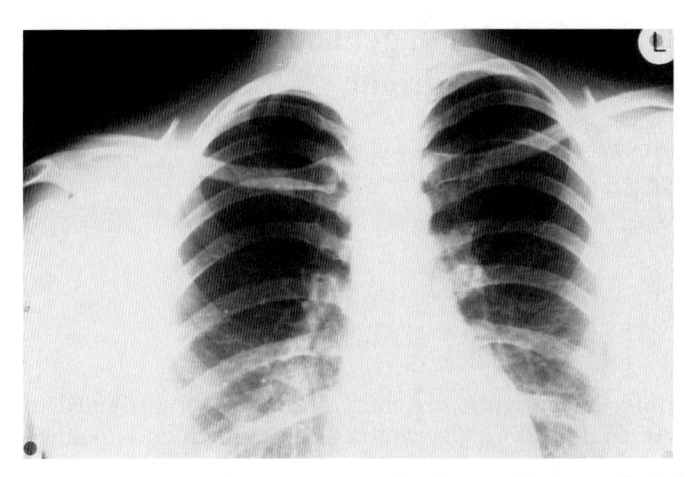

Fig. 2. Preoperative thorax X-ray examination revealing a cervical rib on the right side

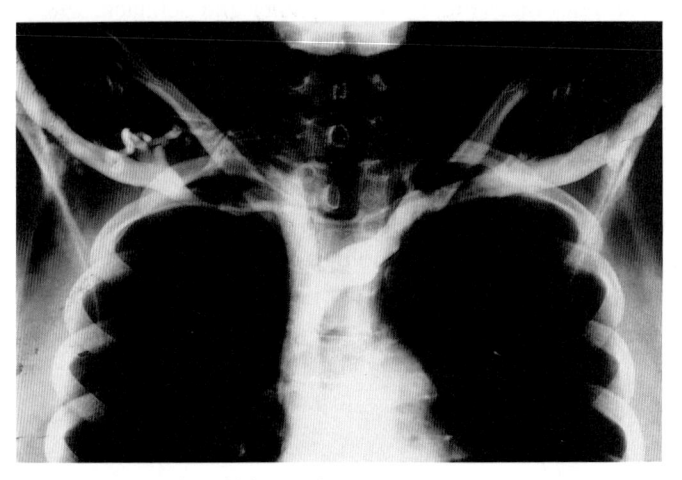

Fig. 3. Preoperative phlebography

Clinical Material

Case 1. An 18-year-old woman complained of diffuse hypoesthesia and paresthesias in the right upper extremity and weakness of the right hand. These complaints were confirmed by neurological examination. An X-ray examination revealed the presence of a cervical rib which caused compression of the right subclavian vein, as confirmed by phlebographic examination. Intraoperatively, the subclavian vein and artery as well as the brachial plexus were found to be compressed by the cervical rib and by ligamentous structures. The cervical and first thoracic ribs were resected using a transaxillary approach (see Figs. 2–6).

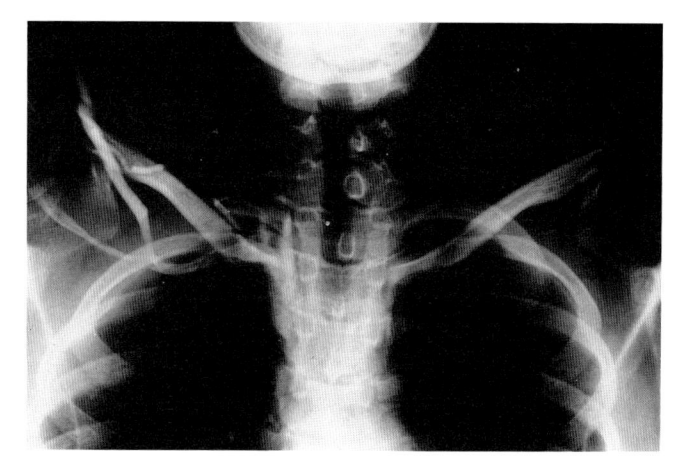

Fig. 4. Postoperative phlebography

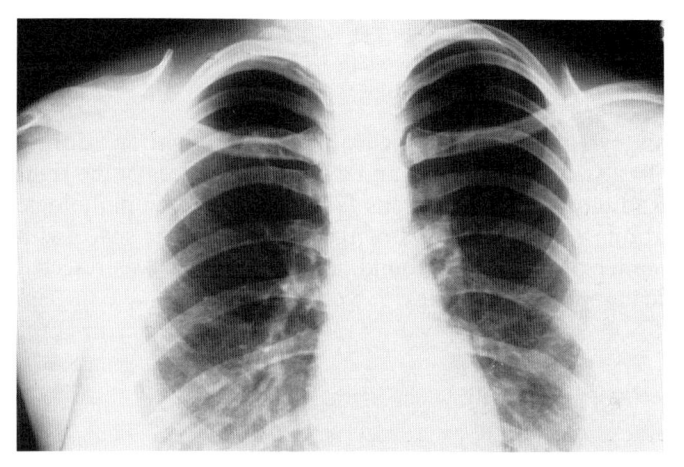

Fig. 5. Postoperative thorax after resecting the cervical rib

Case 2. A 16-year-old girl had a history of pain and cyanosis of the left hand. Neurological examination revealed hypoesthesia and paresthesias along the distribution of C7 and C8 dermatomes on the left side. The left radial pulse could no longer be felt upon abduction of the left arm. Neither X-ray nor phlebographic examination showed an abnormality. The operative findings showed compression of the left subclavian, axillary, and brachial artery as well as the brachial plexus by ligamentous structures. The first rib was resected using again a transaxillary approach.

Case 3. A 34-year-old man complained of diffuse pain in the right hand. He had previously undergone a carpal tunnel release for the same complaints,

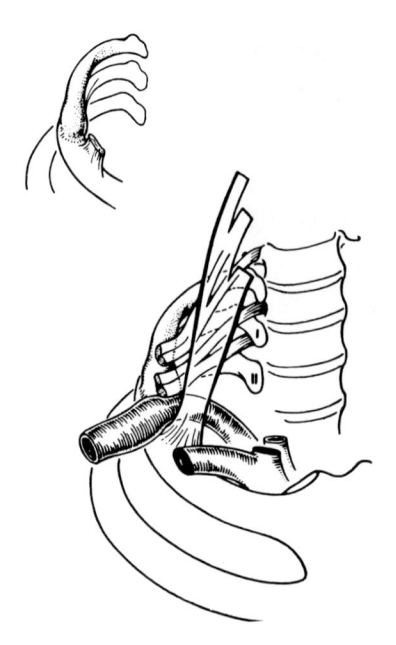

Fig. 6. Narrowing by a cervical rib. (From Mumenthaler and Schliack 1982)

without relief of his symptoms. Upon neurological examination, diffuse hypoesthesia of the first two radial fingers and a motor weakness of the right hand were found. Radiological examinations failed to show any pathologic condition. At operation, a lateral stenosis of the costoclavicular space with compression of the brachial plexus was found, and the first rib was resected using the transaxillary approach (see Figs. 7, 8).

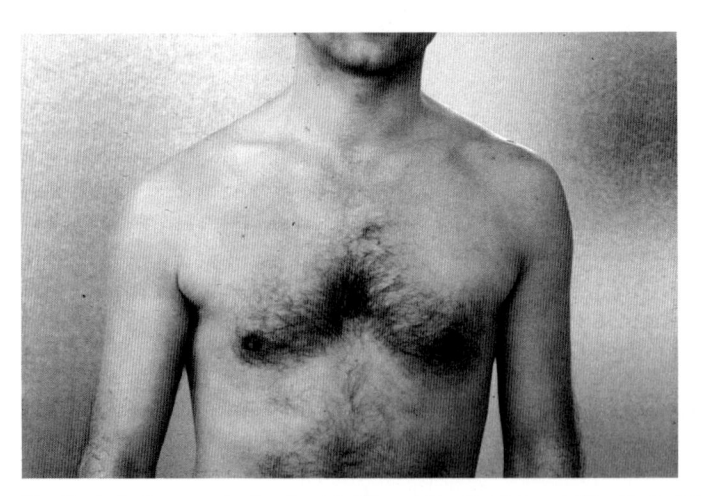

Fig. 7. Anterior aspect of patient 3. The asymmetry is caused by the habitually hanging right shoulder

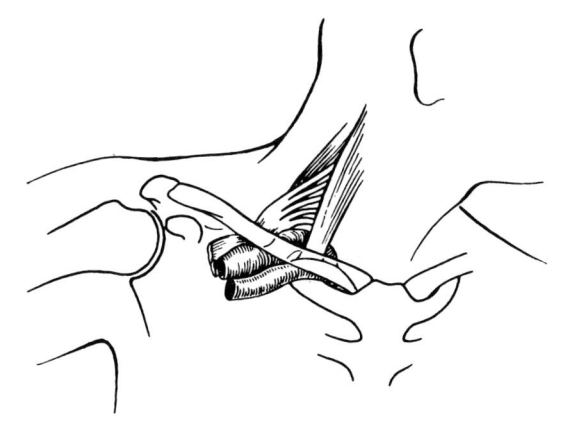

Fig. 8. The costaclavicular space is narrowed. (From Mumenthaler and Schliack 1982)

Case 4. A 44-year-old woman had a history of paresthesias of the left hand and diffuse motor weakness of the left upper extremity. Neurologically, hypoesthesia and hypoalgesia as well as motor weakness of the left hand were found. Upon inspection, a prominence of the middle portion of the clavicle was seen. Radiological examinations showed no pathologic variant. Intraoperatively, we noticed a broadened insertion site of the medial scalene muscle and compression of the brachial plexus by the latter, as well as by ligamentous structures (see Figs. 9, 10).

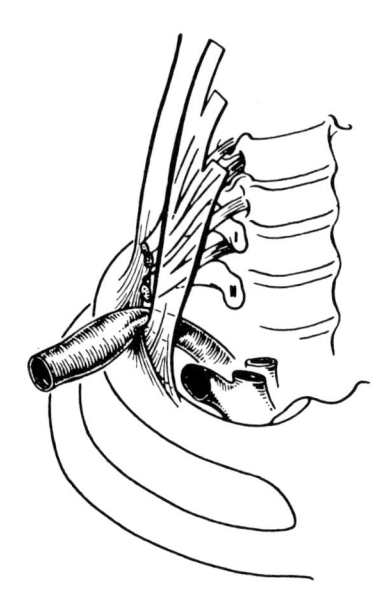

Fig. 9. Narrowing by a broadened insertion site of the medial scalene muscle. (From Mumenthaler and Schliack 1982)

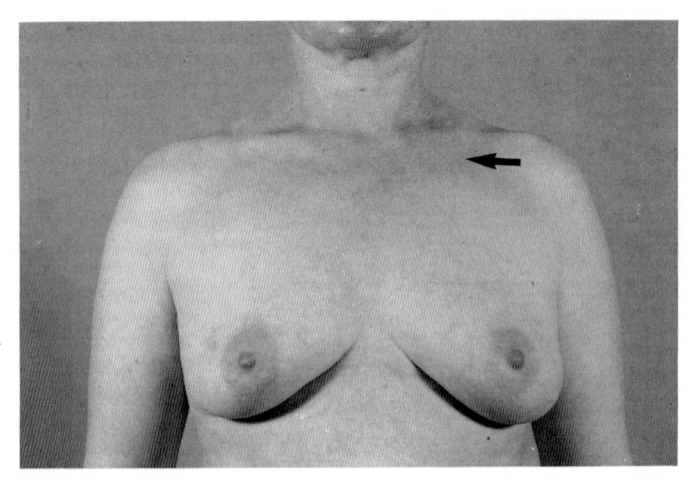

Fig. 10. Anterior aspect of patient 4. Note the swelling of the left infraclavicular space (*arrow*)

Results

In all cases complete relief of symptoms and reversal of neurological findings were obtained. In fact, in all cases, operative management of the compression syndromes prevented an impending change of profession of the patient.

Discussion

TOS clinically is characterized by the sequela either of (a) a compression of the subclavian vessels, i.e., edema, venous dilatation, thrombosis, loss of pulse, or claudication; or (b) a compression of the brachial plexus, i.e., pain, paresthesias, motor weakness; the two may also be found in combination (Fig. 11; see Jaeger et al. 1986). The anatomical basis of these findings may be attributed to the scalene muscles, first rib, clavicle, cervical ribs, or hypertrophic ligamentous structures. These compression mechanisms were illustrated in the cases described above. In the first two cases compression of the subclavian vessels and the brachial plexus by the cervical ribs and by hypertrophic ligamentous structures was the source of patients' complaints. In the third patient, neurological symptoms could be attributed to a stenosis of the costoclavicular space (involvement of scalene muscles). The fourth case was characterized by compression of the brachial plexus due to the combined effects of the scalene muscles, clavicle, and hypertrophic ligamentous structures.

The third case in particular illustrates the necessity of a thorough examination of all patients presenting signs of peripheral neuropathy in order to make the correct diagnosis and apply the correct management. In any suspected case of TOS, a preoperative examination (Table 1) should be

Diagnosis and Surgical Management of the Thoracic-Outlet Syndrome 313

```
                              Compression
                             ↙         ↘
               Subclavian vessels      Brachial plexus
                      ↓                      ↓
                Vascular RCS          Neurological RCS
                 ↙      ↘               ↙        ↘
        Subclavian v.  Subclavian a.  Sympathetic n.  Peripheral n.
                           ↘           ↙
                              Pain
                             Ischemia
                          Trophic change
             ↓             ↓              ↓             ↓
           Edema      Loss of pulse   Sympathetic      Pain
                                       dystrophy
       Venous dilation  Claudication  Raynaud's bodies  Paresthesias
       Paget-Schroetter  Thrombosis                    Motor weakness
         syndrome
```

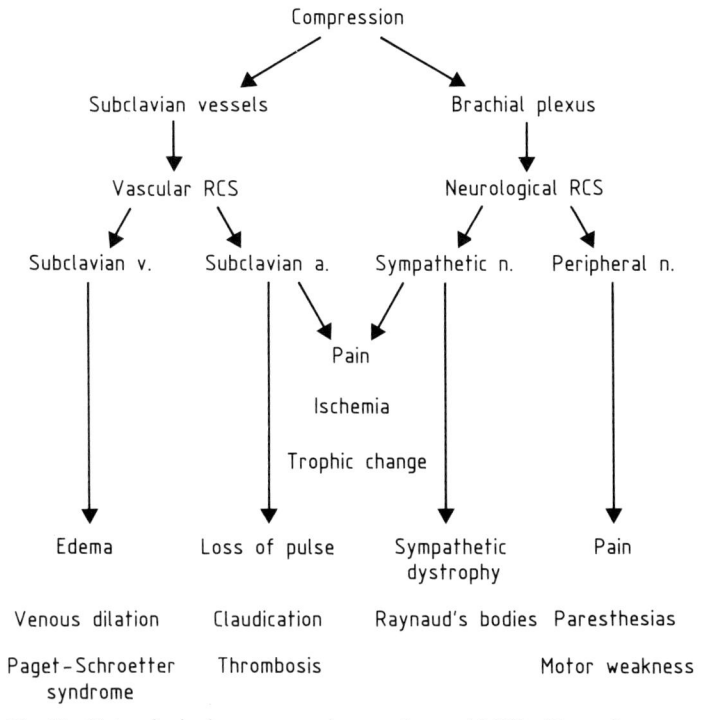

Fig. 11. Retroclavicular compression syndrome (*RCS*). (From Jaeger et al. 1986)

performed. Once the diagnosis of TOS is confirmed, the compressing structures must be resected to prevent irreversible lesions of the brachial plexus or the compressed vessels. As indicated in the literature and confirmed by our experience, two important points must be considered in the surgical management of TOS: (a) A transaxillary approach should be chosen regardless of the etiology of the compressing structure. (b) Not only the primary cause of the

Table 1. Preoperative examination of thoracic-outlet syndrome. (From Wilhelm and Wilhelm 1985)

1. Case history
2. Inspection
3. Determination of skin temperature
4. Examination of peripheral pulses
5. Bilateral determination of blood pressure
6. Auscultation of the subclavian artery
7. Stress abduction test
8. Neurological examination
9. X-ray examination of the chest
10. Phlebography of the subclavian vein
11. Arteriography of the subclavian artery
12. Doppler ultrasound examination

compression but in all cases also the first rib must be resected, otherwise complete relief of neurological signs cannot be expected.

The cases described here should provide a better understanding of the differential diagnosis of peripheral neuropathies and show the necessity of a careful examination in order to provide optimal treatment for each patient.

References

Bonnel F, Rabischong P (1981) Anatomy and systematization of the brachial plexus in the adult. Anatomia clinica 2:289–298
Calen S, Pommexeau X, Gbikpi-Benissen AM, Videau I (1986) Morphologic and functional anatomy of the subclavian veins. Surgical and Radiologic Anatomy 8:121–129
Cooley DA, Wukasch DC (1979) Techniques in vascular surgery 385–391
Jaeger SH et al. (1986) Hand clinics, vol. 2, No. 1, 217–234
Mumenthaler M, Schliack H (1982) Läsionen peripherer Nerven, 4. Aufl. Thieme, Stuttgart, S 180–187
Nguyen H, Vallée B, Person H, Nguyen HV (1984) Anatomical bases of transaxillary resection of the first rib. Anatomia clinica 5:221–233
Roos DB (1976) Congenital anomalies associated with thoracic outlet syndrome – anatomy, symptoms, diagnosis and treatment. Am J Surg 132(6):771–778
Roos DB (1980) Recurrent thoracic outlet syndrome after first rib resection. Acta Chir Belg 79:363–372
Roos DB (1982) The Place for scalenectomy and first rib resection in thoracic outlet syndrome. Surg 97:1077–1085
Wilhelm A, Wilhelm F (1985) Das Thoracic Outlet-Syndrom und seine Bedeutung für die Chirurgie der Hand. Handchirurgie 17:173–187

Retroperitoneal Hematoma with Femoral Neuralgia

S. C. TINDALL, Atlanta/USA

Experience in the treatment of five cases of retroperitoneal hematoma with associated femoral neuralgia forms the basis for this report. In our series, spontaneous retroperitoneal hematoma occurs most often in patients taking anticoagulants. Symptoms generally follow minor trauma to the leg or hip such as stepping into a hole. Patients complain of inability to walk, severe deep aching pain in the hip and thigh, and paresthesias in the distribution of the

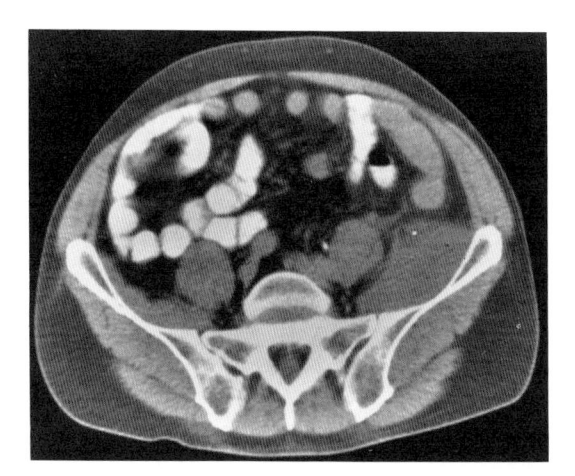

Fig. 1. Intramuscular hematoma within iliacus muscle

femoral nerve. Examination discloses inability to extend the leg at the hip, diminished knee jerk, and variable hypoesthesia in the thigh and anterior foreleg. Quadriceps function is difficult to assess due to patient discomfort. A bruise may appear in the flank. CT scanning demonstrates hematoma in a characteristic location beneath the iliacus muscle posteromedial to the hip joint (Fig. 1).

Of the treatment options available experience has shown that surgery provides the most effective relief of symptoms and potential for recovery of neurological function. Following reversal of anticoagulation, surgical treatment is indicated for evacuation of the hematoma and decompression of the femoral nerve which may be entrapped beneath the inguinal ligament.

The surgical treatment involves exploration of the femoral nerve in the retroperitoneal space and beneath the inguinal ligament. Evacuation of the hematoma within the iliacus muscle is accomplished through a linear incision within the muscle mass immediately lateral to and parallel to the course of the femoral nerve.

Timing Surgery in Nerve Lesions

G. BRUNELLI and L. MONINI, Brescia/Italy

We have always been concerned with the problem of timing surgery in peripheral nerve repair. Immediate repair seemed the best solution when we started peripheral nerve surgery, long before microsurgery. Results were so poor that, even when considering that many other factors were affecting the results, we wondered whether some biological factors could suggest a different surgical therapy, namely a delayed repair. Starting with microsurgery in the 1960s, having read all that was available at the time, we became a supporter of delayed repair, mainly for two reasons: the cell response to the lesion which takes days to become effective and the scar forming at the site of the lesion which can be removed during a more or less early secondary operation. This was our philosophy for several years.

Nevertheless, we noted the differential behavior in recovery related to various factors, such as the level of the lesion, type of trauma, surrounding tissue, time of surgery, general condition of the patients, and many more.

In these years several papers were presented, some in favor and many more against delayed repair. However, in the best, most meticulous papers comparing immediate and delayed repair, the immediate repair had generally been done for less severe lesions while delayed surgery had been performed for worse, more complex, more proximal wounds, also including late (and not slightly delayed) surgery, so that these clinical series were not significant in this respect.

Taking into consideration the bibliography and our clinical notes taken during these years and having done repeated research on motor neuron reaction and nerve behavior at the site of severance and below in different conditions, we arrived at a compromise. Aside from neurapraxia and axonotmesis which do not require surgery, in neurotmesis we must consider the parent cell reaction which (in rats) takes 15–18 days to activate fully the cell organelles. Already at 2 days we can see the so-called satellitosis and the beginning of cromatolysis, which means dilatation of the rough endoplasmic reticulum (RER) cisterns, but it takes 15–18 days to activate fully the smooth endoplasmic reticulum (SER) and Golgi's apparatus. At 20 days the cell reaction is at its maximum, and we have seen this lasting up to 60–90 days.

Figure 1 shows a schematic representation of cell reaction at 20 days. Cromatolysis has taken place, the cell body has swollen, the nucleus has been pushed to the periphery, and the nuclear membrane has enlarged its pores. The RER has enlarged its cistern, the ribosomes have scattered, the SER has

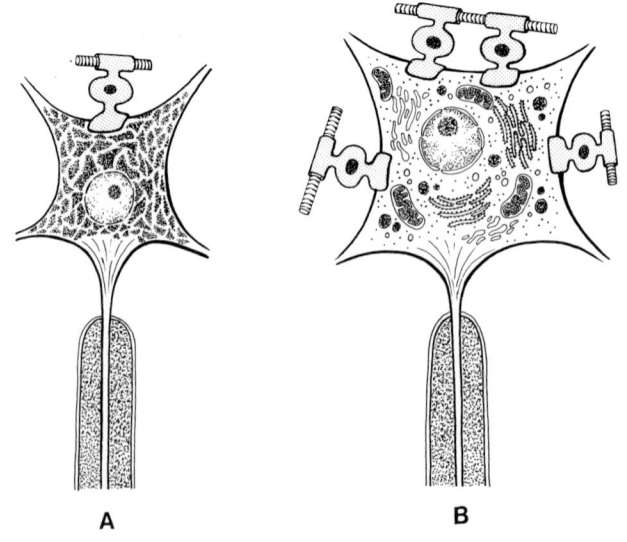

Fig. 1. A Parent cell of an axon at rest. **B** After activation due to peripheral neurotmesis (see text)

dilated, the Golgi's apparatus has been activated, the mitocondria are bigger, etc. This is the best time for the cell to produce all the substances required to reconstruct the cytoskeleton of the axon.

At the severance site (and below) wallerian degeneration takes place followed by sprouting (which is stronger after some days) and invasion by fibroblasts. Schwann's cells proliferate (Fig. 2). Many small axons take the place of the former ones in the so-called regenerating bundles which, later on, will lose the former basal lamina, constituting the endoneural tube, to form new smaller tubes. Eventually at the lesion site we have more numerous, smaller sprouts (the earlier of which are less vital) and scar formation.

Therefore, in timing sutures we should delay surgery (at least from the biological point of view):

1. To wait for healthier sprouts.
2. To remove the scar which has formed in the meantime, thus having the sprouts immediately advancing inside the distal stump to reconstruct the distal cytoskeleton.

But the problem is not as simple as this. Many other factors interfere, for instance, the adoption phenomenon (with the ability to improve the surgical matching) and the internal arrangement of fibers which is different proximally and distally, and these factors must be considered in timing surgery.

In the brachial plexus the roots are either motor or sensory pure nerves, but immediately in the spinal nerves there is an anteroposterior mingling of fibers (Fig. 3). A few millimeters apart, spinal nerves form the trunks, and a craniocaudal mingling takes place (in a plane perpendicular to that of the

Timing Surgery in Nerve Lesions

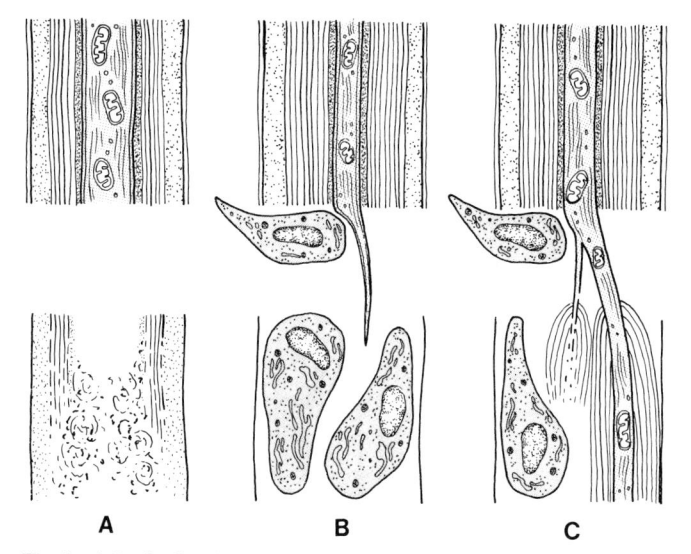

Fig. 2. A In the first hours the axoplasm coagulates. In the distal stump it disappears, as well as the myelin sheet, with fragmentation and reabsorption. **B** One early sprout is shown, thin, poor in amino acids; Schwann's cells proliferate. Fibroblasts enter in the site of the lesion and stop new sprouts. **C** Later, when the cell produces enough amino acids, new sprouts originate, which are sound and reach the distal target while the first thin sprouts degenerate

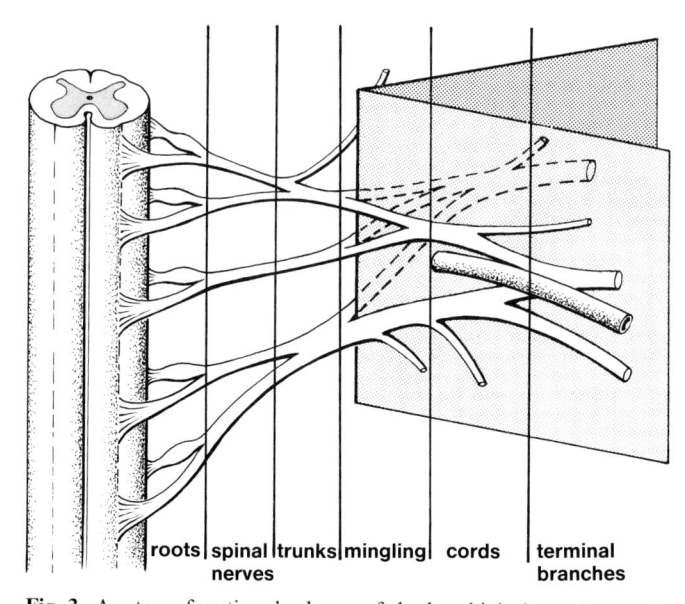

Fig. 3. Anatomofunctional scheme of the brachial plexus (see text)

mingling of fibers in spinal nerves). At this point trunks contain fibers for collateral and terminal branches, both long and short, both volar and dorsal. Next, decussatio takes place giving origin to cords with a first functional separation, as flexor pronator fibers stay in front while extensor supinator fibers go to the rear, the former serving to take the latter to leave. But cords again include fibers to proximal and distal muscles and skin. In turn, a peripheral nerve can be divided into precollateral, collateral, preterminal, and terminal sections (Fig. 4).

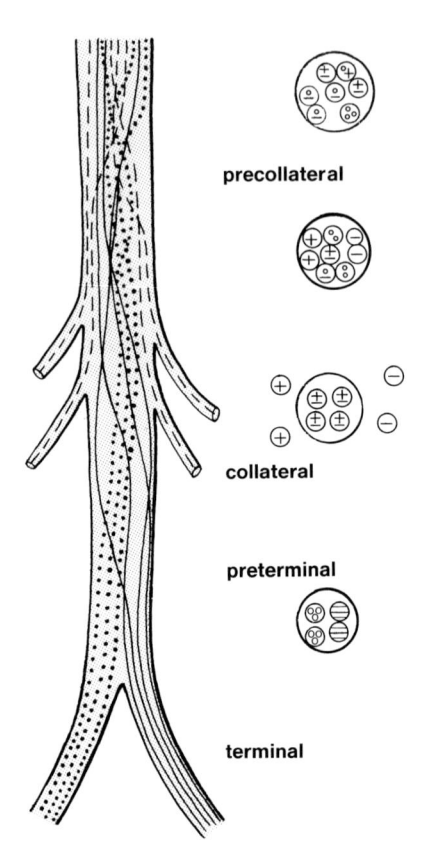

Fig. 4. Internal arrangement of a peripheral nerve (see text)

Collateral and terminal branches have a precise functional arrangement and destiny while the internal precollateral and preterminal parts of the nerve still undergo several exchanges of fibers of different functions. This internal arrangement of fibers favors an immediate repair of the collateral and terminal branches as well as of the preterminal tract of the nerve, as the functional meaning of the structures can be better recognized in emergency; conversely, a nerve the internal pattern of which is not functionally defined has no acute indication for surgery.

In distal lesions there are several other factors favoring an immediate repair. The amount of cytoskeleton to reconstruct is small and does not require a strong activation of the cell. In digits and hand (where there are no or few muscles) the scarring reaction is more severe, and a secondary repair can be difficult and recovery worse due to the summing up of scars. The association with an arterial lesion requires immediate repair, as it has been demonstrated that the nerve function (or the function of muscles and skin depending on the nerve) is much better if the vessels are repaired, and these cannot be repaired late.

On the other hand, a complex lesion is better treated repairing all the damaged structures and performing only an epineural approximation of the nerve to avoid retraction and returning to repair the nerve (if Tinel's sign does not advance distally) when the other structures have healed, thus allowing a nerve surgery with removal of the scar and the damaged portion of the nerve itself. This hardly can be recognized in emergency and is not affected by the treatment of other lesions such as tendon surgery, which with the modern treatment requires immediate mobilization.

Taking into account all these factors (and others) our strategy today is to divide the limb into three sections: Distal, intermediate, and proximal (Fig. 5). Immediate repair is done in the distal section, which makes bad scars, does not need to reconstruct very much cytoskeleton, and has functionally well-defined arrangement. Delayed repair is done in the proximal section, which needs a strong activation of the mother cell, in which nerves are surrounded by soft tissues, and the internal functional arrangement is still so mixed that there is no difference in matching it sooner or later. With regard to the intermediate section we perform immediate or early repair in cases of neat, isolated nerve lesion but wait in those of complex fractures, tendon lesions, bad surrounding tissue, etc.

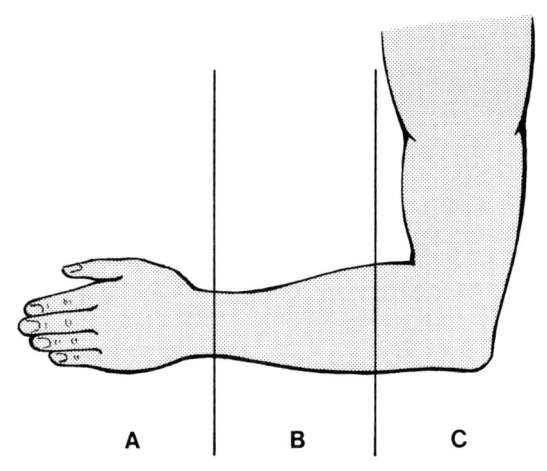

Fig. 5. Division of the limb into three sections: *A*, distal; *B*, intermediate; *C*, proximal

Several factors must be considered: regarding graft timing. First, the graft is not a nerve; it consists of endoneural tubes filled with Schwann's cells serving only as a guide and support to the regrowing axons. It needs to be revascularized (unless it is a vascular graft) so that a good recipient bed is provided. If it is not good, it must be treated and changed (by means of local, pedicled, or free microvascular flaps). Added lesions (tendon, bones, etc.) should have healed. If joints are stiff, they must be mobilized; muscles must be still in a condition to accept reinnervation, which means they must retain some trophism and show fibrillation upon EMG.

As regards entrapments, these initially produce only axonostenosis, which is followed by axonal suffering which involves more and more fibers.

What happens in entrapments? An axon flow dam phenomenon occurs above the entrapment with arterial blood supply obstacle and edema while below it some edema can occur due to the compression of the veins. This is due to the fact that an alteration in the equilibrium of liquid pressure occurs. In normal tunnels the equilibrium should be as follows: the arterial pressure higher than the capillary, the capillary higher than the intraneural, the intraneural higher than the venular, and the venular higher than the tunnel general pressure. Due to alterations in this equilibrium axonostenosis takes place, followed by axonal suffering of a progressively greater number of fibers.

In timing surgery one should not wait for clinical signs of palsy, as the adoption phenomenon masks the lesions. The fibers which have not yet suffered adopt the orphan muscular fibers (and perhaps also some sensory corpuscles), thus constituting giant motor units. Later, when the fibers responsible for giant motor units have also suffered, the palsy develops dramatically, and at this time surgery may prove ineffective because it is too late. Therefore, in entrapments as soon as EMG shows augmented distal latency or giant motor units, surgery must be carried out.

References

Brunelli G (1978) In: Microchirurgia. Pelizza, Brescia
Brunelli G et al. (1980) Influenza dei gangliosidi sulla rigenerazione nervosa. Riv It Chir Mano 17:1
Brunelli G, Fontana G, Jager C et al (1987) Chemotactic arrangement inside and distal to a venous graft. Jour of Rec Micros 2
Comtet JJ (1983) Les greffes nerveuses vascularisées. Acta Chir Belgica 83:293–297
Omer GE (1972) Evaluation d'une lesion nerveuse peripherique posttraumatique from "les lesions traumatiques des nerves peripheriques", Expansion Ed, Paris, pp 63–70
Seddon H (1972) Surgical disorders of the peripheral nerves. Churchill Livingstone, London
Sunderland S (1978) Nerve and nerve injuries. Churchill Livingstone, London

Neurolysis

M. SAMII, Hannover/FRG

Literally speaking, neurolysis means liberation of a nerve from compression. Before the microscope was incorporated into surgical procedures, surgeons were only able to grossly release the major nerve trunks from possible surrounding compressive factors or tissues. The general belief was that if the nerve was in continuity, the function would be restored. From the experimental work and clinical experiences of Seddon and Sunderland, we deepened our understanding regarding different possible lesions of nerves in continuity. The Grade I and II injuries of Sunderland, equivalent to Neurapraxia and Axonotmesis as described by Seddon, represent the lesions. Nevertheless, the most important aspect of Sunderland's classification was the introduction of a *third* degree of lesion, which is a combination of neural and connective tissue lesion. This type of lesions demonstrated that even after external decompression of a nerve lesion in continuity, the functional outcome was not predictable. With the introduction of the operating microscope, we have become able to virtually dissect the major nerve trunk into its smaller anatomical units, namely the fascicular groups by removing the fibrotically altered epineural tissues surrounding the fascicles. I have already designated this technique "fascicular perineural neurolysis" (Samii 1970). This technique allowed us to go a step further eliminating the extrafascicular compression. However, as Sunderland mentioned regarding the grade III type of injuries, one cannot be sure of what is happening within the fascicles, which means that even a fascicular neurolysis may not be sufficient.

Taking into account the condition of the individual fascicles of an involved or affected nerve trunk, we have found three distinctively different types of nerve lesions in continuity which can only be differentiated intraoperatively.

First Type

The fascicles are all intact and may be of normal size or slightly narrowed by an epineural thickening. This sounds simple but in reality we cannot be sure what kind of injury each fascicle has suffered. Was it a simple neurapraxia, or was it axonotmesis with development of epineural fibrosis hindering conduction and therefore causing clinical and functional loss? If it was axonotmesis, has the strangulation blocked the axonal growth and remyelinisation, or are we dealing with a good regeneration of the distal segment with just a conduction block due to the surrounding fibrosis? This phenomenon can sometimes be detected prior to or during surgery by means of neuroelectrophysiological studies. The functional recovery after fascicular neurolysis is variable: there may be an immediate intraoperative response, or recovery may take as much time as the entire process of regeneration needs following wallerian degeneration.

Second Type

In the second type of nerve injury there is a variable pathological change of all fascicles associated with epineural fibrosis. The fascicles as such are in continuity but they may be interrupted with neuromas bridging the gap. This demands for resection and coaptation with or without a nerve graft. The other pathological change is the hardening or thickening of the fascicles with perhaps some deformity. This situation must be considered as a pitfall, and if there is no conduction across the pathological segment, there is no way to know the exact morphological alteration. This may eventually correspond to Sunderlands's grade III injury. In view of the above mentioned dilemma or doubt, when faced with clinical functional loss, my strategy is resection and reconstruction of the segment.

Third Type

The third type of lesion represents a combination of the first and second types. We are therefore dealing with a nerve trunk having varying grades of injury to its different fascicles.

Summary

A classification of nerve injuries is useful, but it yields only an approximation of the true degree of nerve involvement or alteration. A lesion will seldomly produce a single pattern of nerve fiber damage and therefore in one fascicle, different fibers may suffer different grades of injury. A classification will guide us towards a better understanding of nerve injuries and help us standardize treatment protocols.

The aims of neurolysis are the following: on one side it will allow us to evaluate the extent, type and nature of the lesion, on the other side it permits us to liberate the compressed fascicles restoring nerve function. A classification of nerve injury from a surgical point of view could be as follows:

Type 1

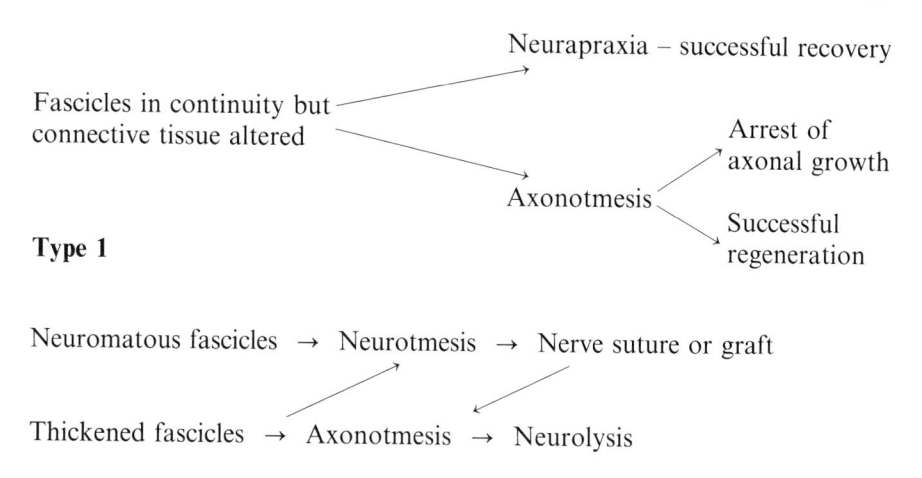

Fascicles in continuity but connective tissue altered
— Neurapraxia – successful recovery
— Axonotmesis
  — Arrest of axonal growth
  — Successful regeneration

Type 2

Neuromatous fascicles → Neurotmesis → Nerve suture or graft
Thickened fascicles → Axonotmesis → Neurolysis

Type 3 is a combination of Type 1 and 2.

References

Kahl RI, Samii M, Willebrand H (1972) Clinical results of perineural fascicular neurolysis. Excerpta Medica, International Congress Series No. 306:209–212
Samii M (1975) Modern aspects of peripheral and cranial nerve surgery. In: Advances and Standards in Neurosurgery 2, Springer Verlag: 33–85
Samii M (1975) Use of microtechniques in peripheral nerve surgery – experiences with over 300 cases. Microneurosurgery, Igaku Shoin Ltd., Tokyo: 85–93
Samii M, Willebrand H (1970) The technique and indication for autologous interfascicular nerve transplantation. Excerpta Medica, International Congress Series No. 217:39
Seddon HJ (1943) Three types of nerve injury. Brain, 66:237
Sunderland S (1951) A classification of peripheral nerve injuries producing loss of function. Brain, 74:491

Free Vascularized Nerve Grafts

A. BERGER, P. MAILÄNDER, and E. SCHALLER, Hannover/FRG

The ideal nerve graft may be that which is already vascularized immediately after transplantation. The classic nerve graft (Millesi et al 1972; Settergreen and Wood 1984) must be vascularized by the recipient bed and autonomic blood supply of the reconstructed nerve stumps. In recent years many investigations have been carried out to obtain further information on vascularized nerve grafts (Taylor and Ham 1976; Breidenbach and Terzis 1984; Fachinelli et al. 1981; Doi et al. 1984; Restrepo et al. 1985; Berger 1987). However, for clinical use the question remains open regarding the place of the vascularized nerve graft in reconstruction of peripheral nerve lesions. It is necessary to ascertain how much we gain by this method, and how much we lose in taking a vascularized graft at the donor site.

A second problem seems to lie in the blood supply and anatomy of the available free grafts. Are these really as constant as sometimes maintained, or are only some grafts available and reliable in constant anatomy? Otherwise, some grafts could be problematic due to sacrificing a major artery and vein or to the inconstant blood supply and the possible length of the vascular pedicled nerve graft.

A number of papers have already been published, as mentioned above, and in our clinic we have also investigated special nerves in cadavers when these have been available and useful for grafting procedures. The following questions arise: (a) how many donor sites are available at the time; (b) how many nerves and of what length can be obtained; (c) how reliable is the anatomy of the blood supply of the investigated nerves; and (d) how important is the loss of function at the donor site?

Strange in 1947 used the ulnar nerve and Taylor and Ham in 1976 the superficial branch of the radial nerve as a vascularized nerve graft. Breidenbach and Terzis (1984) have also published investigations of different types of blood supply to the different nerves. We have had to consider only the extrinsic and the intrinsic blood supplies, that is, the para- and epineural vessels and the epi-/perineural and endoneural capillaries and vessels. We found that a compromise of the two systems is useful. This has been published elsewhere (Millesi 1972).

We began this program in Hanover in 1981. The vascularized nerve graft is a fascinating additional method, but the question of the regeneration of such a graft, whether this is really much better and faster, has not yet been completely answered. Most papers on the topic demonstrate a faster regeneration at the

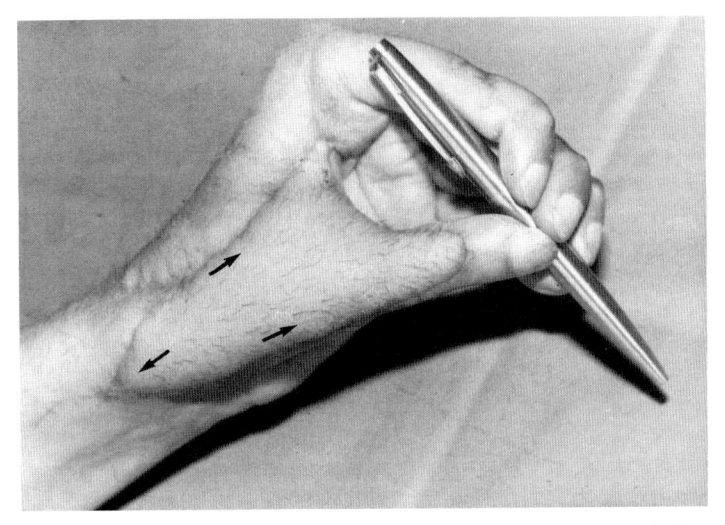

Fig. 1. Reconstruction of the soft-tissue defect and the dorsal digital nerves with a radial artery flap and antebrachii medialis nerve for sensibility

beginning. This means a distal progression of Tinel's sign, but in the end comparison of a classic nerve graft with a vascularized one reveals no significant difference in regained function. This should be considered in larger series. We never use a vascularized nerve graft, when we can use a classic one.

Therefore, only a small number of nerves may be useful because of blood supply and donor site morbidity. We consider now what type of nerves in our experience are the useful ones. First is the superficial branch of the radial nerve. The anatomy is 100% constant (Taylor and Ham 1976). The blood supply is provided by the radial artery and the concomitant veins. The length which can be gained is 24 cm. The vessels are useful for a microvascular anastomosis. The loss of function is very small and only sensitive in nature. The nerve can be folded to provide three or more grafts for a shorter distance. A disadvantage is the sacrifice of a major artery. An advantage is that one can even include this nerve in a lower arm flap for reconstructing a complex area (Fig. 1).

The next interesting one is the ulnar nerve. This is a very useful graft even as a pedicled vascularized nerve in brachial plexus lesions when roots C 8 and T 1 are out of function, and no further recovery in the ulnar muscles (Fig. 2) can be expected. The ulnar nerve has two major vascular pedicles (Künzel et al. 1986), and the anatomy is in 96% constant. It is possible to gain grafts of 30–50 cm length in the upper arm region and 24–30 cm in the lower arm region. The loss of function in a healthy nerve would be a very important factor, but in our opinion this is no indication for using this graft.

Other nerves such as the cutaneous antebrachial and the cutaneous antebrachial dorsalis have smaller sensible fibers with an anatomy reliable

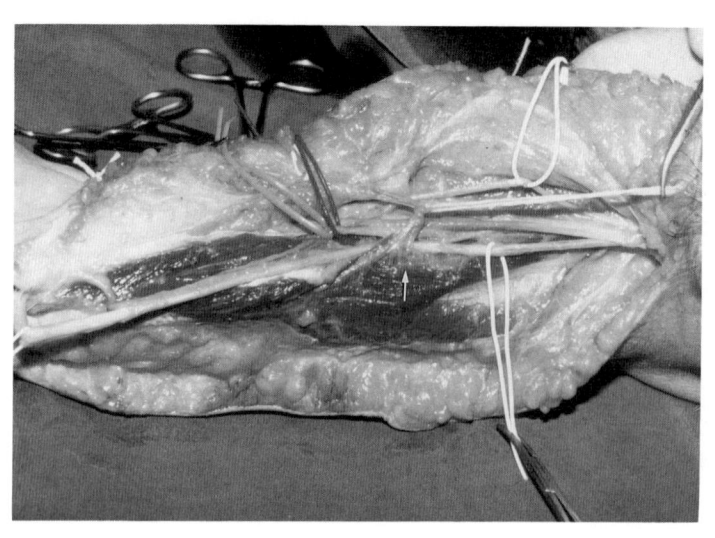

Fig. 2. An ulnar nerve as vascularized graft

only to 60% and very small vessels. The palmar and digital nerves in our material have proven very useful because replantation surgery often provides the opportunity to obtain this type of vascular nerve graft when reconstructing major injuries of a hand, and the replantation of some digits may not be useful. The anatomy in these cases is in 100% constant, and a loss of function is negligible. The *intercostal nerves* are possible vascularized grafts. We have used them only in combined transfers and not as simple grafts alone. In the lower extremity there is the *saphenus nerve*, with a constant anatomy of 80% and a possible length of 40 cm (Fig. 3). This is a very small nerve, and it must therefore be folded, which in our experience is not without problems, especially when this nerve is needed for a lower arm area. The functional loss is not very important.

Our classic nerve graft, the *sural nerve*, can also be used as a vascularized one, but the anatomy in the sural nerve is constant to only 30%, and many variations in the blood supply are seen (Fig. 4). It is a small nerve and presents the same problems as does the saphenus nerve. The length of the graft can be 25–35 cm. The sensible loss is insignificant. A more interesting nerve is the *peroneus profundus*, with an anatomy that is 100% reliable. However, this involves the sacrifice of a major artery, the anterior tibial artery. The functional loss is not very important when taking only the nerve distal to the muscle branches. For a combined tissue transfer (Rose and Kowalski 1985) the branches of the peroneus profundus in the dorsal foot area are very interesting. Not much in length can be gained, usually 5–7 cm, but these nerves can be included in a neurovascular flap pedicled on the dorsalis pedis artery (Fig. 5). It is very useful for reconstruction in the hand and digital areas.

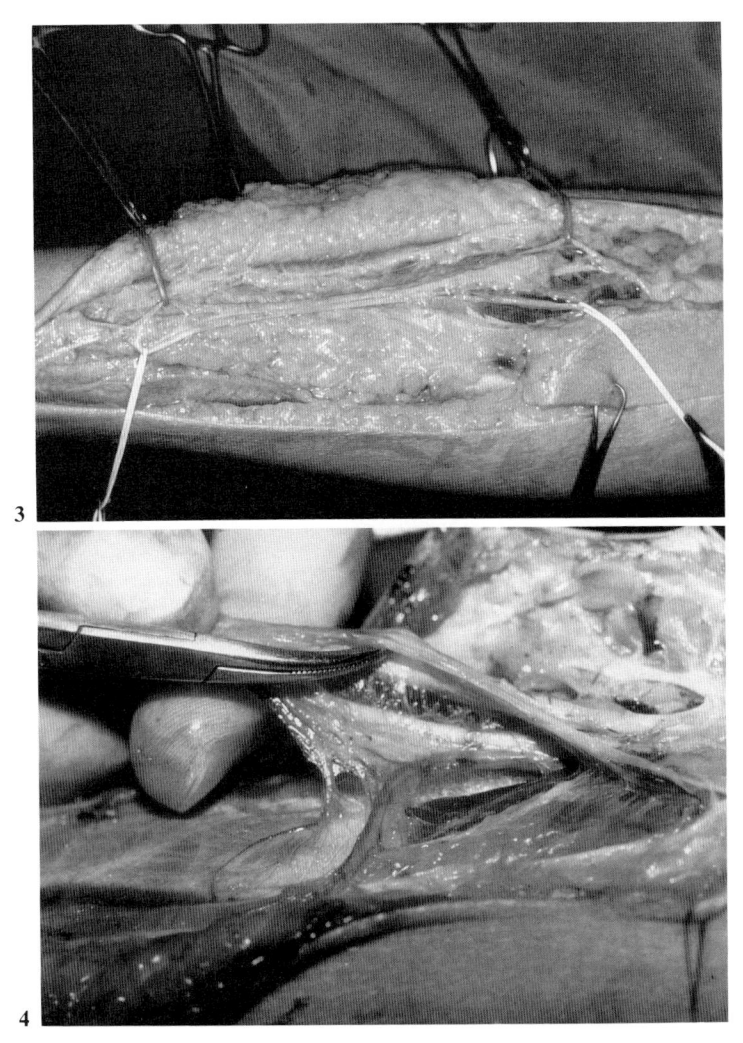

Fig. 3. The saphenus nerve which in 80% has a constant anatomy

Fig. 4. A sural nerve showing a variation of its blood supply

In rare occasions, when the patient has suffered an amputation on one side and reconstruction, for instance of a lower peroneal nerve, is required, one can obtain a part of a major trunk. In our experience the peroneus communis with its vascular pedicle could be used because there is no loss of function in the amputated lower extremity. In one case we reconstructed a gap of 18 cm on the right leg, obtaining the rest of the peroneus communis nerve from the left side. The patient suffered an amputation at the upper third of his lower leg some years ago (Fig. 6).

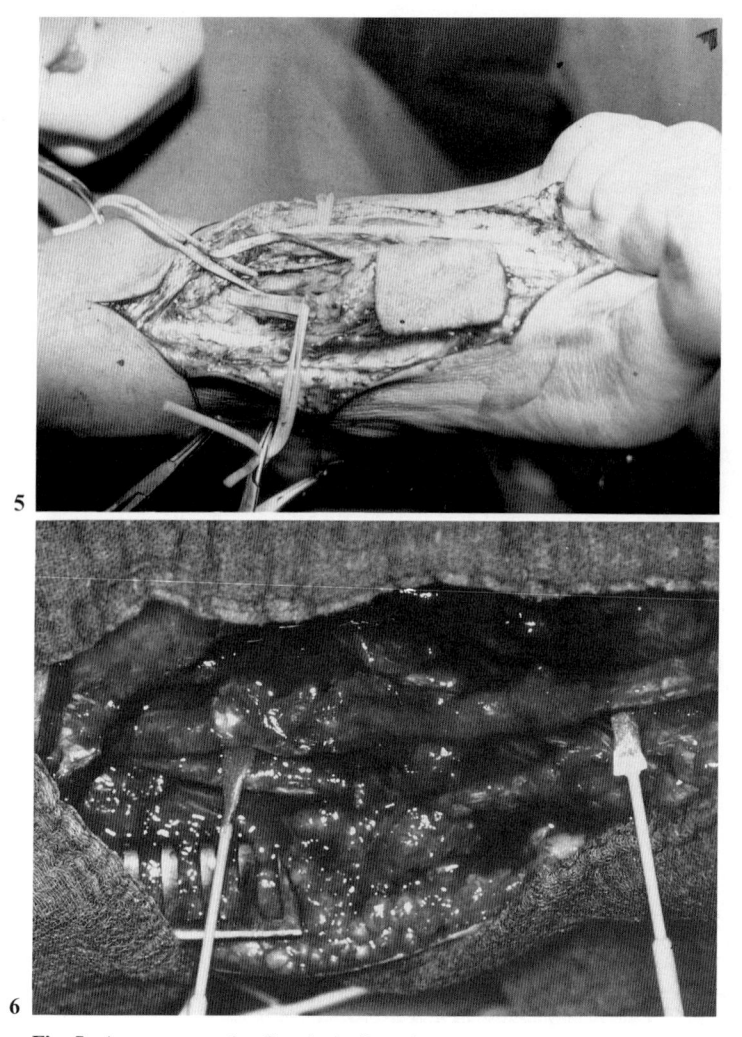

Fig. 5. A neurovascular flap including the peroneus superficialis for finger reconstruction

Fig. 6. A peroneus communis nerve obtained for reconstruction of the peroneus profundus

Discussion

At present we observe two indications for the use of vascularized nerve grafts. The first is when it is not possible to create a good blood supply and bed for a classic nerve graft, or a long distance must be bridged, which may be problematic for classic grafts (Fig. 7). The second indication is in combined injuries, for example, high-voltage burn cases, degloving injuries or similar problems when soft tissue and sensibility must be restored at once. Here in a

Free Vascularized Nerve Grafts 331

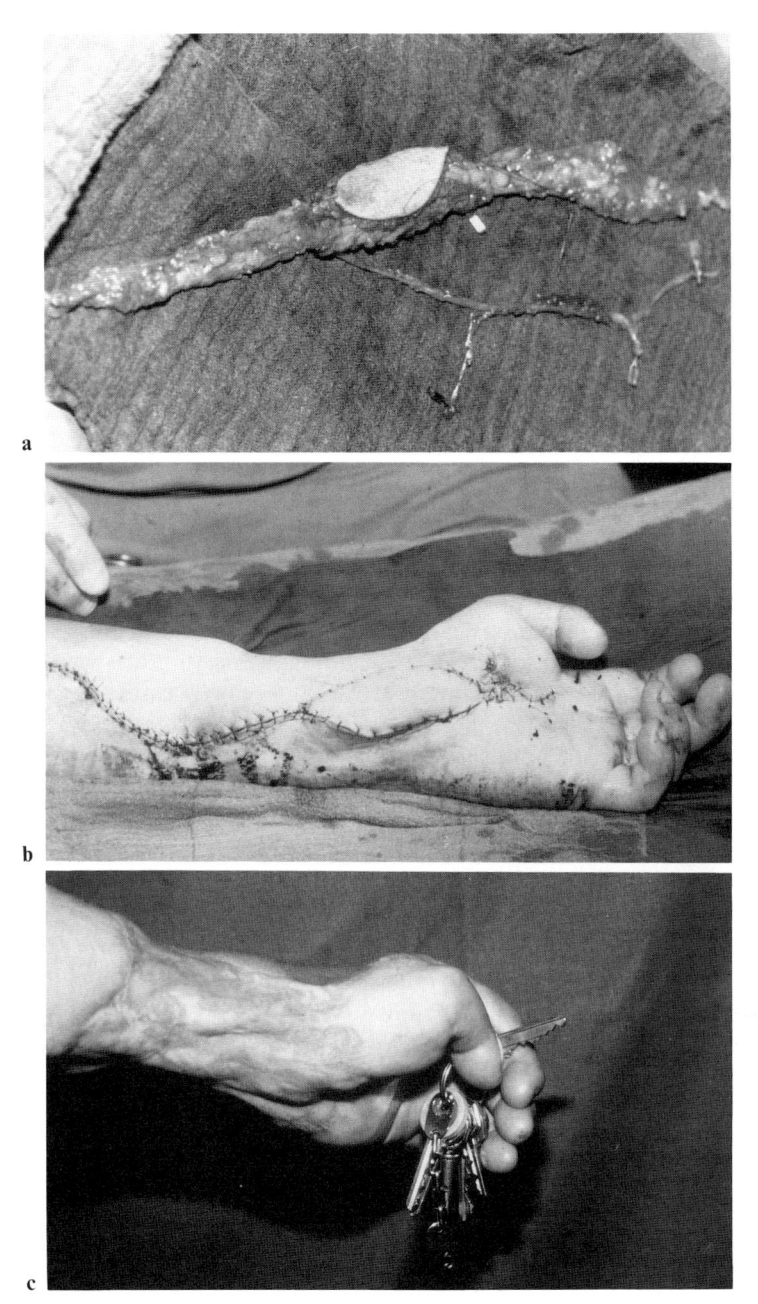

Fig. 7. a A sural nerve with vascular pedicle and skin island. **b** Median nerve repaired in a severe burn case by vascular nerve graft, nerve folded. **c** Result 1 year later showing a useful function

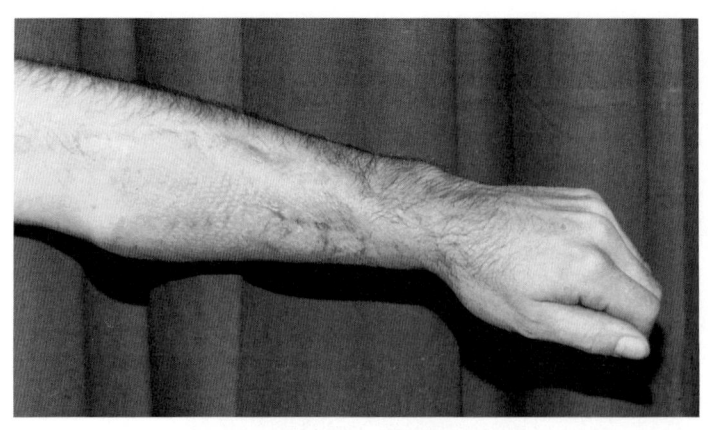

Fig. 8. Combined tissue transfer to reconstruct skin and median nerve. N. Cutaneous brachialis medialis nerve as graft

free-tissue transfer one may include branches of the nerves mentioned above to reconstruct the median, ulnar, or digital nerve (Fig. 8).

In the past 7 years we have repaired nerve lesions with primary suture under ideal conditions without tension in 215 cases. Autologous nerve grafts were used in 310 cases. Vascularized nerve grafts were used in only 39 cases; 14 of these were vascularized nerve grafts alone, and in 15 patients a nerve was included in a combined tissue transfer. Neurovascular flaps are a special indication and are not included in this group. At the same time, 152 plexus cases have been repaired by nerve grafts.

The ulnar nerve was used only three times in brachial plexus lesions. In our material the sural nerve was also used three times for reconstruction of the median nerve in electrical burn cases in the wrist area. In these cases free-tissue transfer was needed additionally for other soft-tissue problems. The palmar and digital nerves were used eight times in replantation cases. The antebrachii medialis nerve was included in radial artery flaps 13 times for reconstruction, the median nerve or ulnar nerve also in combination with classic grafts. In one case the same procedure was used to reconstruct a tibialis posterior nerve. The peroneal profundus dorsalis was included twice in a dorsalis pedis artery flap for reconstruction of digital nerves and soft-tissue problems, including in one case also tendon grafts in the middle phalanx area of the hand (Fig. 9). In one case a vascularized graft from the peroneal communis of the right leg as described above was used to reconstruct the peroneal communis nerve on the left leg.

A sufficiently long follow-up of 12 cases has been evaluated. Our findings in these cases does not differ from the experiences reported in the literature. The regeneration, i.e., the distal progression of Tinel's sign, was faster compared with a classic graft by an average of $1-2$ months. The quality of the regeneration after $1-2$ years was at least at the same level as in the classic grafts depending on the type of injury.

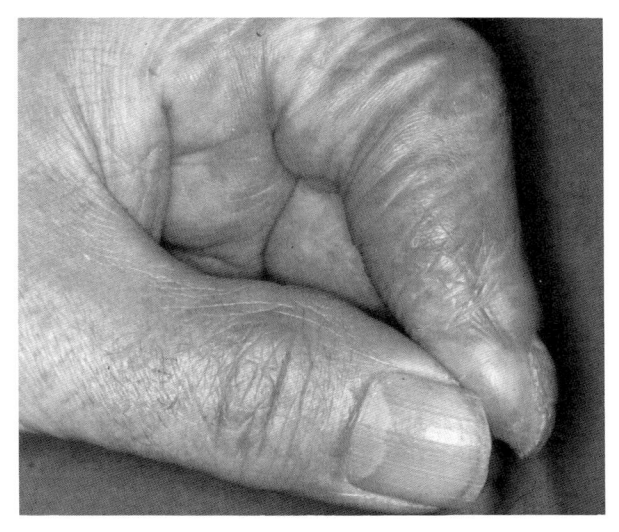

Fig. 9. Dorsalis pedis artery flap including the peroneal profundus dorsalis nerve and a tendon. Result 1 year later

With a clear indication vascularized nerve grafts are an additional tool in cases in which there is a need for a very long graft and a chance to obtain a trunk graft or to include the nerve in a combined vascularized tissue transfer. These are cases in which classic nerve grafts cannot be used.

Thus, if a good soft-tissue bed for the nerve graft can be provided, the classic nerve graft is the method of choice (Millesi et al. 1972; Samii 1980). The indication for a vascularized nerve graft and combined tissue transfer is the indication for a reconstruction of the blood supply and the nerve in one stage, in case no other methods are available. The vascularized nerve graft is therefore an additional method of choice for reconstruction of peripheral nerve gaps.

Summary

In 462 reconstructions of brachial plexus and peripheral nerve lesions by autologous nerve grafts during the past 7 years vascularized nerve grafts or combined tissue transfer including vascularized nerve grafts were used in 29 cases. The nerves used were the ulnar nerve, the palmar and digital nerves, the antebrachii medialis nerve, the sural nerve, the peroneus profundus nerve, and in one special case the peroneus communis nerve. The vascularized nerve graft in our opinion is an alternative to conventional nerve grafts in special indications, such as are disturbed blood supply in the recipient bed where the nerve graft is to be placed, the length of a graft, the trunk graft, or especially a combined tissue transfer which offers the possibility to solve two problems in one operation. The vascularized nerve graft therefore widens the range of possibilities for reconstructing nerve gaps in peripheral nerve lesions.

We thus consider the primary suture as the first choice, the autologous graft as the second, and the vascularized graft as the third choice. This is supported by the concept that when reconstructing a lost function on one side, it must be comparable to the loss of function on the donor site where the graft is obtained.

References

1. Berger A (1984) Fortschritte in der Versorgung verletzter Nerven. Hefte Unfallheilk 164:531–535
2. Berger A (1987) Freie vaskularisierte Nerventransplantate, Spendernerven, geeignete Spenderzonen. Handchirurgie 19
3. Breidenbach W, Terzis JK (1984) The anatomy of free vascularized nerve grafts. Clin Plast Surg 11(1):65–71
4. Daly PJ, Wood MB (1985) Endoneural and epineural blood flow evaluation with free vascularized and conventional nerve grafts in the comine. J Reconstr Microsurg 2(1):45–49
5. Doi K, Kuwata F, Kawakami F, Tamaru K, Kawai S (1984) The free vascularized sural nerve graft. Microsurgery 5:175–184
6. Fachinelli A, Masquelet A, Restrepo J, Gilbert A (1981) The vascularized sural nerve. Int J Microsurg 3(1):57–62
7. Künzel KH, Fischer C, Anderl H (1986) The ulnar nerve as vascularized nerve transplant. J Reconstr Microsurg 2(3):175–179
8. Millesi H, Berger A, Meissl G (1972) Experimentelle Untersuchungen zur Heilung durchtrennter peripherer Nerven. Clin Plast 1:174–206
9. Moura W de, Gilbert A (1984) Surgical anatomy of the sural nerve. J Reconstr Microsurg 1(1):31–39
10. Restrepo Y, Merle M, Michon J, Folliguet B, Barrat E (1985) Free vascularized nerve grafts. Microsurgery 6:78–84
11. Rose EH, Kowalski TA (1985) Restoration of sensibility to anesthetic scarred digits with free vascularized nerve grafts from the dorsum of the foot. J Hand Surg 10(A):514–521
12. Samii M (1980) Fascicular peripheral nerve repair. Modern techniques in surgery. Neurosurg 17:1–22
13. Settergreen CR, Wood MB (1984) Comparison of blood flow in free vascularized versus nonvascularized nerve grafts. J Reconstr Microsurg 1(2):95–101
14. Strange FG (1947) An operation for nerve pedicle grafting: preliminary communications. Brit J Surg 34:423
15. Taylor IG, Ham FJ (1976) The free vascularized nerve graft. Plast Reconstr Surg 57:413

Caution in the Evaluation of Results of Peripheral Nerve Surgery *

D. G. KLINE, New Orleans/USA

Introduction

There are few topics that require more objectivity or attention to detail than analysis of the results of peripheral nerve surgery. The reader is no doubt familiar with how the level of the lesion, nerve involved, mechanisms of wounding, severity of associated injuries, and sometimes age of the patient can affect outcome. As with most surgical procedures, every operation on a nerve, whether repair is done or not, is a little different. What did intraoperative stimulation and nerve action potential studies show? If a neurolysis was done, how far along the length of the nerve did it extend, and to what level of the nerve did it penetrate? Before end-to-end suture how much nerve was resected, how was the repair done, and how much tension was there at the repair site? If grafts were placed, what was the donor source, how many were used and with what technique, and how long were they? Interval between injury and operative repair is important, as is how complete the loss was distal to the lesion at the time the operation was done. Since eventual outcome depends in large measure on the usefulness of the limb to the patient, the latter's educational and work skill levels as well as motivation to recover are especially important factors in determining success.

If all of these variables were not enough, length of follow-up and even its frequency are important in determining results. Critical is how the function, both motor and sensory is graded, and how knowledgeable and experienced the examiner is, as well as whether or not he or she is free of bias.

Needless to say, to document let alone present all of the above concerning a series of nerve injuries, is a very large task. In addition, this may be not only difficult to do but close to impossible to present in a readable and understandable fashion.

One of the few documents to attempt to present enough detail for close analysis concerning peripheral nerve injuries is the monograph of the United States Veterans Administration concerning American cases from World War II entitled "Peripheral Nerve Regeneration: A Follow-up Study of 3,656 World War II Injuries." This is a lengthy and at times difficult to assimilate work but a valuable one, for it provides most of the detail necessary for the

---

* From Department of Neurosurgery, LSU Medical Center, 1542 Tulane Avenue, New Orleans LA 70112, and Charity and Ochsner Hospitals of New Orleans, USA.

reader to draw conclusions. By definition, the great majority of cases reported in this well-documented work were due to gunshot (GSW) or missile fragments. Similar convincing data for civilian cases require a large number of cases, and this is harder to achieve in times of peace than in times of war. Despite this, several centers in Europe, Canada, and the United States may have accumulated enough cases to begin such a comprehensive approach. This is extremely important because mechanisms in peacetime are different, and available techniques have changed.

Methods

What follows is a presentation of the criteria used at the Louisiana State University Medical Center (LSUMC) for evaluation of results and some samples of data obtained from patients with radial and median nerve lesions with 2 or more years of follow-up. Rather than comparing two nerves with

Table 1. Grading individual muscle (LSUMC system)

Grade	Evaluation	Description
0	Absent	No contraction
1	Poor	Trace contraction
2	Fair	Movement against gravity only
3	Moderate	Movement against gravity and some (mild) resistance
4	Good	Movement against moderate resistance
5	Excellent	Movement against maximal resistance

Table 2. Sensory grading (LSUMC system)

Grade	Evaluation	Description
0	Absent	No response to touch, pin, or pressure
1	Bad	Testing gives hyperesthesia or paresthesias: deep pain recovery in autonomous zones
2	Poor	Sensory response sufficient for grip and slow protection, sensory stimuli mislocalized with overresponse
3	Moderate	Response to touch and pin in autonomous zones, sensation mislocalized and not normal with some overresponse
4	Good	Response to touch and pin in autonomous zones; response localized but not normal; however, no overresponse
5	Excellent	Normal response to touch and pin in entire field of nerve including autonomous zones

Caution in the Evaluation of Results of Peripheral Nerve Surgery 337

Table 3. Overall grading (LSUMC system)

Grade	Evaluation	Description
0	Absent	No muscle contraction; absent sensation
1	Poor	Proximal muscles contract but not against gravity; sensory grade 1 or 0
2	Fair	Proximal muscles contract against gravity, distal muscles do not contract, sensory grade if applicable usually 2 or lower
3	Moderate	Proximal muscles contract against gravity and some resistance, some distal muscles contract against gravity, sensory grade usually 3
4	Good	All proximal and some distal muscles contract against gravity and some resistance; sensory grade 3 or better
5	Excellent	All muscles contract against moderate resistance; sensory grade 4 or better

expected differences in results such as radial versus ulnar or tibial versus peroneal, the two selected – radial and median, were chosen to determine whether differences would be brought out by our grading system.

Tables 1–3 depict the methods currently used at LSUMC to grade function in patients with peripheral nerve injuries. The nerve grading scheme for motor and sensory testing have been altered somewhat to permit as accurate as possible an evaluation for grade 3 (moderate) and grade 4 (good) results. Table 3 outlines the system used for giving a grade to a whole nerve or plexus element. This scheme incorporates motor and sensory grades and hinges on a correlation of function in proximal and distal muscles.

Results

As an example of the detail necessary in order to judge results, the LSUMC radial nerve series of cases has been compared to the median nerve series. Table 4 shows upper arm level radial and median lesions listed by etiology of injury and numbers of those operated on. Not too surprisingly, lacerations and GSW were the largest categories for upper arm median lesions while fractures accounted for half of the radial lesions seen and 46% of those operated upon.

Table 5 depicts the operations done, broken down in terms of whether the lesions were in continuity or not. For those not in continuity, the experience with primary and secondary repair at the upper level is provided. For lesions in continuity, results of nerve action potential (NAP) recordings are provided along with outcome of operations done as a result of this observation.

Table 6 shows the results for operated and unoperated radial nerve lesions by etiology of lesion at the upper arm level. Results were very good when cases were properly selected for either operation or conservative management. Thus,

Table 4. Upper arm: cases by etiology

	Radial nerve		Median nerve	
	Seen	Operated	Seen	Operated
Laceration	9	8	18	15
GSW	9	5	22	12
Fracture	36	23	5	5
Contusion/Stretch	7	4	5	4
Compression/Disloc	1	0	7	4
Injection	7	7	1	1
Tumor	3	3	4	4
Total	72	50	62	45

Table 5. Radial and median operations: number operated on (numerator) and number with ≧3 result (denominator)

	Radial	Median
Not in continuity	10	12
Primary repair	3/3	3/2
Secondary repair	7/5	9/5
Suture	4/3	1/1
Graft	3/2	8/4
In continuity	40	29
+NAP, Neurolysis	19/19	17/17
−NAP, Repair	21/15	12/10
Suture	10/8	5/5
Graft	11/7	7/5

Three radial tumors resected without deficit; four median tumors removed with minimal deficit.

Table 6. Results in radial upper arm: operated cases (unoperated in parentheses)

	5/5	4/5	3/5	2/5	1/5	No follow-up
Laceration	3(1)	4(0)	0(0)	0(0)	0(0)	1(0)
Fracture	4(7)	10(2)	3(3)	2(0)	0(1)	4(0)
GSW	1(3)	2(0)	2(1)	0(0)	0(0)	0(0)
Injection	4(0)	2(0)	1(0)	0(0)	0(0)	0(0)
Contusion	1(2)	1(1)	2(0)	0(0)	0(0)	0(0)
Dislocation	0(1)	0(0)	0(0)	0(0)	0(0)	0(0)
Tumor	2(0)	0(0)	0(0)	0(0)	0(0)	1(0)
Total	15(14)	19(3)	8(4)	2(0)	0(1)	6(0)

Grading based on Tables 1–3.

42 of 50 (84%) operated on gained a grade 3 or better result while 21 of 22 (95%) not operated on did well. Table 7 includes similar results for median upper arm lesions. Laceration, GSW, and fracture-associated lesions did not fare quite as well as in the radial series. There were fewer grades 5 and 4 and more grades 3 and 2 results than in the radial series. Nonetheless, 38 of 45 (84%) reached grade 3 or better, a figure identical to that for the radial nerve. When one looks at the detail of Table 7, the subtle differences between the radial series (Table 6) and the median series can be appreciated.

Tables 8 and 9 show information about associated operations and thus severity of injury as well as injury to operative intervals. These tables are

Table 7. Results in median upper arm: operated cases (unoperated in parentheses)

	5/5	4/5	3/5	2/5	1/5	No follow-up
Laceration	1 (0)	6 (2)	4 (1)	4 (0)	0 (0)	0 (0)
GSW	2 (3)	6 (5)	3 (1)	1 (0)	0 (1)	0 (0)
Fracture	0 (0)	1 (0)	3 (0)	1 (0)	0 (0)	0 (0)
Contusion	0 (1)	1 (0)	3 (0)	0 (0)	0 (0)	0 (0)
Compression	2 (2)	0 (1)	1 (0)	1 (0)	0 (0)	0 (0)
Injection	0 (0)	1 (0)	0 (0)	0 (0)	0 (0)	0 (0)
Tumor	3 (0)	1 (0)	0 (0)	0 (0)	0 (0)	0 (0)
Total	8 (6)	16 (8)	14 (2)	7 (0)	0 (1)	0 (0)

Grading based on Tables 1–3.

Table 8. Median upper arm: other operations in operated cases ($n = 45$)

	Laceration	GSW	Fracture	Contusion/stretch	Injection
Vascular repair	8	7	0	1	0
Fracture	0	2	1	1	0
Fasciotomy	0	1	0	0	0
Prior operation, nerve	3	1	1	0	0
	11	11	2	2	0

Table 9. Median upper arm: operative interval (months)

	0	1	2	3	4	5	6	7	8	9	12	>12
Laceration	3	1	4	5	0	1	1	0	0	0	0	0
GSW	0	0	5	3	2	2	0	0	0	0	0	0
Fracture	0	0	0	1	2	0	0	1	0	0	1	0
Contusion	1	0	0	1	1	0	0	1	0	0	0	0
Compression	1	0	1	2	0	0	0	0	0	0	0	0
Injection	0	0	0	0	0	1	0	0	0	0	0	0
Total	5	1	10	12	5	4	1	2	0	0	1	0

(Four tumors were operated on shortly after their discovery, which brings the total number of cases to 45.)

included to point out the importance of details sometimes neglected or not emphasized enough when nerve repair results are presented. In the median upper arm group of injuries, lacerations and GSW had a high incidence of prior operation especially for vascular repair. Not shown in this table or subsequent ones is the incidence of associated ulnar or radial palsies, incidence of primary wound infection, or age of the patient, any or all of which factors may have the potential to affect eventual outcome. Table 9 is important because it gives an idea of the timing of the operations by category of injury. Despite this, it must be kept in mind that many of these cases were seen on referral so there were inevitable delays in operation. For the more blunt injuries where continuity was likely to be maintained, delay was purposeful so that stimulation and recording studies could be used to separate those with meaningful, early regeneration from those without this. In other cases, such as lacerations to the limb with serious proximal median loss, delay was due to late referral. It will be important to correlate those intervals with results, a task not yet done.

Tables 10–12 summarize results by level, by operation done, and by lesion in each case comparing radial results to median results. Table 10 includes figures for distal posterior interosseous nerve (PIN) and wrist level medial lesions. Table 11 includes all radial and median nerve lesions irrespective of level of injury or mechanism and presents the results of neurolysis, suture, and graft. Table 12 presents the summarized results by type of injury for each nerve as well as the totals for the 197 lesions operated upon and evaluated with 2 or more years of follow-up.

Elbow level radial nerve lesions did not fare as well as elbow level median lesions or more distal radial PIN lesions. This is probably because this series included several contusions associated with Volkmann's as well as two prior

Table 10. Results by level, radial versus median: number of cases (numerator) and number with ≥ 3 result (denominator)

	Radial	Median	Total
Upper arm	50/42 (84%)	45/38 (84%)	95/80 (84%)
Elbow/forearm	26/20 (77%)	45/39 (87%)	71/59 (83%)
PIN/wrist	26/25 (96%)	49/45 (92%)	75/70 (93%)
Total	102/87 (85%)	139/122 (87%)	241/209 (86%)

Table 11. Results of operation, radial versus median: number of cases (numerator) and number with ≥ 3 result (denominator)

	Radial	Median	Total
+NAP, neurolysis	68/65 (95%)	67/66 (98%)	135/131 (97%)
Suture	34/28 (82%)	30/25 (83%)	64/53 (83%)
Graft	31/23 (74%)	34/24 (70%)	65/47 (72%)

sutures while the median elbow level series included eight injected nerves, most with partial deficits to begin with. These details and similar ones are not presented since there is space only for a relatively close analysis of the upper arm level lesions. This does point out, however, how much care one must take in interpreting results. As expected, Table 11 shows how well patients undergoing neurolysis fare when partial injury or early adequate regeneration is proven by NAP studies. It also shows that a sutured nerve does slightly better than a grafted nerve, which is as one would expect, as those having grafts had larger gaps to be made up either due to stump retraction after transection or due to resection of a lesion in continuity large enough not to be comfortably repaired by suture.

Table 12. Results by lesion, radial versus median: number of cases (numerator) and number with ≧3 result (denominator)

	Radial	Median	Total
Laceration	23/19 (83%)	54/46 (85%)	77/65 (84%)
GSW	10/9 (90%)	22/19 (86%)	32/28 (88%)
Fracture	34/27 (79%)	11/10 (91%)	45/37 (82%)
Contusion/stretch	9/8 (89%)	18/15 (83%)	27/23 (85%)
Injection	7/7 (100%)	9/9 (100%)	16/16 (100%)

Table 12 presents results by mechanism of injury and combines those having neurolysis, suture, and graft repairs for radial and median nerve. When analyzed in this relatively crude fashion, few significant differences can be seen except for those nerves injured by injection, and many of these had incomplete lesions to begin with and were operated upon in most cases to try to help pain. Again, this table illustrates the need for detailed analysis if reasonable conclusions are to be drawn.

In this paper we have not addressed the use of the limb for daily acts of living, degree of residual pain, or occupational use. All of these are important determinants for success.

References

1. Bowden RE, Napier JR (1961) The assessment of hand function after peripheral nerve injuries. J Bone Joint Surg 43(B):481
2. Kline D, Nulsen F (1981) Acute injuries of peripheral nerves. In: Youmans J (ed) Neurological Surgery, 2nd ed. Saunders, Philadelphia
3. Kline D, Judice D (1983) Operative management of selected brachial plexus lesions. J Neurosurg 58:631
4. Nicholson O, Seddon H (1957) Nerve injuries and repair in civilian practice. Results of treatment of median and ulnar nerve lesions. Br Med J 2:1065
5. Omer G (1980) The evaluation of clinical results following peripheral nerve suture. In: Omer G, Spinner M (eds) Management of peripheral nerve problems. Saunders, Philadelphia

6. Sakellarides H (1962) A follow-up study of 172 peripheral nerve injuries in the upper extremity in civilians. J Bone Joint Surg 44(A):140
7. Seddon H (1972) Surgical disorders of the peripheral nerves. Williams & Wilkins, Baltimore
8. Sunderland S (1978) Nerves and nerve injuries. Churchill Livingstone, New York Edinburgh
9. Woodhall B, Beebe G (eds) (1956) Peripheral nerve regeneration: a follow-up study of 3,658 WW II injuries, VA Monograph. US Gov Print Office, Wash 25 DC

Microsurgical Repair of Peripheral Nerve Lesions: A Study of 150 Injuries of the Median and Ulnar Nerves

J. MICHON (†), P. AMEND, and M. MERLE, Nancy/France

Since 1964 microsurgical techniques have found increasing use for repair of severed peripheral nerves (Michon 1964; Michon et al. 1977; Michon and Möberg 1979; Smith 1964). However, as recently as 1958, Gosset expressed an attitude toward these injuries typical of those times; "Early or delayed repair of divided nerves has a poor prognosis" and "sutures and grafts often fail." In 1967 and 1976 Millesi et al. emphasized the detrimental role of tension at the repair site and advocated the use of interfascicular nerve grafts using microsurgical techniques whenever tension was a problem, as did Samii and Scheinpflug (1974). Over the past 20 years, a variety of experimental and clinical studies have been reported with a wide disparity of results. In many of the studies small series were examined; many different surgeons treated the patients, and rigorous postoperative evaluation or assessment was not always carried out. It is therefore difficult to define realistic postoperative expectations. Indeed, one could be erroneously convinced that a secondary repair is preferable to a primary repair, and that a fascicular nerve graft should be preferred to a direct suture.

Since 1977, our results have been evaluated by one person (Amend 1982) who did not operate on any of the patients reported, as recommended by Chanson et al. (1977) in the interest of a strict evaluative objectivity. We here report on our results in a comparative study of 150 median and ulnar nerve injuries at the wrist or forearm level, which were repaired by our unit (Merle et al. 1984). Five senior surgeons with a sound training in neurovascular microsurgery, operated on these patients in the unit "Assistance Main" of the academic teaching hospital of Nancy. Our aim was to correlate the results of the nerve repairs with factors related to the condition of the patient, the type of accident, and the different microsurgical techniques utilized.

Material and Methods

From 1977 to 1982, more than 500 repairs of peripheral nerves were performed in our unit. Only injuries of the median and ulnar nerves at the forearm level or at the wrist level were analyzed. All lesions of other nerves were excluded from this study because they could alter the significance of the results. A total of 131 patients with 150 nerve injuries (19 patients sustained multiple ipsilateral or bilateral nerve injuries) were analyzed by one individual (P. Amend) who was not directly involved in the treatment of any of the patients. The follow-up period varied from 2 to 7 years. There were 89 men (68%) and 42 women (32%); their age ranged from 2 to 90 years, the majority of patients being 20–30 years old.

Statistical analysis was carried out using the χ^2 test and Cramer's test.

Techniques for Nerve Repair

Secondary suture was performed in 12 patients (9.3%), with 14 nerve repairs; fascicular graft was performed in 44 patients (33.3%), with 50 nerve repairs; and primary suture was performed in 75 patients (57.4%), with 86 nerve repairs. The specific technique for microsurgical repair varied according to the type of nerve injury.

In patients with a sharply cut nerve, visualized clearly, a mixture of fascicular repair (with interfascicular epineural sutures as guiding sutures) and epiperineural repair was performed. This technique is chosen because we believe that the isolation of the repaired site and the presence of vascularized epineurium help decrease excessive scarring around the neurorrhaphy site. A fascicular (funicular) repair was performed, on the other hand, for a partial laceration of a nerve. Immediate repair is preferable in such cases because the fascicular characteristics and orientation are obvious early after injury.

When the injury had led to a limited fascicular avulsion, fascicular repair was preferred to interfascicular epineural repair to avoid the overturning of fascicles at the repair site. When dealing with a nerve laceration with significant contusion, an epiperineural suture was performed, bearing in mind that within 6–8 weeks a secondary suture or a nerve graft would be performed. However, this primary suture has the advantage of maintaining the overall orientation of the nerve with the likelihood of reducing neuroma formation. When the neuroma measured less than 1.5 cm in length, it was possible to perform a secondary suture after its resection with a minimal degree of tension. An interfascicular nerve graft was performed according to the principles of Millesi et al. (1976), using the sural nerve or the medial cutaneous nerve of the arm as a graft. This technique was performed when injury caused a partial or total laceration of a peripheral nerve resulting in a gap which could not be repaired by a tension-free secondary suture. Primary suture of severed nerves was performed at the same time as the repair of other lesions (such as tendons, bones and arteries) according to the principle "the treatment of all the lesions in one stage followed by early mobilisation" (Michon et al. 1977). Secondary nerve grafts were more often performed as a single-goal operation to avoid excessive fibrous reaction around the grafts.

Evaluation of Results

Physical examination and electromyographic studies were performed. The minimum follow-up period in our series was 2 years. Chanson's method (Chanson et al. 1977) was used to evaluate motor and sensory functions and to determine patients' satisfaction (Table 1).

Table 1. Chanson's method of evaluation

Patient's satisfaction	Manual muscle test	Sensory evaluation
G4 No discomfort, no pain	M4 Possible contraction	S4 Weber's test < 5 mm
G3 Slight discomfort with no restraint of normal activity	M3 Possible contraction against low resistance	S3 Weber's test < 10 mm
G2 Discomfort with little restraint of normal activity	M2 Possible contraction against gravity	S2 Weber's test < 20 mm
G1 Permanent pain or discomfort with difficult use of hand	M1 Possible contraction with gravity eliminated	S1 Weber's test < 20 mm or protective sensation
G0 Very severe pain or discomfort with a useless hand	M0 No contraction	S0 Anesthesia or dysesthesia with loss of protective sensation

Results			Evaluation		
			G	M	S
Useful	Excellent	>	4	4	4
	Very good	>	4	3	3
	Good	>	3	2	2
Fair	3 2 2 > fair	>	2	1	1
Bad	2 1 1 > poor	>	1	0	0
	Useless	<	1	0	0

Results

The overall results (all types of nerve repair) are described in Table 2. Useful results (good, very good, excellent) were obtained in 49.3% of the nerve repairs.

Effect of Factors Related to Patient Condition

The sex of the patient did not directly influence the results (Table 3). However, it seemed that the type of nerve injury varied according to the sex of the patient; compound wounds were more often observed in men, usually following accidents at work. Women, on the other hand, more often sustained housework-related, sharp lacerations and therefore had a better prognosis. The age of the patient was a relevant factor (Table 4). Excellent results were observed in patients under 30 years of age, good and fair results in patients aged 30–60, and poor and totally unsatisfactory results in patients over 60 years old. These findings urge caution concerning elderly patients when considering a secondary repair after an acceptable primary repair. Moreover, the age factor should be borne in mind when a series of nerve repairs is considered, for excellent results appear sometimes because sampling is heterogeneous.

The results also appeared to be correlated with the type of the accident sustained. The patients were divided into three groups, depending on the etiology of the accident: industrial, attempted suicide, or an accident linked with housework or a light task. Table 5 show that in patients who had sustained an industrial accident 15.6% of the results were good, 44.4% were fair. In patients who had attempted suicide (sharp wound in female patients), 44.5% of the results were very good or good; and in patients who had sustained housework or odd-job accidents 67.8% were very good, good, or excellent. This group consisted mainly of patients of under 15 years of age, and this may explain the high rate of success. It would appear, therefore, that the type of trauma, the physiological context in which the accident occurred (suicide attempt, for example), and the disability claims filed after accidents at work are important factors to be considered when studying the postoperative results of nerve repair.

Effect of Factors Related to the Type of Nerve Injury

The level of the injury (Table 6) of the median and ulnar nerve definitely affected the prognosis. More proximal lesions were associated with poorer results. We attributed this to the greater distances traveled by regenerating axons after proximal lesions and to the fact that the more proximal lesions were associated with more severe trauma. Thus, useful results (good, very good, excellent) were noted in 53.5% of injuries at the wrist whereas only 36.8% of useful results were observed after repair of a severed nerve at the forearm level.

The type of trauma (Table 7) also modifies the quality of recovery. Results were useful (good, very good, excellent) after repair of a clean sharp laceration

Table 2. Overall results of the series of 150 median and ulnar nerve repairs

Results	Failures			Fair results	Useful results			
	Useless	Poor	Total		Good	Very good	Excellent	Total
Sutures + grafts	7 4.7%	35 23.3%	42 28.0%	34 22.7%	53 35.3%	12 8.0%	9 6.0%	74 49.3%	150 Cases 100%

Table 3. Results of median and ulnar nerve repairs according to sex

Sex	Failures			Fair results	Useful results			
	Useless	Poor	Total		Good	Very good	Excellent	Total
Men	4 (3.9%)	24 (23.5%)	28 (27.4%)	22 (21.6%)	41 (40.2%)	6 (5.9%)	5 (4.9%)	52 (51%)	102 (100%)
Women	3 (6.3%)	11 (22.9%)	14 (29.2%)	12 (25%)	12 (25%)	6 (12.5%)	4 (8.3%)	22 (45.8%)	48 (100%)
									150 Cases

$\chi^2 = 5.114$, df = 5, no statistically significant correlation.

Table 4. Results of median and ulnar nerve repairs according to age

Age	Failures			Fair results	Useful results					
	Useless	Poor	Total		Good	Very good	Excellent	Total		
0–9		1 (8.3%)	1 (8.3%)		4 (33.3%)	2 (16.7%)	5 (41.7%)	11 (91.7%)	12 (100%)	
10–19	2 (5.7%)	4 (11.4%)	6 (17.1%)	6 (17.1%)	18 (51.4%)	3 (8.6%)	2 (5.7%)	23 (65.7%)	35 (100%)	
20–29	1 (1.8%)	6 (11%)	7 (12.8%)	18 (32.7%)	22 (40.0%)	7 (12.7%)	1 (1.8%)	30 (54.5%)	55 (100%)	
30–39	1 (4.7%)	6 (28.6%)	7 (33.3%)	8 (38.1%)	6 (28.6%)	0	0	6 (28.6%)	21 (100%)	
40–49	2 (14.3%)	5 (35.7%)	7 (50%)	4 (28.6%)	2 (14.3%)	0	1 (7.1%)	3 (21.4%)	14 (100%)	
50–59	0	2 (40.0%)	2 (40%)	2 (40.0%)	1 (20.0%)	0	0	1 (20.0%)	5 (100%)	
60–69	1 (16.7%)	4 (66.6%)	5 (83.3%)	1 (16.7%)	0	0	0	0	6 (100%)	
Over 70	0	2 (100%)	2 (100%)	0	0	0	0	0	2 (100%)	
									150 Cases	

$\chi^2 = 72.31$, df $= 35$, $p < 0.001$; Cramer $= 0.31$, significant correlation.

Table 5. Effect of type of accident on results

Type of accident	Failures			Fair results	Useful results			Total
	Useless	Poor	Total		Good	Very good	Excellent	
Accident at work	3 (6.7%)	15 (33.3%)	18 (40.0%)	20 (44.4%)	7 (15.6%)	0	0	7 (15.6%)	45 (100%)
Suicide attempt	2 (11.1%)	3 (16.7%)	5 (27.8%)	5 (27.8%)	5 (27.8%)	3 (16.6%)	0	8 (44.4%)	18 (100%)
Housework and odd jobs accident	2 (2.5%)	17 (19.5%)	19 (22.0%)	9 (10.3%)	41 (47.1%)	9 (10.3%)	9 (10.3%)	59 (67.7%)	87 (100%)
									150 Cases

$\chi^2 = 42.39$, df $= 10$, $p < 0.001$; Cramer $= 0.38$, very significant correlation.

Table 6. Effect of the injury level on the results

Injury level	Failures			Fair results	Useful results			Total
	Useless	Poor	Total		Good	Very good	Excellent	
Wrist	4 (3.6%)	21 (18.7%)	25 (22.3%)	27 (24.1%)	41 (36.6%)	11 (9.8%)	8 (8.1%)	60 (53.5%)	112 (100%)
Forearm	3 (7.9%)	14 (36.8%)	17 (44.7%)	7 (18.5%)	12 (31.6%)	1 (2.6%)	1 (2.6%)	14 (36.8%)	38 (100%)
									150 Cases

$\chi^2 = 7.10$, df $= 2$, $p < 0.025$; Cramer $= 0.217$, significant correlation.

Table 7. Effect of type of trauma on results

Type of trauma	Failures			Fair results	Useful results			Total
	Useless	Poor	Total		Good	Very good	Excellent	
Sharp laceration	1 (0.9%)	24 (22.0%)	25 (22.9%)	27 (24.8%)	41 (37.6%)	10 (9.2%)	6 (5.5%)	57 (52.3%)	109 (100%)
Crushed laceration	5 (16.7%)	7 (23.3%)	12 (40.0%)	6 (20.0%)	7 (23.3%)	2 (6.7%)	3 (10.0%)	12 (40.0%)	30 (100%)
									139 Cases

$\chi^2 = 16.06$, df = 2, $p < 0.001$; Cramer = 0.33, significant correlation.

Table 8. Effect of type of nerve injury on results

Type of nerve injury	Failures			Fair results	Useful results			Total
	Useless	Poor	Total		Good	Very good	Excellent	
Complete lesions	5 (4.5%)	32 (28.6%)	37 (33.1%)	23 (20.5%)	39 (34.8%)	6 (5.4%)	7 (6.2%)	52 (46.4%)	112 (100%)
Partial lesions	0	2 (6.5%)	2 (6.5%)	9 (29.0%)	12 (38.7%)	6 (19.3%)	2 (6.5%)	20 (64.5%)	31 (100%)
									143 Cases

$\chi^2 = 12.9$, df = 5, $p < 0.05$; Cramer = 0.30, significant correlation.

in 52.3% of the cases, whereas only 40% of repaired crushed nerves achieved a useful result. This difference can be explained by the difficulty involved in accurately delineating the area of nerve contusion during an immediate repair. This type of injury may, in fact, require a secondary nerve grafting procedure. The prognosis for functional recovery was very poor when the nerve was avulsed or crushed.

The extent of nerve lesion also plays a role (Table 8). Fascicular suture of a partial nerve laceration performed immediately after injury resulted in a rate of 64.5% excellent, very good, or good results, whereas useful results were observed in only 50% of patients presenting a complete transection of a nerve. This difference was probably related to the fascicular orientation achieved in cases of partial nerve laceration, which was more accurate than in cases of total nerve severance. The capability of the intact fascicles of a partially lacerated nerve to compensate for an insufficiency of axonal regeneration of the repaired fascicles may also play an important role. However, poor results were observed when secondary repair was selected for partial nerve injuries. This probably depends on the fact that, following injury, accurate identification of healthy nerve fascicles becomes increasingly difficult with time.

Effect of the Surgical Technique

Because of the multiple factors related to the patient's condition and to the type of nerve injury it is difficult to report on the actual contribution of each different microsurgical technique utilized in nerve repair. Thus, to estimate the influence on the results of both the microsurgical techniques and the simultaneous repair of one or two main arteries, we selected 119 comparable cases in which the nerves were completely severed at the wrist level or at the forearm level. In this group of patients of 20–49 years of age, there were 38 primary neurorrhaphies performed on an emergency basis, 21 secondary interfascicular nerve grafts, and 8 secondary neurorrhaphies.

It was evident, as shown in Table 9, that better results were achieved by primary repair than by secondary repair, and that the technique of interfascicular grafting was clearly less successful. Statistical analysis confirmed that there is a significant correlation between the method of treatment and the result. Four observations in this group of patients are of particular interest. (a) There were neither excellent nor very good results when the nerve repair was delayed. (b) Primary neurorrhaphy gave 50% useful results. (c) Secondary neurorrhaphy gave 50% fair results, and interfascicular grafting gave a poor result in 57% of cases. (d) The percentage of failures found after nerve repair performed on an emergency basis was higher than the percentage of failures observed after secondary repair; it should be noted, however, that this group of patients was small. This observation may reflect the difficulties involved in assessing the degree of nerve contusion in cases of emergency, as well as the fact that the fresh nerve laceration may pose more technical difficulties as far as instrumentation and future placement are concerned.

Table 9. Effect of type of microsurgical repair on results

Type of repair	Failures			Fair results	Useful results				
	Useless	Poor	Total		Good	Very good	Excellent	Total	
Immediate suture (emergency)	2 (5.3%)	7 (18.4%)	9 (23.7%)	10 (26.3%)	15 (39.5%)	3 (7.9%)	1 (2.6%)	19 (50.0%)	38 (100%)
Secondary suture	0	1 (12.5%)	1 (12.5%)	4 (50.0%)	3 (37.5%)	0	0	3 (37.5%)	8 (100%)
Fascicular graft	2 (9.5%)	10 (47.6%)	12 (57.1%)	4 (19.1%)	5 (23.8%)	0	0	5 (23.8%)	21 (100%)
									67 Cases

$\chi^2 = 10.15$, df $= 4$, $p < 0.05$; Cramer $= 0.275$, significant correlation.

Table 10. Effect of arterial repair on results of nerve repair (immediate suture)

Type of art. lesion	Failures			Fair results	Useful results				
	Useless	Poor	Total		Good	Very good	Excellent	Total	
No arterial injury	0	0	0	3 (23.1%)	7 (53.8%)	2 (15.4%)	1 (7.7%)	10 (76.9%)	13 (100%)
Repaired art. lesion and patent art.	0	2 (14.3%)	2 (14.3%)	3 (21.5%)	8 (57.1%)	1 (7.1%)	0	9 (64.2%)	14 (100%)
No repaired art. lesion or not pat.	2 (18.2%)	5 (45.4%)	7 (63.6%)	4 (36.4%)	0	0	0	0	11 (100%)
									38 Cases

$\chi^2 = 22.25$, df $= 1$, $p < 0.01$; Cramer $= 0.541$, very significant correlation.

Effect of Vascular Repair

Complete lacerations of the median or ulnar nerve were often complicated by injuries of the radial artery and/or the ulnar artery. The effect of the arterial repair on the results of nerve repair is shown in Table 10. There was a statistically significant correlation between arterial repair and functional return following nerve repair. In fact, in isolated nerve lacerations without arterial lesions, useful results (good, very good, excellent) were observed in 76.9% of cases. In cases of arterial injury it was noted that where the artery was repaired and remained patent, the rate of useful results was 64.2%, but where the artery was not repaired or did not remain patent, no useful results were obtained.

Discussion

From this study, which considers the surgical treatment of 150 median and ulnar nerve injuries and uses a rigorous method of evaluation, clear conclusions can be drawn concerning the role of factors related to the patient's condition, the type of nerve trauma sustained, and the microsurgical techniques used in nerve repair. Our findings confirm that good results in children and poor results in the elderly are likely. The type of accident causing the nerve injury alters the prognosis. Patients who sustained accidents at work had the more complex type of trauma. It is interesting that of these patients who underwent a primary repair, 46% were back at work by the 6th postoperative month. When reconstruction by nerve grafting was performed, only 30% returned to work within 6 months. Furthermore, after a direct nerve suture, 70% of patients returned to their previous jobs, whereas only 59% of the patients treated with a nerve graft did so.

Finally, it is important to bear in mind that a simple tendon opponensplasty can transform a fair result into a good or a very good one. In Fig. 1 seven such cases are reported. It may of course be pointed out that the secondary nerve grafts were performed to repair more complex nerve injuries. However, in our 10 years of clinical experience, we have favored primary nerve repair, when feasible. This study highlights the benefit of arterial repair with regard to the quality of neurologic recovery after nerve suture. We have systematically repaired a significant arterial lesion on an emergency basis, and the conclusions of this study confirm that this is a well-founded principle.

The frequent association between arterial injuries and nerve lacerations should make the surgeon consider this type of lesion a microsurgical emergency. It is on such an emergency basis that the surgeon, using microsurgical techniques, should repair sharp laceration of nerves. Moreover, this notion of emergency treatment is also pertinent for crush injuries because simultaneous vascular repair may be an essential factor for the maintenance of tissue viability. Even if vascular repair is not required for tissue viability, it is likely to improve the quality of the soft-tissue bed for nerve grafting of secondary nerve suture following neuroma resection.

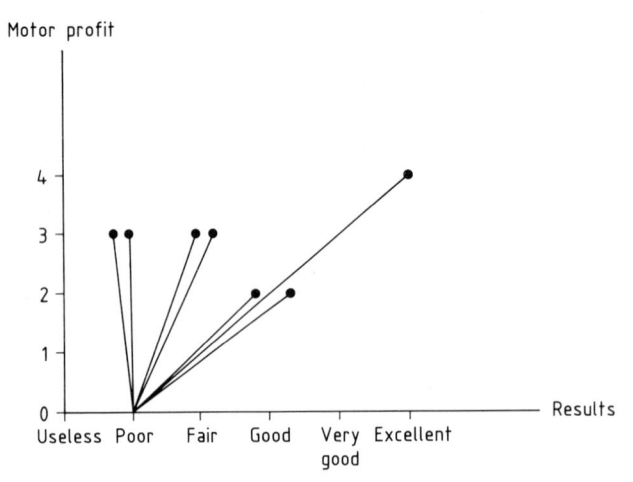

Fig. 1. Comparison of results in nerve repair surgery between 1976 and 1984

While performing an immediate nerve repair under magnification, the epineurial vessels and the surrounding tissues help in the overall nerve orientation. This difficult process is governed by chance after resection of a neuroma and secondary repair. The data on the advantages of primary repair of sharp injuries of peripheral nerves will hopefully modify the surgeon's approach to this problem and may support the concept that the results following primary nerve repair are superior to those following secondary nerve repair.

Figure 2 clearly demonstrates that results of nerve grafts and secondary nerve repair have improved little since 1977 (Chanson et al.). The only improvement to be noticed in the quality of function occurred when nerve repair was carried out on an emergency basis. To accomplish this, surgical teams trained in microsurgery are required. Every surgeon trained in microsurgical techniques agrees that primary nerve repair is challenging and perhaps even more difficult than microvascular anastomosis. The nerve ends of a fresh laceration are very gelatinous and have ill-defined fascicular margins. This makes accurate end-to-end fascicular coaptation technically difficult. The surgeon is unable to distinguish morphologically between the different fibers (sensory, motor, and sympathetic) in a mixed nerve and we are of the opinion that over the past decade, the only real progress made in the field of peripheral nerve repair can be attributed to microsurgical techniques used on an emergency basis and the systematic repair of associated vessel injuries. It is evident that microscopes, microsurgical instruments, sutures and microneedles have been improved upon. The surgical teams have likewise perfected their skill in repairing vessels of very small diameter, as well as in epiperineural neurorrhaphy and interfascicular nerve grafting.

Of course, surgery does not suffice in the treatment of peripheral nerve injuries. Postoperative splints must be used to avoid or to correct claw-hand

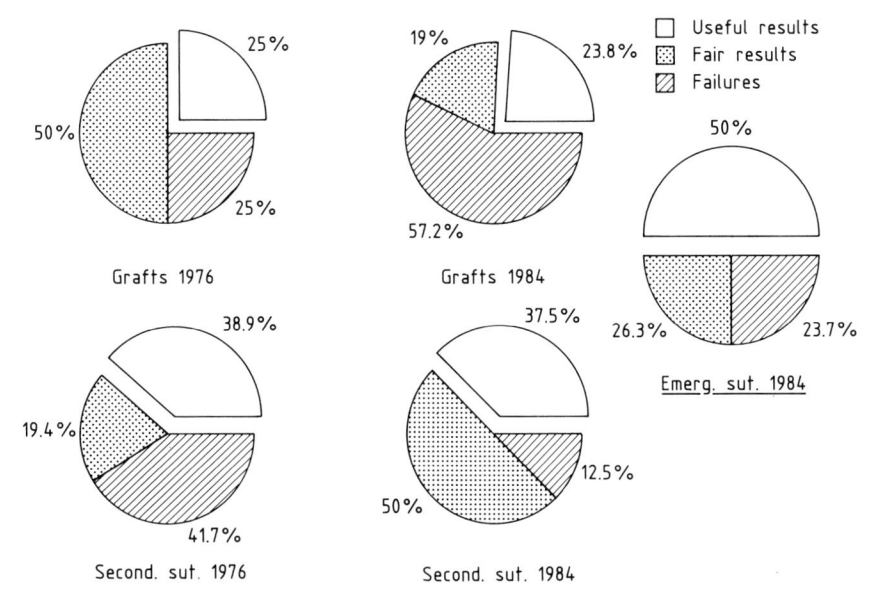

Fig. 2. Effect of opponensplasty on motor function

deformities. Recovery of sensation must be monitored and reeducated and a well-oriented physiotherapy carried out if maximal qualitative improvement in functional results is to be attained (Wynn Parry 1984).

Conclusion

A partial or complete sharp laceration of a peripheral nerve (median and ulnar nerves) should be repaired on an emergency basis using microsurgical techniques.

The frequent association between arterial injuries and nerve lacerations may call for repair as an emergency microsurgical procedure. Primary repair of a sharply severed nerve using microsurgical techniques gives better results than secondary repair either by suturing or by interfascicular nerve grafts.

References

Amend P (1982) Réparation microchirurgicale des nerfs périphériques. A propos des 100 cas de plaies du nerf médian et du nerf cubital revus après un délai supérieur à 2 ans 1/2. Thèse de Médicine (Nancy)

Chanson J, Michon J, Merle M, Delagoutte P (1977) Etude des résultats de la réparation de 85 nerfs dont 49 gros nerfs. Rev Chir Orthop 63:153–160

Merle M, Amend P, Foucher G, Michon J (1984) Plaidoyer pour la réparation primaire microchirurgicale des lésions des nerfs périphériques. Etude comparative de 150 lésions du nerf médian et du nerf cubital avec un recul supérieur à deux ans. Chirurgie 110:761–771

Merle M, Foucher G, Van Genechten F, Michon J (1984) Repair of peripheral nerve injuries in emergency. Bulletin of the hospital for joints diseases orthopaedic institute 44(2):338–346

Michon J (1964) Le moment optimum de la suture nerveuse dans les plaies du membre supérieur. Rev Chir Orthop 50:205–212

Michon J, Möberg E (1979) Les lésions traumatiques des nerfs périphériques. Monographie du GEM, 2ème éd. Expansion Scientifique, Paris

Michon J, Merle M, Foucher G (1977) Traumatismes complexes de la main. Traitement tout en un temps avec mobilisation précoce. Chirurgie 103:956–964

Millesi H, Meissl G, Berger A (1976) Further experience with inter-fascicular grafting of the median, ulnar and radial nerves. J Bone Joint Surg 58(A):209

Millesi M, Gangelberger J, Berger A (1967) Erfahrungen mit der Mikrochirurgie peripherer Nerven. Chir Plast Reconstr 3:47–55

Samii M, Scheinpflug W (1974) Clinical electromyographic and quantitative histological investigations following nerve transplant. An experimental study. Acta Neurochirurgica 30:1–29

Smith JW (1964) Microsurgery of peripheral nerves. Plast Reconstr Surg 33:317–329

Wynn Parry CB (1984) Symposium on Sensation. J Hand Surg 1:4–6

Brachial Plexus Lesions

Operative Experience with Tumors of the Brachial Plexus*

D. G. KLINE, M. LUSK, and C. GARCIA, New Orleans/USA

During a 20-year period at Louisiana State University Medical Center (LSUMC), 77 patients with tumors arising from or compressing the brachial plexus were seen. Seventy-four of these patients had operations for removal of 75 plexus tumors. These 75 lesions involving the plexus form the basis for this report, which includes 22 cases in addition to the 57 lesions reported by the same authors in October 1987 [7]. This series is the largest reported in the literature to date concerning tumors of neural sheath origin involving plexus [1, 2, 3, 6, 8, 9]. Other reports also indicated that our experience with various other tumors involving plexus is also very large [4, 5]. The case material was collected between January 1968 and March 1987. Each patient has had at least 6 months of follow-up; the average follow-up was a little over 3 years.

Tumors of Neural Sheath Origin

Tumors of neural sheath origin were by far the largest category in our experience; the various forms are listed in Table 1. We have encountered 32 neurofibromas in patients either with or without von Recklinghausen's disease (VRD), 2 meningiomas, 11 schwannomas, and 7 tumors of sheath origin which were malignant.

Neurofibromas

The largest subset of plexus tumors was that of neurofibromas (Figs. 1, 2). These tumors can be divided into two categories, those associated VRD and those not. Patients with neurofibromas of the plexus associated with VRD had café-au-lait spots, often but not always subcutaneous tumors, and usually a history of tumors elsewhere. Four of these patients had laminectomies as well as tumor excision from plexus, in three cases to remove the spinal portion of the same neurofibroma as involved plexus but in another instance to resect meningioma at the midthoracic level. In six cases only an incomplete removal

---

* From Departments of Neurosurgery and Neurology/Neuropathology, LSUMC 1542 Tulane Avenue, New Orleans LA 70112, and Charity and Ochsner Hospitals of New Orleans, USA.

Table 1. Tumors of brachial plexus: LSUMC series 1968–1987

Neural sheath origin	
Neurofibromas[a]	
With VRD	11
Without VRD	19
Lengthy solitary plexiform	2
Schwannomas[b]	
With VRD	0
Without VRD	11
Meningiomas	2
Malignant sheat tumors	
Malignant schwannoma with VRD	3
Malignant schwannoma without VRD	2
Lengthy solitary plexiform	1
Fibrosarcoma	1
Non-neural sheath origin	
Benign tumors	
Desmoid	2
Myoblastoma	2
Lymphangioma	2
Lipoma	3
Myositis ossificans	1
Branchial cleft cyst	1
Malignant secondary tumors	
Breast cancer	5
Lung extension (Pancoast)	4
Melanoma	2
Malignant thymoma	1
Total	75

[a] Prior attempt at removal in 11 (resultant deficit in 6); prior biopsy in 12 (resultant deficit in 5).
[b] Prior attempt at removal in 4 (resultant deficit in 3); prior biopsy in 4 (resultant deficit in 1).

of the plexus tumor could be achieved, and in two of these function was considerably worse postoperatively than preoperatively. More complete removal was gained in five cases, and functional loss increased in only one of these. Despite the presence of VRD, these latter patients had more of a solitary and less of a plexiform or "up and down" lesion. These tumors could be resected by tracing proximal and distal fascicles into and around the tumor sacrificing those without a nerve action potential (NAP) across the lesion and sparing those with NAP. Thus, these more solitary lesions associated with VRD could be managed surgically just as the solitary neurofibromas unassociated with VRD. Where elements as well as tumor had to be resected because of severe pain and progressive deficit, repair was seldom possible because of the extensive "up and down" nature of the lesion(s). This was especially so in the two cases of regionalized VRD in which neurofibroma(s)

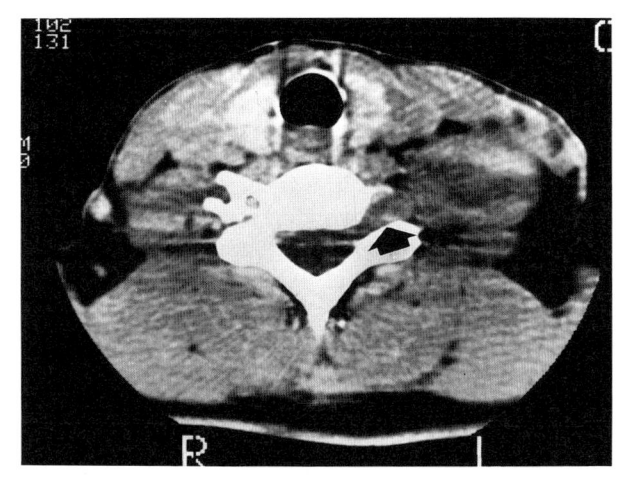

Fig. 1. CAT scan of a relatively large neurofibroma intrinsic to C 7 and middle trunk. *Arrow*, involvement of interforaminal portion of the root. Tumor was removed and function spared

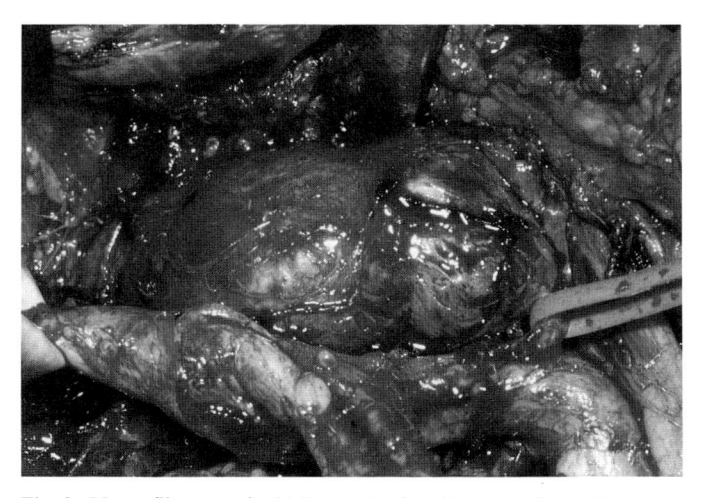

Fig. 2. Neurofibroma of middle trunk after dissection free of fascicle and before sacrifice of nonfunctional fascicle

involved plexus in one limb without neurofibromas or evidence of VRD elsewhere. In one instance, a patient with extensive regionalized VRD who had subtotal removal by laminectomy as well as plexus resection underwent malignant change in her residual tumor. Response to irradiation has been partial. Nonetheless her course, to date, has extended for 8 years.

In the 19 patients with solitary neurofibromas not associated with VRD complete resection without further significant deficit could be gained in 11 instances. This was despite the fact that many of these lesions were quite large, and most had been either biopsied or operated on beforehand. Wide exposure of the lesion and fascicular dissection under magnification both distal and, where possible, proximal to the lesion was of help. Fascicles were traced into and usually around the bulk of the lesion. Stimulation of those entering and recording from those leaving the lesion usually gave a flat trace (no NAP). This permitted proximal as well as distal section of these fascicles and a total tumor removal. The posterior subscapular approach was definitely of help in exposing proximal tumors, especially those involving the C7, C8, and T1 roots, and was used in five neurofibroma cases. There have been no known recurrences in this group of patients as yet, but average follow-up is only 40 months.

Only nine patients with neurofibromas either with or without VRD had not had a prior operation. Pain was still a complaint in four of these, but preoperative deficit, if any, was minimal. By comparison, 11 patients had had prior attempts at removal of the tumor. Eight of these patients presented with severe deficits requiring graft repair, and six also had severe pain prior to our operation. Of those patients biopsied before definitive operation (12 instances), nine presented to us with deficit. In five cases, deficit had not been present prior to biopsy, and four of these patients had complete loss in the distribution of one or more elements and requried graft repair.

Of great interest is that patients with solitary neurofibromas not associated with VRD were twice as likely to have their tumor on the right side than the left side and were also three times as likely to be women. These characteristics were not present in the patients with neurofibromas that were associated with VRD.

Schwannomas

Eleven patients with schwannomas were operated upon. None of these cases was associated with VRD. This was a less complicated group than that of neurofibromas. Resection was easier since fascicles were displaced to the circumference of the tumor and seldom intrinsically involved (Fig. 3). Nonetheless, several of these lesions were quite large and for this reason were technically difficult although not impossible to remove. Despite this, in four instances, prior partial removal had led to deficit in three and severe pain in two. Repair of lost element(s) and resection of residual tumor was necessary in these cases. Surgical approach included dissecting away adjacent uninvolved elements and then opening the capsule between the fascicles encompassing the schwannoma. The fascicles were gradually dissected away so that the tumor could be enucleated. The capsule was then teased away from the fascicles in order to complete the procedure. The posterior subscapular approach was used in three cases in which tumor involved proximal, lower elements. There was no propensity to right-side involvement nor preponderance among women as had been seen in solitary neurofibromas not associated with VRD.

Meningiomas

It was surprising that two meningiomas were found involving plexus since these lesions are almost invariably more centrally located. One of these lesions was

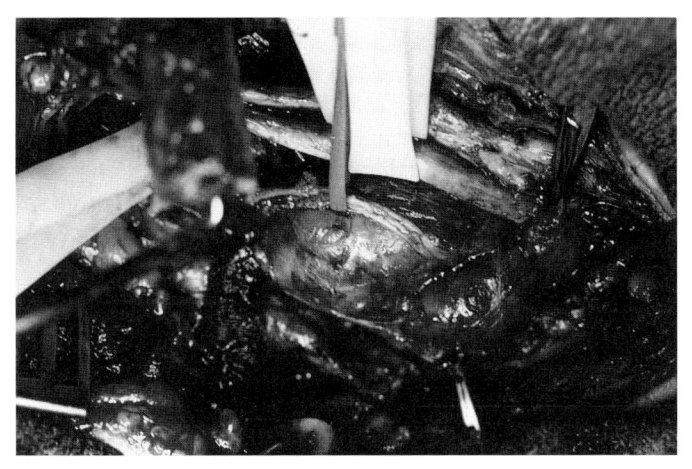

Fig. 3. Schwannoma of supraclavicular plexus element extending below clavicle and requiring its section. One of the peripherally displaced elements has been dissected free and is partially suspended by the narrow rubber band

massive and very aggressive, having been operated on at four prior occasions. It required an extensive operation with resection of C7 to middle trunk and a portion of C6 and upper trunk to control pain (Fig. 4). Fortunately, graft repair of these elements has led to partial recovery, but follow-up is only a little more than 1 year.

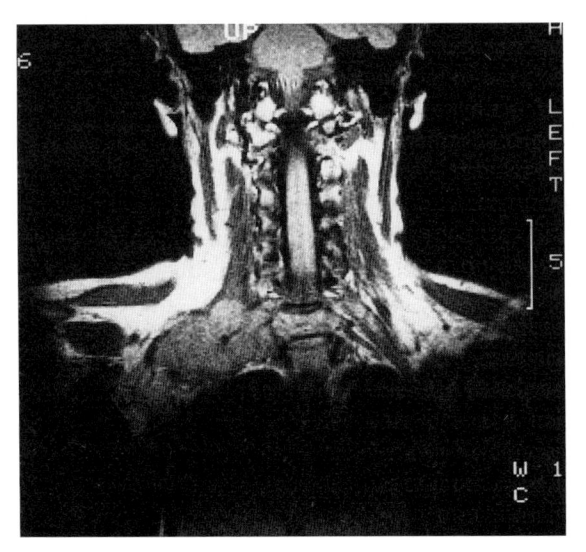

Fig. 4. Magnetic resonance scan showing large tumor in right supraclavicular, axillary, and anterior mediastinal space. Resection required removal of C7 to middle trunk and a portion of the upper trunk with subsequent graft repair. Lesion proved to be a benign but very aggressive meningioma

Malignant Neural Sheath Tumors

This difficult to manage group of patients included three neurogenic sarcomas or malignant schwannomas associated with VRD and two without VRD. An additional patient had a lengthy plexiform but solitary neurofibroma not associated with VRD which became malignant; a further patient had a fibrosarcoma. Tumors at an infraclavicular level initially had a local resection. After histologic confirmation forequarter amputation was offered. Even though there was some delay on the patient's part in two cases, all four patients with neurogenic sarcoma at an infraclavicular level subsequently had a proximal amputation. One died 1 year postoperatively while the others have now survived 1, 8, and 12 years postoperation. The two patients with supraclavicular neurogenic sarcomas have had as thorough removals as possible (one by an anterior and one by a posterior approach) followed by irradiation. Both patients are still alive at 2 and at 1.5 years postoperation. The patient with the supraclavicular fibrosarcoma had two operations, one by a posterior approach and one followed by irradiation anteriorly and is known to have survived with only winging of the scapula for 5 years but has subsequently been lost to follow-up.

Tumors of Non-Neural Sheath Origin

Benign Tumors

This category contained 11 tumors which were operated on (see Table 1). Two of these benign tumor were desmoids felt to arise from muscle and fascial structures adjacent to plexus but involving plexus. Both were extensive lesions, – one supraclavicular and one infraclavicular. Their removal required lengthy dissection, and the supraclavicular lesion has already recurred and required reresection at 2 years postoperatively. The other patient had had a chest wall desmoid resected in 1984, and recurrence with involvement of plexus at the cord level required reresection in 1986. Three patients had lipomas and scar from prior biopsy or subtotal removal. Both had secondary plexus involvement. In another case, myositis ossificans encased the distal subclavian artery as well as plexus cords and cord to nerve level. Operation for this lesion was lengthy and required several repairs of the axillary artery during the dissection. Because of its adhesive and somewhat invasive nature, removal of the myoblastoma from upper supraclavicular plexus elements and accessory nerve was also tedious but was accomplished without deficit. Other less complicated operations were required for a lymphangioma and a branchial cleft cyst involving plexus.

Malignant Secondary Tumors

We encountered five cases with breast carcinoma compressing plexus usually at the axillary level, four plexus cases due to pulmonary or Pancoast's tumor at a supraclavicular level, two melanomas metastatic to plexus, and one malignant thymoma arising at a mediastinal level and involving plexus secondarily. Four of the breast carcinoma patients were surgically approached anteriorly with an infraclavicular and axillary approach. The tumor, although adherent to plexus, could be dissected free from the elements. Pain but not deficit was helped. In one case, the deficit progressed 6 months later despite the decompression. One breast carcinoma patient had supraclavicular involvement by tumor as well as irradiation change and was only temporarily helped by a posterior subscapular approach to the plexus with as thorough a clean-up of the area as possible. Survival times following plexus decompressions for breast carcinoma were 3.5 years, 2.5 years, and 1 year. One patient died 10 months after decompression from pulmonary spread.

The four patients with Pancoast's tumor experienced significant amelioration of pain by a posterior subscapular approach. After resection of the first rib, plexus (usually C8-T1, and lower trunk) was cleaned of tumor and secondary scar. One of these patients also had a high thoracic laminectomy for epidural carcinoma and then a high open cervical cordotomy. Survival times are 2.5, 3.5, 4, and 1.5 years in these patients. The malignant thymoma has done well in terms of survival (4.5 years) but developed a more complete plexus palsy 3 years after plexus decompression. This was felt to be secondary to irradiation fibrosis.

The two melanomas involving plexus were of interest because both were metastatic. An instance is offered by the following case report. A 36-year-old right-handed athletic instructor and active amateur athlete had a history of melanomas at multiple sites which had been resected over a 15-year period. Despite this he remained in splendid physical condition. He was referred with a 6-month history of paresthesias in the right forearm and hand accompanied by radicular pain. Both CAT scan and MRI showed a massive right supra- and infraclavicular mass. At operation, melanoma was investing subclavian vessels, supraclavicular and infraclavicular plexus and had even extended into superior mediastinum. Nonetheless, it could be readily dissected from vessels and plexus. A gross total but certainly not microscopic resection was possible. Postoperatively, the patient was free of pain and had no deficit. Unfortunately, because of previous radiotherapy for a lower chest wall lesion, he was a candidate only for chemotherapy. It remains to be seen whether the tumor will recur at this site.

Summary

Our 20-year operative experience with 75 tumors in 74 patients is reviewed. Included were 52 tumors of neural sheath origin, of which seven were malignant. Also included were 11 benign tumors and 12 malignancies arising elsewhere and secondarily involving plexus. Surgical results were surprisingly good.

Many solitary neurofibromas could be completely resected without producing deficit especially if there had not been a prior attempt at removal. Even some of the neurofibromas in VRD patients could be removed without additional deficit. Nonetheless, there were exceptions, and in these repair was not always possible because of proximal root involvement and lengthy plexiform lesions. Where prior partial removal or biopsy had led to serious deficit, repair usually by grafts as well as removal of residual tumor was necessary. Schwannomas were readily managed, but in several cases because of prior operative procedures, repairs were necessary. The posterior approach was useful for both neurofibromas and schwannomas involving proximal C 7, C 8, and T 1 roots and their trunks. Intraoperative NAP studies were also of value in selecting fascicles for resection especially in the neurofibromas. This often permitted total tumor removal. Malignancies of neural sheath origin were most difficult to manage. Forequarter amputation was carried out where tumor was infraclavicular. Resection of tumor without sacrifice of plexus elements followed by irradiation was used for the supraclavicular malignancies. Survival rates to date have been good but larger follow-up is necessary.

A variety of benign tumors of non-neural sheath origin involved plexus. Two of these cases were meningiomas involving supraclavicular plexus. One had no evidence at all of a central nervous system component. Tumors spreading or metastatic to plexus included five breast carcinomas, four Pancoast's tumors, two melanomas, and one malignant thymoma. Some amelioration of pain was afforded by operation, but deficit was seldom reversed, and subsequent mortality in the breast and Pancoast's tumor categories remains high.

References

1. Dart L, MacCarty C, Love J et al. (1970) Neoplasms of the brachial plexus. Minn Med 53:959–964
2. Fisher R, Tate H (1970) Isolated neurilemmomas of the brachial plexus. J Neurosurg 32:463–467
3. Goodwin JT (1952) Encapsulated neurilemmoma of the brachial plexus. Report of 11 cases. Cancer 5:708–720
4. Hudson A, Gentilli F, Kline D (1987) Peripheral nerve tumors. In: Schmidek H, Sweet W (eds) Operative neurosurgical techniques, 2nd ed. Grune & Strattoh, Orlando
5. Kori S, Foley K, Posner J (1981) Brachial plexus lesions in patients with cancer: 100 cases. Neurology 31:45–50
6. Kragh L, Soule E, Masson J (1960) Benign and malignant neurolemmomas of the head and neck. Surg Gynecol Obstet 11:211–218
7. Lusk M, Kline D, Garcia C (1987) Tumors of the brachial plexus. Neurosurgery 21(4):439–453
8. Noterman J, Dittaens J, Nubourgh Y, Colle H (1982) Les tumeurs du plexus brachial. Neurochirurgie 28(2):139–141
9. Whitaker W, Droulias C (1976) Benign encapsulated neurolemmomas. A report of 76 cases (4 of brachial plexus). Am Surg 42:675–678

Neurotization of the Avulsed Brachial Plexus

G. Brunelli, L. Monini, and F. Brunelli, Brescia/Italy

Avulsion of the motor and sensory roots of the brachial plexus is a very severe lesion which cannot be repaired by means of classical techniques (Jaeger and Whiteley 1953; Mendelsohn et al. 1957; Sunderland 1978). As it is impossible to reimplant the avulsed roots in the spinal cord, neurotization by means of foreign nerves is the only operation which can supply some innervation to the muscles and the skin depending on the brachial plexus (Alnot 1977; Alnot et al. 1977; Gilbert et al. 1980; Millesi 1977).

The intercostal nerves have been used, but results have not been satisfactory even with the most sophisticated techniques (such as taking the nerves posteriorly to have a greater number of fibers, using the lower nerves, utilizing the pedicled ulnar nerve as graft). This is due to several reasons (Seddon 1963; Tsuyama et al. 1968; Kotami et al. 1971; Narakas 1972; Millesi 1973; Allende and Mana 1977; Allieu 1977; Sedel 1977; Celli and Bonola 1975):

(a) They bring a small number of fibers (about 4000 for four nerves). (b) The fibers of intercostal nerves are mixed (motor and sensory) so that mismatching is a real danger which can cause a loss of fibers of up to 50%. (c) The function of the motor fibers is semiautomatic and can supply a movement only together with breathing. (d) As the impulse of the intercostal nerves is simultaneous, the intercostal nerves can be used for only one muscle; if two muscles are innervated by different intercostal nerves, they co-contract with severe impairment of the function in both. (e) The corticalization of the new movement is difficult. In addition to the intercostal nerves, the accessory nerve has also been used; results here have been good, if used to reinnervate only one function.

Due to these limitations we have considered the possibility of using the anterior nerves of the third cervical ansa, namely the motor nerves for the sternocleidomastoid, trapezium, levator scapulae, rhomboid muscles and the sensory nerves for the supraclavicular and supraacromialis skin. This surgical technique innervates part of the brachial plexus by using these anterior nerves in combination with the accessory nerve.

We have checked on cadavers and in vivo (by means of electrical stimulation during the operation) the existence and characteristics of these nerves and have counted their fibers. On average these four motor nerves can supply 4000 motor fibers and the sensory nerves some 2500 sensory fibers. From the theoretical point of view, as well as from the practical results, there are several advantages to using the anterior nerve of the third cervical ansa. These include the following: (a) the greater quantity of fibers; (b) the fact that the fibers of these nerves are either pure motor or pure sensory fibers; (c) the motor nerves are voluntary nerves; (d) the fact that each nerve receives autonomous impulses without danger of co-contraction; (e) the facility of cortical adaptation; and (f) the possibility for the sensory nerves to be transferred to the receiving structures without grafts.

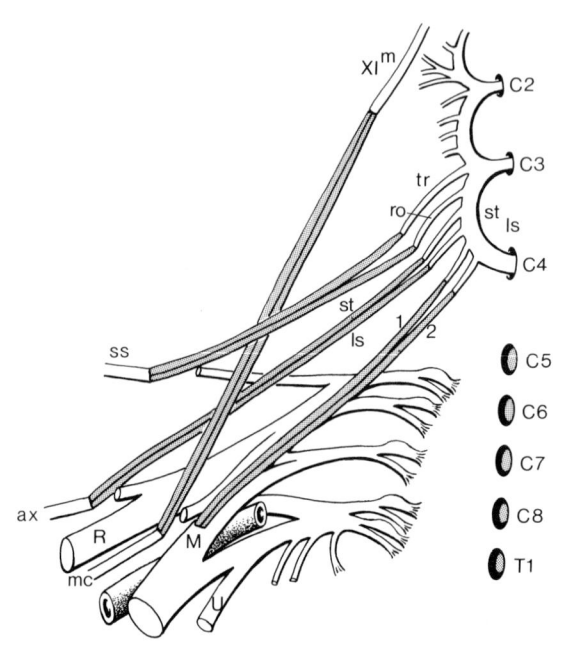

Fig. 1. Scheme of the neurotization of part of the totally avulsed brachial plexus by means of grafts from the XI cranial nerve and the anterior nerves of the third ansa of the cervical plexus. *XI*, Accessory nerve; *tr*, nerve for the trapezius muscle; *ro*, nerve for the rhomboid muscle; *st*, nerve for the sternocleidomastoid muscle; *ls*, nerve for the levator scapulae muscle; *1, 2*, grafts from supraacromialis and supraclavicular nerves to the lateral origins of the median nerve

By using also the accessory nerves (Allieu et al. 1982; Kotami et al. 1971; Brunelli 1979, 1980; Sedel 1982; Narakas 1982) we have at our disposal 2000 more fibers. When neurotizing a brachial plexus which contains more than 120 000 myelinated fibers, the 6000 motor fibers and the 2500 sensory fibers that we have at our disposal must be used very carefully without dispersion. These fibers must therefore be led only onto terminal branches (Figs. 1, 2). Loading them onto trunks or cords leads to dispersion and loss of the fibers.

In a total palsy, limited aims can be pursued: moderate abduction of the arm, stabilization of the shoulder by means of extrarotator muscle reinnervation, flexion of the elbow, and some sensation in the finger. This can be obtained by neurotizing the suprascapularis, the axillary, the musculocutaneous, and median nerves.

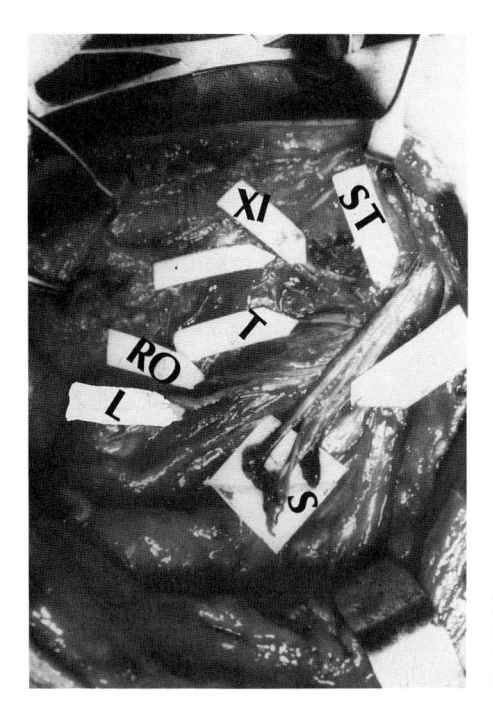

Fig. 2. Preparation of the donor nerves. Sensory nerves: *RO*, rhomboid nerve; *T*, trapezius nerve; *ST*, sternocleid omastoideous nerve; *L*, levator scapulae nerve

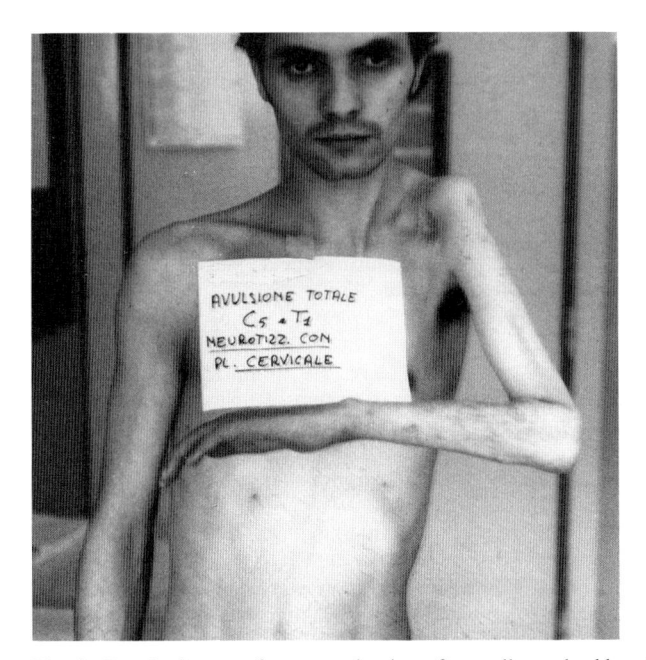

Fig. 3. Results 2 years after neurotization of a totally avulsed brachial plexus by means of the personal technique

After several trials our preferred scheme is now to graft the accessory nerve onto the musculocutaneous, the nerves to the rhomboid and levator scapular muscles onto the suprascapularis nerve, the nerve for the trapezius and sternocleidomastoid muscles onto the axillary nerve, and all the sensory nerves onto the external contingent of the median nerve (Fig. 1).

We have operated on 36 cases. The first 10 cases had poor results because we grafted the motor nerves onto trunks or cords, however the last 26 operations have achieved their goal. If the lower plexus is spared, the results are good, while if the palsy is total, a subsequent arthrodesis of the wrist can supply an elementary, firm, slightly sensory tool. This is a substantial achievement for young men starting from a total palsy (Fig. 3).

References

Allende BT, Mana YE (1977) Trasferencia de nervios intercostales a plexo braquial. Rev ortoped Traumatol Latino-Am 16:79–82

Allieu Y (1977) Exploration et traitement des lésions nerveuses dans les paralysies traumatiques par élongation du plexus brachial chez l'adulte. Rev Chir Orthop 63:89–107

Allieu Y, Privat JM, Bonnel F (1982) Les neurotisations par le nerf spinal (nerf accesorius) dans les avulsions radiculaires du plexus brachial. Neurochirurgie 28:115–120

Alnot JY (1977) Etude clinique et paraclinique plus evaluation spontanée des paralysies du plexus brachial. Rev Chir Orthop 63:58–64

Alnot JY, Mansat M, Huten B, Bonnel F, Narakas A, Cadre N, Sedel L et al. (1977) Symposium sur la paralysie traumatique de plexus brachial chez l'adulte. Rev Chir Orthop 63(1):19–126

Brunelli G (1979) In: Microsurgery. Edited and published by Pelizza. Brescia, Italy.

Brunelli G (1980) Neurotization of avulsed roots of the brachial plexus by means of anterior nerves of the cervical plexus. Int J Microsurg 2 (1):55–58

Celli L, Bonola A (1975) Intercostal nerve transplant in brachial plexus lesions with tearing of the nerve root. Surgical technique. Proceedings of the 13th Congress of the Société Internationale de Chirurgie Orthopédique et Traumatologique. Copenhagen, July 6–11

Gilbert A, Khouri N, Carlioz H (1980) Exploration chirurgicale du plexus brachial dans la paralysies obstétricale. Rev Chir Orthop 66(1):33–42

Jaeger R, Whiteley WH (1953) Avulsion of the brachial plexus. J Am Med Assoc 153:633–635

Kotami PT, Toyoshima Y, Matsuda H, Suzuki T, Ishikazi Y, Iwani H, Yamano K et al. (1971) The postoperative results of nerve transfer of the brachial plexus injury with root avulsion. Proceedings of the 14th Annual Meeting of the Japanese Society for Surgery of the Hand, Osaka

Mendelsohn RA, Weiner JH, Keegan JM (1957) Myelographic demonstration of brachial plexus root avulsion. Arch Surg (Chicago) 75:102–107

Millesi H (1973) Résultats tardifs de la greffe nerveuse interfasciculaire. Chirurgie réparatrice des lésions du plexus brachial. Rev Méd Suisse Romande 93:7, 511–519

Millesi H (1977) Surgical management of brachial plexus injuries. J Hand Surgery 2, 367–378

Narakas A (1972) Plexo Brachial. Terapeutica quirurgica directa. Tecnica. Indication operatoria. Resultados. Rev Orthop traumat 16:855–921

Narakas A (1982) Les neurotisations ou transferts nerveux dans les lesions du plexus brachial. Ann Chir Main 1:101–118

Seddon H (1963) Nerve grafting. J Bone Joint Surgery 45(B):447–461
Sedel L (1977) Traitement palliatif d'une serie de 103 paralysies par élongation du plexus brachial. Rev Chir Orthop 63(7):651–677
Sedel L (1982) The results of surgical repair of brachial plexus injuries. J Bone Joint Surg 64:54–66
Sunderland S (1978) Brachial plexus lesions due to compression, stretch and penetrating injuries. In: Nerve and Nerve Lesions. Churchill Livingstone, London
Tsuyama N, Sakaguchi RT, Hara T, Kindo S, Kaminuma M, Ljichi M, Ryn D (1968) Reconstructive surgery in brachial plexus injuries. Proceedings of the 11th Annual Meeting of the Japanese Society for Surgery of the Hand, Hiroshima 39–40

Special Considerations Regarding the Treatment of Brachial Plexus Lesions

M. SAMII, Hannover/FRG

Introduction

Brachial plexus lesions constitute, due to the anatomical characteristics, the most serious lesions affecting the peripheral nervous system. The reason for this lies not only in the complicated anatomical relationships at the time of surgery, but, even more, in the metabolic environment of the damaged nerves. The region of damage is localized in the proximity of the cell body, and as a result of retrograde degeneration, a considerable amount of neurons can be lost which no longer regenerate. In comparison with lesions of peripheral nerves, such as the median nerve at the wrist, the neurons in the plexus have considerably more difficult tasks to perform in the case of lesions or interruptions. The cell body must render a higher metabolic activity. While in the case of a median nerve lesion at the wrist approximately 10% of the intracellular substance of the altered neuron must be rebuilt, more than 50% of the intracellular substance is lost in brachial plexus continuity lesions (Fig. 1).

Many therapeutic failures independent of optimally performed surgical procedures can be explained by the fact that the cell bodies are unable to compensate the demands of regeneration or only to a limited extent thus remaining insufficient for a satisfactory function. The results are furthermore influenced by the fact that due to the long nerve regeneration time the muscles atrophy and finally undergo fibrotic changes, this is most prominent in the small muscles of the hand. Therefore, an early diagnosis and a correct operative indication is of fundamental relevance (Samii 1975, 1980).

Unfortunately, the majority of these lesions occur during polytraumas. In our material, about 50% of all patients also had head injuries with loss of consciousness, so that in many of these cases the primary diagnosis of a plexus lesion was overlooked or was difficult to make in the initial patient evaluation.

Etiology

With 85%, traffic accidents constitute the most frequent cause of brachial plexus lesions. Motor-cyclists are the most endangered, representing more than 50% of the total of brachial plexus lesions. The average age of the patients is between 16 and 25 years. Other causes are industrial accidents, for example, when the hand is caught in the gears of a machine and traction is exerted on the

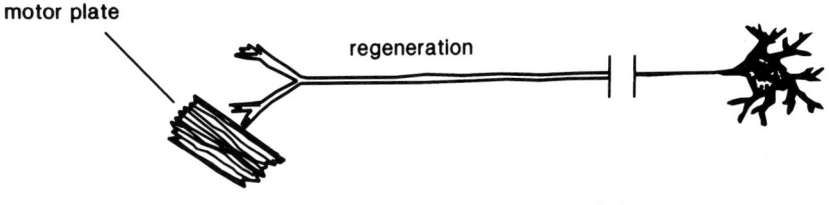

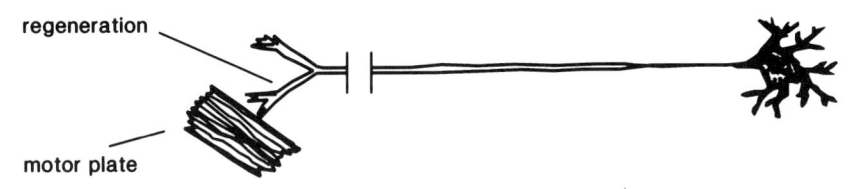

Fig. 1. Schematic representation of the regeneration segment of a damaged neuron in a brachial plexus lesion and, as comparison, a more peripheral lesion affecting the median nerve at the wrist

extremity. Firearm lesions were often seen during the world wars, and still constitute the leading etiological factor in patients coming from the different conflict areas around the globe. Blunt trauma as well as iatrogenic lesions occur less often.

Basically, open and closed plexus lesions should be differentiated. Open lesions result, for example, from gunshot wounds or penetration by sharp objects. Due to their usually clear localization after diagnosis and the ability to quantify exactly the impairment of function, they should be primarily treated; in our experience the results are good.

The closed plexus trauma occurs due to blunt injuries or compression and/or traction lesions. In 80% of this type of plexus lesions, we find associated osseous damage of the shoulder, chest, arm and/or cervical vertebrae.

Anatomy

For the differential diagnosis of supra- and infraclavicular plexus lesions the knowledge of the anatomical characteristics is extremely important.

The brachial plexus is formed of five cervical nerves and one thoracic nerve. Each of these nerves contain motor and sensory as well as sympathetic fibers. After leaving the spinal canal through the intervertebral foramen, the spinal nerves divide into anterior branches constituting the brachial plexus and posterior branches for the innervation of the posterior neck muscles and dorsal cutaneous region. Lesions proximal to this division, for example in cases of nerve or root avulsion, will cause complex deficits involving both types or modalities of innervation.

The ventral branches of the spinal nerves form three primary trunks: The superior trunk originates from C5 and C6, perhaps also from C4. The median trunk is supplied by C7, and C8 and Th1 form the inferior trunk. Each of the primary trunks divides also into a dorsal and a ventral branch, of which three secondary trunks or fasciculi are formed and are grouped in a characteristic way around the axillary artery. The posterior fascicle unites the different dorsal primary trunks (C5–Th1). The ventral branches of the superior and medial trunks go into forming the lateral fascicles. Those from the inferior trunk form the medial fascicle. From these fasciculi the long arm nerves originate: from the posterior fascicle the axillary and radial nerves, from the lateral fascicles the median and musculocutaneous nerves and from the medial fascicle the following nerves: median, ulnar, cutaneus brachii medialis and cutaneus antebrachii medialis.

The costoclavicular passage represents the origin of the secondary trunks, and also the point of demarcation between supraclavicular and infraclavicular plexus portions.

Clinical Evaluation of a Plexus Lesion

The first evaluation must differentiate between supra- and infraclavicular lesions. The infraclavicular lesions usually occur during closed traumas involving the secondary trunks. Common causes are shoulder luxation and luxation fractures of the proximal humerus or scapula. These lesions are of a more favorable prognosis than the supraclavicular lesions produced by traction trauma, so it is of great clinical value to differentiate correctly between them. Helpful differentiation criteria can be:

1. Evidence of damage to supraclavicular branches, for example the dorsalis scapulae nerve, the suprascapularis nerve and the subscapulares thoracicus longus and thoracodorsalis nerves
2. Thickening or hardening of the suprascapular area
3. Horner syndrome
4. Fractures affecting the clavicular or transverse process of the cervical vertebrae

Combined supra- and infraclavicular lesions occur quite frequently.

In case of the supraclavicular lesion, the correct therapeutic step depends first on the answer to the question: Does a root avulsion exist or not? As direct treatment is practically impossible, root avulsion has been considered for a long time as a contraindication to surgery.

To the etiology of root avulsion belongs the traction traumas. Experimental studies on cadavers have clearly demonstrated the effect of the pulling force when the arm, head and shoulder are pulled away from each other. If the arm

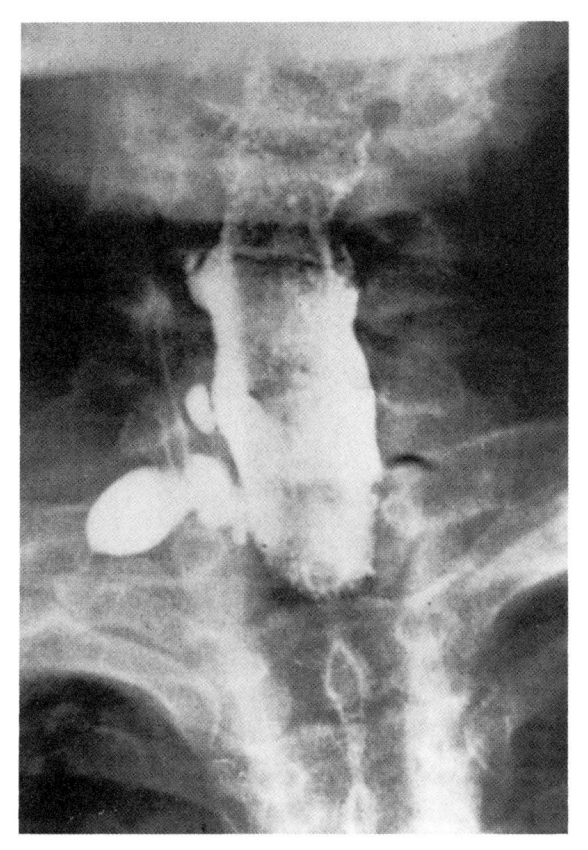

Fig. 2. Myelographic representation of root avulsions affecting C7 and Th1 in a traction trauma of the brachial plexus

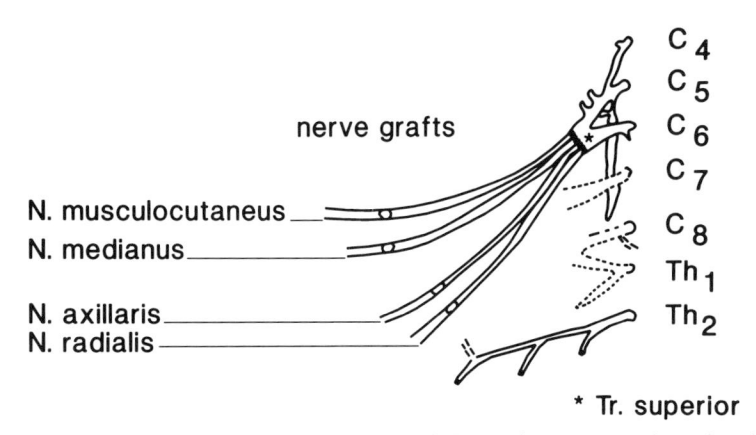

Fig. 3. Scheme showing the operative technique of nerve transplantation for a complete brachial plexus lesions with C7, C8 and Th1 root avulsion

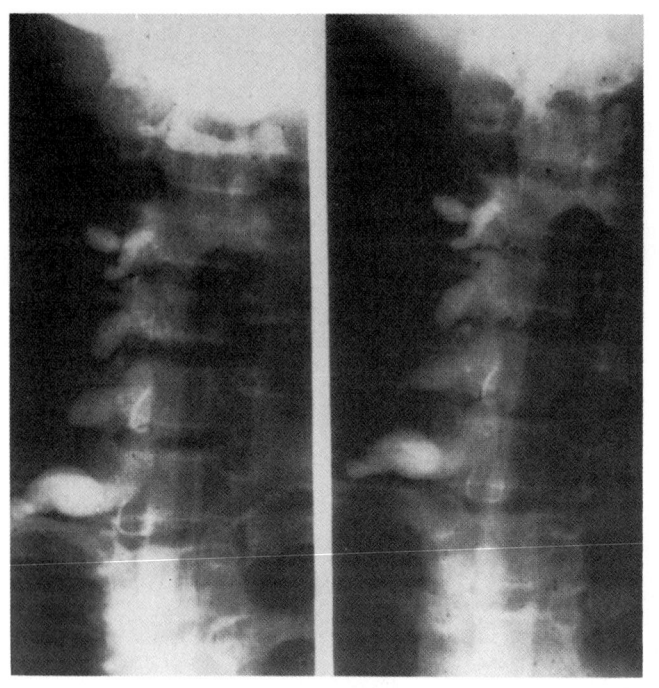

Fig. 4. X-ray film of a cervical myelography showing root avulsion at the level of C4–C7, by traction trauma of the brachial plexus

is in an extreme abducted position, the lower roots will be affected first. A halfway position of the arm and a considerable traumatic force may lead to root avulsions in all segments.

Clinical, electromyographic and radiological examinations can demonstrate the existence of a root avulsion: in an acute phase, the evidence of blood in the cerebrospinal fluid can be considered when an associated cerebral or medullary lesion is excluded as pathognomonic. At the same time, medullary symptoms prove that the damage lies not only peripherally in the plexus. The avulsion of the root from the medulla can determine intramedullar hemorrhages. Even temporary medullary symptoms such as commotio spinalis can be manifest. Therefore, a mandatory search is indicated for dissociated sensibility of the caudal segments, pyramidal signs or alterations of the sphincters when confronted with these serious traumas.

Avulsions of the roots C8 and Th1 cause a more or less apparent Horner syndrome. The syndrome may also be present in traumatic brachial plexus paresis through a direct lesion of the sympathetic trunk. These root lesions can also lead to altered thermoregulatory sweat secretion of the head and neck (not of the arm), although pilocarpine sweat reaction is preserved. This is due to the anatomical fact that the vegetative efferent supply which runs via the sympathetic trunk within the roots C1 to C7 is not preserved and that deeper emerging fibers will first be switched in the sympathetic trunk ganglion to the

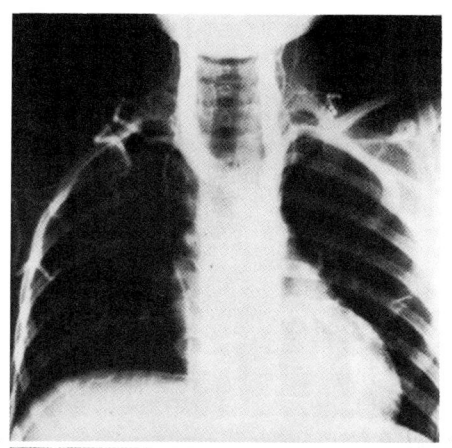

Fig. 5. a Preoperative angiography in a case of combined lesion of the brachial plexus and the axillary artery (note the collateral circulation). b Surgical view of the brachial plexus with the intervertebral foramen and the individual peripheral nerve branches for the arm. c Same case, now demonstrating the area after resection of the neuromas, preparation of the nerve stumps, interposition of several nerve transplants and reconstruction of the vascular deficits using a venous interpositional graft

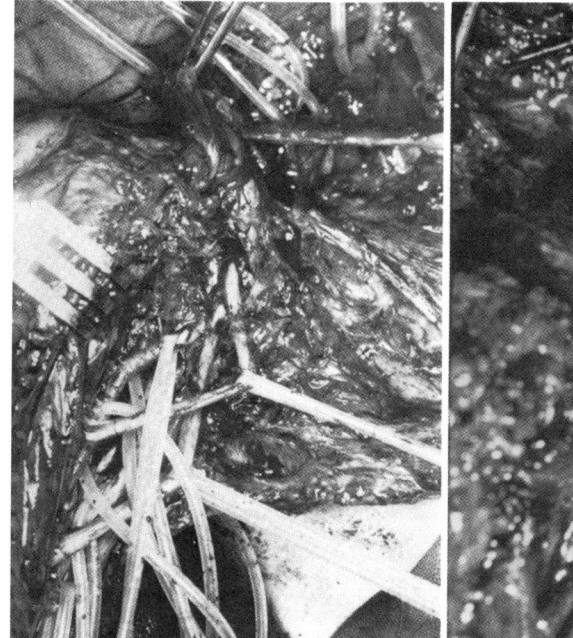

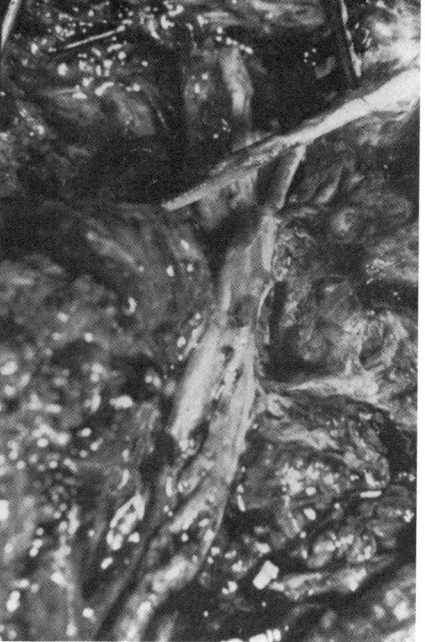

last peripheral neuron. The vegetative efferent fibers for the arm originate at Th4 or lower, and therefore remain intact in pure root lesions from C4 to Th2, as they connect to the brachial plexus more distally at the passage through the sympathetic trunk ganglions. In such cases of root lesions the sweat secretion of the arm remains preserved, even if the avulsion of C4 to Th1 has determined sensory and motor deinnervation. If clinically a deficit of the sweat secretion and missing reaction to thermoregulatory and pharmacological stimuli of the area of sensitive deficit is found, one can be sure that the interruption of the conduction is distally located.

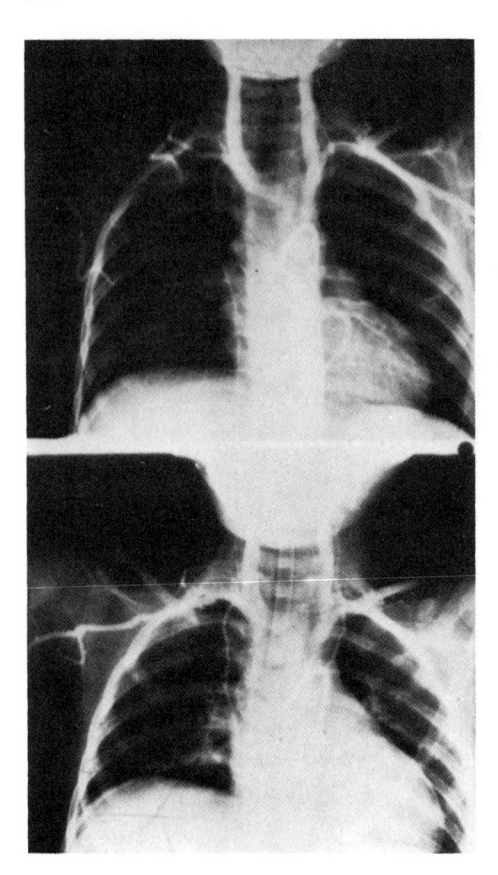

Fig. 5. d Postoperative control angiography 4 weeks after surgery. In comparison to the preoperative findings, vascular patency is present in the area of the axillary artery

Another examination which can be employed in the differential diagnosis of a root avulsion is the histamine test or axon reflex (Mumenthaler, 1987). As in root avulsions the damage is preganglionic in location, and the peripheral neuron remains intact, the histamine test will be positive. After intracutaneous application to a normal innervated area a large red macular papula results which also appears when the connection with the medulla is blocked by regional anesthesia. This is, therefore, not a reflex. The cutaneous reaction also develops when the posterior roots are sectioned proximally to the spinal ganglion, but not when they are distally sectioned, when a wallerian degeneration originates. It is assumed that the histamine determines impulses within intact afferent fibers which by the next possible bifurcation of the axons are centrifugally directed to nearby arterioles, causing vasodilatation. The preservation of the histamine reaction in a totally anesthetic dermatome can only be explained by posterior root avulsion, as long as the anesthesia is not caused by a neurapraxia. When the red macular papula does not appear in a lesion peripheral to the spinal ganglion, a degenerative nerve lesion must exist, although an associated nerve root avulsion is always possible.

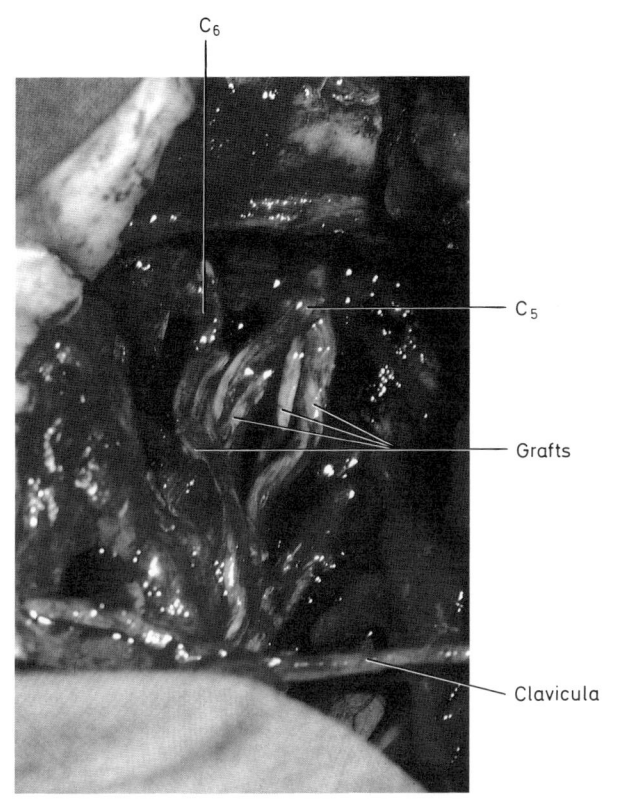

Fig. 6. Supraclavicular exposure of the brachial plexus and reconstruction of the C5 and C6 nerve roots with several free transplants

The electromyographic examination may also deliver valuable information. In root avulsion a sensitive nerve action potential is still recordable, because the lesion lies proximal to the spinal ganglion and therefore the peripheral portion of the sensitive neurons remains intact. In lesions distal to the spinal ganglion, the axon degenerates and the sensitive pathway becomes extinct.

Another electromyographic proof of nerve avulsion is denervation of the dorsal paravertebral neck muscles; already in the area of the intervertebral foramen the dorsal branches of the spinal nerves have set out to innervate the neck muscles. If the muscles are affected in a brachial plexus lesion, then it can be assumed that the damage is located proximal to the intervertebral foramen, i.e., in the area of the nerve roots.

Fractures affecting the transverse processes of the cervical bodies on the side of the plexus lesion can point to possible or probable root involvement. Therefore, X-ray films of the cervical spine are indicated in every case of plexus lesions. So are thorax X-rays in inspiration and expiration for functional evaluation of the diaphragm.

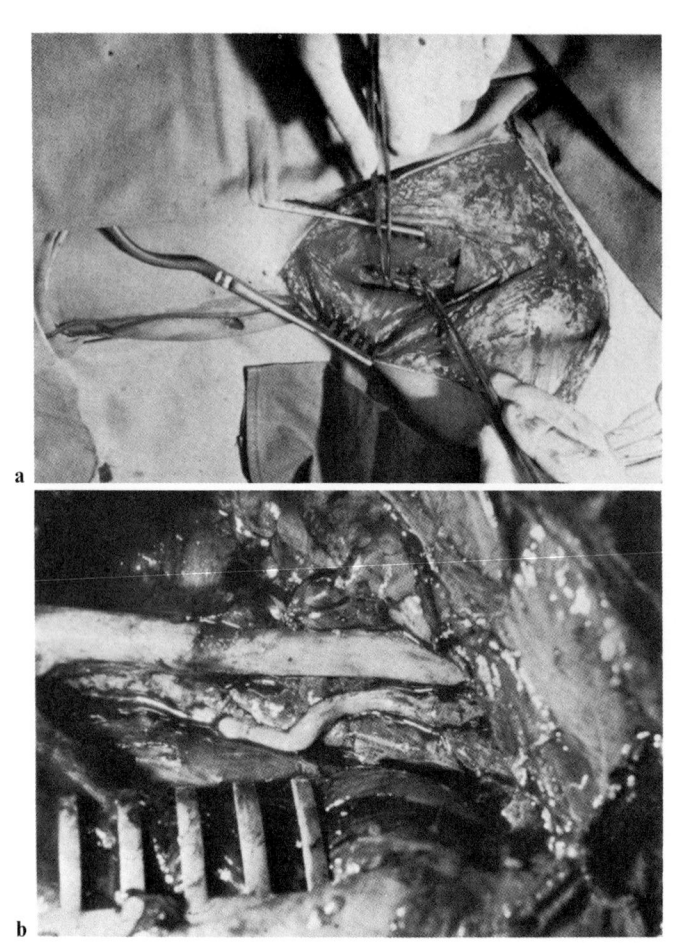

Fig. 7. a Brachial plexus lesion combined with an interruption of the axillary nerve's continuity. To bridge the axillary nerve, the cutaneus brachii medialis nerve is exposed. **b** Same case after neurolysis of the brachial plexus and transplantation of the axillary nerve (exposure by ventral approach)

Most important is radiological examination with contrast medium. With myelography, one can demonstrate the large empty root pockets, a direct sign of root avulsion (Fig. 2). This sign is, nevertheless, not absolutely reliable, as the root pockets can still be filled with the distal root stumps or secondary arachnoiditic growth or scars. Therefore one can demonstrate the root avulsions, but not exclude their presence. This generalized view can only be accepted with certain restrictions, as we have had two cases with manifest contrast medium spillage outside the spinal canal along the root pockets where intraoperatively there was no root avulsion. The clinical course with good reinnervation of the affected segments has supported this observation.

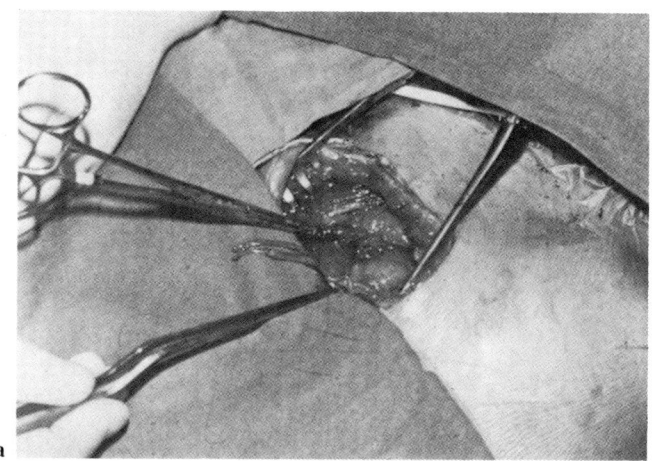

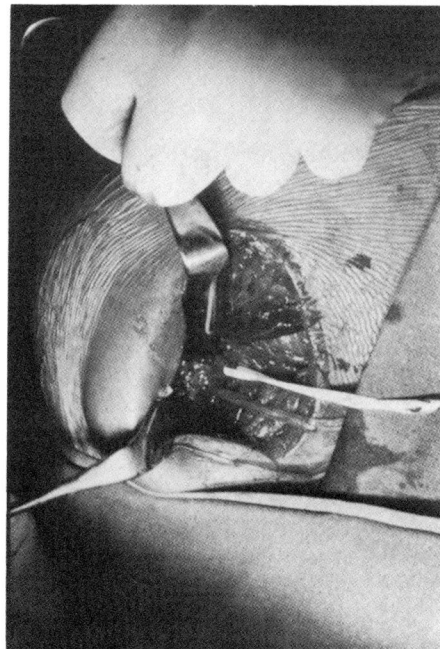

Fig. 8. a Example of an axillary nerve injury after shoulder luxation. Even though the proximal nerve stump was exposed ventrally, the distal stump had to be approached by means of a dorsal exposure. **b** The dorsal exposure in the same case. Identification of the axillary nerve before penetration of its fascicles in the deltoid muscle

Indications for Surgery

Through continuous clinical and electromyographic control studies during the first 3 months the question of whether a neurapraxia or an axonotmesis exists has to be resolved. If during this time signs of reinnervation appear in the affected arm muscles, we can then pursue intensive conservative treatment and await the further clinical development.

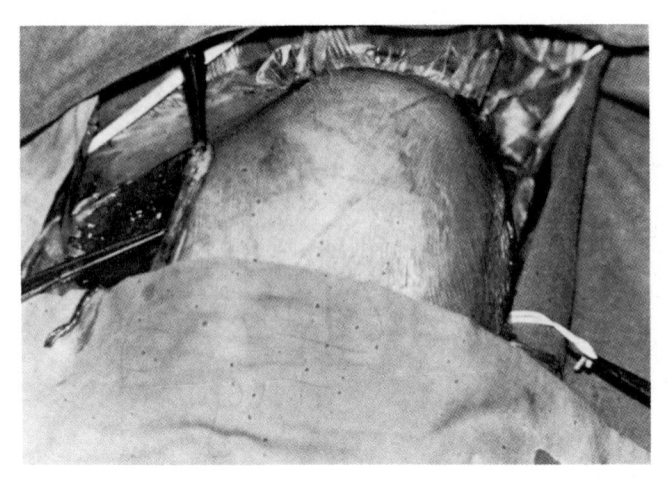

Fig. 8. c Overview of the same case showing the ventral and dorsal exposures. The approximately 10 cm long transplant was passed through the axilla so that proximal and distal stumps could be coadapted

If no functional improvement appears within the first 6 months, then surgical exposure is indicated. For surgical procedures the preoperative demonstration of a root avulsion is extremely important. Proven root avulsion has a poor prognostic value but does not contraindicate surgery, even if a complete plexus paresis exists.

In root avulsions affecting C7/C8/Th1 with complete plexus damage, by means of neurolysis and free autologous nerve transplants we can possibly achieve an anastomosis between the still intact upper primary trunk (C4, C5, C6) and the most important arm nerves. The choice of those nerves which can bring about reinnervation of the upper plexus is schematically represented in Fig. 3.

If all the nerve roots of the brachial plexus are involved (Fig. 4), we can then arrange for connections between intercostal nerves and the musculocutaneous nerve for isolated flexion of the arm (Seddon 1963; Bonnel et al. 1979).

To achieve an adequate reinnervation of the biceps muscle, at least four intercostal nerves will be needed for regeneration of the musculocutaneous nerve. As the musculocutaneous nerve holds an average of 6000 nerve fibers and the intercostal nerves approximately 1300 each, we routinely use the third, fourth, fifth and sixth intercostal nerves to obtain approximately the necessary number of nerve fibers.

When there is no root avulsion or vascular damage as a result of a serious traction trauma, the results of microsurgical procedures for brachial plexus lesions are particularly satisfactory. In these cases the extension of the lesion to the supra- or infraclavicular area can be determined intraoperatively, and by means of specific microsurgical neurolysis, neurosuture and neurotransplantation it is possible to obtain successful decompression or reconstruction of the nerve structures (Samii 1982) (Fig. 5a–d).

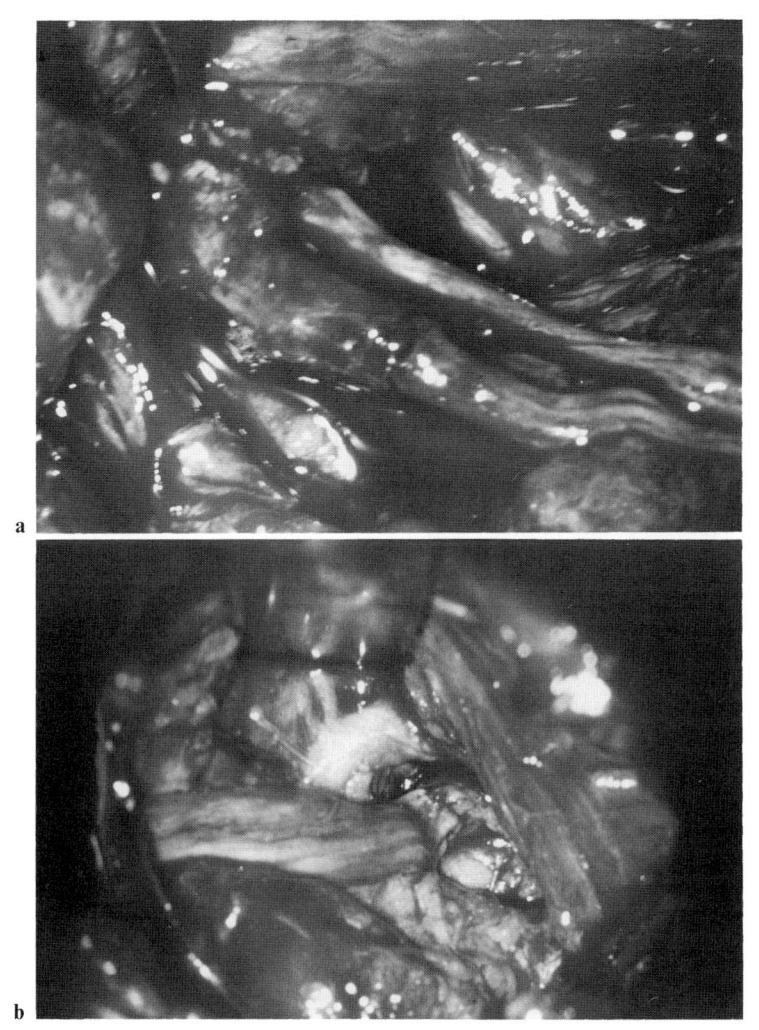

Fig. 9 a, b. Reconstruction of the axillary nerve by interposition of two sural nerve grafts. **a** View of the proximal stump after suture. **b** View of the distal stump of the axillary nerve in the same patient

When faced with penetrating open lesions in the supraclavicular region, at the level of C5 and C6, a reconstruction with satisfactory functional results can be obtained when after resection of the damaged portions intact nerve stumps are available (Fig. 6). The nerve deficits can then be bridged by means of free nerve transplants.

As the primary trunk of the plexus in the area of the costoclavicular passage proceeds into secondary trunks with exchange of numerous fibers, in the case of further distal extension of the lesion the dissection of this area is not advisable due to the risk of an additional lesion of the nearby intact trunks. In

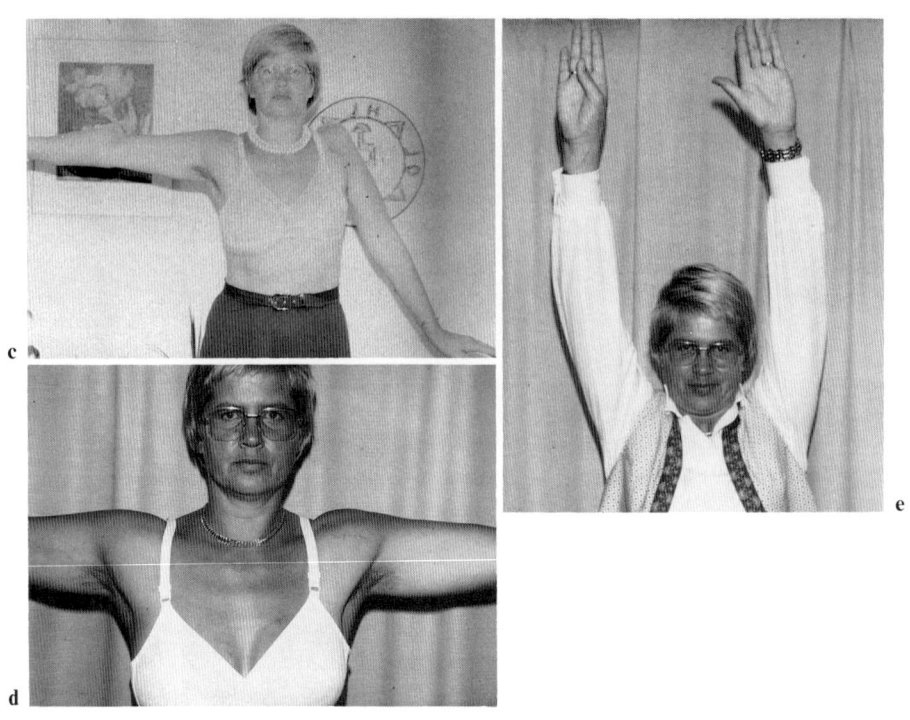

Fig. 9. c Before surgery: paresis and hypotrophy of the left deltoid muscle. **d, e** Eighteen months after the operation. Good recovery of the deltoid function

such a situation with an isolated C5 lesion the complete restitution of the missing deltoid muscle function can be achieved by anastomosis with the axillary nerve, using two transplants of 15 cm length each (Fig. 7a, b).

In closed osseous lesions of the shoulder with infraclavicular damage, the secondary trunks will be involved. The posterior fascicle is especially affected, and very often there is a lesion of the axillary nerve. The exposure of the proximal stump of the axillary nerve, if necessary, can be unproblematic, whereas due to progressive damage a ventral exposure of the distal stump through the axilla is sometimes impossible. Here the dorsal exposure of the axillary nerve before its penetration through the deltoid muscle is necessary. After suture to the proximal stump the approximately 10 cm long nerve transplant has to be passed through the axilla and dorsally joined with the intact distal stumps of the axillary nerve (Figs. 8a–c, 9a–e).

References

Bonnel F (1980) Bases anatomiques et histologiques de la chirurgie du plexus brachial de l'adulte. Rev Readapt prfo soc 6:36–41

Bonnel F, Allieu Y, Sugata Y, Rabischong P (1979) Anatomico-surgical bases of neurotization for root-avulsion of the brachial plexus. Anatomia Clinica 1:291–296

Mumenthaler M (1987) Vegetative Innervation der Haut. In: Läsionen peripherer Nerven. Georg Thieme Verlag Stuttgart, New York, 5. Auflage 67–73

Mumenthaler M (1987) Die topische Diagnostik bei Armplexusläsionen und die Diagnostik der Wurzelausrisse. In: Läsionen peripherer Nerven. Georg Thieme Verlag Stuttgart, New York, 5. Auflage 174–178

Samii M (1974) Indication and operative technique of birth injuries of the brachial plexus. Progress in Pediatric Neurosurgery, Hippokrates Verlag Stuttgart 243–245

Samii M (1974) Verletzungen der Hirnnerven und des Plexus brachialis. Hefte zur Unfallheilkunde, Springer Verlag 117:372–378

Samii M (1975) Use of microtechniques in peripheral nerve surgery – experiences with over 300 cases. Microneurosurgery, Igaku Shoin Ltd, Tokyo 85–93

Samii M (1979) Die Versorgung offener Nervenverletzungen (technisches Vorgehen, Prognose, Ergebnisse). Hefte zur Unfallheilkunde 138:68–72

Samii M (1980) Fascicular peripheral nerve repair. Modern Technics in Surgery, Neurosurgery, 17, Futura Publishing Company New York

Samii M (1982) Revision und operative Behandlung bei Verletzungen am Plexus brachialis. Schriftenreihe Unfallmedizinische Tagungen der Landesverbände der gewerblichen Berufsgenossenschaften, Heft 49, Bonn 155–176

Samii M, Penkert G (1986) Verletzungen der peripheren Nerven. In: Lehrbuch der Chirurgie. Hrsg.: Koslowski L, Irmer W, Bushe K-A, F. K. Schattauer Verlag Stuttgart New York

Samii M, Penkert G (1986) Chirurgie bei peripheren Nervenverletzungen. In: Lehrbuch der Chirurgie. Verlag Urban und Schwarzenberg, München

Samii M, Wagner D (1975) Ergebnisse der autologen Nerventransplantationen bei Läsionen kranialer und peripherer Nerven. Therapeutische Umschau, 32(7):453–460

Schliack H (1962) Zum Problem der Schweißdrüsensekretion. Nervenarzt 33:421–423

Schliack H (1976) Ninhydrin-Schweißtest nach Moberg, Dtsch med Wschr 101:1336

Seddon HJ (1963) Nerve Grafting. J Bone Jt Surg 45B:447–461

Schwannomas of the Brachial Plexus

A. ALEXANDRE, P. CISOTTO, D. BILLECI, S. CUSUMANO, F. DI PAOLA, and A. CARTERI, Treviso/Italy

Neurogenic tumors of the brachial plexus are very rare lesions. A few reports are found in the literature, and they concern a small number of cases. Excluding cases of von Recklinghausen's disease, the total number of surgically treated cases that have undergone pathological evaluation is 171. Das Gupta et al. [1] presented in 1969 the pathological features of 60 neurilemmomas of the neck, but they did not specify the exact site of implantation. Horak et al. [4] in 1983 reviewed 11 neurofibromas and 5 schwannomas. Only the other 95 cases [2, 5, 7] of solitary schwannomas are clearly diagnosed and described in their clinical and pathological features.

Patients and Methods

Patients. This study analyzes a series of patients with neurogenic tumors admitted to the Division of Neurosurgery at Padua University in Treviso from 1 January 1985 to 2 January 1987. The classification of Seddon, drawn up by the World Health Organization in 1969 on the basis of the proposal by Russel and Rubinstein [11], is the most commonly employed. On this basis our series includes the following cases: two solitary schwannomas, two solitary neurofibromas, two neurofibromas with von Recklinghausen's disease, two schwannomas with von Recklinghausen's disease, and one malignant schwannoma. The typical clinical presentation of primitive benign neurogenic tumors of the brachial plexus was in this series a visible and palpable mass in the supraclavicular (five cases) or axillary (three cases) fossa. Generally no neurological deficit was present.

We agree with the observation that rapidly evolving neurological deficits and severe pain must be considered as signs of possibly malignant lesions. Each neurogenic tumor causes the so-called pseudo-Tinnel's sign, that is, the sensation of electricity when the mass is gently hit. The sign may also give information as to which nerve trunk is involved.

Each patient underwent careful anamnestic and clinical study, and complete electrophysiological investigation of nerve and muscular functions. Moreover, a careful radiological study of the shoulder girdle was performed by means of CT scan (Figs. 1, 2). This allowed definition of the probable site of implantation of the tumor, of its anatomical relationship with the surrounding vascular, nerve, muscular, and bony structures.

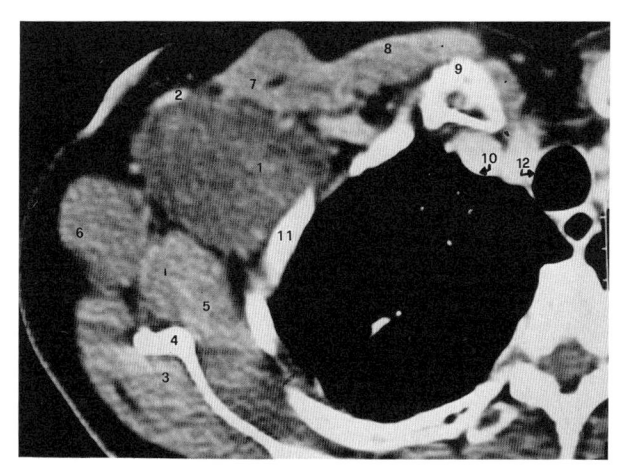

Fig. 1. Cross-section of the chest at T3 level. *1*, Brachial plexus schwannoma; *2*, brachial plexus and vessels on the lesion; *3*, infraspinous; *4*, scapula; *5*, subscapularis; *6*, teres major; *7*, pectoralis minor; *8*, pectoralis major; *9*, sternal extremity of the clavicle; *10*, lung; *11*, ribs; *12*, trachea

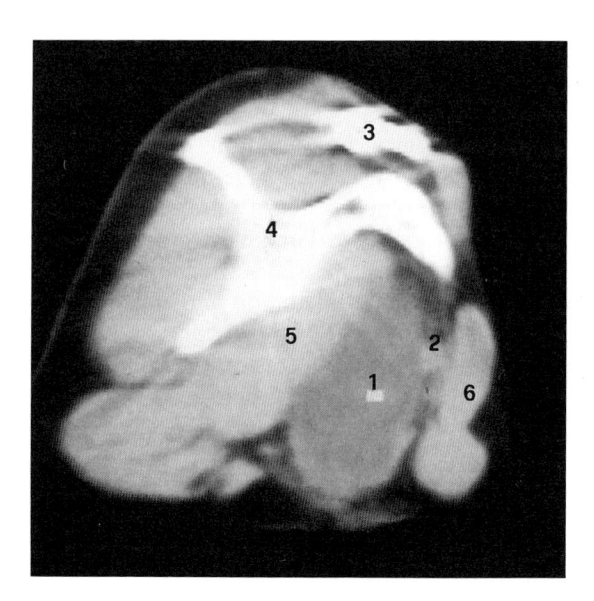

Fig. 2. The arm is introduced in CT gantry. *1*, Schwannoma of the brachial plexus; *2*, brachial plexus and vessels; *3*, clavicle; *4*, scapula; *5*, subscapularis muscle; *6*, pectoralis muscles

Surgical Approach. We have employed the classical supra- and/or infraclavicular routes owing to the anatomical features of the lesion [6, 8]. In our series it was not necessary to resect either the clavicular insertion of the sternocleidomastoid muscle or the clavicle itself, as proposed by Millesi [9]. Microsurgical techniques were employed in all cases to obtain complete removal of the tumor and absolute preservation of nerve structures. In the case of malignant lesions or nerve infiltration, grafts of sural nerve were employed to perform interfascicular nerve grafting.

Pathology. Specimens were embedded in paraffin and stained with hematoxiline-eosin. Diagnosis was confirmed in all cases by immunohistochemical staining of S100 protein, which is specific for Schwann's cells.

Results and Discussion

When a space-occupying lesion is met in the anatomical region of the brachial plexus, clinical and instrumental examinations have two goals: definition of the exact location of the mass and probable pathological diagnosis. The latter may be suggested by anamnestic and clinical data. For example, it was possible to screen the patients with neurofibromatosis, who subsequently underwent a series of examinations in order to confirm the diagnosis and to provide genetic information to the relatives.

On clinical evaluation all our patients showed a palpable, solid mass which was fixed along the axis of the plexus and slightly movable transversely. In four cases motor and sensitive deficit of the involved nerve trunk was observed. Severe pain was always absent in benign lesions and present in the malignant ones.

Electrophysiological and neuroradiological investigations were not conclusive for the pathological diagnosis. Only CT scans give an indication of probable malignancy if areas of dishomogeneous density are seen inside a lesion with shaded margins. Both neuroradiological and electrophysiological data, and especially the relationship between them, were extremely useful for obtaining a preoperative anatomical view of the tumor and surrounding tissues. Measurements of conduction velocity and EMG provide a description of the altered nerves and the location of the compression. Five of the six patients with benign lesions showed no neurological deficits, but in four of them sensitive conduction velocity was slackened, and mild neurogenic alterations of the muscles were observed. For the purpose of localizing the lesion, CT scan is the method of choice. The tumor's shape is visualized, its exact dimensions are indicated and anatomical relationships with pleura, brachial plexus, vessels, muscles, and bones are clearly outlined.

The excision of a schwannoma is a rather delicate surgical procedure, and the result is improved by microsurgery, which allows an absolute consideration of nerve structures. In our two cases of neurofibroma removal imposed sacrificing a part of a trunk which was infiltrated; the nerve defect was filled by a sural nerve graft. An entire primary trunk had to be removed together with the malignant schwannoma; it was replaced by three interfascicular nerve grafts.

Once the problem of von Recklinghausen's disease is excluded, pathological classification of these tumors originating from peripheral nerve sheets, is not unanimous. Das Gupta [1] asserts that the terms solitary neurilemmoma, schwannoma, and solitary neurofibroma refer to the same clinical entity, and that the difference is only histological and does not alter the management. Consequently the terms are used interchangeably in his series. Inoue et al. [5] distinguish neurinomas (also called schwannomas or neurilemmomas, as tumors originating from Schwann's cells) from neurofibromas, which originate from fibroblasts. Fisher and Tate [2] do not make a clear distinction between the two entities; Gullotta [3] is of a similar opinion. Palladini [10] maintains a distinction because of the rich fibroblastic component of neurofibromas but admits that not all authors agree with him. Kline [7] maintains the distinction, most of all for the implications at surgery. We agree with him, and we think it correct to maintain the distinction between the two forms, as proposed by Russel and Rubinstein [11]. While the schwannoma is perfectly enucleated from the parent nerve, the neurofibroma penetrates among the fascicles. Its complete removal requires sacrificing the parent nerve and inserting an autologous graft.

Table 1. Three cases of solitary benign tumors

Patient	Sex	Age (years)	Clinical manifestation	Site and size	Histology
L.S.	M	40	Ulnar hypoesthesia, infraclavicular mass	Anterior cord, 2×3 cm	Schwannoma
P.T.	F	32	Infraclavicular mass	Posterior cord, 6×8 cm	Schwannoma
S.B.	M	44	Median hypoesthesia, supraclavicular mass	Upper trunk, 2×2 cm	Neurofibroma

Localization at the brachial plexus is a rare event in cases of neurofibromatosis, the so-called solitary lesions of both histological types are particularly rare in this anatomical region. Kline [7] has carefully reviewed the literature on brachial plexus tumors of neural sheath origin and finds, as we did, approximately 130 cases (some reports are not precise in specifying the number or the location of cases). He adds, in a paper which has been published in October 1987 in *Neurosurgery*, his own series of 40 neural sheath tumors: 26 neurofibromas, 8 schwannomas, 4 malignant neural sheath tumors, one fibrosarcoma, and one meningioma. Of these, 15 were solitary neurofibromas, 8 were solitary schwannomas, and 2 were malignant schwannomas without von Recklinghausen's disease. Thus, the total number of solitary benign tumors is 23, which are to be added to the 55 reported in the preexisting literature, giving a total number of 78 cases reported in the world literature. The three cases reported in this paper are in addition to the previously 78 collected cases (Table 1).

References

1. Das Gupta T, Brasfield RD, Strong EW, Hajud SI (1969) Benign solitary schwannomas (neurilemmomas). Cancer 24:355–366
2. Fisher RG, Tate HB (1970) Isolated neurilemmomas of the brachial plexus. J Neurosurg 32:463–467
3. Gullotta F (1971) Compendio di Neuropatologia. Piccin, Padova
4. Horak E, Szentirmay Z, Sugar J (1983) Pathologic features of nerve sheath tumors, with respect to prognostic signs. Cancer 51:1159–1167
5. Inoue M, Kawano T, Matsumura H, Mori K, Yoshida T (1983) Solitary benign schwannoma of the brachial plexus. Surg Neurol 20:103–108
6. Kline DG, Judice DJ (1983) Operative management of selected brachial plexus lesions. J Neurosurg 58:631–649
7. Kline DG (1987) personal communication
8. MacCarty CS (1984) Surgical exposure of the brachial plexus. Surg Neurol 21:593–596
9. Millesi H (1980) Traumatic lesions of the brachial plexus. In: Omer GE, Spinner M (eds) Management of peripheral nerve problems. Saunders, Philadelphia
10. Palladini G (1983) Neurinoma. In: Encicl Med Ital vol X. Milano, p 746
11. Russel DS, Rubinstein LJ (1963) Pathology of tumors of the nervous system. Williams & Wilkins, Baltimore

Results of Brachial Plexus Surgery

G. Brunelli, L. Monini, and F. Brunelli, Brescia/Italy

Evaluation of the results of brachial plexus surgery is very difficult. This is due to a number of factors, the first of which is the site of the lesion. Results are worst in the more proximal lesions, because of the greater amount of cytoskeleton to reconstruct, the longer time of denervation of the muscles, and the higher difficulty in matching the fibers, as proximal fibers are still very mixed. Therefore, results improve starting with root lesions and extending down to those of spinal nerves, trunks, cords, and terminal branches. The second factor is the type of the lesion. Brachial plexus can be damaged to a varying severity: neurapraxia (types 1 and 2 by Sunderland), axonotmesis, neurotmesis, axonostenosis, and axonal suffering. Of course the worst result is in neurotmesis with loss of substance, especially if combined with internal scar and cachexia.

The first practical prognostic division can be made between supraganglionic and infraganglionic lesions. In fact, supraganglionic lesions are due to avulsion of the roots from the spinal cord and cannot as yet be repaired but only treated by means of neurotization with other nerves. Supraganglionic (i.e., root avulsion lesions) can be diagnosed before surgery by means of myelography and EMG of paraspinal muscles and during the operation by means of evoked potentials. The second practical division is that between supraclavicular and infraclavicular lesions, the latter corresponding to cord and terminal branch lesions and having a better prognosis. A further division is that which considers the involvement of the superior roots, spinal nerves or trunks, or the inferior elements of the brachial plexus: Duchenne-Erb type (C5/C6), Dejerine-Klumpke type (C8/T1), intermediate trunk, or total involvement.

Involvement of the lower part of the plexus is associated with the worst prognosis, probably due to the longer course which the regenerating axons must travel, the longer denervation time of the hand muscles, and the greater amount of cytoskeleton which the parent cells must reconstruct. Prognosis is also worsened by the type of traumatic agent (missiles, for instance) and by scar. Also the length of time elapsed from the occurrence of the lesion worsens the prognosis.

We have reviewed our cases according to the level and type of lesion and the types of traumatic agents. A series of 364 cases of brachial plexus have been operated on by us. Cases of Duchenne-Erb syndrome due to a lesion limited to C5/C6 spinal nerves and/or upper trunk have been operated on by means of grafts taken from the sural nerve. Results of these cases vary from very good to poor, the latter in general being those treated late or due to gunshot wounds (two cases). (There are cases treated late with good results and others treated early with bad results, probably due to surgical mismatching which at the moment cannot be avoided). In few cases (five) there was an isolated lesion of C7 by an anteroposterior trauma (two of these cases were avulsion). The avulsion of C5/C6 in general gives poor results, which are less poor if only C5 is avulsed. The rupture or avulsion of the roots of C7 are generally associated with (a) upper trunk lesions, (b) avulsions of C8/T1 and ruptures of the upper trunk, (c) lower trunk ruptures, or (d) ruptures of upper and lower trunks.

In all these cases results depend mainly on the associated lesions. In the lower trunk or C8/T1 spinal nerve ruptures with Dejerine-Klumpke syndrome results were so poor that a difference between spinal nerve or lower trunk rupture and C8/T1 root avulsions was not distinguishable. Total palsy due to rupture of all the trunks is also a very severe lesion with very poor results, the severity of which varies slightly according to several factors. In root avulsions the prospects for repair are very limited. Only by neurotizing two or three branches (in particular the suprascapularis, axillary, and musculocutaneous nerves) by means of the anterior nerves of the cervical plexus and the spinal nerve some limited function of the shoulder and elbow can be regained.

The lesions of the cords give better results, which of course are related to the number of injured cords, the type of lesions, the size of the gap after dissection, and the associated lesions. Terminal branches behave as peripheral nerves, but results are poorer due to the longer course of the regrowing axons in reaching their targets and to the undetermined function in terms of quadrantic location as a result of the mixing of fibers in the large precollateral zone of the nerves. Results in double-level lesions are in general also poor, with severity related to the number of double lesions and the distance between the upper and lower ruptures.

The evaluation of results is very difficult. The upper limb contains 50 muscles, and each muscle can recover from M0 to M5, i.e., from 0% to 100%. The sensory recovery can be very good, good, fair and poor in the same patient for different skin areas, related either to roots or trunks or to terminal branch innervation. Furthermore, up to now the final result cannot be related to single factors; these are so numerous and interactive with one another that even with a special program in our computer we have not been able to correlate results with single factors. The pathological type of the lesion, its extent, the time elapsed from the onset of the lesion, and the personal factors such as age, general condition, alcohol, smoking, and drug addiction interfere, as well as the type of surgery, the training of the surgeon, and the time and constancy of medical and physical postoperative treatment and re-education.

After having tried several ambitious means to evaluate the results, none of which has proved to our satisfaction, we are now trying to use an evaluation scheme that we find as useful as it is simple (Table 1). This scheme has the merit of presenting the results in figures. We divided the upper limb into the following sections: (a) shoulder, elbow, and wrist regions, (b) digital extension and flexion (those related to median or ulnar functions), and (c) the intrinsic muscle

Results of Brachial Plexus Surgery

Table 1. Tentative evaluation scheme for brachial plexus lesions

Upper Limb
Very difficult to classify the results (50 muscles)
Each muscle can recover M0 to M5, i.e., 0% to 100%
       (× 50)
       plus sensory function

Classification by function	Sensory function
Shoulder: abduction – external rotation	Protection
Elbow: flexion – extension	Discrimination
Wrist: extension	Total
Digit: extension – flexion (median) – flexion (ulnar)	Partial
Intrinsic: – median – ulnar	Joint stiffness

Shoulder:	abduction:	perfect	10[a]
		valid	5
		paralytic	0
	external rotation:	perfect	10
		valid	5
		paralytic	0
Max. 20			
Only brachiothoracic pliers: 5			
Elbow:	flexion:	perfect	10
		valid	5
		paralytic	0
	extension:	perfect	10
		valid	5
		paralytic	0
Max. 20			
Wrist:	extension:	perfect	10
		valid	5
		paralytic	0
Finger:	extension:	perfect	10
		valid	5
		paralytic	0
Max. 20			
Digit flexion:		perfect	10
(median)		valid	5
		paralytic	0
Digit flexion:		perfect	10
(ulnar)		valid	5
		paralytic	0
Max. 20			

Pain must be evaluated separately as in general it is not affected by surgery done on the elements of the brachial plexus.

[a] Perfect, M5; valid, M3+. It is understood that abduction 10 and external rotation 10 imply good function also of the other muscles of the shoulder.

Table 1 (continued)

Intrinsic muscles: (median)		perfect	10
		valid	5
		paralytic	0
Intrinsic muscles: (ulnar)		perfect	10
		valid	5
		paralytic	0
Max. 20			
Sensory function:		2PD < 15 – All the digits 20 (4 × digit)	
		2PD > 15 – All the digits 10 (2 × digit)	
Max. 20			
Joint stiffness:	severe:	minus 20	
	mild:	minus 10	
Wrist and hand (sensation included) Max. 80			
Global evaluation	shoulder	0– 20/20	
	elbow	0– 20/20	
	wrist and hand	0– 80/80	
	Total limb	0–120/120	

function and sensory function. All these sections can give a figure from 0 to 20 according to the perfect, valid, or paralytic function of the muscle or to the two points' discrimination. Perfect is scored 10 when reaching M 5, valid is scored 5 when reaching M 3+, and paralytic 0. Arbitrary scores between 0 to 10 are left to the examiner. For instance, it is understood that abduction 10 and external rotation 10 imply good function also of the other muscles of the shoulders. These scores can reach a total of 120 and may be lowered if there is stiffness of joints.

In cases of total palsy, any improvement is worthwhile. In young, healthy patients operated on early, good and very good results can be achieved with a good technique, better still in cord lesions. Nevertheless, exceptionally good results can be obtained even in severe cases, whereas complete failures may occur in easy cases.

References

Alnot JY (1984) Infraclavicular lesions. Clin Plast Surg 11:121
Bateman JE (1962) Trauma to nerves in limbs. Saunders, Philadelphia
Bonnell F (1984) Microscopic anatomy of the adult human brachial plexus: an anatomical and histological basis for microsurgery. Microsurgera 5:107
Bonney G, Birch R, Jamieson AM, James RA (1984) Experience with vascularized nerve grafts. Clin Plast Surg 11:137
Breidenbach W, Terzis JK (1984) The anatomy of free vascularized nerve grafts. Clin Plast Surg 11:65

Brunelli G, Monini L (1984) Neurotization of avulsed roots of brachial plexus by means of anterior nerves of cervical plexus. Clin Plast Surg 11:149

Brunelli G (1980) Neurotization of avulsed roots of the brachial plexus by means of anterior nerves of the cervical plexus. Int J Microsurg 2:55–58

Celli L (1978) Conference at the Giornata Internazionale di Chirurgia Taranto, Italy

Clark JPM (1946) Reconstruction of biceps brachii by pectoral muscle transplantation. Br J Surg 34:180

Kline DS, Judice DJ (1983) Operative management of selected brachial plexus lesions. J Neurosurg 58:631

Koshima I, Harii K (1983) Experimental study on vascularized nerve grafts: morphometric and biochemical analysis of axonal regeneration of nerves transplanted into scar. Paper presented at the 7th Symposium on Microsurgery

Kotani PT, Matsuda H, Suzuki T (1972) Trial surgical procedures of nerve transfer-to-avulsion injuries of plexus brachialis. Abstracts of the 12th Congress of the Société International de Chirurgie Orthopédique et Traumatologique, Israel

Lundborg G (1975) Structure and function of the intraneural microvessels as related to trauma neuroma formation and nerve function. J Bone Joint Surg 57(A):938

Millesi H (1973) Resultats tardifs de la greffe nerveuse interfasciculaire. Chirurgie réparatrice des lesions du plexus brachial. Rev Méd Suisse Romande 93:7, 511

Narakas AO (1984) Thoughts on neurotization or nerve transfer in irreparable nerve lesion. Clin Plast Surg 11:153

Sedel L (1951) The management of supraclavicular lesions. Clin Plast Surg 11:121

Seddon HJ (1963) Nerve grafting. J Bone Joint Surg 45(B):447

Seddon HJ (1975) Surgical disorders of the peripheral nerves, 2nd ed. Churchill Livingstone, Edinburgh, p 194

Taylor IE, Ham FJ (1976) The free vascularized nerve graft. Plast Reconstr Surg 57:413

Terzis JK, Dykes RW, Hakstian RW (1976) Electrophysiological recordings in peripheral nerve surgery. A Review. J Hand Surg 1:52

Tsuyama N, Sakaguchi RT, Hara T, Kondo S, Kaminuma M, Ijichi M, Ryn D (1968) Reconstructive surgery in brachial plexus injuries. Proceedings of the 11th Annual Meeting of the Japanese Society for Surgery of the Hand, Hiroshima, pp 39–40

Zancolli E, Mitre E (1973) Latissimus dorsi transfer to restore elbow flexion. J Bone Joint Surg 55(A):1265

Selection of Brachial Plexus Cases for Operation – Based on Results*

D. G. KLINE, New Orleans/USA

Introduction

The amount of literature on the surgical management of plexus injuries has grown logarithmically in the past decade. In great part this is due not only to improved intraoperative electrodiagnostic and repair techniques such as grafts but also to a greater appreciation of the range of electrodiagnostic and radiologic studies available to evaluate plexus lesions preoperatively. Not to be minimized is the willingness of a number of European [1, 2, 5, 7, 9, 17, 18, 22, 24, 27] and a few North American surgeons to undertake these difficult operations [10, 13, 16, 30]. As might be expected under these circumstances, many questions still remain to be answered. Among these is whether all serious plexus injuries require operation, and, if not, how does one select those for operation? Closely related to these questions are those concerning timing for operation.

Table 1. Serious brachial plexus injuries

	Evaluated	Operated
Lacerations	47	45
GSW	141	90
Stretch/Contusion	283	190
Iatrogenic	36	30
Total	507	355

This analysis is part of an on-going study concerning brachial plexus lesions at the Louisiana State University Medical Center (LSUMC) in New Orleans. It is based on a 19-year period ending in early 1986, so that a follow-up of at least 2 years is available (See Table 1). Excluded from the analysis are minor plexus injuries, plexus tumors, birth palsies, and thoracic outlet cases. The questions of selection for and timing of operation are addressed here regarding lacerating injuries, gunshot wounds (GSW), stretch/contusion injuries, and iatrogenic injuries.

---

* From Department of Neurosurgery, LSU Medical Center, 1542 Tulane Avenue, New Orleans LA 70112, and Charity and Ochsner Hospitals of New Orleans, USA.

Lacerating Injuries

Not too surprisingly, almost all lacerating injuries to the plexus seen in our clinic were operated upon. There were a number of reasons for this. Because of the nature of the mechanism, plexus loss was usually complete in the distribution of one or more elements. Such loss was frequently but not necessarily due to transection of those elements involved, and transected nerves in humans seldom recover spontaneously. In addition, these injuries were usually relatively focal in nature, were seen or referred to us relatively early, and seldom involved damage close to spinal cord. As a result, these lacerating injuries readily lent themselves to repair. The two cases not operated on both had from the onset partial loss in the distribution of two elements due to knife wounds; since loss was partial, these were followed and improved in the early months after wounding.

Lacerating injuries can be placed into two categories – sharp injuries usually due to knives or glass, and blunt injuries due to auto metal, fan or propellar blades, chain saw, or animal bites. In the sharp-injury category, primary repair within 72 h was carried out if referral was timely enough. If referral was late, delayed or secondary repair was necessary. Comparison of results in these two subsets of sharp injuries was interesting. End-to-end suture with little tension could be readily achieved in all those receiving primary repair. Of the elements repaired 65% achieved a grade 3 or better result (0 to 5 basis) [13]. In those sharp injuries receiving secondary repair because of delayed referral, most elements required graft repair because of retraction and scar formation. Few of the sharp injuries referred late and thus repaired after a delay could be sutured end-to-end. Results dropped to a little better than 50% of elements recovering to grade 3 or better. The few sharp injuries capable of repair by end-to-end suture fared well. The implications seem clear. Sharp and thus neat transections of the plexus are best repaired within 72 h if possible [3, 13, 25, 27].

In the blunt-injury category, where neural transection was ragged or irregular, secondary or delayed repair was undertaken. Only a few of these lesions could be repaired by end-to-end suture. Most required grafts, and again results were at the 50% level if a grade 3 or higher function was used as an index of a good result. It must be kept in mind that this figure includes elements not usually considered favorable for repair, such as lower spinal nerves, lower trunk, and medial cord. Thus, it may be worthwhile to "tack down" the stumps of bluntly transected elements to adjacent facial planes while awaiting secondary repair. That blunt as well as sharp lacerating injuries to the plexus can be associated with vascular injury requiring acute repair is a point to the kept in mind by those repairing the vessel(s) as well as those asked to look at the bluntly torn or raggedly transected neural elements.

In both the sharp- and blunt-injury categories, some elements (10%) which had serious loss were found in continuity at exploration. These elements had been contused and/or stretched by the wounding instrument. If discovered in the early weeks after injury such elements received only an external neurolysis.

Table 2. Lacerating injuries to plexus

Most require repair

Sharp (neat) transection
  Primary (within 72 h) repair best
  End-to-end suture can be done with good results (65%)

Blunt (ragged) transection
  If seen acutely, tack down stumps to maintain length
  Secondary or delayed repair best (several weeks)
  Grafts likely unless stumps tacked down; results with grafts a little better than 50%

Some elements with serious loss due to lacerating injury are not transected but are contused and/or stretched (10%).

If operation was 6 weeks or more after injury, intraoperative stimulation and recording of nerve action potentials (NAPs) were used to decide whether the contused segment of the element needed resection (Table 2).

Gunshot Wounds

Decisions whether to operate and when to operate on plexus GSWs are much more pressing than those for lacerating injuries, in part because of a greater number of cases in some parts of the world even in peacetime. In addition, GSWs usually (85% of the time) leave the injured element(s) in continuity rather than transecting them; thus there is a possibility, but an extremely variable one, for spontaneous recovery. The older literature concerning GSWs to the plexus favors for the most part a nonoperative, expectant approach or operation only for very favorable elements. Much of this work was based on wartime experience, some of which was very closely analyzed particularly by the allies [6, 21]. More recently, even a report on a small number of cases seen in Vietnam urged a conservative approach to the neural portion of the injury [20].

In the interim, it has become clear that many plexus GSWs with complete loss in the distribution of one or more elements do not improve to the level that timely exploration and repair using intraoperative electrophysiologic assessment and microscopic techniques can currently achieve. The criteria currently used at LSUMC to select patients with GSWs to the plexus for operation and the timing for the procedures are outlined in Table 3. In a 19-year period at LSUMC, 90 patients with GSW to the plexus were operated on. In 75 of these, follow-up has been at least 2 years, the average length of follow-up being 46 months. The average interval from injury to operation in those not requiring immediate operation on the plexus was 17 weeks. Those selected for operation were seriously injured, as indicated by the fact that 30 required initial vascular repair, usually by grafts. In addition, eight patients had acute thoracotomies for pulmonary injury. Six patients required repair of a false or pseudo-aneurysm, usually in the early days or weeks after wounding. Neural loss as well as pain was progressive in most of these aneurysm cases. Of the 75 plexus

Table 3. GSWs to the plexus

Usual indications for operation

Immediate: Occluded or transected major vessel, open pulmonary wound, compression by clot, associated aneurysm or A-V fistula, and/or orthopedic shoulder injuries requiring immediate stabilization.[a] External neurolysis of those elements in continuity. Tack up stumps of elements transected to maintain length.

Delayed (2–5 months after GSW):
   Persistent complete clinical and EMG loss in the distribution of one or more elements
   Severe noncausalgic pain resistant to medication in less complete injuries

Usual indications for not operating
   Improved complete or incomplete loss in the early months after GSW
   Loss restricted to lower elements unless pain difficult to control
   Referral 1 year or more after GSW

---
[a] Four patients in our series required relatively acute sympathectomy for true causalgia.

operative cases with adequate follow-up, lesions were centered at a truncal level in 19, cord level in 21, and cord to nerve level in 35.

If clinical and EMG deinnervational change did not begin to reverse in the early months after wounding, the injuries were explored usually by a supra- and/or infraclavicular approach. Occasionally, a posterior subscapular approach was used [12]. A total of 22 elements were found transected and were repaired usually by grafts. Results in this relatively small subset were best with upper elements such as C5, C6, or C7, upper or middle trunks, or their more distal outflows. The majority of injured elements were found in continuity and were evaluated intraoperatively by stimulation and stimulation and recording studies (NAPs) [11, 13]. As can be seen in Table 4, 47 of 164 lesions to elements considered complete by both clinical examination and EMG were found intraoperatively to have NAPs across their lesions and were spared resection or had a "split" or partial repair. Grade 3 or better results in those spared resection based on NAP recordings were 95%. Of the 96 elements repaired by grafts, 51 recovered to grade 3 or better while 13 of the 20 sutured end-to-end reached a grade 3 or better level. Although not shown in tabular form in this paper, only 7 of 56 elements felt to be incomplete or recovering preoperatively did not show response to stimulation or NAPs. These required resection and repair. One such element was a C7 to middle trunk injury. Other "incomplete" lesions found not to be regenerating included those to lateral and posterior cords and lateral cord to median and medial cord to median injuries. Six of these seven "unexpected" lesions were relatively focal and could be repaired by end-to-end suture. Five of these recovered significant function. The one C7 to middle trunk lesion felt to be incompletely injured preoperatively but having absence of NAPs at operation was repaired by grafts and fortunately recovered to a grade 3 level.

The 51 cases which did not have plexus exploration showed a relatively low incidence of severe vascular and/or pulmonary injuries acutely and usually had incomplete loss which improved with time. Pain was usually well controlled by

Table 4. Results of GSWs in continuity with complete loss

	NAP		Results			
	P	Ab	Neurolysis	Suture	Graft	Imp
Roots to Trunk						
C5–C6 to UT (13)	3	10	3/3	0/0	10/7	0/0
C7 to MT (10)	1	9	1/1	0/0	9/4	0/0
C8–T1 to L.T. (12)	3	9	3/3	0/0	8/2	1/0
Divisions to Cords						
Lateral (9)	3	6	3/3	1/1	5/4	0/0
Medial (13)	5	8	5/5	1/0	4/1[a]	3/0
Posterior (12)	3	9	3/3	2/1	7/5	0/0
Cords to Nerves						
Lat. to M.C.N. (10)	3	7	3/3	2/2	5/5	0/0
Lat. to med. (28)	10	18	9/7	5/4	14/9[b]	0/0
Med. to med. (19)	3	16	2/2	4/2	13/7	0/0
Med. to ulnar (20)	6	14	5/5	2/0	12/2[a]	1/0
Post. to radial (16)	7	9	6/6	2/2	8/4	0/0
Post. to axillary (2)	0	2	0/0	1/1	1/1	0/0
Total (164)	47	117	43/41	20/13	96/51	5/0

NAP, Nerve action potential; P, present distal to lesion; Ab, absent distal to lesion; Imp, repair impossible due to lesion length.
[a] One split or partial graft repair with grade 3 or better results.
[b] Two split or partial graft repairs with grade 3 or better results.

pharmacologic means although one patient with causalgia required a sympathectomy. Six patients with more severe loss were unfortunately referred much to late for a direct repair of their plexus lesions.

Stretch/Contusion Injuries

Controversy concerning the value of operation, its timing, and patient selection remains maximal for these lengthy and usually proximal lesions. Some consider few or none of these patients to be candidates for operation whereas others feel all should be explored despite variations in the extent and level of their injury. For purposes of this discussion, the less severe plexus stretch lesions producing sensory symptoms without motor loss and those with a relatively rapid reversal of motor loss are excluded. The latter are usually neuropraxic lesions such as are sometimes seen in sports injuries. Nonetheless, even some stretch injuries of a more serious nature recover spontaneously with time. Table 5 presents data collected by Wynn Parry and published in 1980 [32]. It is unclear how many patients had absolutely complete loss in the distribution of the roots noted. The LSUMC data would indicate that if complete initial loss persisting for several months is used as a criterion, not quite as many patients spontaneously

Table 5. Nonoperative management of stretch contusion. (From [32])

Location	Results
C5–C6	2/3 recovered biceps, 1/3 some shoulder (36 patients)
C5, C6, C7	1/3 recovered biceps and some shoulder (50 patients)
C5, C6, C7, C8, T1	20% recovered biceps, 16% triceps, 7% finger flexion (84 patients)

regain useful recovery. Nonetheless, the point made by Wynn Parry is still a very important one because some patients do recover significant function with time and without the help of surgery. It is also equally clear that a number of severe stretch injury patients are not candidates for direct repair of their plexus. The most frequent reason is that some stretch injuries are very proximal involving roots close to the spinal cord and/or the cord itself. In the case of the sensory roots, this presents a preganglionic level of injury. If the sensory root has such a proximal level of injury, usually the anterior or motor root does as well. Successful direct repair of the motor root at such a proximal level is technically difficult even though it may in some cases be achievable [26].

Direct repair is impossible if roots are avulsed from cord, or secondary cord damage makes regeneration through the grafts unlikely. Some of these patients may be candidates for substitutive or neurotization procedures, but most are not candidates for direct repair [18, 19]. Other nonoperative stretch cases include those confined to lower elements such as C8, and T1 or lower trunk to medial cord where results with repair except in children or infants are poor. A third group of plexus stretch injuries which seldom benefit from direct repair comprises those adults seen 1 year or later after injury. Time limitations are very real particularly when one needs to place relatively lengthy grafts, as is the case with most operated stretch injuries.

Specific Points about Selection of Patients for Operation

The initial question to be answered is whether or not loss is complete in the distribution of one or more plexus elements. Thus, a patient with absent supraspinatus, infraspinatus, biceps/brachialis, and brachioradialis but spared forearm and hand muscles has in one sense incomplete brachial plexus palsy but in another sense has complete loss in the distribution of two elements, C5 to upper trunk and C6 to upper trunk. *Complete loss in the distribution of one or more elements may reverse with time but is much less likely to do this than incomplete loss.* This makes the patient with complete loss a more likely candidate for surgery than one with incomplete loss.

The next question to be answered is, if loss is complete in the distribution of one or more elements, does it begin to reverse clinically or on EMG in the early months following injury? Particularly important is whether motor rather than sensory loss reverses, since sensory "improvement" may be due to overlap from adjacent normally innervated territories. In addition, true sensory regener-

Table 6. Selection of stretch injuries for operation

Clinical questions
  Is lesion complete or incomplete in distribution of one or more elements?
  Does significant motor (not sensory) improvement occur in first 4 months?
  If at a root level, how proximal?
Relative "stops"
  Winging of scapula – long thoracic nerve
  Rhomboid paralysis – dorsal scapular nerve
  Diaphragm paralysis – phrenic nerve
  Extensive paraspinal deinnervation by EMG
  Sensory potentials (C7, C8, T1); higher roots may still be operable
  Myelopathy and/or fracture/dislocation of spine
Less certain "stops"
  Total flail arm
  Sensory improvement without motor improvement
  Horner's syndrome
  Meningoceles at some (usually lower levels) but not all levels
    False positive and negative rates are significant
    Levels above those with meningoceles may or may not be reparable

---

ation, although suggesting the possibility of subsequent motor recovery, does not guarantee it. If the stretch injury is supraclavicular and thus most likely at a spinal nerve or root level, one needs to try to determine how far proximally the lesion extends. Such an approach requires a combination of preoperative clinical, electrodiagnostic, and radiologic studies [29].

Few of the individual "stops" listed in Table 6 are absolute in the sense of negating the possibility of a successful operation. On the other hand, if a number of them are present, they suggest very strongly a proximal lesion. Such lesions are usually irreparable, at least by direct repair of the root related to the finding. Presence of a "stop" related to one root suggests *but does not prove* proximal injury to other roots as well. It suggests such but does not prove it.

Long thoracic nerve has a variable origin but is usually contributed to by C5, C6, and C7, and sometimes even C8. The nerve itself originates from the posterior aspect of the C6 or C7 root, so loss of serratus anterior indicates a very proximal injury to one or more of these roots. A similar analogy may be used for dorsal scapular loss to rhomboids since input to form this nerve comes from the proximal portions of C5 and C6. Although the phrenic arises from C2, C3, and C4, it travels close to and is usually adherent to C5. As a result, diaphragmatic paralysis in the absence of a penetrating wound to the neck indicates a proximal, and thus most likely irreparable, injury to the C5 root. Since the paraspinal muscles receive input from multiple roots, deinnervation does not mean that all plexus roots have a proximal injury. However, extensive deinnervational changes in an "up and down" fashion does suggest this.

Another indication of proximal and thus irreparable root damage is presence of sensory potentials even though sensation is clinically absent in the distribution of the nerve being tested. This test works best for the lower (C7, C8, T1) roots since precise input points and recording sites that are specific for

C6 and especially C5 are not available, at least to noninvasive testing. However, at operation, recording of cortical somatosensory potentials and NAP studies can be used to test the preganglionic status of the sensory root [13, 28]. Positive sensory potentials in the lower root distribution suggests the possibility that damage to upper roots may be proximal also, but again does not prove it. Indeed, a number of patients with such positive studies for C8 and T1 have had successful repair of C5 and/or C6 level injuries.

Myelopathy with or without fracture and/or dislocation of the spine augers poorly for successful repair of any portion of the plexus. Fracture of a portion of the cervical spine including those of the facets, laminae, and transverse processes make it unlikely that repair will be successful, at least at the fractured level. Less certain "stops" for repair include total flail arm, Horner's syndrome, and meningoceles and other myelographic abnormalities. Patients with total paralysis due to stretch/contusion are very difficult to salvage at least by direct repair. To date, the LSUMC series includes 72 such patients, and a little over half of these have regained some useful upper arm and shoulder function from repair. It has been very difficult to recover distal forearm and hand function in this group of patients with flail arms. Thus, many of these patients had "salvage" type operations in an attempt to regain some proximal function. Success has been variable in those patients in whom repair of C7 and middle trunk was possible. In the few patients whose injury was not very proximal on C8 and T1, repair of these elements was usually unsuccessful. A few exceptions were provided when significant regeneration was shown by intraoperative electrical studies, and as a result lower element(s) were spared resection and subsequently regrew enough axons to restore hand function.

Unfortunately, improvement in sensory examination especially in the shoulder and upper arm does not mean that motor recovery will necessarily follow. Thus, such "apparent" improvement should not be used to deny operation. Presence of Horner's syndrome, although an indication of proximal T1 and/or C8 root injury, does not necessarily mean that roots at higher levels are damaged at such a proximal level.

Myelography

Use of myelography and interpretation of results referable to stretch injuries is a large topic requiring a lengthier discussion [4, 8]. Suffice it to say here, that with myelography as well as scanning techniques there is both a false positive and false negative incidence which is significant (see Fig. 1–3). A meningocele at a given level does strongly suggest that at least enough force was applied at a proximal root level to tear the arachnoid and produce a leak of contrast. It does not necessarily mean that the root is avulsed or pulled apart. More commonly, in our experience, a meningocele means that although the root may still be in gross continuity, it has significant internal damage at a very proximal level. Nevertheless, normal or very mildly damaged roots have been seen at levels with meningoceles, and conversely irreparable roots have been found at levels

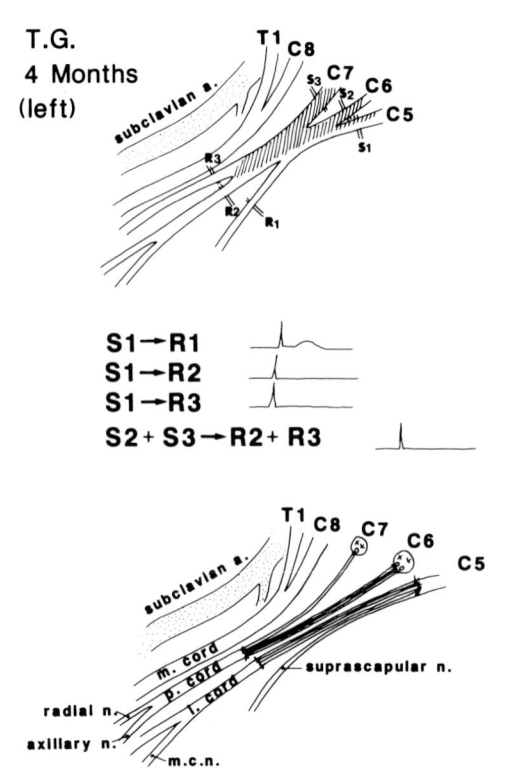

Fig. 1. Left plexus of patient 4 months after severe stretch injury in C5, C6, and C7 distribution. Loss was complete clinically and by EMG at these levels. There was no winging of the scapula or phrenic paralysis, and paraspinal muscles were only partially deinnervated on EMG. Myelography showed a meningocele at C7. Intraoperative NAP recordings were flat for most of C5, C6, C7 outflows except for suprascapular nerve which was split away from upper trunk and a portion of C5 and was preserved. Most of C6 and almost all of C7 were damaged at an intraforminal level close to dura although a small part of both could be used to lead out grafts. C5 was trimmed back to healthier tissue at a foraminal level and could be used to lead out three sural grafts

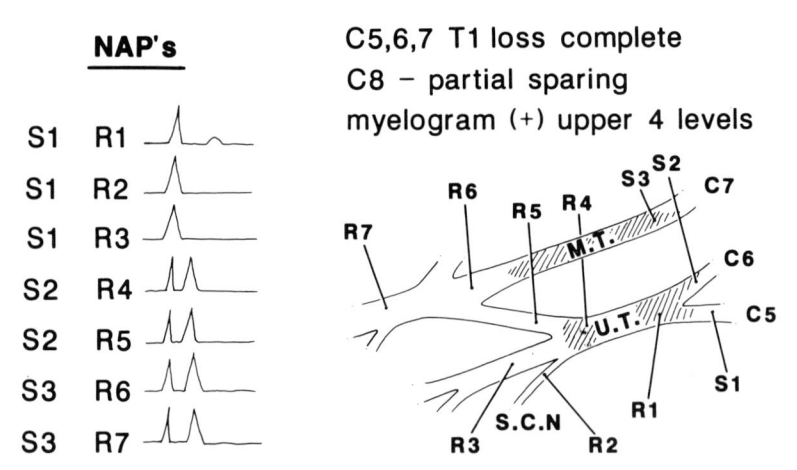

Fig. 2. In this patient operated on 5 months after injury, the myelogram was positive at C5, C6, C7, and C8 even though C8 had partial function in its distribution. Operative NAP recordings confirmed a preganglionic lesion at C6 and C7 since potentials were large and relatively rapid in conduction when recorded from their distal outflows. An early regenerative potential was recorded from C5, C8 had a NAP recorded from lower trunk, and T1 was damaged right up to spinal dura despite absence of a meningocele at this level. As a result, only a neurolysis could be done on this plexus

C.D.
C5,6,7 Loss(C)
6 Months
Stretch

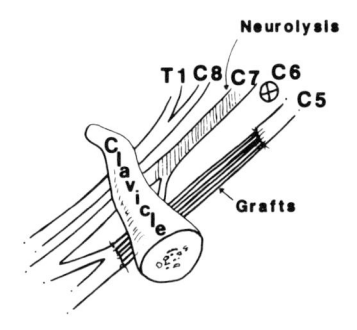

Fig. 3. Despite complete clinical and EMG loss in the distribution of C5, C6 and C7, one element, C7 to middle trunk, was found to be regenerating. C6 which had a meningocele by myelography preoperatively was irreparable. C5 was not regenerating well and was used to lead out sural grafts to the anterior and posterior divisions of the upper trunk

where there have been no meningoceles. Certainly, a number of our patients have now had successful repair of roots at levels where there have not been meningoceles (usually upper levels). This is despite the fact that there have been meningoceles on other roots (usually lower roots) found at operation to have proximal irreparable damage. Nonetheless, if weighed appropriately, myelography is still a useful adjunct in the decision-making process. If a meningocele is present, it is more likely than not, even though not necessarily so, that a root has proximal and thus irreparable damage not reparable by direct repair.

CAT and NMR Studies

CAT scans with intrathecal contrast are of interest in stretch injuries, but unless many cuts are made at each root level, an abnormality can still be missed [8]. Several patients referred to us with CAT scans that have been performed with intrathecal contrast and interpreted as negative have been shown by subsequent myelography to have meningoceles. For this reason, myelography is still preferred in this clinic. NMR has also been of interest for the reason that in some cases one can actually visualize the root. However, this and CAT scan studies are only adjunctive. Information gleaned from them must be weighed accordingly.

**A.J.
5 Months
(right)**

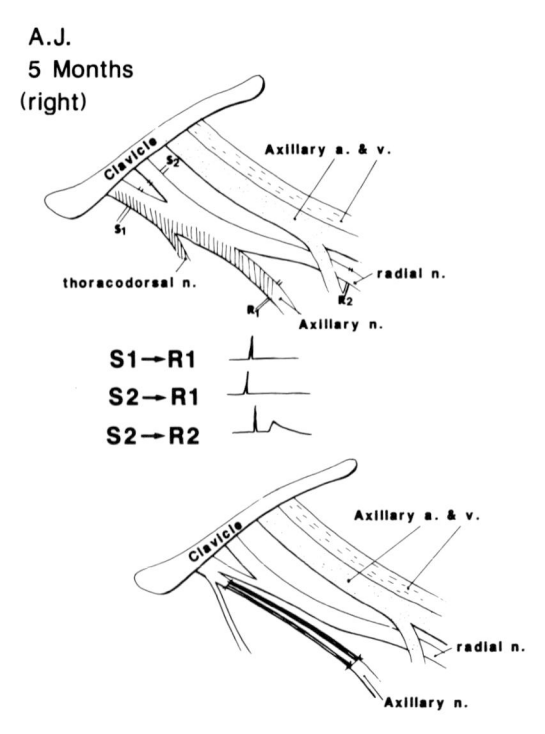

Fig. 4. Axillary nerve stretch injury involving posterior cord. Thoracodorsal nerve could be spared. Grafts for axillary outflow had to run from proximal posterior cord to distal axillary branches near the quadralateral space

Operative Correlations

Even with a selective approach as outlined above, some elements were found to be irreparable because of proximal damage or in a few cases because of loss extending over a substantial length of the plexus. Once the selective process was followed, it was unusual, however, not to find two or more roots or elements which were reparable (see Figs. 1–3). Often, C8 and T1 and sometimes C7 were not reparable, but C5 and C6 were. As can be seen in Figs. 1–4, intraoperative stimulation as well as recording of NAPs was used [13, 15, 33]. Operations in this category of injury were done 4 or more months after the accident (mean, 23 weeks). As a result, 20% of the elements so evaluated showed evidence of early regeneration by presence of a NAP and/or distal muscle contraction on stimulation of the element. This was despite the fact that preoperative clinical and EMG evaluation indicated complete deinnervation. Although regenerating well, axons had either not reached distal inputs or had not done so in enough numbers to reverse either clinical loss or deinnervational change by EMG. In addition, based on preoperative studies, some roots considered to have postganglionic injuries were proven by NAP and evoked cortical studies to have preganglionic injuries. In these instances, NAP recordings showed a relatively large fast-conducting response inconsistent with regeneration (Fig. 2). Moreover, evoked cortical responses obtained by stimulating proximal root(s) and recording from contralateral parietal scalp

Table 7. LSUMC surgical results: stretch contusion (percentage attaining a grade 3 or better result)

Elements with best results (C5, C6, U.T., lateral and posterior cords)	
Neurolysis	90%
Direct suture	71%
Grafts	50%
Elements with worse results (C8, T1, L.T., medial cord)	
Neurolysis	86%
Direct suture	29%
Grafts	28%

On exploration, repair found to be limited or impossible in 17% of elements.

were absent (Fig. 2). There were also a few instances in which loss was in the C5 and C6 distribution but at operation C7 was found to be involved and electrically silent. More common with C5, C6, and C7 loss was the finding by intraoperative studies that C7 was regenerating (Fig. 3). In other cases, the supraclavicular portion of the C5 to upper trunk outflow was recovering and was spared resection (Fig. 1).

In patients with flail arms selected for surgery, it was unusual not to be able to repair one or more roots. Elements thought to be reparable by preoperative studies were usually at an upper root level and usually required grafts. There were important exceptions, however. In these cases one or more roots were found to be regenerating by intraoperative electrical studies and were spared resection (Fig. 2).

Table 7 outlines results to 1980 (as reported in 1983) with 163 elements operatively evaluated in 60 stretch/contusion cases selected for operation [13]. In the next 6 years another 130 cases were selected for operation, and results, although not as closely analyzed as for the 1983 paper, have kept pace. It should be kept in mind that we have attempted direct repair whenever possible or feasible. Neurotization by transfer of intercostal nerves, accessory nerve, or descending cervical plexus has not been attempted [19, 31]. Patients not considered operative candidates for direct repair have had this option explained to them. Some of our patients have had shoulder fusions and/or muscle or tendon transfers, but indications and results of these reconstructive procedures are not assessed in this paper.

Iatrogenic Injury

Between 1968 and 1985, 36 patients with iatrogenic injuries were seen, and 30 of these came to operation. Five of the six not operated on were seen 1 year or later after injury and were thus felt to be unsuitable for repair or had partial injuries which improved with time. The sixth case was a lower trunk to medial cord injury secondary to a thoracic-outlet procedure in an older adult.

Table 8. Iatrogenic injuries of the plexus

Timing
    Undue delay in operation if loss is complete or severe, is unwarranted despite origin of injury.
    Use same guidelines as for lacerating injuries or contusive/stretch injuries.
Operations and results
    Surprisingly good since some are focal.
    Lengthy lesions requiring grafts have limitations just as in other injury categories.

Although loss was complete, the patient did not have a significant pain problem, and it was felt that repair at this level of such elements would not be of great benefit in a patient of this age.

Included in those cases that were operated on were injuries due to first rib resection or scalenectomy for presumed thoracic-outlet syndrome, Putti-Platt or other orthopedic procedures on the shoulder, and lymph node removal or other tumor operations on the neck [23]. Other iatrogenic mechanisms included pseudoaneurysm and/or clot compressing the plexus due to axillary angiography, and plexus injury and/or compression secondary to construction of axillary A-V fistula for renal dialysis or injury associated with transaxillary vascular bypass. Although timing of operation depended more on the timeliness of referral in this category than in others, operation was usually worthwhile. As pointed out by Hudson as well as Kline, delay beyond the usual guidelines applied to other noniatrogenic sharp or blunt injuries is not warranted [14, 22]. As indicated in Table 8, results to date suggest surgical exploration rather than an expectant attitude.

A group of 30 patients were not included in this analysis since they had specialized injuries due to irradiation plexitis. As discussed in earlier papers, operative experience in 14 indicated that pain was sometimes helped. Functional loss was reversed only in cases seen relatively early or in a few instances where tumor external to the plexus and complicating the plexitis could be decompressed. Many more cases were referred late in their course. Severe loss accompanied by lymphedema minimized the likelihood of decompression and neurolysis reversing the loss. Nonetheless, a few of those chosen for operation had severe loss but because of intractable pain were operated on anyway. Several of these had significant improvement in their pain patterns, but others did not. Despite operation, loss tended to progress except in those operated on relatively early in their course. We have not had experience with other surgical approaches to this severe disorder [7].

Summary

Indications and thus the selection process for operation on 355 serious plexus injuries have been discussed. An attempt was made to individualize this process as well as the timing for operation, based on results over a 19-year period with

507 patients with lacerating, gunshot, stretch/contusion, or iatrogenic injuries. The conclusions hinge on two premises. Some serious injuries improve significantly with time and do not require operation. Secondly, some plexus lesions cannot be improved or have minimal return of function as a result of direct repair. In this regard, no attempt was made to analyze the role of secondary procedures such as neurotization or reconstructive procedures such as shoulder fusion or tendon and muscle transfers. It must also be emphasized that the criteria proposed here have evolved over a period of years, have often been proposed previously by others, and have sometimes been arrived at and simultaneously put to use by others. As a result, it should be understood that not all of the operative or nonoperative patients in this series met the proposed criteria. Most of the patients reported here did meet these, but there were exceptions. Hopefully, such patients will meet these guidelines in the future, but even this may be subject to change since plexus injury management has been evolving relatively rapidly over the past 20 years and will undoubtedly continue to change. Nonetheless, patients in the LSUMC series meeting the criteria outlined here have fared well to date. Such a selective approach, especially when properly timed, seems to make sense especially in our present setting in North America.

References

1. Allieu Y, Privat J, Bonnel F (1980) L' exploration chirugicale et le traitement des paralysies du plexus brachial. Réunion annuelle de la Societe' Française de Neurochirurgie. Paris
2. Alnot JY, Augereau B, Frot B (1977) Traitement direct des lesions nervuses dans les paralysies traumatiques por elongation du plexus brachial Chez l'adulte. Chirurgie 103:935–947
3. Amine AR, Sugar O (1976) Repair of a severed brachial plexus, A plea to emergency room physicians. JAMA 235:1039
4. Armington W, Harnsberger H, Osborn A, Seay A (1987) Radiographic evaluation of brachial plexopathy. Am J Neurorad 8:361–367
5. Bonney G (1977) Some lesions of the brachial plexus. Ann R Coll Surg Eng 59:298–306
6. Brooks DM (1949) Open wounds of the brachial plexus. J Bone Joint Surg (Br) 31:17–33
7. Brunelli G (1980) Neurolysis and free microvascular omentum transfer in treatment of post actinic palsies of the brachial plexus. Int Surg 65:515–519
8. Gebarski K, Glazer G, Gebarski S (1982) Brachial plexus, anatomic radiologic, and pathologic correlation using computed tomography. J Comput Assist Tomgr 6:1058–1063
9. Gilbert A, Khouri N, Carliozz H (1980) Birth palsy of the brachial plexus. Surgical exploration and attempted repair in 21 cases. Rev Chir Orthop 66:33–42
10. Hudson AR, Trammer B (1985) Brachial plexus injuries. In: Wilkins RH, Rengachary SS (eds) Neurosurgery. McGraw Hill, New York, pp 1817–1832
11. Hudson AR, Dommisse I (1977) Brachial plexus injury, due to GSW. Canad Med Assoc J 117:1162–1164
12. Kline DG, Kott J, Barnes G, Bryant L (1978) Exploration of selected brachial plexus lesions by the posterior subscapular approach. J Neurosurg 49:872–880
13. Kline DG, Judice DJ (1983) Operative management of selected brachial plexus lesions. J Neurosurg 58:631–649

14. Kline DG, Hudson AR (1984) Complications of nerve injury and nerve repair. In: Greenfield L (ed), Complications in surgery and trauma. Lippincott, Philadelphia, pp 695–708
15. Landi A, Copeland SA, Wynn-Parry CB, Jones SJ (1980) Role of somatosensory evoked potentials and nerve conduction studies in the surgical management of brachial plexus injuries. J Bone Joint Surg (Br) 62:492–496
16. Leffert RD (1985) Brachial plexus injuries. Churchill Livingstone, London
17. Millesi H (1984) Brachial plexus injuries – management and results. Clin Plast Surg 11:115–120
18. Narakas A (1981) Brachial plexus surgery. Orthop Clin North Am 12:303–323
19. Narakas A (1984) Thoughts on neurotization or nerve transfers in irreparable nerve lesions. Clin Plast Surg 11:153–159
20. Nelson KG, Jolley PC, Thomas PA (1968) Brachial plexus injuries associated with missile wounds of the chest: report of nine cases from Vietnam. J Trauma 8:268–275
21. Nulsen FE, Slade WW (1956) Recovery following injury to the brachial plexus. In: Woodhall B, Beebe G (eds) Peripheral nerve regeneration: a follow-up study of 3,656 WW II injuries. Veterans Administration, Washington DC, pp 389–408
22. Samii M (1975) Use of microtechniques in peripheral nerve surgery – experience with 300 cases. In: Handa H (ed) Microneurosurgery, Univ Park Press, Baltimore
23. Richards R, Hudson A, Bertoia, Urbaniak J, Waddell J (1987) Injury to the brachial plexus during Putti-Platt and Bristow procedures. Am J Sports Med 15:374–380
24. Sedel L (1982) The results of surgical repair of brachial plexus injuries. J Bone Joint Surg (Br) 64:54–66
25. Seddon H (1972) Surgical disorders of peripheral nerves. Williams & Wilkins, Baltimore, pp 174–198
26. Smith B, Hurst J, Kline D, Richter H (1986) Posterior laminotomy approach to brachial plexus roots in primates. Surgical Forum 37:487–489
27. Solonen K, Vastamaki M, Strom B (1984) Surgery of the brachial plexus. Acta Orthop Scand 436–440
28. Sugioka H, Tsuyamu N, Hora T (1982) Investigation of brachial plexus injuries by intraoperative cortical somatosensory evoked potentials. Arch Orthop Trauma Surg 99:143–151
29. Sunderland S (1978) Nerves and nerve injuries. Churchill Livingstone, New York
30. Terzis J (1987) microreconstruction of peripheral nerve injuries. Saunders, Philadelphia
31. Tsuyama J, Hura T, Nagano A (1987) Intercostal nerve crossing as a treatment of irreparably damaged brachial plexus. In: Recent developments in orthopedic surgery. Noble J, Galasko C (eds) Manchester Univ Press, Manchester
32. Wynn Parry CB (1980) The management of traction lesions of the brachial plexus and peripheral nerve injuries in the upper limb: a study in teamwork (The Roscoe Clarke Memorial Lecture, 1979). Injury 11:265–285
33. Zalis A, Rodriquez A, Oester Y, Mains D (1972) Evaluation of nerve regeneration by means of evoked potentials. J Bone Joint Surg 54(A):1246–1253

Free Greater Omentum Transfer After Neurolysis for Actinic (X-Ray) Lesions of the Brachial Plexus

G. BRUNELLI, L. MONINI, and F. BRUNELLI, Brescia/Italy

X-ray radiation is still in use, mainly after mastectomy for breast cancer to avoid recurrence in lymphnodes, axilla, and supraclavicular fossa but also for other conditions (e.g., Hodgkin's disease, hemangiomas). Radiation causes severe devascularization and paraneural sclerosis (Fig. 1) that result in chronic nerve compression, axonostenosis, and axonal suffering with progressive palsy, which in more than 50% of cases is associated with severe pain, often so excruciating that it may lead to suicide.

Simple neurolysis is not at all effective as it is followed by a new scar, generally worse than before. Local skin and muscular flaps as well as pedicled greater omentum flap (Kirikuta 1963) have been suggested and tried, with fair and with poor results. Clodius et al. (1973) suggested using the free greater omentum flap to improve the big lymphatic arm. Since 1977 we have used a free microvascular greater omentum flap to wrap around the elements of the brachial plexus in the axilla and supraclavicular fossa after neurolysis. We consider this operation the only useful one because the pedicled greater omentum does not reach the supraclavicular fossa, and very often this area is

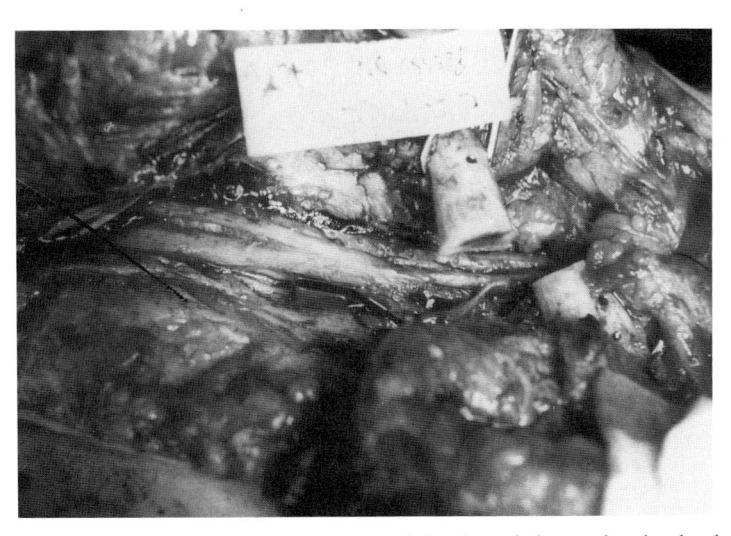

Fig. 1. Severe sclerosis of the tissue around the plexus below and under the clavicle in a patient treated with 7000 rad 13 years ago

severely affected by radiations. An operation for radiation plexitis must provide a good padding protection and blood supply while avoiding a new scar in contact with the neurolyzed structure. This is the only way to stop pain and avoid recurrence. When we originally introduced this operation it was hoped also to improve the palsy. We now know, however, that this surgery does not affect the palsy. Even if in some cases a very slight improvement may be seen for a short time, the palsy very soon resumes, if also at a slower rate. Pain, on the other hand, is always relieved and in the majority of cases disappears completely. Therefore, indications for neurolysis with free greater omentum transfer are limited to pain in established palsy, severe radiodermatitis with pain, and beginning palsies in order to prevent the onset of pain.

We have treated 86 cases of actinic brachial plexus lesions in 11 years; 37 were not operated on either because there was no pain, or because it was very mild; 3 underwent simple neurolysis (in the earliest days); 2 received local flaps after neurolysis; 38 had greater omentum transfer after neurolysis; and in 6 the operation was interrupted (with regard to greater omentum transfer) due to the finding of cancer metastasis in the axilla. After the first cases, in which we searched for local recipient vessels only to realize that no sound vessels could be found in the radiated area, we have routinely used facial artery and branches of the external jugular vein as recipient vessels.

The greater omentum is taken in a convenient size (not too large), in general with two radiating vascular axes coming from the right gastroepiploic artery. Also, the donor vein is the right gastroepiploic vein because in one case we have seen no connection between the right and left blood supplies of the greater omentum (Fig. 2). The operation is carried on by two teams, one taking the greater omentum through a xiphoumbilical incision and the other starting

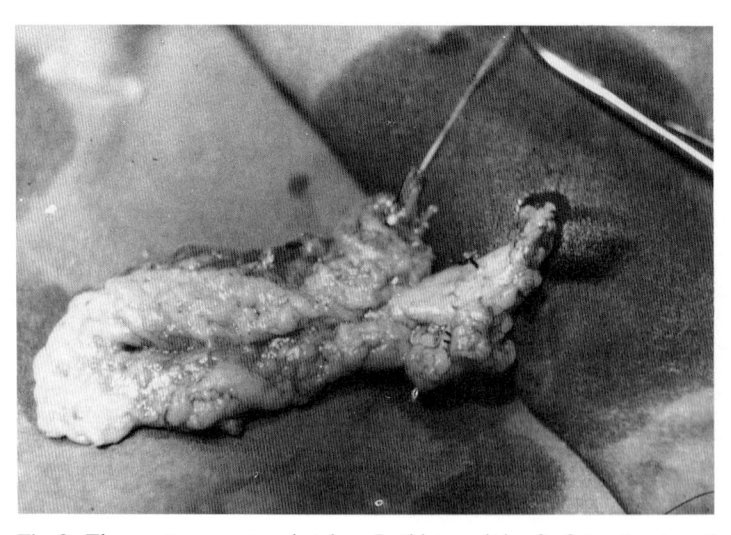

Fig. 2. The greater omentum is taken. In this case it is of a fatty structure (in other cases it is much thinner). Perfusion of the right gastroepiploic artery is in progress

slightly earlier and freeing all the constricted elements of the brachial plexus by means of a careful neurolysis below and above the clavicle. Neurolysis can be very difficult in certain cases in which all the tissues are very severely damaged, and cleavage planes cannot be found. In two cases we removed en bloc such a piece of scar; we then grafted several nerves and padded them with the omentum. The omentum may be difficult to draw in case of previous abdominal surgery. It may be thin or very fat. After neurolysis the omentum is wrapped around the elements of the brachial plexus passing under the clavicle and trying to adapt it to the single terminal branches, cords, and, if necessary, trunks.

Microsurgical suture of the right gastroepiploic artery is performed with the homolateral facial artery under the angle of the mandible. The right gastroepiploic vein is sutured either end-to-end to a branch of the jugular vein or end-to-side to the vein itself (Fig. 3). We have encountered two complications consisting of the worsening of the radiodermatitis with skin sores; both of these healed quickly by means of local rotatory flaps. The mistakes that are possible in this surgery include (a) a neurolysis which is too limited, (b) the use of an oversized greater omentum flap, (c) an anastomosis with damaged receiving vessels, and (d) the removal of the clavicle.

Results depend on several factors, in particular the dose of radiations, the severity and age of the lesion, the patient's individual response, and the quality of surgery. Our results are shown in Table 1.

The repeated objections that it is a time-consuming and risky operation, and that muscle flaps could be used with simpler surgery leading to the same

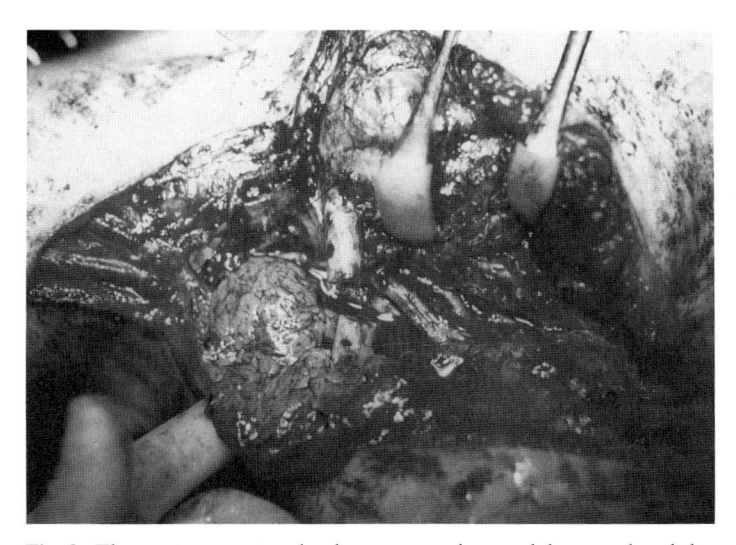

Fig. 3. The greater omentum has been wrapped around the neurolyzed elements of the plexus, and anastomosis was performed of the right gastroepiploic artery to the facial artery and of the gastroepiploic vein to the external jugular vein. The finger is showing the revascularization

Table 1. Results in actinic brachial plexus operations (n = 42)

	Pain		Palsy		Radiodermatitis		Sensation		ROM	
Neurolysis (n = 3)	Severe	2	Unchanged	3	Unchanged	2	Unchanged	2	Worsened	3
	Worsened	1			Worsened	1	Worsened	1		
Neurolysis and skin flap (n = 2)	Severe	2	Unchanged	2	Improved	2	Unchanged	1	Worsened	2
							Worsened	1		
Neurolysis and greater omentum microvascular graft (n = 34)	Disappeared	28	Temporarily improved	1	Improved	21	Improved	2	Improved	11
	Much improved	3	Slightly, temporarily improved	3	Unchanged	11	Temporarily improved	4	Unchanged	19
	Improved	3	Unchanged	20	Worsened	2	Unchanged	19	Worsened	4
			Immediately worsened	5			Worsened	4		
			Tardily worsened	5						
Metastasis (n = 3)	Closure									

414   G. Brunelli et al.

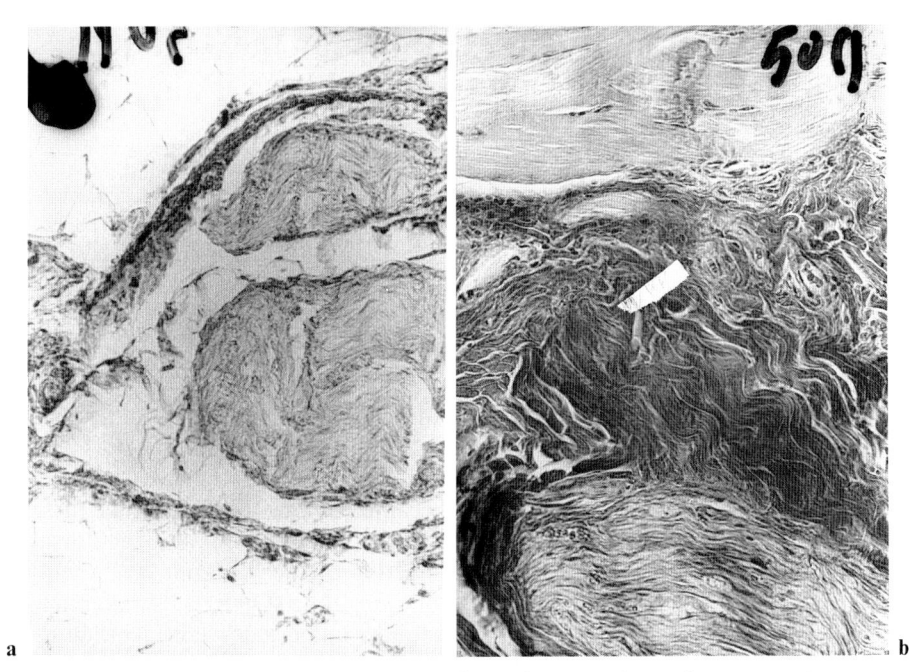

Fig. 4. Experimental wrapping around the femoral nerve of rats by means of greater omentum (**a**) and of muscles (**b**). Note the thin connective tissue around the nerve with use of the greater omentum but the great amount of scar formation with use of the muscle

results led us to carry out an experimental study on 40 rats. In 20 we wrapped the femoral nerve with the greater omentum while in the others the nerve was wrapped with the abdominal wall muscles. Wrapping with muscles produced a large scar between the muscle and the nerve while use of the greater omentum caused only a thin collagen tissue around nerve, which is practically the epineurium of the nerve (Fig. 4).

This demonstrates the superiority of padding with the greater omentum and reassures that in clinical surgery the free greater omentum transfer is also the best method.

References

Brunelli G (1978) Lesioni del plesso brachiale in microchirurgia. Pelizza Brescia, pp 78–97
Brunelli G (1980) Neurolysis and free microvascular omentum transfer in the treatment of postactinic palsies of the brachial plexus. Int Surg 65:6
Clodius O, Uhlschmid G, Madridtsch W (1973) Chirurgische Möglichkeiten der Lymphödembehandlung. Folio Angiol 21:304–313
Dupot C, Menard Y (1972) Transposition of greater omentum for reconstruction of the chest wall. Plast Reconstr Surg 49:263
Kirikuta I (1963) L'emploi du grand epiploon dans la chirurgie du sein cancereux. Presse Medicale, pp 71:1

Dorsal Root Entry Zone Lesions for the Treatment of Post-Brachial Plexus Avulsion Injury Pain

A. H. Friedman, B. S. Nashold, and J. Carter, Durham NC, USA

Introduction

The pain which occurs concomitant to a brachial plexus avulsion injury has proven to be recalcitrant to most conventional forms of therapy. In 1976, Nashold et al. proposed destruction of the substantia gelatinosa as possible therapy for this type of pain [6]. It soon became obvious that in practice these surgical lesions destroy not only the substantia gelatinosa but also the dorsal horn, Lissauer's tract, and the adjacent portion of the posterior and lateral funiculi, and thus were termed dorsal root entry zone (DREZ) lesions. Early reports of this form of therapy with short follow-up periods were encouraging [5], but we know from our experience with other neuroablative procedures such as percutaneous cordotomy and trigeminal rhizotomy that immediate pain relief does not necessarily portend long-term relief of pain. In order to assess the long-term efficacy of DREZ lesions, we undertook this retrospective analysis of 56 patients who had undergone DREZ lesions for the treatment of intractable pain secondary to a brachial plexus avulsion.

Patient Profile

Fifty-six patients who had sustained a brachial plexus avulsion underwent DREZ lesions at the Duke University Medical Center for the treatment of intractable pain. This group comprised 54 men and 2 women with a mean age of 27 years. Of these, 18 incurred the injury in an automobile accident, 21 in a motorcycle accident, and 17 in a fall or industrial accident. In all but two patients, the pain began within 4 months of the accident responsible for the avulsion. Approximately one-third of the patients noted that their pain was present within hours of the injury.

Patients described two distinct components of their pain. In any particular patient both elements of pain may be manifest equally, or one component may be prevalent. The first component of the pain that most patients note is constant and persistent. This pain is most often burning in nature but is sometimes described as the sensation of intense needles and pins, an abnormal uncomfortable posturing of the finger and wrist joints or rarely a throbbing sensation. Most frequently, this pain is most intense in the hand or fingers, but it is occasionally confined to one side of the patient's forearm. The pain does not respect dermatomal boundaries, but it always resides in a portion of the anesthetic region. Unlike causalgia, it is not associated with hyperesthesia and is not aggravated by severe cold. This pain is often ameliorated by distraction and exacerbated by boredom.

The second component of the pain is not persistent but appears in paroxysms. The pain is usually crushing in nature with each paroxysm lasting up to 5 min. The paroxysms are not triggered or alleviated by any particular activity although some patients report that manipulation of the analgesic extremity causes the pain to subside more quickly. The paroxysms do not follow any particular time pattern, and thus the patients cannot anticipate their onset.

All patients in this series had suffered pain for at least 5 months prior to their DREZ lesion procedure. The diagnosis of brachial plexus avulsion was usually strongly suspected from the patient's neurologic examination, and in most cases it was corroborated by meningoceles seen on cervical myelogram. Early in the series, all patients underwent psychiatric evaluation, a trial of biofeedback, a trial of transcutaneous nerve stimulation, and an extensive trial of medication. Selected patients had undergone a spinothalamic tractotomy, a mesencephalotomy, or placement of a dorsal column stimulator. Once DREZ lesions proved to be an effective and safe procedure, patients were given only a trial of transcutaneous nerve stimulation and a trial of selected medications prior to surgery.

Of our patients 80% were either examined or contacted by telephone at the time of this analysis. Follow-up ranged from 1 to 13 years following surgery (Fig. 1). Patients who were lost to follow-up were rated as poor results if their hospital records recorded a return of pain at any time following surgery. Patients lost to follow-up were considered to have good results only if pain relief was documented to have lasted more than 1 year. Six patients who were documented to have had pain relief 3 months following surgery, but who had no further documented follow-up were excluded from this series.

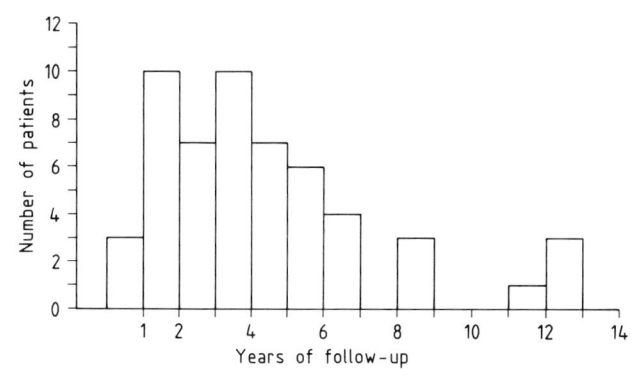

Fig. 1. Duration of follow-up (1–13 years). Three patients with early pain recurrence were lost to follow-up within 1 year of surgery

Procedure

The general method for making DREZ lesions has been well described [1]. Although the lesions in the cervical spinal cord can be made through hemilaminectomies, full laminectomies are generally used so that the contralateral DREZ with intact nerve roots can be viewed to assist in localization. Our technique for lesioning the DREZ has evolved. Early in our experience, the posterior lateral sulcus was localized using low-power loupe magnification and lesions were made using up to 70 mA current held for 15 s. These large lesions were spaced approximately 13 mm apart so that relatively few lesions covered the area of the avulsions. More recently the posterior lateral sulculi has been defined using the operating microscope, and lesions have been produced using a 0.25-mm diameter electrode with a 2-mm uninsulated tip. The lesions have been spaced approximately 1 mm apart and produced by heating the electrode to 75 °C for 15 s. Using our initial technique, an avulsion involving the C5-T1 nerve roots would be treated with 16–25 lesions. Using our present size lesions, 50–80 lesions were needed to lesion the same area.

Results

Results were graded employing a scale which took into account the patient's postoperative functional impairment and need for analgesic agents. The patient's outcome was considered good if the patient was either completely free of pain, or if the residual pain did not require analgesics and did not interfere with the patient's daily activities. Pain relief was judged to be fair if the patient required nonnarcotic analgesics, and poor if the patient was taking narcotic analgesics, or if the residual pain interfered with the patient's normal activities or employment. Although this rating system relegates several patients with significant pain relief to the poor result category, it yields a measure of the functional status of our patients.

By these criteria 33 (59%) patients were rated as having received good pain relief, 7 (12%) were rated as having obtained fair pain relief, and 16 (29%) were rated as having obtained poor pain relief.

Of the 16, who were not afforderded pain relief from surgery, 14 noted the pain to return within 7 months of surgery. Of these 14 patients, 10 noted the pain to return within 2 months of surgery. Two patients noted a recurrence of significant pain more than 1 year after surgery. One of these patients noted his burning elbow pain to have returned 13 months following his surgery, and a second noted that his burning pain had returned 2 years following his surgery. Three additional patients noted a partial recurrence of their pain that was not severe enough to require narcotic analgesics or limit their activity. Two noted a partial recurrence of their burning pain 1 year following surgery, and one noted the appearance of burning pain which replaced her preoperative stabbing pain 6 months following her surgery. During our survey, only one patient reported that his pain was worse following surgery than before surgery. In this patient, the character of the pain was unchanged by the procedure.

There appears to be a correlation between the number of lesions made and the effectiveness of the procedure. Of those patients treated early in our series with a small number of large lesions 6 (31%) reported good results, 2 (11%) reported fair results, and 11 (57%) reported poor results. Of the patients treated with multiple small lesions 27 (73%) reported good results, 5 (13.5%) reported fair results, and 5 (13.5%) reported poor results. Although the average period of follow-up was longer in those patients treated with larger lesions, the patients treated with smaller lesions were followed well beyond the period of time at which pain was most likely to recur (Fig. 2).

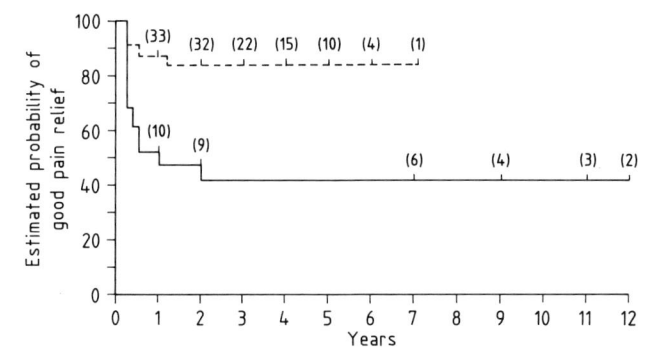

Fig. 2. Kaplan-Meiers curves comparing probability of pain relief following dorsal root entry zone lesions. *Upper curve*, patients receiving more than 40 lesions; *lower curve*, patients receiving fewer than 40 lesions; *numbers in parenthesis*, number of patients at risk for a recurrence at any given time

Minor neurological deficits were not uncommon following surgery. Some 50% of patients (27/56) were noted to have a new subjective or objective neurological deficit following cervical DREZ lesions. Even using multiple smaller lesions, 40% of patients (15/37) were found to have some new minor neurological deficit. Some 25% of patients (9/37) noted a change in sensation over their ipsilateral lower extremity. Although their neurological examination remained normal, the patients noted a "tight" sensation over the ipsilateral lower extremity. Of the patients treated with multiple small lesions 27% were noted to have an ipsilateral lower extremity motor deficit. Some patients noted clumsiness or easy fatigability of the ipsilateral lower extremity while others noted no deficit but were found to have increased deep tendon reflexes. No patient was unable to ambulate or needed support to ambulate.

Discussion

Persistent pain, which is recalcitrant to most forms of therapy, is a common sequelae of a brachial plexus avulsion injury [13, 14]. Despite the constant burning pain noted by most patients, sympathetic blocks, stellate ganglion blocks, intravenous guanethidine, and narcotic medications have little effect [13, 14, 15]. Transcutaneous nerve stimulation has been reported to afford good pain relief in 34 of 56 patients in one series [14, 15]. Deep brain stimulation has been reported to be effective in alleviating pain in a small number of isolated cases [3, 4, 10]. Despite these encouraging reports of pain relief from electrical stimulation, a relatively high percentage of patients are left with a significant amount of pain.

In 1977, Nashold and Ostdahl reported that DREZ lesions effectively alleviated pain associated with a brachial plexus injury [5]. Their series was small, and they had followed these patients for only a short time. Our experience with other neuroablative procedures such as spinal tractotomy and rhizotomy indicates that short-term pain relief does not automatically imply long-term pain relief. Since most brachial plexus injuries occur in young men with a long life expectancy, we undertook this study to investigate the long-term effects of this procedure. A portion of these results have been published elsewhere [2].

Our data indicate that DREZ lesions afforded patients long-term relief from pain associated with a brachial plexus avulsion injury. Almost all patients who experienced recurrent pain experienced this pain within the 1st year following the surgery. Because this study follows patients for as long as 13 years postoperatively, late recurrence of pain must be rare. Our results are in keeping with other small series of patients reported in the literature [8, 9, 12].

Our data also indicate that the geometry of the DREZ lesion is important in determining long-term outcome. Our patients who were treated with multiple small DREZ lesions had a significantly better outcome ($p \leq 0.02$) than those treated with a few large DREZ lesions. Successful pain relief has been reported following DREZ lesions performed with a laser and partial DREZ lesioning performed by sectioning the anterior aspect of the dorsal root and the lateral portion of Lissauer's tract [7, 11]. How these lesions compare with DREZ lesions produced with an electrode awaits larger series and longer follow-up.

Although minor neurological deficits have become rarer as our DREZ lesions have become smaller, they still may be detected in 40% of patients who undergo a careful postoperative neurological examination. In most cases, the deficit is of no functional detriment to the patient. No patient needs support to ambulate, and the most impaired patients note fatigue only on walking a long distance.

References

1. Friedman AH, Nashold BS Jr (1986) DREZ lesions for relief of pain related to spinal cord injuries. J Neurosurg 65:465–469
2. Friedman AH, Nashold BS Jr, Bronec PR (1988) Dorsal root entry zone lesions for the treatment of brachial plexus avulsion injuries: A follow-up study. Neurosurgery 22:369–373
3. Loeser JD, Ward AA Jr (1967) Some effects of deafferentation on neurons of the cat spinal cord. Arch Neurol (Chicago) 17:629–636

4. Mundinger F, Salamão JF (1980) Deep brain stimulation in mesencephalic lemniscus medialis for chronic pain. Acta Neurochirurgica (Suppl) 30:245–258
5. Nashold BS, Ostdahl RH (1977) Dorsal root entry zone lesions for pain relief. J Neurosurg 51:59–69
6. Nashold BS Jr, Urban B, Zorub DS (1976) Phantom relief by focal destruction of substantia gelatinosa of Rolando. In: Bonica JJ, Albe-Fessard D (eds) Advances in pain research and therapy, vol 1. Raven Press, New York, pp 959–963
7. Powers SK, Adams JE, Edwards MSB, Boggan JE, Hosobuchi Y (1984) Pain relief from dorsal root entry zone lesions made with argon and carbon dioxide microsurgical lasers. J Neurosurg 61:841–847
8. Richter HP, Seitz K (1984) Dorsal root entry zone lesions for the control of deafferentation pain: experiences in ten patients. Neurosurgery 15:956–959
9. Samii M, Moringlane JR (1984) Thermocoagulation of the dorsal root entry zone for the treatment of intractable pain. Neurosurgery 15:953–955
10. Siegfried J, Hood T (1983) Current status of functional neurosurgery. In: Kragenbühl (ed): Advances in technical standards in neurosurgery, vol 3. Springer, Wien, pp 147–185
11. Sindou M, Mifsud JJ, Boisson D, Goutelle A (1986) Selective posterior rhizotomy in the dorsal root entry zone for treatment of hyperspasticity and pain in the hemiplegic upper limb. Neurosurgery 18:587–595
12. Thomas DGT, Jones SJ (1964) Dorsal root entry zone lesion (Nashold's procedure) in brachial plexus avulsion. Neurosurgery 15:966–968
13. Wynn-Parry CB (1984) Brachial plexus injuries. Br J Hosp Med 32:130–139
14. Wynn-Parry CB (1984) Pain in avulsion of the brachial plexus. Neurosurgery 15:960–965
15. Wynn-Parry CB (1974) The management of injuries of the brachial plexus. Proc Royal Soc Med 67:488–490

Dorsal Root Entry Zone Coagulation for Control of Intractable Pain Due to Brachial Plexus Injury

M. SAMII, E. KOHMURA, H. KHALIL, and C. MATTHIES, Hannover/FRG

Introduction

Severe intractable pain is an extremely difficult problem in managing patients with brachial plexus avulsion injury. Pain usually appears within some weeks after a root avulsion. Wynn Parry [7] observed a significant degree of pain in 98 out of 108 patients with root avulsion. Nashold and Ostdahl [4] described the incidence of intractable pain requiring surgical intervention in 20% of plexus avulsion injuries, while pain is an early symptom in 70% of patients. Many attempts – including medication, psychotherapy, acupuncture, cordotomy, mesencephalotomy, thalamotomy, transcutaneous nerve stimulation, dorsal column stimulation, deep brain stimulation – have been tried to relieve the deafferentation pain, however most of them failed to help the patients satisfactorily. Since the successful reports on dorsal root entry zone (DREZ) coagulation by Nashold et al. in 1976 [3] and Nashold and Ostdahl in 1979 [4] the operation has been tried in our clinic [5]. This paper presents indication, surgical technique and results including follow-up series of over 3 years.

Patients and Methods

From March 1980 to March 1987, 32 patients with brachial plexus injuries were treated in our clinic for intractable pain. There were 29 men and 3 women; ages ranged from 18 to 64 years (mean, 35.5). All but one had a traumatic plexus lesion. The cause of injury was a traffic accident in 23, sporting accident in 3, work-related accident in 2, an explosion in 2, and a missile injury and radiation therapy in one each.

Severe intractable pain had begun within some weeks after the injury. Patients usually complained of continuous pain with paroxysmal exacerbation on emotional stress and on weather change. They described the pain as burning, pulling, electric shock, boring, or crushing in the hand. Pain was localized in the dermatomes of the avulsed roots, where anesthesia or severe hypesthesia was commonly found. All patients were disabled, not only due to the flaccid arm but also due to the severe intractable pain. In most of them analgesics, antidepressants, and/or carbamazepine had proven ineffective. Some had already received other surgical intervention without success. The mean duration of pain was 4.4 years. This was 4 months to 1 year in 15, 1–2 years in 7, 2–5 years in 4, 5–10 years in 4, and over 10 years in 2 (longest duration, 41 years).

The first 11 patients were operated on in the semisitting position. Thereafter, the prone position was preferred because of its greater comfort and of its lesser risk. Laminectomy or hemilaminectomy is completed throughout the corresponding cervical segments to the pain distribution. The dura is opened under the microscope. In none of the cases did the spinal cord appear normal. Scarring between the spinal cord and its surrounding, atrophy of the injured side of the cord, or distortion of the cord was found. It is usually difficult to identify the intermediolateral sulcus on the injured side where the sensory roots have been avulsed. One can compare both sides, and the intermediolateral sulcus on the uninjured side is identified without difficulty. The other method is to expose the next intact root both cranially and caudally on the injured side. We now prefer this exposure because electrocoagulation should be made till just adjacent to the intact nerve roots. A hemilaminectomy is sufficient in this instance so that postoperative neck pain can be reduced. Radiofrequency lesions must be made exactly on the imaginary intermediolateral sulcus. The electrode was introduced at an angle of 25° into the spinal cord in the lateromedial direction. Lesions were made at intervals of 1–2 mm with 35–110 mA for 15 s each to produce a circular whitened area extending 1–2 mm beyond the electrode. The dura was closed in a water-tight fashion. Antiedema therapy was started during the operation.

Results

Results were evaluated according to the subjective score of the patients: excellent, pain relief over 75% without need of analgesics; good, pain relief 50%–74% without need of analgesics; fair, pain relief 25%–49% without need of analgesics; poor, pain relief under 25% with analgesics perhaps necessary. At discharge from our clinic, which was usually 2 weeks after the operation, the results in 12 patients were excellent, in 11 good, in 2 fair, in 4 poor, and 3 patients could not score the change exactly as it was fluctuating.

No significant correlation was found between the number of coagulated segments and the result. Pain duration before the DREZ lesion was found to be a significant factor. Excellent or good results were obtained in 23 patients with mean duration of 2.5 years and an average 3.2 coagulated segments, while fair or poor results were found in 6 patients with mean duration of 13 years 11 months and an average 3.1 coagulated segments. Two patients with over 10-year pain duration did not respond to DREZ coagulation (Fig. 1).

Follow-up evaluation was done in March 1987 by means of a questionnaire sent to the patients with at least 3-year follow-up after the operation. Subjective pain was compared to that before operation. Of the 32 patients, six had changed their address, two lived in a foreign country, four gave no answer, one had died of cancer, and five were too early to evaluate; thus 14 patients could be analyzed. The follow-up period ranged between 3 and 6.6 years (mean, 4.5).

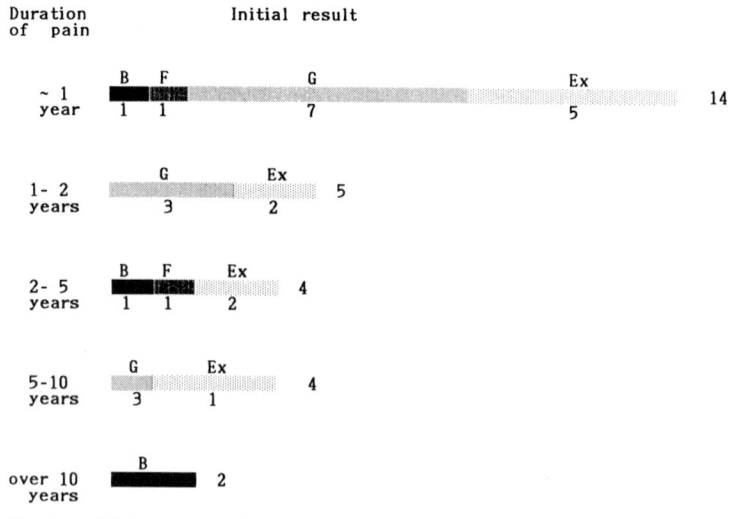

Fig. 1. Initial results and results at various stages of follow-up after DREZ coagulation treatment. *B*, Bad; *F*, fair; *G*, good; *Ex*, excellent

Eight patients reported excellent (two) or good (six) results (57.1%); the results in two were fair and in 4 poor. Seven patients reported no change during the follow-up period (two excellent, four good, one poor); the score in four fell by one grade, in one by two grades, and in one by three grades. In one case the rating rose from poor to good; here an additional procedure had been used. Return of pain after an initial relief has occurred between 3 weeks and 1.5 years.

With regard to morbidity 14 patients were free of complications. Sensory disturbance and/or motor disturbance was the major postoperative complication; 13 patients complained of some kind of sensory disturbance of the ipsilateral leg, i.e., paresthesia or disturbed position sense, immediately after surgery. In nine of these the disturbance has persisted but in a mild form. Nine patients showed moderate weakness of the ipsilateral leg postoperatively, and in three of these minimal weakness has persisted. Four patients complained of neck pain due to the surgical intervention. In one patient anterior cervical fusion was performed due to the neck deformity, and in one patient wound revision was needed to repair a CSF fistula.

Discussion

The severe intractable pain in patients with brachial plexus avulsion injury is believed to be based on the central changes caused by deafferentation. Even now one can only speculate as to the mechanism of the pain. Hypersensitive neuronal pools of the injured DREZ due to deafferentation, injury to spinothalamic and spinoreticular pain pathway, and local dysfunction of the neuronal pools of the DREZ due to facilitatory or inhibitory influences of

Lissauer's tract were suggested by Nashold and Ostdahl [4]. However, one cannot exclude a more central disturbance.

It is not our purpose to discuss the pain mechanism further. The clinical problem is how one can save patients from this disastrous situation. Previous experiences had revealed disappointing results. The results of DREZ lesion reported by Nashold et al. [3] and Nashold and Ostdahl [4] were fascinating. Ten of the 18 patients (56%) with avulsion injury found over 75% pain relief with a follow-up period ranging from 6 months to 3.5 years. In our series, 72% of the patients obtained sufficient pain relief initially, and 57% retained the pain relief even at 3-year follow-up (mean, 4.5; range, 3–6.6). All of the patients with over 50% pain relief reported that they were no longer disabled by the pain, although they have still some kind of pain.

Analysis of the failing results shows that pain duration before the surgical intervention plays a major role. It is reasonable to suppose that another factor, perhaps a psychological change, complicates the pain mechanism further in these patients. Early recurrence of pain after initial success can be explained due to an imperfect lesion.

With regard to morbidity we should be very strict, as the operation is functional in nature. We recorded all the complaints of the patients, even if they were very subtle. In nine patients mild sensory deficit persisted, and in three minimal weakness of the ipsilateral leg. These complications are explained as involvement of the long tracts neighboring to the DREZ. In the series of Thomas and Jones [6] minor deficits were found in 50% and significant change in 12%. Compared to the early reports by Nashold et al. [3] and Nashold and Ostdahl [4], the morbidity seemed to be high. In fact, however, all patients are ambulant, and none is disabled by complications. Special care should be taken to make exact coagulation in the DREZ. Under the microscope DREZ should be carefully identified and appropriate lesions made. Use of a laser instead of a radiofrequency coagulation [2] or use of a neurophysiological monitoring during the operation [1] may help to reduce morbidity.

Due to the destructive nature of the DREZ lesion and the possible morbidity the indication should be carefully considered. The procedure must be reserved in the early stage, as spontaneous relief of pain is not rare [4, 7]. Other types of pain, such as stump pain or causalgia, should be differentiated. Careful analysis of the pain character is necessary to exclude them. Psychological analysis is also important. Before the DREZ coagulation is performed, all possible surgical complications must be well explained to the patient.

Our study confirms the DREZ lesion as a reliable procedure with long-lasting effect. It is the best choice today to save patients from intractable pain following a brachial plexus avulsion injury. Studies examining the mechanism of deafferentation pain could lead to further improvements.

References

1. Campbell JA, Miles J (1984) Evoked potentials as an aid to lesion making in the dorsal root entry zone. Neurosurgery 15:951–952
2. Levy WJ, Nutkiewicz A, Ditmore M (1983) Laser-induced dorsal root entry zone lesions for pain control. J Neurosurg 59:884–886
3. Nashold BS Jr, Urban B, Zorub DS (1976) Phantom relief by focal destruction of substantia gelatinosa of Rolando. In: Bonica JJ, Albe-Fessard D (eds) Advances in pain research and therapy, vol 1. Raven Press, New York, pp 959–963
4. Nashold BS Jr, Ostdahl RH (1979) Dorsal root entry zone lesions for pain relief. J Neurosurg 51:59–69
5. Samii M, Moringlane JR (1984) Thermocoagulation of the dorsal root entry zone for the treatment of intractable pain. Neurosurgery 15:953–955
6. Thomas DGT, Jones SJ (1984) Dorsal root entry zone lesions (Nashold's procedure) in brachial plexus avulsion. Neurosurgery 15:966–968
7. Wynn Parry CB (1980) Pain in avulsion lesions of the brachial plexus. Pain 9:41–53

Postoperative Treatment in Nerve Lesions

G. Brunelli and F. Brunelli, Brescia/Italy

Surgical treatment represents only a part, albeit a significant one, of nerve repair and recovery. In addition, several forms of physical and medical treatment can improve results in diminishing scar formation, encouraging regeneration, maintaining muscle trophism or joint mobility during denervation, and re-educating the sensory and motor functions. Among those that we routinely use are the following:

- Steroids: against scar-formation
- X-ray therapy: against scar formation
- Magnetic therapy: to reduce fibrosis and improve elastic tissue
- Orthosis: to avoid deformities, subluxation, and muscle exhaustion
- Electrotherapy: to maintain muscle trophism (used on nerves and on muscles)
- Physiotherapy: to maintain muscle trophism and joint mobility
- Gangliosides: to improve nerve regeneration
- Re-education: motor and sensory

Against scar formation, which is the worst enemy of nerve recovery, we routinely use steroids (moderate doses of steroids starting on the 10th day and extending to the 30th day) and X-ray therapy. The tractofibroblasts which are responsible for scar formation strangulating the fibers of the nerve may be blocked or dramatically reduced by means of these treatments.

As regards X-ray therapy, we have carried out research on animals which demonstrate the almost total absence of collagen fibrils among the nerve fibers after surgery in the treated animals, while in the control group there was an enormous amount of scar. For many years now we have therefore been routinely using a 1000-rad treatment, which is considered the best antifibroblastic dose for all patients having undergone nerve surgery. This treatment starts on the 12th or the 15th day and is performed administering 100 rad every 2 days for 20 days (Fig. 1).

Magnetic therapy in animal experiments has also proven capable of reducing scar reaction. Both in vessels and in nerves after surgery the magnetic fields reduce collagen production while increasing the number of elastic fibrils.

Orthoses are used both to avoid joint subluxation or stiffness in bad positions and to help re-education, especially for radial and peroneal nerve palsies. They also prevent muscle exhaustion resulting from fibrillation due to continuous traction.

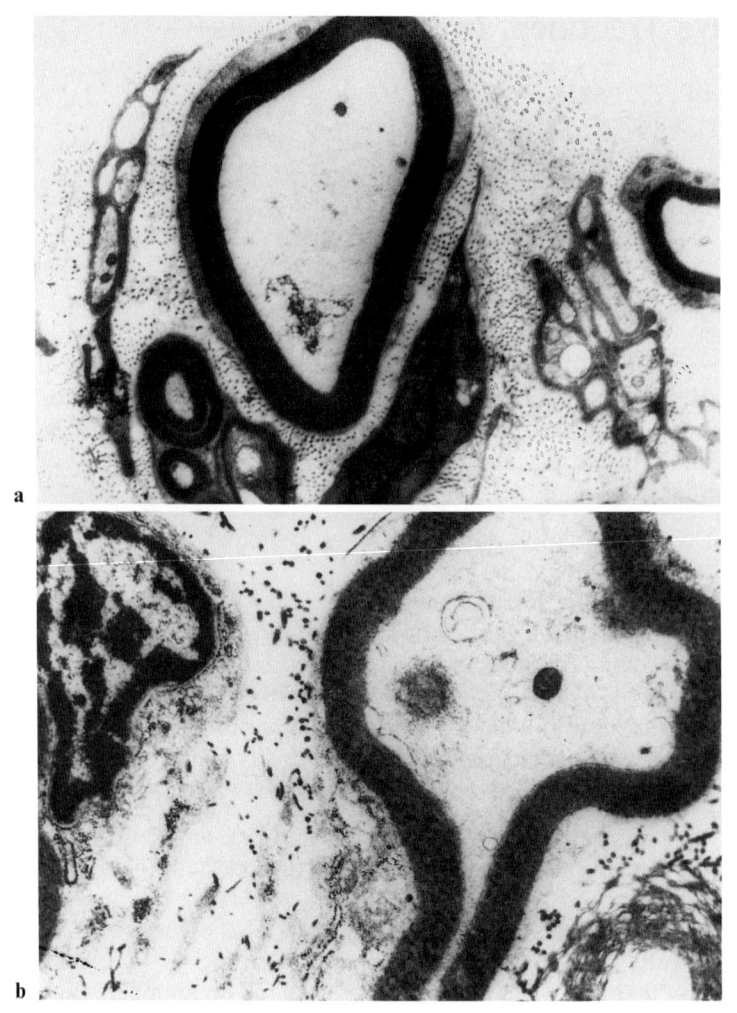

Fig. 1. a After nerve repair a large number of collagen fibrils form around the suture. **b** If X-ray therapy is used (at a dose of 900–1000 rad), the amount of scar reaction (collagen fibrils) is much reduced

Electrotherapy – although possibly dangerous for nerves, in which it provokes internal fibrosis – is very useful for muscles, helping here to reduce degeneration and atrophy. Exponential waves must be used, and their parameters must be adjusted according to muscle response, which varies according to the state of recovery. Electrotherapy, to be effective, must be used every day for several hours; this means at home by the patient with an individual apparatus such as is available at a reasonable price.

Physiotherapy has two main aims: (a) to maintain muscle trophicity (or better to delay and diminish its atrophy) by means of massages, stretch exercises, and various types of gymnastics as soon as the innervation occurs; and (b) to avoid joint stiffness by means of daily, passive mobilization.

Gangliosides are used to improve nerve regeneration. Our experiments on animals showed a quicker sprouting with a greater number of sprouts. For over 10 years now all our patients have undergone this treatment; in addition to the good results achieved, we have experienced no instance of intolerance. We use a mixture of several gangliosides at the dose of 100 mg per day for 1 month after surgery and 20 mg per day from then until recovery.

Re-education is a very important part of postoperative therapy. In fact, surgery may result in a lesser or greater mismatching so that sensations may be referred in wrong areas, and motor functions may activate wrong muscles (or part of them). If corticalization of the new pathways is not obtained, the functional disuse will lead to a very poor result. Re-education can improve and accelerate the reorganization of both sensory (afferent) and motor (efferent) impulses.

References

Bednar JM et al. (1986) Prosthetic nerve grafts: the use of a resorbable tube as an alternative to autogenous nerve grafting. Paper presented at the 41st Annual Meeting of the American Society for Surgery of the Hand, New Orleans

Brunelli G (1986) Paper presented at a course in microsurgery at Louvain University. Organized by Prof. De Conninck

Brunelli G, Fontana G, Jager C et al. (1985) Tropismo elettivo delle fibre nervose e motrici e sensitive dentro e distalmente uno spazio vuoto endoteliale (innesto venoso). Congresso Società Ricerche in Chirurgia, Como/Italy

Chiu DT, Janecka I, Krizek TJ et al. (1982) Autogenous vein graft as a conduit for nerve regeneration. Surgery 91 (2):226

Fontana G, Milanesi S, Brunelli G, Bartolaminelli P (1983) Invaginamento in segmenti venosi di lesioni nervose. Atti dell'VIII Congresso della Società di Ricerche in Chirurgia. Il Policlinico

Lundborg G, Hansson HA (1981) Nerve lesions with interruption of continuity: studies on the growth pattern of regenerating axons in the gap between the proximal and distal nerve ends. In: Gorio A, Millesi H, Mingrino S (eds) Posttraumatic peripheral nerve regeneration. Raven Press, New York

Karnowsky MJ, Roots L (1964) A direct coloring thiocholine method for cholinesterase. J Histochem Cytochem 12:219

Koelle GB, Fridenwald JS (1949) A histochemical method for localizing cholinesterase activity. Proc Soc Exp Biol Med 70:617

Strauch B, Rosenberg B, Brunelli F et al. (1983) Autogenous vein graft as a graft substitute in long vein segment nerve defects. Presented at the Plastic Surgery Research Council, Durham/NC

Tountas CP et al. (1986) Peripheral nerve repair by tubulization. Paper presented at the 41st Annual Meeting of the American Society for Surgery of the Hand, New Orleans/LA

Tsuji S (1974) On the chemical bases of thiocholine methods for demonstration of acetylcholinesterase activity. Histochemistry 69:42

Tsuji S (1983) A modification of the thiocholine-feracynamide method of Karnovsky and Roots for localization of acetylcholinesterase activity without interference by Koelle's copper thiocholine iodide precipitate. Histochemistry 78:317

Results of Brachial Plexus Surgery: Secondary Reconstruction

U. LAUMANN, Borken/FRG

Introduction

Formerly, poliomyelitis was the main cause of brachial plexus palsy. As a solely motor paralysis with maintained cutaneous and deep sensibility, this is an ideal basis for reconstructive surgery, such as muscle and tendon transference, tenodesis, and arthrodesis. Accordingly, all reconstructive operations used at the present time were developed in patients with poliomyelitis.

The brachial plexus palsies that we see today are usually of traumatic origin. These differ from poliomyelitis in showing disturbed sensitivity and often osseous and vascular injuries in addition to the loss of motor function. Under these conditions, the basis for reconstructive procedures is less favourable. A special group among traumatic brachial plexus palsies is birth palsy. In this case the growing organism is affected and responds with abnormal skeletal growth to persistent fixed deformity. Consequently, reconstructive procedures should be completed before such deformities become developed. Correct timing is therefore important.

Reconstruction Principles

General Reconstruction Principles

In general, orthopaedic reconstructive surgery starts only when spontaneous remissions are no longer expected, and when neurosurgical interventions have been completed. On the other hand, we must consider that a patient with extensive brachial plexus palsy becomes one-handed within 1 year. Any cooperation, whether by means of a prosthesis or by a more or less satisfactorily reconstructed upper extremity, is then definitely abandoned. Reconstructed motor functions can be utilized completely only in cases of permanent training; for this reason reconstructive procedures should be started before the patient becomes one-handed.

Also for social reasons, particularly with respect to rehabilitation, reconstructive procedures should be completed after an adequate period, in general not exceeding 2 years. A close collaboration between the neurosurgeon and the orthopaedic surgeon is therefore important. The aim of all reconstruction procedures is dynamic repair of the lost function. This is possible by transposing muscles with good function to paralyzed muscles. Tenodesis and arthrodesis are always procedures of second choice. Muscle transposition combined with tenodesis or arthrodesis is permitted; the operation can be carried out in one or two steps. Special conditions must be fulfilled to complete the reconstructive procedure successfully. These are classified into general and specific conditions:

General conditions
− Infection-free operation area.
− Free joint passive mobility, stable articulation, ossified fractures.
− Scar-free sliding areas of the tendons.

Specific conditions
− The muscle used for transposition must have at least grade M4 strength, according to the grading system of Daniels et al. (1966).
− Adequate tension of the tendon must be chosen to gain a sufficiently wide contraction amplitude.
− The acting direction of the transplant should be approximately the same as the paralyzed muscle.
− The anastomosis should be end-to-end without interposition of a transplant.
− The patient's mental state must permit him to use the transpositioned muscle in terms of the new function. Here, children succeed better than adults.

Special Reconstruction Principles

With regard to these conditions we treated 34 patients with brachial plexus palsy during the past 12 years, and we now consider the following reconstruction procedure to be best.

Complete Brachial Plexus Palsy. In complete brachial plexus lesion with preserved residual sensitivity at the inner side of the upper arm – in terms of the segmental sensory nerve supply from D2 – several procedures can be considered. (a) In the case of fibrous ankylosis of the glenohumeral joint, the state can be maintained, or under certain circumstances the joint can be fitted with a splint (Fig. 1). (b) For the unstable glenohumeral joint, the flail arm syndrome with preserved active stabilization of the scapula, we prefer arthrodesis of the joint in order to coordinate the uncontrolled pendular movements of the arm, especially when the patient is running. (c) To restore function in the injured extremity we consider the amputation of the upper arm at the border of sensitivity combined with glenohumeral arthrodesis and a varus osteotomy to be a very good method. The varus osteotomy widens the axillary space, thus giving an optimum basis for fitting a prosthesis and for good care of the axilla (Fig. 2). Another means is the amputation through the forearm after reconstruction of flexion ability in the elbow joint by myoplasty according to Clark (1946) or Hovnanian (1956) or by neurotonization of the musculocutaneous nerve. This type of reconstruction is also combined with a shoulder arthrodesis. A disadvantage of this method is the loss of sensitivity in

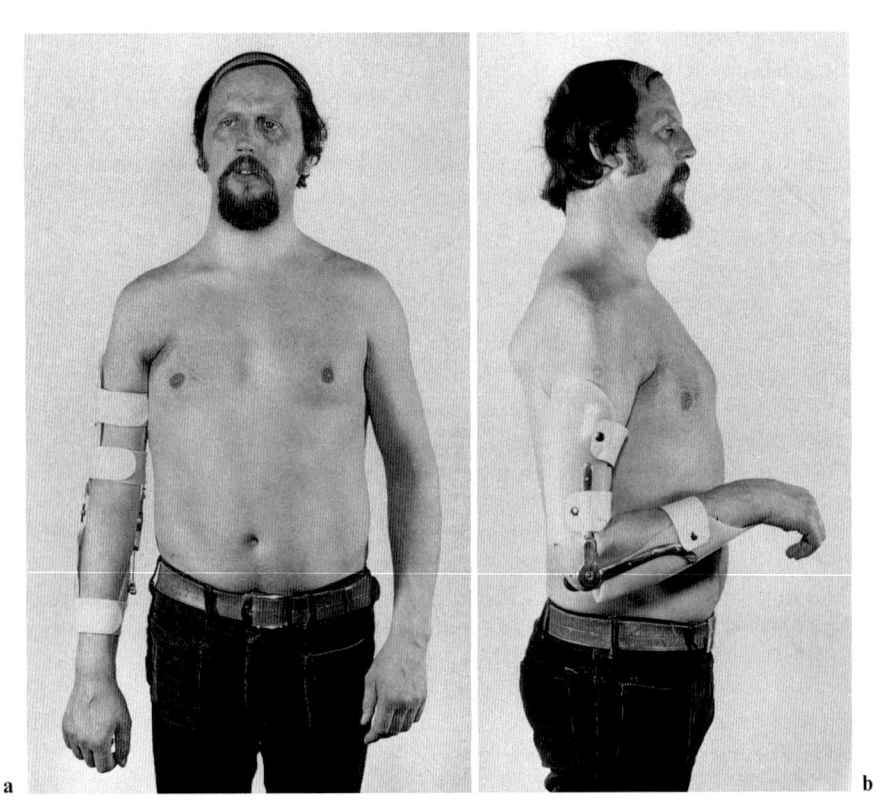

Fig. 1a, b. Splint for elbow joint and hand in a case of complete brachial plexus palsy with stable shoulder joint, self-locking elbow joint, and splint that holds the hand extended

the amputation stump. Most young patients refuse amputation although it brings the best functional results in the flail arm. Reconstructive procedures of the flail arm are therefore usually restricted to shoulder arthrodesis.

Incomplete Brachial Plexus Palsy. After the flail arm, the most frequent form is the injured brachial plexus lesion of C5/C6/C7. For this type we emphasize the following reconstruction procedure: (a) Stabilization of the glenohumeral joint, (b) Reconstruction of active flexion in the elbow joint, and (c) Reconstruction of extension ability of hand, fingers and thumb (Table 1). To stabilize the glenohumeral joint we prefer arthrodesis to myoplastic reconstruction because the final results are more reliable. Saha's muscle transfer for poliomyelitic flail shoulder (1967) can obviously not be readily applied in traumatic brachial plexus palsy. Our results after such muscle transfers have been poor (Fig. 3). For reconstruction of elbow flexion we use Clark's and Steindler's (1944) procedure. With both surgical techniques we have obtained a mean active elbow flexion of grade MIII or MIV. The pronated position of the forearm and the hand could not be improved by any of

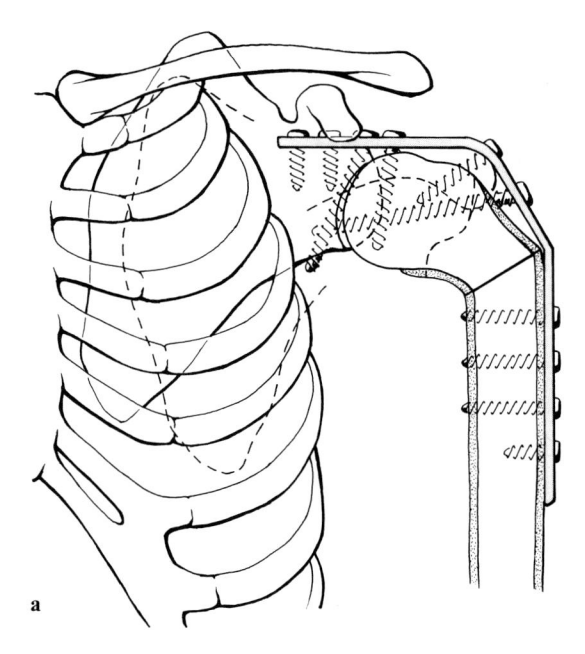

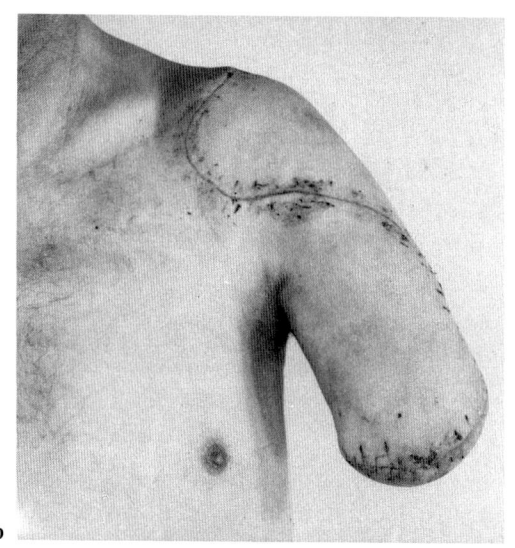

Fig. 2. a Combined glenohumeral arthrodesis, varus osteotomy, and amputation through upper arm with AO technique. **b** Postoperative amputation stump with widened axilla and sensitive stump end

these procedures. We observed after the Steindler operation a progressive pronation and flexion of the hand when flexing the elbow. After Clark's procedure this functionally unfavorable complex movement did not occur to the same extent.

We do not have experience with transfer of the triceps (Bunell 1951) or the latissimus dorsi muscle (Hovnanian 1956) for elbow flexion. To reconstruct the

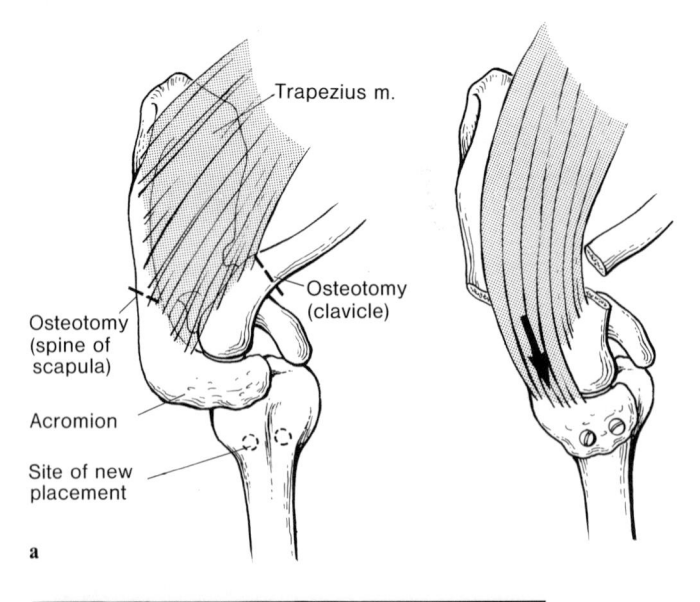

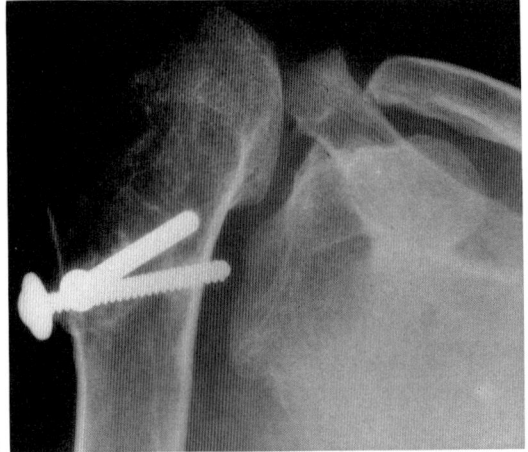

Fig. 3. a Saha's transfer of trapezius for paralysis of the deltoid muscle. **b** Bad result after Saha's muscle transfer with dislocation of the humeral head in cranial direction. In addition to transposition of the trapezius muscle the paralyzed muscles of the rotator cuff were reconstructed as follows: supraspinatus by levator scapulae and infraspinatus by latissimus dorsi

hand, finger, and thumb extension we usually perform the Perthes (1918) plasty, in some cases combined with wrist arthrodesis; occasionally we use the technique of Boyes (1960); both of these methods have proven quite successful (Fig. 4).

Brachial Plexus Birth Palsies. In brachial plexus birth palsies we perform the procedure according to Zachary (1947). This involves Z-shaped lengthening of the tendons of the pectoralis major and subscapularis muscles, anterior capsulotomy, transfer of latissimus dorsi and teres major muscles from the ventral to the dorsal side of the upper arm in order to obtain active external rotation. This is performed at the age of 3 or 4 years, before secondary bone

Table 1. Secondary reconstruction in incomplete brachial plexus injury

Shoulder joint: stabilization
Muscle transfer
    Deltoideus – trapezius
    Supraspinatus – levator scapulae
    Infraspinatus – latissimus dorsi + teres maior
Arthrodesis
Elbow joint: flexion
Muscle transfer
    Pectoralis major

    Flexor carpi radialis
    Palmaris longus
    Pronator teres
    Flexor digitorum sublimis
    Flexor carpi ulnaris

    Triceps

    Latissimus dorsi

Hand and finger joints: extension of wrist, fingers, thumb
Muscle transfer
    Flexor carpi ulnaris
    Palmaris longus
    Flexor carpi radialis
    Pronator teres
(+) Arthrodesis of wrist
    Flexor digitorum sublimis III + IV

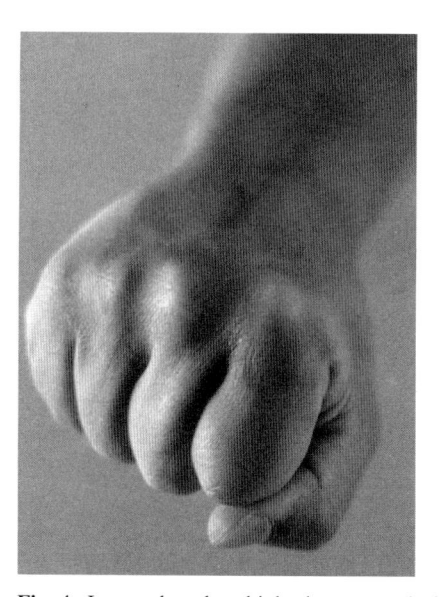

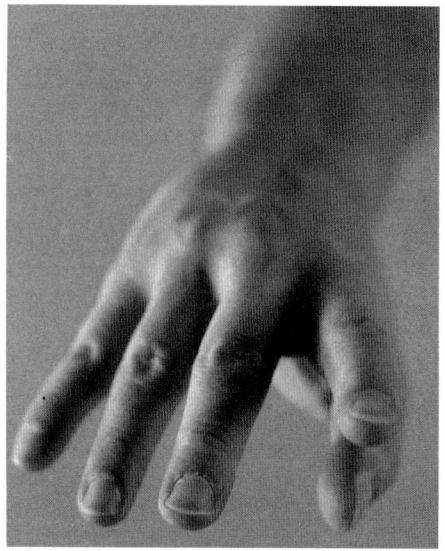

Fig. 4. Incomplete brachial plexus paralysis (C5, C6, C7) with high radial nerve palsy reconstructed with wrist arthrodesis and Perthes procedure: transposition of flexor carpi radialis to abductor pollicis brevis and extensor pollicis brevis; palmaris longus to extensor pollicis longus; flexor carpi ulnaris to extensor digitorum 2–5

changes develop. If secondary osseous alterations are present, a derotational humeral osteotomy is carried out. Pronation contractures of the forearm need rarely correction. Supination contractures are often found in Klumpke-Erb palsy. Such deformities of the hand are cosmetically striking. However, they are functionally very valuable as an opposite support. For this reason, surgical corrections should be carefully considered.

Conclusions

Secondary reconstructive surgery for brachial plexus lesions must be carefully considered with regard to the timing as well as to the indication. Amputations are seldom accepted by the patients; pain attacks cannot be eliminated by amputation. An important condition for reconstruction of active elbow flexion is a stable shoulder. In our case material shoulder arthrodesis proved to be superior to muscle transposition in stabilizing the shoulder joint. We use the procedures of Clark and Steindler to reconstruct active elbow flexion. Both of these procedures give satisfactory active elbow flexion. A disadvantage of Steindler's technique is the progressive pronation and flexion posture of the hand with increasing active elbow flexion. Satisfactory reconstruction of hand, finger, and thumb extension is reached by Perthes and Boyes procedures with or without wrist arthrodesis. In brachial plexus birth palsies myoplastic procedures should be performed early, before secondary osseous changes occur.

References

Alnot JY (1977) Paralysie traumatique du plexus brachial chez l'adulte. Rev Chir Orthop 63:17
Boyes JH (1960) Tendon transfers for radial palsy. Bull Hosp Joint Dis 21:997
Boyes JH (1964) Bunnell's surgery of the hand, 4th edn. Lippincott, Philadelphia
Bunnell S (1951) Restoring flexion to the paralytic elbow. J Bone Joint Surg 33(A):566
Clark JMP (1946) Reconstruction of biceps brachii by pectoral muscle transplantation. Brit J Surg 34:180
Daniels LV, Williams M, Worthingham C (1966) Muskelfunktionsprüfung. 2. Aufl. Fischer, Stuttgart
Dautry P, Apoil A, Moinet F, Koechling P (1977) Paralysie radiculaire supérieure du plexus brachial. Traitement par transposition musculaires associées. Rev Chir Orthop 63:399
Harmon PH (1950) Surgical reconstruction of the paralytic shoulder by multiple muscle transplantations. J Bone Joint Surg 32(A):583
Hardy AE (1981) Birth injuries of the brachial plexus. J Bone Joint Surg 63(B):98
Hoffer M, Wickenden R, Roper B (1978) Brachial plexus birth palsies. J Bone Joint Surg 60(A):691
Hovnanian AP (1956) Latissimus dorsi transplantation for loss of flexion or extension at the elbow. A preliminary report on technic. Ann Surg 143:493
Laumann U, Schilgen L (1977) Varisierende subkapitale Osteotomie in Verbindung mit Schulterarthrodese und Oberarmamputation bei Plexusparese. Z Orthop 115:787
Perthes O (1918) Über Sehnenoperationen bei irreparabler Radialisparese. Beitr Klin Chir 113:289

Post M (1978) The shoulder. Lea & Febiger, Philadelphia
Rorabeck CH, Harris WR (1981) Factors affecting the prognosis of brachial plexus injuries. J Bone Joint Surg 63(B):404
Saha AK (1967) Surgery of the paralyzed and flail shoulder. Acta Orthop Scand (Suppl) 97:1967
Schottstaedt ER, Larsen LJ, Bost FC (1958) The surgical reconstruction of the upper extremity paralyzed by poliomyelitis. J Bone Joint Surg 40(A):633
Sedel L (1982) The results of surgical repair of brachial plexus injuries. J Bone Joint Surg 64(B):54
Steindler A (1944) Muscle and tendon transplantation at the elbow. American Academy of Orthopaedic surgeons Instructional Course Lectures, vol 2. Edwards, Ann Arbor MI
Tsuyama N, Hara T (1973) Über die Wiederherstellungsoperation der gelähmten Ellenbogenflexoren. Z Orthop 111:600
Wynn Parry CB (1980) The management of traction lesions of the brachial plexus and peripheral nerve injuries in the upper limb; a study in teamwork. Injury 11:265
Zachary RB (1947) Transplantation of teres maior and latissimus dorsi for loss of external rotation at shoulder. Lancet 2:757

Subject Index

acetylcholinesterase
   posttraumatic changes 181, 183
acromio-clavicular joint
   rupture, paralysis of brachial plexus 230, 231
acute nerve compression
   block of impulse conduction 32
allodynia
   ulnar nerve transection 44
amputation
   lower leg, peroneus nerve graft 330
amputation neuroma
   causalgia, lumbar canal stenosis, laminectomy 241
   Livingstone's plexus brachial resection 239
   prognosis, after microsurgical procedure 239, 240
amputation stump
   brachial plexus palsy, special reconstruction 433
anatomy
   axillary nerve 261
   brachial plexus 373, 374
   brachial plexus roots: $C_{5/6}$ Duchenne-Erb, C_8/Th_1 Déjerine-Klumpke 391, 392, 404
   C_2-C_4, C_5-C_7 roots, brachial plexus 402
   canal of Gujon 262
   canalis obturatorius 264
   costoclavicular passage 260
   entrapment sites, thoracic outlet 260
   forearm, nerve branches, division 249
   incisura scapulae syndrome 260, 261
   inguinal ligament 264
   median nerve 262, 263
   nerve transplantation, brachial plexus, root avulsion, operative technique 375
   peripheral nerve vasculature 130
   physiological, sensory evoked potentials 214
   quadrilateral space 261
   radial nerve ramifications 248, 249
   saphenous nerve 265
   scalenus passage 260
   spinal nerves 373
   supinator space 261
   thoracic outlet structures 307
   ulnar nerve 262, 298
anesthetic agents
   intrafascicular injection, pathology 135
aneurysm
   axillary artery, gunshot wounds, brachial plexus 398
angiography
   axillary, plexus injury 408
   free autologous nerve graft 145–148
   pre-, postoperative, brachial plexus, root avulsion 377, 378
anterior interosseus nerve
   entrapment neuropathy, Kiloh-Nevin syndrome 263
arterial injuries
   nerve lacerations, association, prognosis 353
astrocytes
   glial fibrillary acidic protein (GFAP) synthesis 4
   motoneuron axotomy, postoperative changes 2, 3, 4
autografting methods
   repair of peripheral nerve injury 88–95
autopsy
   entrapment syndromes 279
avulsion
   brachial plexus, pain, dorsal root entry zone lesions 416–421
axillary artery
   pseudoaneurysm, brachial plexus lesion 408
axillary nerve
   entrapment neuropathy 259, 261
   injury, shoulder luxation, ventral, dorsal surgical view 381, 382
   intraoperative somatosensory evoked potential 227
   reconstruction, sural nerve graft, technique of Samii 383

440 Subject Index

axillary nerve
 stretch injury 406
 transplantation, brachial plexus injury 380, 381, 382
axon
 cells, at rest, after peripheral neurotmesis 318
 colonization of vein graft, mechanism 102
 conduction velocity, normal, after resuture of median and ulnar nerves 219
 degeneration, nerve compression 32
 diameter, histograms, centrocental anastomosis 77
 diameter, histograms, control nerves and centrocentral anastomosis grafts 17
 growth, allogenic nerve graft 108
 injury, metabolic changes 175, 185
 injury, production of sprouts, presumption 14
 interruption, cellular biology 1–6, 15
 outgrowth, stimulation by neuropeptides 73, 74
 reflex, brachial plexus root avulsion, differential diagnosis 378
 regenerating, orthograde growth, microsurgically performed nerve suture 121
 regeneration, inhibiting effect of fat tissue 124–129
 sprouts, after laser assisted nerve transplantation 170
 stenosis, entrapment neuropathy, electrophysiology 32, 36
 transection, Wallerian degeneration 33, 34
axonal growth
 allogenic, autologous grafts 108–110
axonostenosis
 X-ray radiation, brachial plexus lesion 411
axonotmesis
 blood-nerve barrier, disruption 138
 brachial plexus lesions 381
 carpal tunnel syndrome 272
 classification 324
 excitability, impulse conduction 33, 34
 ischiadic nerve compression 64
axons
 capable of regeneration, intraoperative analysis 216
 conduction velocity, after nerve suture 219, 221
 damaged, positive feed back circle of pain 55
 demyelination, remyelination, carpal tunnel syndrome 280, 283, 284
 diameter, after compression 198

 myelinated, after muscle transplantation, histology 68
 myelinated, ultrastructure 283
 protein transport, molecular biology 15
 regenerating, after nerve suture 121
 regenerating, limitation of outgrowth by fat tissue 124–129
 regeneration after laser assisted nerve suture 142
 regeneration, laser irradiation 173
 sprouting, presupposition for nerve injury recovery 14
 Wallerian degeneration, electrophysiology 33, 34
axotomy
 molecular biological changes, microglia 16, 17
 NGF-mRH, changes, sciatic nerve 31

biology
 cellular, peripheral nerve lesion 1
biopsy
 carpal tunnel syndrome 281, 284
 skeletal muscle, after denervation 8
 sural nerve, regeneration, morphometric data 23, 24, 25
biothesiometry
 carpal tunnel syndrome, findings before and after surgery 271
blood-nerve barrier
 disruption, anesthetic agents 135
 function, nerve grafting, autografts, allografts 139, 140
 investigation methods, physiology 132, 133
 nerve injury, repair, regeneration 130–142
brachial plexus
 actinic (X-ray) lesions, greater omentum transfer 411–415
 amputation neuroma, resection, prognosis 239
 anatomofunctional scheme 319
 anatomy 373, 374
 avulsion, injury pain, dorsal root zone lesions 416–421
  intraoperative somatosensory evoked potential 232
  neurotization 367–371
  severe pain, operative results 423, 424
  treatment 416–421
 birth palsies, surgical treatment 434, 435
 damage, intraoperative monitoring of sensory evoked potentials 217
 dorsal root entry zone lesions 416–421
 entrapment neuropathy, thoracic outlet

Subject Index

syndrome 260
greater omentum flap, radiation damage, surgical view 411, 412
injuries, blunt, indications for surgery 397
  gunshot wounds, indication for surgery, results 373, 396, 398, 399, 405
  iatrogenic, operation results 407, 408
  incomplete, secondary reconstruction 435
  intractable pain, dorsal root entry zone coagulation 422–429
  lacerating, indications for surgery, results 397
  neurolysis 380
irradiation plexitis, operative treatment 408
lesions, actinic, operative treatment, results 412, 414
  dorsal root entry zone 416–421
  Duchenne-Erb type, Déjerine-Klumpke type 391, 392
  electroneurography, electromyography, MRI, indications 205
  etiology 372
  fractures 374, 379
  Horner syndrome 374, 376
  indications for surgery 381, 382, 396–410
  intraoperative somatosensory evoked potential 227–232
  medullary symptoms 376
  root avulsion, etiology 374
    myelography 375, 376
    pre-, postoperative angiography 377, 378
    surgical view, reconstruction, venous interpositional graft 379
  secondary reconstruction, results 430–437
  selection for operation 396–410
  tentative evaluation scheme 393, 394
  treatment 372–385
  ulnar nerve graft, transplantation 332
neurofibroma, CAT scan, operative situs 361
neurogenic tumors, surgery 386–390
palsy, poliomyelitis 430
palsy, special reconstruction 431, 432
Recklinghausen's disease, diagnosis, operative results 252, 386–390
reconstruction, free vascularized nerve grafts, results 333
  indications 218
root lesions, thermoregulation, sweat secretion 377
schwannoma 386–390

stretch contusion, nonoperative management 400, 401
structures, anatomy 307
surgery, results 391–395
  secondary reconstruction, results 430–437
tumoral lesions, computed tomography 201
tumors, operative experience 359–366
X-ray lesion, tissue sclerosis, operative situs 411
brachial cleft cyst
  compression, brachial plexus, operation 360, 364
brachialgia paresthetica nocturna
  carpal tunnel syndrome, differential diagnosis 289
  prognosis 274
brain
  somatosensory cortex, functional changes after peripheral nerve transection 55
breast cancer
  metastases, brachial plexus compression 360, 365

C_2–C_4 roots
  brachial plexus, topography 402, 404
C_5-, C_6-roots
  brachial plexus, avulsion, intraoperative somatosensory evoked potential 232
C_5–C_6 roots
  brachial plexus lesions, Duchenne-Erb type 391, 392, 404
  brachial plexus, reconstruction 383, 402
C_5–C_7 roots
  brachial plexus, avulsion, operative situs, results after neurotization 369
  brachial plexus paralysis, incomplete 435
  brachial plexus, topography 374
  long thoracic nerve, topography, brachial plexus injuries 402
C_7 radiculopathy
  differential diagnosis 289
  neurofibroma, CAT scan, operative situs 361
C_8-Th_1 roots
  brachial plexus, lesions, Déjerine-Klumpke type 391, 392
café-au-lait spots
  neurofibromatosis 251
canal of Gujon
  anatomy 262
canalis obturatorius
  anatomy 264
carbonic anhydrase
  sensory ganglion cells, enzyme 15

carpal canal
  pressure inside, Phalen test 263
carpal ligament
  self-regulation system 284
carpal tunnel syndrome
  a new surgical approach 292–294
  circulatory disorders, prognosis 275, 276, 286
  complete conduction block 233, 235
  complications 288
  computed tomography 201–203
  depression, normalization of nerve conduction velocity 286
  diagnosis, differential diagnosis 289
  diagnosis, neurophysiological parameters 270–272
  distal motor latency, muscular response potential, pre-, postoperative findings, comparison 233–238, 271
  electroneurographic findings 214
  electrophysiological confirmation 233, 271
  entrapment neuropathy 201, 202, 212, 214, 233, 235, 238, 258, 259, 260, 263, 270, 273, 278, 288, 292
  etiology: degenerative, traumatic, inflammatory 284
  median nerve, entrapment neuropathy 259, 263
    Renaut's bodies 280
    sensory evoked potentials 213
  morphologic considerations 278
  neurological deficit, long-standing 288, 289
  neurophysiologic parameters before and after surgery 270–272
  pathogenetic considerations 278
  Phalen test 258, 263
  preoperative symptoms, electrophysiology, intraoperative findings, prognosis 273–277
  provocational tests, prognosis 274, 276
  reoperations, reasons 289
  sensory evoked potentials 212
  surgery, pitfalls, reasons 288–291
    skin incision 289, 290
    transverse carpal ligament, extent of transection 289
  surgical decompression, postoperative nerve conduction times 233, 234
caudal thoracic nerves
  entrapment neuropathy 264
causalgia
  amputation, neuroma, lumbar canal stenosis, laminectomy 241

  morphological changes 286
  pathogenesis 52, 53
cellular biology
  peripheral nerve lesion 1–6
central nervous system
  basic functions 45
  capacity for regrowth 52
  changes following peripheral nerve injury 54, 55
  large fiber sensory tracts, sensory evoked potentials 214
  nerve trauma, regenerative processes 42
  pain following peripheral nerve injury 51–57
  specific pain pathways 51
  transsynaptic plasticity after a peripheral lesion 48
central synaptic transmission
  sensory ganglion cells, short-term changes 14
centrocentral anastomosis
  operative photographs 76
cervical rib
  brachial plexus entrapment 260
  thoracic-outlet syndrome, pre-, postoperative X-ray examination, phlebography 308, 309
chest
  cross section, T 3 level: Brachial plexus schwannoma 387
  see thoracic-outlet syndrome
  wall, desmoid, operative treatment 360, 364
children
  nerve injuries, operative repair, prognosis 353
circulatory disorders
  carpal tunnel syndrome, prognosis 275, 276, 286
classification
  neurogenic tumors, World Health Organization 386
clinical aspects
  entrapment neuropathies 258–269
clinical pain
  pathogenesis 51
clinical picture
  brachial plexus lesions 374
  ischiadic nerve compression 58–65
  sensory disturbance, patterns 43, 44
  thoracic-outlet syndrome, topographic relations 307, 312
clinical testing
  sensory system of peripheral nerves 42, 43

Subject Index

colchicine
  nerve growth factor, interruption of retrograde transport 29
commotio spinalis
  brachial plexus, root avulsion 376
complications
  carpal tunnel syndrome, surgery 288
  dorsal root entry zone coagulation 424
  hip surgery, nerve lesions 243
computed tomography
  neurofibroma at the head of fibula 206
  peripheral nerve pathology 201–203
conduction block
  carpal tunnel syndrome, muscular action potential 235
  electrophysiology 38
  Guillain-Barré syndrome, electrophysiology 32, 33
conduction velocity
  after anastomosis with venous graft 93
  facial nerve, Bell's palsy 33
  laser assisted nerve suture 161, 162
  motor, after nerve section 35
  postoperative, carpal tunnel syndrome, preoperative DML, relationship 234
  thoracic-outlet syndrome 302, 303
cordotomy
  relief of pain 416
corrosion cast technique
  epi-, perineural vessels newly developed 151
cranial nerves
  retrograde changes in motoneurons 1–5
crush lesions
  peripheral nerves, increased activity of pentose phosphate pathway enzymes 177
    metabolic responses, reinnervation changes 175–188, 189–196
    posttraumatic changes in capillary number in extensor hallucis longus muscle fibers 192
    posttraumatic changes in fast glycogenolytic muscle fiber size 191
    posttraumatic changes in fast oxidative glycogenolytic muscle fiber size 190
    posttraumatic changes in histochemical profile of extensor digitorum longus muscle fibers 192
    posttraumatic changes in mitochondrial fraction 193
    posttraumatic changes in number of nuclei 193
    posttraumatic changes of acetylcholinesterase 181
    posttraumatic changes of cytochrome oxidase 179, 180
    posttraumatic activity of G 6 PDH 178, 179
CT
  brachial plexus, schwannoma 386, 387
  ganglion, elbow joint 208
  neurofibroma, tibialis anterior muscles 206
  retroperitoneal hematoma 315
  stretch injuries 405
  wristdrop syndrome 207
cubital tunnel syndrome
  entrapment neuropathy 299
cutaneous receptors
  examination, microelectrode techniques 46
cyclosporin A
  suppression of nerve graft rejection 105, 111, 140
cytophotometry
  normal spinal motoneuron, measurement of G 6 PDH activity 176
  spinal cord segments L 3, L 4 177

definition
  neurolysis 323
  pain, physiological, inflammatory, neuropathic 51, 52
deltoid muscle
  paresis, function before and after surgery 384
dendrites
  regeneration, alterations, loss of synaptic contacts 5, 99, 101
denervation potentials
  nerve compression 62
desmoid
  chest wall, recurrence, operative treatment 360, 364
diabetes mellitus
  neuropathy, sensory evoked potentials, carpal canal syndrome 212
diagnosis
  aneurysm, brachial artery, digital subtraction angiography 209
  brachial plexus lesions 372
  carpal tunnel syndrome, false-positive 289
    neurophysiological parameters 270–272
  footdrop syndrome 210
  ganglion, CT 208
  modern imaging procedures 206–211
  peripheral nerve lesions, MRI 204, 205
  plexus brachialis entrapment neuropathy, thoracic outlet syndrome 205, 260

diagnosis
  thoracic outlet syndrome 302–306
  wristdrop syndrome, ganglion, CT 207
diagnostic criteria
  entrapment neuropathies 258
differential diagnosis
  brachial plexus, root avulsion 378
  brachial plexus lesions, proximal, distal 377
  C7 radiculopathy 289
  carpal tunnel syndrome 201, 273, 289
  entrapment neuropathies 258, 259
  Morton's toe 265
  nerve lesions, computed tomography 201–203
  obturator nerve entrapment 264
  pain, hand, forearm 263
digital nerves
  free vascularized grafts, transplantation 328
digital subtraction angiography
  aneurysm of brachial artery 208, 210
digitales plantares communes nerves
  chronic compression syndrome, entrapment neuropathy 265
distal motor latency (DML)
  carpal tunnel syndrome, decompression effect 237
    findings before and after surgery 271
    postoperative conduction velocity, relationship 234
dopamine β-hydroxylase
  neurotransmitter, sympathetic neurons 29
dorsal root entry zone
  avulsion injury pain, treatment 416–421
  coagulation, intractable pain, technique of Samii 422–429
  lesions, definition 416
Duchenne-Erb-, Déjerine-Klumpke types
  brachial plexus lesions, results of surgery 391, 392

electromyography (EMG)
  brachial plexus, gunshot wounds 399
    lesions, indications for surgery 381
    root avulsion 376, 379
  carpal tunnel syndrome, findings before and after surgery, prognosis 263, 271, 273, 275, 276
  evoked, facial nerve, excitability test, Bell's palsy, prognosis 34, 35
  findings, after nerve suture, clinical function, correlation 224
  peripheral nerve conduction studies 212
  thoracic-outlet syndrome 303, 304

electromyoneurography
  before and after vein graft, nerve regeneration 98, 99, 100
  brachial plexus lesions 205
  carpal tunnel syndrome, prognosis 213, 273, 275
  ischiadic nerve, compression 61, 62
  nerve suture, results, comparison with clinical function 224
  peroneal nerve, after neuronal anastomosis 91
electron microscopy
  astrocytes, glial fibrillary acidic protein (GFAP) 4
  axon terminals, degenerative changes 15
  cross section, myelinated, amyelinated nerve fibers 101
  endoneurium, vascular architecture 131
  myelin sheaths, structure 231
  nerve compression 136
  perineurium 133
  sciatic nerve suture 139
electrophysiology
  after peripheral nerve suture, comparison with clinical function 224–226
  carpal tunnel syndrome, delayed distal latency of muscular responce potential 233
    differential diagnosis 289
    prognosis 273–277
  changes after motor nerve injury 32–41
  evoked compound muscle response (ECMR) 32, 34
  motor nerve injury 32–41
  nerve conduction block 38
  nerve conduction velocity, suturless laser-assisted nerve anastomosis 162
  neurogenic tumors, brachial plexus 386, 388
  reinnervation potentials after laser-assisted nerve anastomosis 166, 167
  sensory system of peripheral nerves, investigation 42
  tests, brachial plexus entrapment 260
endoneurium
  architecture, regeneration of nerve graft 143
  injury, blood-nerve barrier, disruption 138
  intact structures, precondition for regenerating autologous grafts 143
  plexus, anatomy, scheme 149
  vascular architecture, electron-microphotography 131
  vascular permeability, regenerating

Subject Index

growth cone, effect 138
vessels, corrosion cast specimen 157
entrapment neuropathy
  anterior interosseus nerve 263
  axillary nerve, quadrilateral space 261
  axon stenosis 32
  brachial plexus, thoracic outlet 259, 260
  carpal tunnel syndrome 201, 212, 214, 233, 235, 238, 258, 259, 260, 263, 270, 273, 278, 288, 292
  clinical characteristics 258
  cubital tunnel syndrome 299
  diagnostic criteria 258, 270
  digitales plantares communes nerves 265
  femoral nerve 264, 265
  frequency 259
  gonalgia paresthetica 265
  Guyon's tunnel syndrome 299
  Howship-Romberg syndrome 264
  ilioinguinal nerve 264
  incisura scapulae syndrome 260
  Kiloh-Nevin syndrome 263
  median nerve 262, 263
  Morton's toe 265
  neuropathia patellae 265
  obturator nerve, canalis obturatorius 264
  peroneal nerve 265, 266
  radial nerve, supinator canal 261
  scalenus syndrome 260
  suprascapular nerve 260, 261
  tarsal tunnel syndrome 259, 265, 266
  thoracic spinal nerves 263, 264
  tibial nerve 265
  ulnar nerve 262
    neurolysis 298–301
entrapment syndromes
  morphological and pathogenetic considerations 278–287
epineurium
  blood supply 130, 131
  fibrosis, ulnar nerve entrapment neuropathy 300, 301
  fibrotic, operative removal, technique of Samii, nerve compression syndrome 301
  peripheral nerve, anatomy, scheme 149
  ultrastructural aspects after laser assisted transplantation 172
  vascular architecture, sciatic nerve 149
    suture region, sciatic nerve, micro-angiogram 151, 152
  vascular corrosion cast specimens 155, 156, 157
  vessels, newly developed, corrosion cast 151
evoked compound muscle response (ECMR)
  conduction block 32

extensor digitorum longus muscle
  fiber diameters, reinnervation with and without suture of spinal nerve 120
facial nerve
  Bell's palsy, conduction velocity 33, 35
  trauma, functional recovery, delay 4
fat tissue
  neuroma formation, limitation 124
femoral nerve
  entrapment syndrome 259, 265
  lesion, hip surgery 243–247
  neuralgia, retroperitoneal hematoma 315, 316
  Recklinghausen's disease 252
  wrapping by greater omentum 415
fibrosarcoma
  operative experience 360
finger amputation
  centrocentral nerve anastomosis 75
finger reconstruction, neurovascular
  flap 330
flexion/extension tests
  carpal tunnel syndrome, prognosis 274
fluorescence microscopy
  blood-nerve barrier, examination 133
  microvessel containing EBA tracer 137
  sciatic nerve, compression 137
fluoride-resistant acid phosphatase (FRAP)
  sensory ganglion cells, enzyme 15
foot
  entrapment syndromes 265
footdrop syndrome
  calcified tendon of gastrocnemius muscle, CT 210
fractures
  brachial plexus injury 374, 379
  nerve lesions, results of therapy, critical review 337, 341
function
  central nerve stump, intraoperative analysis, sensory evoked potentials 216
  changes, single motor units after nerve suture 219–223
  clinical, after traumatic nerve transection, electroneurographical parameters comparison 224
  dorsal horn cells, alteration by peripheral nerve section 54
F-wave measurement
  thoracic-outlet syndrome 304

ganglion
  elbow joint, CT 208
  sensory, response to injury 14–21
  wristdrop syndrome, CT diagnosis 207

ganglion cells
  sensory, fluoride-resistant acid phosphatase (FRAP), carbonic anhydrase 15
  sensory, injury, cell death, range 16
    short term, long term changes 14, 16
gastrocnemius muscle
  fiber diameters, histogram, reinnervation with and without spinal nerve suture 119, 120
gastroepiploic artery
  microsurgical suture, actinic lesion, brachial plexus 413
"gate-control therapy"
  traumatic peripheral neuroma 239
glenohumeral arthrodesis
  brachial plexus palsy, special reconstruction 432
glia
  cellular reactions, postoperative 2, 3, 4
glial cells
  reaction of sensory neurons to peripheral axotomy 16
gonalgia paresthetica
  saphenous nerve entrapment 265
graft
  allogenic, genetic model 104–112
  coagulated epineurium, laser assisted 171
  colonization by axons and Schwann's cells, mechanism 102
  free autologous, revascularization 143–148
  free vascularized, hand surgery 326–334
  homologous, retrograde atrophy 25, 26
  interfascicular, microsurgical technique of Samii 343
  laser assisted, ultrastructural aspects 169–174
  membrane enclosement, lateral, longitudinal revascularization 144
  nerve implantation, regeneration types 22, 23
  nerve, repair, after extirpation of neurofibroma 255
  radial, median nerves, results, comparison 340, 341
  regeneration, isomorphic conditions 143
  schwannoma, supraclavicular plexus 363
  successfully regenerated nerve fibers, sural nerve biopsy 23
  sural nerve, brachial plexus injury, surgical view 383
    neurofibromatosis, microsurgical reconstruction 251
  venous, brachial plexus lesions 377
  venous, regeneration 88–95, 96–103

grafting
  brachial plexus, stretch injuries, results 407
  centro-central anastomosis, histograms 77
  nerve autografts, allografts, blood barrier function 139
  peripheral nerve, clinical investigation 43, 44, 45
  radial nerve, secondary reconstruction 250
  sudomotor activity, Ninhydrin finger printing test 44, 45
  traumatic lesions of radial nerve ramifications 248–250
  venous, nerve regeneration 88–95, 96–103
  venous, technique of neural anastomosis 89, 90
growth-associated proteins
  fast axonal transport 15
Guillain-Barré syndrome
  conduction block 33
gunshot wounds
  brachial plexus, indications for surgery, results 372, 396, 398, 399, 400
Guyon's tunnel syndrome
  entrapment neuropathy 299

hand
  nerves, sensory disturbances, patterns 43, 44
  painful, entrapment syndrome 278
  single fiber recording, microelectric technique 46, 47
hand surgery
  anterior interosseus nerve entrapment, Kiloh-Nevin syndrome 263
  canal of Gujon, anatomy 262
  finger amputation, centrocentral nerve anastomosis 75
  free vascularized nerve grafts, transplantation 326–334
  median, radial, ulnar nerves, entrapment neuropathy 261, 262
hemangioma
  X-ray radiation, brachial plexus lesion 411
hip surgery
  femoral nerve lesions 243–247
histamine test
  brachial plexus, root avulsion, differential diagnosis 378
histochemistry
  G6PDH activity, normal spinal motoneuron 176

muscle-, nerve transplants 68
profiles of extensor digitorum longus, extensor hallucis longus muscle fibers after crushing and resection of peroneal nerve 190–193
spinal cord segments L_3, L_4 177
histology
  allogenic nerve graft, with and without cyclosporin A suppression 106, 107, 109, 110
  autogenic nerve graft 109, 110
  coagulated graft epineurium, fasciculation of cell processes 172
  ischiadic nerve, changes after compression 197
  malignant schwannoma 254
  myelin sheaths, Renaut's bodies 281
  nerve graft of centrocental anastomosis 78
  nerve regeneration, vein graft 97–101
  nerve repair 428
  nerve transplantation, laser assisted 171
  neurofibroma 253
  neuroma 22
  neuroma, implantation into fat tissue, inhibiting outgrowth of nerve fibers 126, 127
  perineuronal microglial cell 2, 4
  radial nerve, interosseus ramus, primary chronic polyarthritis 280
  radial nerve, Renaut's body 282
  Recklinghausen's disease 252, 253
  Renaut' bodies, median nerve, carpal tunnel 280
  schwannoma 253
  spinal motoneuron, normal 176
Hodgkin's disease
  radiotherapy, brachial plexus lesion 411
Hoffmann-Tinel sign
  carpal tunnel syndrome, prognosis 274
  nerve regeneration, old nerve injuries 216
Horner syndrome
  brachial plexus lesions 374, 376
Howship-Romberg syndrome
  obturator nerve entrapment neuropathy 264

ilioinguinal nerve
  entrapment neuropathy 259, 264
imaging procedures
  planning of microsurgical operations 206–211
immunocytochemistry
  electron microscopique, astrocytes, stimulation by neuroaxotomy 4

melanocyte-stimulating hormone, enolase, nerve regeneration under vein graft 101, 102
immunology
  background, nerve transplantation 104
incidence
  neurofibromatosis 251
incisura scapulae syndrome
  brachial plexus entrapment neuropathy 258, 260
indications
  biopsy, muscle denervation 8
  brachial plexus lesions, surgery 396–410
  dorsal root entry zone coagulation, severe intractable pain 422, 423
  electroneurography, electromyography, MRI 205
  free greater omentum transfer, actinic brachial plexus lesions 411–415
  free vascularized nerve grafts, hand surgery 326–334
  intraoperative monitoring of sensory evoked nerve potentials 218
  microsurgical procedures, neurofibromatosis 252, 255
  operative treatment, neurofibroma 255
  posttraumatic neuroma 240
  radial nerve grafting, secondary reconstruction 250
  surgery, brachial plexus, lesions 381, 382, 396–410
  surgery, brachial plexus stretch injuries 402
inflammatory pain
  pathogenesis 51
inguinal ligament
  lateral femoral cutaneus nerve entrapment 264
innervation
  changes, muscle response 7–13
intercostal nerves
  donors, free vascularized graft, transplantation 328
  transection, cell death, range, time 17
  transplantation, brachial plexus injuries 382
irradiation plexitis
  brachial plexus, operative treatment 408
ischiadic nerve
  compression, clinical picture, pathological findings 58–65
    structural changes 197–200
  neuroma, traumatic, prognosis after microsurgical procedure 240

Kiloh-Nevin syndrome
  anterior interosseus nerve entrapment, forearm fracture 263

laser
  application, coagulation of dorsal root entry zone, severe pain, results 425
    nerve anastomoses 162, 165–168
    nerve transplantation, ultrastructural aspects 169–174
    reduction of suture granulomas 173
lateral femoral cutaneus nerve
  entrapment neuropathy 264
lipoma
  brachial plexus compression, operative treatment 360, 364
  computed tomography, localization 201, 202
localization
  neurofibromatosis 251, 252
lumbar canal stenosis
  laminectomy 241
lymphangioma
  brachial plexus, operative treatment 360, 364

major histocompatibility complex (MHC)
  nerve graft rejection 104
median nerve
  alterations, carpal tunnel syndrome 274, 275
  axonal conduction velocity, after suture 219–223
  compression, carpal tunnel syndrome 259, 263
    pathology 284
    processus supratrochlearis 296, 297
  compression syndrome, sensory nerve action potentials, sensory evoked potentials 212–215
  conduction velocity, thoracic-outlet syndrome 303
  decompression, carpal tunnel syndrome 273, 286
    incomplete, carpal tunnel syndrome 289
  donor, free vascularized graft, transplantation 330, 331
  entrapment neuropathy 262, 263, 296
    autoptic findings 279
  grafting, sensory disturbances, patterns 43, 44, 45
  irritation, processus supratrochlearis 296
  lesions, surgery, results, critical review 336, 337, 341, 346
  microneurography, after suture 46, 47

  microstimulation, interpretation 47, 48
neurinoma, diagnosis, MRI 205
neurofibromatosis 252
neurolysis, carpal tunnel syndrome 292, 293
neurolysis, neurofibromatosis 251
  postoperative nerve conduction times 233–238
neuroma, traumatic, prognosis after microsurgical procedure 239, 240
palsy, aneurysm of brachial artery, digital subtraction angiography 209, 210
polyneuropathy, sensory evoked potentials 213
Recklinghausen's disease 252
regeneration segment of a damaged neuron 372
Renaut's bodies, carpal tunnel 280
resuture, conduction velocity 219
sensory motor fascicle differentiation, intraoperative 217
suture, clinical and electrophysiological procedures 42
  clinical and electrophysiological results, correlations 224–226, 343
  motor units in abductor pollicis brevis muscle 220, 221
  sensory disturbances 43, 44, 45
  transection, grafting, sudomotor activity, Ninhydrin finger printing test 44, 45
magnetic resonance scan
  schwannoma, brachial plexus
Meissner's bodies
  carpal tunnel syndrome 284
melanoma
  metastases, brachial plexus 360, 365
meningioma
  operative experience 360, 362, 363
meralgia paresthetica syndrome
  entrapment neuropathy 264
metabolism
  cell bodies, alteration, peripheral nerve section 53
  injured neurons 29, 53
  peripheral nerves, crush lesion 175–188
microangiography
  graft revascularization, control 143, 145
  vascular architecture, suture region, sciatic nerve 152
microcirculation
  peripheral nerves, "extrinsic", "intrinsic" 154
microelectrode technique
  single fiber recording 46
microglia
  cell numbers after peripheral axotomy 16

Subject Index

cellular reactions, postoperative 2, 3
endoplasmic reticulum cisternae 2, 4
proliferation, "progressive microglia" 2, 3
microneurography
 action potentials of motor units 219
morbidity
 dorsal root entry zone coagulation, severe pain 424, 425
morphology
 entrapment syndromes 278
 ischiadic nerve, normal, after compression 199
 peripheral nerve vasculature 130, 131
 peripheral nerves, cross section, fascicular structures 216
 thoracic-outlet structures 307
morphometry
 spinal nerve fibers, sutured, nonsutured 116–120
Morton's metatarsalgia
 computed tomography 201
Morton's toe
 entrapment syndrome, tibial nerve 259, 265
motoneuron growth factors
 trophic homeostasis, loss after nerve injury 184
motor distal latency
 carpel tunnel syndrome, before and after operation 271
motor endplates
 degeneration, late nerve repair 71
motor nerve
 conduction velocity, carpal tunnel syndrome, before and after surgery 271, 273
 injury, electrophysiology 32–41
MRI
 brachial plexus, stretch injuries 405
 calcified tendon of gastrocnemius muscle, footdrop syndrome 210
 diagnosis, peripheral nerve lesions 204, 205
 schwannoma, brachial plexus 363
muscle atrophy
 electrical stimulation 10, 11
 loss of innervation, regeneration 7, 8
muscle membrane properties
 changes, after loss of innervation 8, 9
muscle response
 after vein graft, electromyography 99
myelin sheath
 after laser assisted nerve anastomosis 162
 allogenic nerve graft, lymphocytic infiltration 108
 alterations, carpal tunnel syndrome, intraoperative findings 276

disrupting neuropathies, sensory evoked potentials, conduction velocity 214
 histology, Renaut's bodies, pathology 281, 285
 lymphocytes, migration and margination, typical signs of rejection 108
 structure, electron microscopy 231
 tumors, operative treatment 359
myelography
 root avulsion, brachial plexus 375, 376
 stretch injuries, cervical roots, brachial plexus 403, 404
myelopathy
 traumatic, cervical spine, prognosis 403
myoblastoma
 operative treatment 360, 364
myositis ossificans
 compression, axillary artery, brachial plexus cords 360, 364
nerve anastomosis
 laser assisted 161–164, 165–168
nerve atrophy
 cell death after injury 7, 25, 26, 29
nerve biopsy
 morphometric data 24
nerve compression
 acute, chronic, pathophysiology 136, 137
 clinical, electrophysiological, morphological findings 58–65
 distal motor latency, before and after 63
 electromyogram 62
 entrapment syndromes 278–287
 impulse conduction block 32, 64
 internal neurolysis 137, 138
 motor functions, reflex disappearance 65
 nerve conduction, disappearance 200
 scar tissue, electrophysiology 32
 structural changes 135, 136, 197–200
 tarsal tunnel syndrome 265
 thoracic-outlet syndrome, topography 310, 311
nerve compression syndrome
 coexistence of conduction block, slowing of conduction velocity, axon degeneration 32
 ulnar nerve, cubital tunnel syndrome 299
nerve conduction
 disappearance after pressure lesion, structural changes 200
nerve conduction block
 carpal tunnel syndrome 233, 234
 Guillain-Barré syndrome 33
nerve conduction times
 after neurolysis 233–238

nerve conduction velocity
  carpal tunnel syndrome, before and after surgery 273
  thoracic-outlet syndrome 302, 303
nerve crush
  acetylcholinesterase, posttraumatic changes 181
  blood-nerve barrier disruption 138
  central regeneration 18, 19
  cytochrome oxidase, posttraumatic changes 179, 180
  double, electrophysiology 32, 37
  fast muscle fibers, reinnervation changes 189–196
  G 6 PDH, posttraumatic activity 178, 179
  mitochondrial fraction, posttraumatic changes 193
  muscle fibers, reinnervation changes 189–196
  neuroma, microsurgical excision 240
  pentose phosphate pathway enzymes 177
  spinal motoneurons, posttraumatic metabolism 175–188
  transection, comparison of effects 17, 18
nerve degeneration
  retrograde fiber atrophy 25, 26
nerve denervation
  early signs, muscle membrane properties 8
nerve entrapment
  clinical aspects 258–269
nerve excitability test
  facial nerve, Bell's palsy, prognosis 34, 35
nerve fascicles
  neurolysis, type I, II, III 323–325
nerve fibers
  minimal outgrowth into fat tissue 126, 127
nerve function
  basic, central nervous system 45
  disturbances, different sites 26
  grading, prognosis 336, 337, 341
  internal arrangement 320
  intraoperative, sensory evoked potentials 216–218
  minor impairment, detection 36
  sensory, recovery after nerve injury, presuppositions 14
nerve graft
  allogenic, rejection, genetic model 104
  allogenic, with and without cyclosporin A suppression, histology 106, 109, 110, 111
  autologous, histology 109
  centrocentral anastomosis, microphotograph 78
  free autologous, revascularization 143–148
  free vascularized 326–334
  homologous, retrograde atrophy 25, 26
  implantation, regeneration types 22, 23
  median nerve, burned hand 331
  microangiography 145–148
  regeneration, autografts, allografts, blood-nerve function 139
    bioptic studies 22, 23, 24
    centrocentral anastomosis 75–80
  rejection, suppression by cyclosporin A 105, 111
nerve grafting
  allogenic 104–112
  allografts, cyclosporin A suppression 140
  autografts, revascularization 139
  centrocentral anastomosis, histograms 77
  clinical investigations 43, 44, 45
  dimensions of regenerated nerve fibers 23
  laser assisted, ultrastructural aspects 169–174
  successfully regenerated nerve fibers 23
  sudomotor activity, Ninhydrin finger printing test 44, 45
nerve growth factor (NGF)
  physiology, pathology 29, 30
  trophic homeostasis, loss after nerve injury 184
nerve injury
  afferent neurons, changes 55
  avulsion, brachial plexus, results after neurotization 369
  blood-nerve barrier, repair, regeneration 130–142
  brachial plexus, traffic accidents 372
  cell death, atrophy 7, 29
  cellular biology 1–6
  classification 323–325
  degenerative axonal alterations 18
  electrophysiology 32–41
  follow-up study of 3656 world war II cases 335
  functional restitution, time 7
  grade I, II, III Sunderland 323
  grading, prognosis 336, 337
  gunshot-, critical review 336
  gunshot wounds, brachial plexus 373
  Hoffmann-Tinel sign 216
  iatrogenic, nerve injection injuries 134, 135
  iatrogenic, results of therapy 338, 339, 340
  mechanisms, operation results 341
  metabolism 29
  microsurgical repair, results 343–356

microvasculature 159
muscle reactions 38
nerve-muscle interaction, disturbance 7
neuroma formation 22, 26, 53, 75, 79, 101, 102, 121, 124–129, 239–242, 248, 249
neuroma, metabolism 29
 microsurgical procedures, prognosis 239–242
 pain, causalgia syndrome 52, 53
 pathogenesis 51–57
 prognosis, effective factors 346–355
 recovery, pathogenetic mechanisms 14
 regeneration, with and without nerve suture 113–123
 repair, blood-nerve barrier 130–142
 repair using venous autograft 88–95
 sensory ganglia, response 14–21
 somatosensory regeneration, clinical testing 42–50
 transsynaptic changes 17
nerve involvement
 Recklinghausen's disease 251–257
nerve lesions
 brachial plexus, root avulsion, etiology 374
  treatment 372–385
 cellular biology 1–6
 categories 32
 central nervous system, transsynaptic plasticity 48
 diagnosis, MRi 204, 205
 hip surgery 243–247
 incomplete, decrease of evoked compound muscle response (ECMR) 32, 34
 microsurgical repair 343–356
 modern imaging procedures 206–211
 pain, general features 53
  pathogenesis 51
 peripheral and central compensating mechanisms 52
 reconstruction, free vascularized graft 326
 sympathetic outflow, disturbances 55
 timing surgery 317–322
 transsynaptic plasticity 48
nerve microcirculation
 models 154–160
 nutritive, epineural, intrafascicular plexus 154
nerve-muscle interaction
 disturbances 7
nerve palsy
 Bell's-, conduction velocity 33
nerve pressure
 intraneural measurement 262

nerve reconstruction
 axillary nerve transplantation, technique of Samii 382
 general principles 430, 431
 sensorimotor, intraoperative analysis, sensory evoked potentials 217
nerve regeneration
 after laser-assisted anastomosis, time course 166
 after neural anastomosis with venous autograft 91
 axon growth 23
 blood-nerve barrier 130
 brachial plexus lesions 372
 centrocentral anastomosis, technique of Samii 75–80
 clinical, electrophysiological results, correlation 224–226
 clinical, electrophysiological testing 42–50
 electrical stimulation 11
 evaluation, somatosensory evoked potentials 226
 follow-up study of 3656 world war II injuries 335
 free vascularized graft, transplantation 326
 graft, free autologous 143–148
  regeneration types 22, 23
  venous 96–103
 histology 97–101
 Hoffmann-Tinel sign 216
 laser-assisted transplantation, ultrastructural aspects 169–174
 microenvironment chambers, experimental work 81–87
 muscle- and nerve transplants 66–69
 myelin sheaths, Lanterman incisures 23
 nerve growth factor (NGF), NGF messenger RNA 29, 30, 31
 nerve stump, neurotrophic biochemical agents 81, 82
 nerve tubulation system 124
 neuromatous type 22, 23
 neuronal metabolism 1, 15, 29
 neurotrophic effect of fat tissue 124
 neurotrophic factors 29–31, 124
 pathomorphology 22–28
 promotion by nerve growth factor (NGF) 73
 somatosensory, following nerve injury 42–50
 sural nerve, biopsy 23
 tubulation, neurotrophic effects 124
 ultrastructural architecture of bridging segment 68

nerve regeneration
  ultrastructural aspects, laser-assisted transplantation 169
  vein graft 96–103
  with gangliosides 429
  with and without suture 113–123
nerve regeneration chambers
  biochemical manipulation of microenvironment 81–87
nerve reinnervation
  cutaneous receptors, fiber recording with microelectrode technique 46
nerve repair
  histology 428
  microsurgical technique of Samii, results 344–356
nerve resection
  posttraumatic changes, fast glycogenolytic muscle fiber size 190, 191
    in mitochondrial fraction 193
    muscle capillary number 192
nerve section
  amputation, pain mechanisms 52
  cell bodies, metabolic alterations 52
  dorsal horn cells, spinal cord, alterations of functional performance 53, 54
  motor nerve velocity, distal latency 35
nerve stenosis
  nerve function, minor impairment, detection 36
nerve stump
  axillary nerve injury, dorsal, ventral surgical view 381, 382
  brachial plexus injury, surgical view 377
  central, function after nerve transection 216
  distal, trophic factors 17, 18
  implanted into fat tissue, minimal outgrowth of nerve fibers 126
  intraoperative somatosensory evoked potentials 227
  neuroma, diagnosis, MRI 205
  regeneration, neuromatous type 22, 23
    neurotrophic biochemical agents 81, 82
nerve suture
  autologous nerve grafts 332
  clinical, electrophysiological procedures, results 42, 224–226
  constriction by scar tissue 32
  delayed motor recovery 70–72
  dimensions of regenerated nerve fibers 23
  electron microscopy 139
  electrophysiological changes 32, 36
  epineural, vascularization 149–153
  fascicular perineural neurolysis (Samii) 323
  functional changes of single motor unit 219–223
  granulomas, reduction by laser application 173
  growth of regenerating axons 121
  histology 428
  laser assisted anastomosis, reinnervation, comparison 161, 167
  microneurography, before and after 46, 47
  microsurgically performed, reduction of neuroma formation risk 121
  radial, median nerves, results, comparison 340, 341
  sensory disturbances, investigation methods 43, 44, 45
  single motor units, functional changes 219
  spinal nerve lesion, results 113–123
nerve transection
  axon outgrowth, stimulation by neuropeptides 73, 74
  blood-nerve barrier disruption 138
  central nerve stump function 216
  centrocentral anastomosis 75, 76
  clinical function, electroneurography, comparison of results 224
  crush, comparison of effects 17, 18
  decline in motor response amplitudes 34
  fiber atrophy, degeneration 25, 26
  fiber regeneration, bioptic studies 23–25
  grafting, sudomotor activity, Ninhydrin finger printing test 44, 45
  increased activity of pentose phosphate pathway enzymes 177
  interruption of axoplasmic transport 29
  ischemic necrosis 26
  neuroma formation, histology 22
    surgical prevention 26
  posttraumatic activity of G6PDH 178, 179
  posttraumatic changes of acetylcholinesterase 181
  posttraumatic changes of cytochromic oxidase 179, 180
  regeneration, neuromatous type 22, 23
  role of distal stump, trophic factors 17, 18
  sensory disturbances, patterns 43, 44, 45
  sudomotor activity, Ninhydrin test 44, 45
  Wallerian degeneration of axons, electrophysiology 33, 34
nerve transplantation
  autologous, regeneration-, degeneration-, rejection phases 104
  axillary nerve, brachial plexus injury 380, 381, 382

Subject Index 453

brachial plexus, root avulsion 375, 377, 378
   reconstruction of C5, C6 nerve roots 379
   free vascularized graft 326–334
   genetic-, immunologic background 104
   laser-assisted, ultrastructural aspects 169–174
   muscle- and nerve transplants 66–69
   ultrastructural aspects 169
nerve transplants
   laser assisted 165–168
   regeneration 66–69
nerve trauma
   changes of cytochromic oxidase 179, 180
   changes of fast cytogenolytic muscle fiber size, capillary number, histochemical profile, mitochondrial fraction 190–193
   changes of G6 PDH activity 178, 179
   histochemical, computer-assisted cytophotometric methods 175
   microreconstruction 175
nerve tubulation
   nerve regeneration, neurotrophic effects 124
nerve tumors
   amputation neuroma, avoiding, microsurgical technique 101, 102
   brachial plexus, computed tomography 201
      operative experience 359–366
   computed tomography, differential diagnosis 202, 203
   neurinoma, diagnosis, MRI 204, 205
   neurofibroma, CT 206
      radial nerve, histology 253
      ultrasound examination 208
   neuroma, acoustic, bilateral, Recklinghausen's disease 251
      histology 22, 126
      limitation by nerve stump implantation into fat tissue 124–129
      pain, centrocentral anastomosis 75, 79
      pathogenesis 53
      prevention methods 121, 124
      radial nerve injury 248, 249
   schwannoma, computer tomography 202
      malignant transformation 251, 252
nerve vascularization
   ischemic neuropathies 154
   laboratory animals 154–160
   normal, pathological 130, 131
neural anastomosis
   technique using venous graft 89, 90
neural sheath
   tumors 359, 360, 364

neurilemmoma
   neck, pathological features 386, 389
neurinoma
   diagnosis, MRI 204, 205
neurite response
   occupation of venous graft by nerve fibers 101
neurofibroma
   computed tomography 206
   indications for surgery 386, 389
   operative experiences 359, 360, 361
   radial nerve, histology 253
   tibialis anterior muscles, CT 206
   ultrasound examination 208
neurofibroma, neurofibrosarcoma
   computed tomography 202
neurofibromatosis
   brachial plexus, diagnosis, operative results 388, 389
   microsurgical reconstruction with sural nerve graft 251
neurolysis
   brachial plexus 380
      stretch injuries, results 407
   definition, types 323
   median nerve, carpal tunnel syndrome 292, 293
   operative techniques, types I, II, III 323–325
   postoperative changes in nerve conduction times 233–238
   radial-, median nerves, results, comparison 340, 341
   specific microsurgical indications 382
   ulnar nerve, entrapment syndrome 298–301
   X-ray radiation, brachial plexus lesion 411, 412
neuroma
   acoustic, bilateral, Recklinghausen's disease 251
   amputation, avoiding microsurgical technique 101, 102
   dorsal fascicle, brachial plexus, intraoperative somatosensory evoked potential 228, 229
   epineural nerve suture technique 153
   formation, limitation by implantation of nerve stump into fat tissue 124–129
      preventive methods 124
      reduced risk, microsurgically performed nerve suture 121
   transection, peripheral nerves, histology 22
   transection, peripheral nerves, surgical prevention 26, 102

neuroma
  histology 22
  nerve fibers, histology 126
  pain, prevention, centrocentral anastomosis 75, 79
  peripheral nerve injury, pathogenesis 53
  radial nerve ramifications, injury with a pointed knife 248, 249
  resection, brachial plexus, surgical view 377
    prognosis 239–242
  therapy, different physical and chemical methods 239
  traumatic, alcohol injection, prognosis 240
    peripheral, outcome after microsurgical procedure 239–242
neurons
  alpha-motoneuron, control of the motor unit's functional properties 219
  axotomized, main priorities, RNA metabolism 15
  cell body, metabolism, injuries 372
  central, capacity not to degenerate after lesions with alteration of function 52
  damaged, regeneration, brachial plexus lesions 373
  degeneration, brachial plexus lesions 372
  dorsal horn, membrane potential, alteration by neurotransmitters and -modulators 53
  metabolism during regeneration 1, 15, 29
  nerve growth factor (NGF), physiology, pathology 29, 30
  regeneration, neurotrophic biochemical agents 85
  sensory, substance P, physiology 29, 30
  sympathetic, neurotransmitters, physiology 29
  synthesis of trophic substances 10
neuropathia patellae
  saphenous nerve entrapment 265
neuropathic pain
  pathogenesis 51, 52
neuropathy
  diabetes mellitus, uremia, sensory evoked potentials 212
  entrapment-, clinical aspects 258–269
  myelin disrupting, conduction velocity 214
neuropeptid hormones
  nerve regeneration, promotion 53, 73
neurophysiology
  anastomosis with venous graft, results 91, 94
  blood-nerve barrier, perineurium 130, 136

  carpal tunnel syndrome, parameters for diagnosis 270–272
  criteria for a successful anastomosis 91, 93
  endoneurium, electron micrograph 131
  histamine test, brachial plexus injuries 378
  intraneural pressure 262
  muscle-, nerve transplantation 67–69
  nerve growth factor (NGF) 29, 30
  neurotransmitters, sympathetic, sensory neurons 29, 30
  neurotrophic factors 29, 53
  perineurium, blood-nerve barrier 130
  radial nerve 261
  Schwann's cells, nerve growth factor, synthesis 30
  thoracic outlet syndrome, diagnosis, surgical management 302–306, 307–314
  ulnar nerve 262
neurotmesis
  activation of axon cells 318
  blood-nerve barrier, disruption 138
  diagnosis, MRI 204
  microsurgical nerve suture, preferable treatment 122
neurotransmitters
  enzyme synthesis, regulation by nerve growth factor 29
  physiological functions 29, 53
neurotrophic biochemical agents
  nerve regeneration 81, 82
neurotrophic factors
  physiology, pathology after surgical, chemical interruption 29
NGF-mRHA
  peripheral nerves, following axotomy 30, 31
notalgia paresthetica
  thoracic spinal nerves entrapment 264

obturator canal
  obturator nerve entrapment neuropathy 264
opponensplasty
  motor function, effect 355

pain
  A-delta, C nociceptors, threshold activation, causes 51
  brachial plexus avulsion 416–421
    lesions, dorsal root coagulation 422–429
  causalgic, pathogenesis 52, 53, 65
  chronic, neuroma, pathogenesis 75, 76
  contribution of both the peripheral and

Subject Index

central nervous system 51–57
entrapment neuropathy 258
general features 53
intractable, dorsal root entry zone coagulation, technique of Samii 422–429
irradiation plexitis, operative treatment 408
Kaplan-Meiers curves 419
neuroma, prevention, centrocentral anastomosis 75, 79
neuropathic, pathogenesis 51, 52
pathogenesis 51
peripheral nerve injury, pathogenesis, contribution of both peripheral and central nervous system 51–57
positive feedback circle, damaged axons 55
postamputation, centrocentral nerve anastomosis 75
post-brachial plexus avulsion, treatment 416–421
relief, after spinal rhizotomy, tractotomy 420
stump-, disappearance after centrocentral anastomosis 75
thoracic-outlet syndrome 305
X-ray radiation, brachial plexus lesions 411
palmar nerves
 free vascularized graft, transplantation 328
Pancoast tumor
 brachial plexus compression 360, 364
pathogenesis
 brachial plexus lesions 372
 carpal tunnel syndrome 275
 causalgic syndrome 52, 53
 entrapment syndromes 278, 284
 pain 51
  chronic, peripheral nerve regeneration 75, 76
  peripheral nerve injury 51–57
 ulnar nerve compression 296
pathology
 brachial plexus lesions 374
 electrophysiology after motor nerve injury 32–41
 entrapment syndromes 278
 intrafascicular injection of anesthetic agents 135
 ischiadic nerve compression 63, 64
 nerve growth factor (NGF) 29, 30
 neurilemmoma 386
 neurotrophic factor, after surgical, chemical transection 29, 30
 peripheral nerves, computed tomography 201–203
 regeneration, peripheral nerves 22–28
pathophysiologic
 brachial plexus lesions, histamine test 378
 carpal tunnel syndrome 263
 chronic peripheral compression neuropathy 135, 136
 entrapment neuropathy 260
 incisura scapulae syndrome 260, 261
 nerve compression 136
 radial nerve, entrapment neuropathy 260, 261
 scalenus syndrome 260
 sensory evoked potentials, findings, fingers, wrist 214
 ulnar nerve, entrapment syndromes 262
pentose phosphate pathway enzymes
 posttraumatic changes 177, 182
perineural sheath
 thickened, carpal tunnel syndrome 281, 282, 283, 284
perineurium
 blood-nerve barrier physiology 130, 136
 blood supply, vascular architecture, electron microphotograph 130, 131
 electron microphotograph, physiology 132, 133
 fascicular perineural neurolysis (Samii) 323
 injury, blood-nerve barrier, disruption 138
 peripheral nerve, anatomy, scheme 149
 sciatic nerve, suture region, vessels, corrosion cast 151
 ultrastructural aspects after laser assisted transplantation 170
 vascular architecture 130, 131, 158
 vessels, suture region, corrosion cast technique 151, 152
peripheral nerves
 allogenic nerve graft 104–112
 anastomosis, CO_3 laser assisted 161–164, 165–168
 atrophy, cell death, after injury 29
  loss of innervation 7
  retrograde, degeneration 25, 26
 axillary nerve transplantation, brachial plexus lesions, surgical view 380, 381, 382
 axonal injury, metabolism 29
  transsynaptic changes 17
 axotomy, changes in glial cells 16
 brachial plexus injuries, etiology, clinical picture, treatment 372–385
  surgical view, venous interpositional graft 377
 Bell's palsy, conduction velocity 33

peripheral nerves
  compression, block of impulse conduction 32, 64
    by scar tissue, electrophysiology 32
    clinical picture, pathology 58–65
    entrapment syndromes 278–287
    injuries 135, 136
    structural changes 197–200
    syndromes, ulnar nerve 298–301
    tarsal tunnel syndrome 265
  compressive scar formation, MRI 205
  conduction times, after neurolysis 233–238
  crush, central regeneration 18, 19
    double, electrophysiology 32, 37
    increased activity of pentose phosphate pathway enzymes 177
    neuroma, prognosis after microsurgical procedure 240
    posttraumatic activity of G 6 PDH 178, 179
    posttraumatic changes in capillary number in extensor hallucis longus muscle fibers 292
    posttraumatic changes in fast glycogenolytic muscle fiber size 191
    posttraumatic changes in fast oxidative glycogenolytic muscle fiber size 190
    posttraumatic changes in histochemical profile of extensor digitorum longus muscle fibers 192
    posttraumatic changes in mitochondrial fraction 193
    posttraumatic changes in number of nuclei 193
    posttraumatic changes of acetylcholinesterase 181
    posttraumatic changes of cytochrome oxidase 179, 180
    reinnervation changes, muscle fibers 189–196
    transection, comparison of effects 17, 18
  disappeance of nerve conduction after compression 200
  endoneural environment 130
  endoneural plexus, electron microscopy 159
  entrapment neuropathies, clinical aspects 258–269
  function, intraoperative analysis with sensory evoked potentials 216–218
    minor impairment, detection 36
  functional arrangement 320
  grafting, centrocentral anastomosis, histograms 77
    clinical investigation 43, 44, 45
    successfully regenerated nerve fibers, sural nerve biopsy 23
  growth of regenerating axons 121
  gunshot injuries, critical review 336, 338
  homologous grafts, retrograde atrophy 25, 26
  injury, blood-nerve barrier 130–142
    by injection of tranquilizers, antibiotica, steroids 134, 135
    cellular biology 1–6
    changes in primary afferent neurons 55
    degenerative axonal alterations 18
    electrophysiological changes 32–41
    follow-up of 3656 cases of world war II 335
    functional restitution, time 7
    Hoffmann-Tinel sign 216
    iatrogenic 159
    microvasculature 159
    muscle reactions 38
    nerve-muscle interaction, disturbance 7
    neuroma, metabolism 29
    neuroma, microsurgical procedures, prognosis 239–242
    pain, pathogenesis 51–57
    recovery, pathogenetic mechanisms 14
    repair, blood-nerve barrier 130–142
    repair using venous autografts 88–95
    short-term-, long-term changes in sensory ganglion cells 14, 16
    somatosensory regeneration, clinical testing 42–50
  intraneural pressure measurements 262
  involvement, Recklinghausen's disease 251–257
  lesions, categories 32
    cellular biology 1–6
    central nervous system, transsynaptic plasticity 48
    computed tomography, differential diagnosis 201, 202
    diagnosis, MRI 204, 205
    hip surgery 243
    modern imaging procedures 206–211
    pain, general features 53
    peripheral and central compensating mechanisms 52
    preoperative diagnosis, MRI 204, 205
    sympathetic outflow disturbances 55
    timing surgery 317–322
  lipoma, brachial plexus 360, 364
    computed tomography 202
  luxation injury, cubital tunnel syndrome 299
  median compression syndrome, sensory

Subject Index

evoked potentials 212–215
metabolism, neuronal, during regeneration 1
microcirculation, microvascularization, models 154–160
microneurography, action potentials of motor units 219
motor endplates, degeneration, late nerve repair 71
motor nerve velocity 35
muscle interaction, disturbances 7
nerve graft implantation, regeneration types 22, 23
nerve-muscle interaction, disturbances 7
neurofibromatosis 251–257
neurofibrosarcoma, computed tomography 202
neurogenic tumors, computed tomography 202
neurolysis, definition, types 323
neuroma formation, preventive methods 124
 painful, excision, centrocentral anastomosis 75
 treatment, difficulties 240, 241
neuronal metabolism 1, 2
pain, contribution of both the peripheral and central nervous system 51–57
pathology, computed tomography 201–203
plexiform neurofibroma, computed tomography 202
pressure lesion, structural changes 197–200
Recklinghausen's disease 251–257
Recklinghausen's disease, operative experiences 359, 360
reconstruction, free vascularized grafts, late results 333
regeneration, after laser-assisted anastomosis 166
 after neural anastomosis, using venous autograft 91
 blood-nerve barrier 130
 centrocentral anastomosis, autologous graft, technique of Samii 75
 clinical, electrophysiological results, correlations 224–226
 clinical, electrophysiological testing 42–50
 electrical stimulation 11
 evaluation by somatosensory evoked potentials 226
 follow-up of 3656 world war II injuries 335
 free autologous grafts 143–148

graft, regeneration types 22, 23
histological specimens 97–101
Hoffmann-Tinel sign 216
laser-assisted transplantation 169–174
microenvironment chambers, experimental work 81–87
muscle and nerve transplants 66–69
nerve growth factor (NGF), NGF messenger RNA 29, 30, 31
neuronal metabolism 1, 15, 29
neurotrophic effect, fat tissue, preatrophied muscle 124
neurotrophic factors 29–31
pathomorphology 22–28
promotion by nerve growth factor (NGF) 73
somatosensory, nerve injury 42–50
sural nerve, biopsy 23
time course after laser-assisted anastomosis 166, 167
ultrastructural architecture of bridging segments 68
ultrastructural aspects, laser assisted transplantation 169
vein graft 96–103
with and without nerve suture 113–123
regeneration chambers, biochemical manipulation of microenvironment 81–87
reinnervation of cutaneous receptors, single fiber recording with microelectrode technique 46
resection, posttraumatic changes in fast glycogenolytic muscle fiber size 190, 191
 posttraumatic changes in capillary number in extensor hallucis longus muscle fibers 192
 posttraumatic changes in histochemical profile of extensor digitorum longus muscle fibers 192
 posttraumatic changes in mitochondrial fraction 193
 posttraumatic changes in number of nuclei 193
schwannoma, computed tomography 202
section, alterations of dorsal horn cells 53, 54
sensory disturbance, patterns 43, 44, 45
sensory evoked potentials 212–215
sensory system, clinical and electrophysiological investigation 42, 43
 lesions, functional disturbances, different sites 26, 27
 microstimulation 47
stenosis, conduction velocity 36
stump regeneration, neurotrophic biochemical agents 81, 82

peripheral nerves
  suture, clinical and electrophysiological results, correlations 42, 224–226
    constriction by scar tissue 32
    delayed motor recovery 70–72
    electron microscopy 139
    electrophysiological changes 32, 36
    epineural, vascularization 149–153
    functional changes of single motor units 219–223
    granuloma, reduction by laser application 173
    laser assisted 161, 167
    microneurography, before and after 46, 47
    microsurgically performed, orthograde growth of regenerating axons, reduction of neuroma formation risk 121
    sensory disturbances, investigation methods 43, 44, 45
    spinal nerve lesions, results 113–123
  transection, axon outgrowth, stimulation by neuropeptides 73, 74
    blood-nerve barrier, disruption 138
    central nerve stump function 216
    centrocentral nerve anastomosis 75, 76
    clinical function, electroneurographical parameters, comparison 224
    crush, differences, comparison of effects 17, 18
    decline in motor response amplitude 34
    fiber atrophy, degeneration 25, 26
    fiber regeneration, bioptic studies 23, 24, 25
    grafting, sudomotor activity, Ninhydrin finger printing test 44, 45
    increased activity of pentose phosphate pathway enzymes 177
    interruption of axoplasmic transport 29
    ischemic necrosis 26
    neuroma formation, histology 22
    neuroma formation, surgical prevention 26
    posttraumatic activity of G 6 PDH 178, 179
    posttraumatic changes of acetylcholinesterase 181
    posttraumatic changes of cytochromic oxidase 179, 180
    regeneration, neuromatous type 22, 23
    role of distal stump, trophic factors 17, 18
    sensory disturbances, patterns 43, 44, 45

  sudomotor activity, Ninhydrin test 44, 45
  Wallerian degeneration of axons, electrophysiology 33, 34
  transplantation, autologous, regeneration-, degeneration-, rejection phases 104
    genetic-, immunologic background 104
    laser-assisted, ultrastructural aspects 169–174
    muscle-, nerve transplants 66–69
    ultrastructural aspects 169
  transsynaptic changes 17
  trauma, changes of cytochromic oxidase 179, 180
    changes of cytogenolytic muscle fiber size, capillary number, histochemical profile, mitochondrial fraction 190–193
    changes of G 6 PDH activity 178, 179
  tubulation, nerve regeneration, neurotrophic effects 124
  tumors, computed tomography 202
    neurinoma, diagnosis, MRI 204, 205
    neurofibroma, radial nerve 253
    neurofibroma, sonography 208
    neuroma, acoustic nerve, Recklinghausen's disease 251
      avoiding, microsurgical technique 101, 102
      histology 22, 126
      limitation, nerve stump implantation into fat tissue 124–129
      pain, centrocentral anastomosis 75, 79
      pathogenesis 53
      preventive methods 121, 124
      radial nerve 248, 249
    schwannoma, computed tomography 202
    schwannoma, malignant transformation 251, 252
  ulnar nerve entrapment syndromes neurolysis 298–301
  ultrastructural architecture, nerve and muscle transplants, regeneration 66–69
  vascularization, ischemic neuropathies 154
    laboratory animals 154–160
  vasculature, normal 130, 131
peripheral nerve surgery
  microtechniques:
    Allogenic nerve graft 104
    Amputation neuroma avoiding 101, 102
    Anastomosis, laser assisted 161, 169–174

Subject Index

Autologous graft, centrocentral anastomosis, technique of Samii 75
Autologous graft, regeneration conditions 143
Brachial plexus, actinic (X-ray) lesions, therapy results 408, 411–415
Brachial plexus lesions, indications 396–410
Brachial plexus lesions, results, evaluation 391–395
Brachial plexus lesions, results of secondary reconstruction 430–437
Brachial plexus, root avulsion neurotization 367–371
Brachial plexus, root avulsion, surgical view, graft interposition 377, 378
Brachial plexus, root avulsion, topography 375
Brachial plexus, secondary reconstruction, results 430–437
Brachial plexus, stretch injuries, results 407
Brachial plexus surgery, results 391–395
Brachial plexus tumors 359–366
Carpal tunnel syndrome, intraoperative findings, prognosis 273–277
Carpal tunnel syndrome, median nerve decompression, incomplete 289
Carpal tunnel syndrome, median nerve decompression, sensory evoked potentials 215
Carpal tunnel syndrome, new surgical approach 292–294
Carpal tunnel syndrome, pitfalls, reasons 288–291
Carpal tunnel syndrome, reoperations, reasons 289
Carpal tunnel syndrome, skin incision 289, 290, 292
Carpal tunnel syndrome, technical problems 289
Carpal tunnel syndrome, transverse carpal ligament, extent of transection 289
Coagulation, dorsal root, for intractable pain 422–429
Compressive scar formation, MRI, diagnosis 205
Dorsal root entry zone, coagulation, technique of Samii 422–429
Dorsal root entry zone, plexus avulsion 416–421
Emergency cases, prognosis 351
Epineural nerve suture, neuroma formation, causes 153
Epineural, perineural fascicular nerve suture 121
Epineural, perineural suture techniques, results 91, 92, 93
Evaluation of results 335–342
Fascicular perineural neurolysis (Samii) 323
Free greater omentum transfer, actinic brachial plexus lesions 411–415
Free vascularized nerve grafts 326–334
Function of central nerve stump, intraoperative analysis 216
Grafting, clinical results 43, 44, 45
Grafting, successfully regenerated nerve fibers 23
Homologous graft 25, 26
Intraoperative analysis of nerve function with sensory evoked potentials 216–218
Laser assisted anastomoses, transplants 161, 165
Laser assisted transplantation, ultrastructural aspects 169–174
Measurement techniques, intraoperative information, functional capacity of the proximal nerve stump 218
Median nerve lesions 343
Median nerve neurolysis, carpal tunnel syndrome 233–238, 292, 293
Median nerve operations, results, critical review 338, 339, 341
Median nerve suture, electrophysiological results 225
Meningioma 360, 362, 363
Microelectrode technique, single fiber recording 46
Microenvironment chambers, regeneration 81–87
Microneurolysis, posttraumatic ulnar compression syndromes 301
Microneurolysis, technique of Samii 301
Microstimulation of sensory system 47
Muscle and nerve transplants, regeneration 66–69
Nerve decompression, carpal tunnel syndrome 215
Nerve growth factor, physiology, pathway 29, 30
Nerve lesions, timing surgery 317–322
Nerve reconstruction, intraoperative monitoring of sensory evoked potentials 217
Nerve suture, functional changes of single motor units 219–223

peripheral nerve surgery
   Nerve trauma 175
   Neural anastomosis using venous graft, results 89, 90
   Neurofibroma, results 360, 361, 362
   Neurofibromatosis 251–257
   Neurogenic tumors, brachial plexus 387–389
   Neurolysis, postoperative conduction times 233–238
   Neurolysis, ulnar nerve entrapment syndromes 298–301
   Neuroma excision, centrocentral anastomosis 75
   Neuroma formation, causes, surgical prevention 26, 102, 153
   Neuroma pain, prevention, centrocentral anastomosis 75, 79
   Neuroma, traumatic, prognosis 239–242
   Neuromas of radial nerve ramifications, nerve grafting 248–250
   Neurorrhaphy, results, prognosis 351
   Neurotrophic biochemical agents, nerve regeneration 85
   Old peripheral nerve injury, intraoperative determination of resection limits 217
   Planning by means of MRI 205
   Postoperative conduction velocity 233–238
   Postoperative treatment 427–429
   Prognosis, effective factors 351
   Radial nerve operations, results, critical review 338, 341
   Recklinghausen's disease 251–257
   Recklinghausen's disease, operative experience 359, 360
   Recklinghausen's disease, removal of neurofibroma, sural nerve grafting 255
   Results, critical review 335–342
   Results, radial versus median nerves, comparison 340, 341
   Schwannoma, brachial plexus 387, 388
   Schwannoma, operative experiences 360, 362, 363
   Stretch injuries, brachial plexus, results 402
   Stump regeneration, neurotrophic biochemical agents 81, 82
   Suture, delayed motor recovery 70–72
   Suture, electrophysiological changes 32, 36
   Suture, epineural, revascularization 149–153
   Suture, free vascularized grafts 326–334
   Suture of spinal nerve lesion 113
   Suture, orthograde growth of regenerating axons 121
   Suture, sensory disturbances, investigation methods 43, 44, 45
   Suture, successfully regenerated nerve fibers 23
   Thoracic-outlet syndrome 307–314
   Thoracic-outlet tumors 359–366
   Transplantation after neuroma resection 240
   Transplantation, autologous, regeneration-, degeneration-, rejection phases 104
   Transplantation, genetic-, immunologic background 104
   Transplantation, laser-assisted, ultrastructural aspects 169–174
   Transplantation, muscle-, nerve transplants 66–69
   Transplantation, ultrastructural aspects 169
   Traumatic neuroma 239–242
   Tumors, brachial plexus 359–366
   Ulnar nerve compression syndromes, late results 301
   Ulnar nerve lesions 343
   Vein graft, regeneration 88–95, 96–103

peroneal nerve
  carpal tunnel syndrome 258, 263
  crush injury, acute posttraumatic changes 189–196
  donor, free vascularized graft, transplantation 328, 330
  entrapment neuropathy 265
  injury, repair using venous autograft 88, 89
  nerve potential, muscle potential, recordings 98
  neurofibromatosis 252
  neuroma, traumatic, prognosis after microsurgical procedure 240
  Recklinghausen's disease 252
  suture, delayed, motor recovery 70

phantom limb pain
  amputation neuroma, lumbar canal stenosis, laminectomy 241

physiological pain
  pathogenesis 51

physiology
  blood-nerve barrier, perineurium 130, 136
  histamine test, brachial plexus fibers 378
  nerve growth factor (NGF) 29, 30
  neurotransmitters, sympathetic, sensory

neurons 29, 30, 53
neurotrophic factors 29, 53
Schwann's cells, nerve growth factor,
  synthesis 30
plexiform neurofibroma
  computed tomography 202
  operative therapy 255
plexus brachialis
  intraoperative somatosensory evoked
  potential 227
plexus lesions
  supra-, infraclavicular 373
poliomyelitis
  brachial plexus palsy, secondary
  reconstruction 430
polyneuropathy
  reduced motor and sensory conduction
  velocities 213
  toxic, sensory nerve action potentials 212
polytrauma
  brachial plexus lesions 372
processus supratrochlearis
  plain X-rays 296
prognosis
  actinic lesions, brachial plexus, operative
  results 412, 414
  brachial plexus lesions, surgery,
  results 391
  carpal tunnel syndrome, preoperative
  symptoms, intraoperative findings 270,
  273–277
  carpal tunnel syndrome, surgery 289
  effect of surgical technique 351
  interfascicular nerve grafting 351
  malignant schwannoma 255
  myelopathy, traumatic, cervical spine 403
  nerve transection, delayed repair 343
  neuroma, traumatic, after microsurgical
  procedures 239–242
  neurorrhaphy 351
  peripheral nerve surgery 335–342
provocation tests
  carpal tunnel syndrome, prognosis 274,
  276

radial nerve
  anatomy, topography, forearm 248, 249
  conduction velocity, after suture 229
  donor, free vascularized graft,
  transplantation 326–334
  entrapment syndrome 259, 261, 278
  grafting, secondary reconstruction 250
  incomplete palsy, brachial plexus
  paralysis 435
  isolated lesions of peripheral muscular
  branches, reconstruction by nerve

graft 248–250
lesions, surgery, results, critical
review 336, 337, 340, 341
neurofibroma, histology 253, 254
neuroma, traumatic, prognosis after
microsurgical procedure 240
ramifications, anatomy 248, 249
Recklinghausen's disease 252, 253
sensory motor fascicle differentiation,
intraoperative 217
radiation plexitis
  brachial plexus, operative treatment 412
Recklinghausen's disease
  brachial plexus, diagnosis, operative
  results 388
  operative experiences 359–361
  peripheral nerve involvement 251–257
rectus abdominis syndrome
  caudal thoracic nerves entrapment 264
renal dialysis
  transaxillary vascular bypass, brachial
  plexus injury 408
Renaut's bodies
  median nerve, carpal tunnel, ultrastructure 280, 282, 285

saphenous nerve
  donor, free vascularized graft,
  transplantation 329
  entrapment syndrome 259, 265
scalenotomy
  brachial plexus injury 408
scalenus syndrome
  brachial plexus entrapment 260
scanning electron microscopy
  ischiadic nerve, after compression 199
  microvasculature of peripheral nerves 159
scapular nerve
  entrapment neuropathy 261
scapular notch syndrome
  plexus brachialis entrapment
  neuropathy 260
scar formation
  diminishing methods 427
Schwann's cells
  after laser assisted nerve anastomosis 162
  autologous nerve graft,
  revascularization 143
  colonization of vein graft, nerve regeneration, mechanism 101
  electron micrograph 131
  growth-supporting influence, posttraumatic nerve regeneration 173
  nerve growth factor, synthesis 30
  physiological function 143–148
  pseudopodic spreading 143

Schwann's cells
  specific chemical staining 388
  ultrastructural aspects after laser assisted nerve transplantation 170
schwannoma
  brachial plexus 386–390
  computed tomography 202
  magnetic resonance scan 363
  malignant, operative situs, histology 254
  malignant transformation into malignant neurilemmoma 251, 252
  operative experience 360, 362, 363
  plexus brachialis 386–390
sciatic nerve
  autologous graft, revascularization conditions 143
  compression injury, fluorescence microscopy 136, 137
  crush, metabolic responses 175
  electron photomicrograph, after compression injury 136
  electron photomicrograph, suture line 139
  epineurium, vascularization 149
  freeze-broken specimen, epineural vessels, corrosion cast 157
  laser-assisted anastomoses, transplants 161, 165–168
  lesion, hip surgery 243
  microvascularization, corrosion casting technique 154, 155
  nerve graft implantation, regeneration 23
  nerve growth factor, synthesis 30, 31
  neuroma formation, inhibition by implantation into fat tissue 125
  neurotomy, cell death, time, range 17
  regeneration-, degeneration-, rejection phases 104
  regeneration, with and without nerve suture 113, 114
  transplantation, laser assisted, ultrastructural aspects 169–174
  suture, electron microscopy 139
  suture, epineural technique, neuroma formation, causes 153
  sutureless laser-assisted nerve anastomosis 161–164
  transection, regeneration, centrocentral anastomosis 75, 76
  vascularization, scheme 149
  vessels, corrosion cast 151
sensory conduction velocity
  carpal tunnel syndrome, before and after surgery 271, 275
sensory evoked potentials (SEP)
  after nerve suture, clinical function, comparison 224–226
  electromyography, after nerve suture, correlations 224–226
  intraoperative analysis of nerve function 216–218
  median nerve, compression syndrome 212–215
  peripheral nerve function, intraoperative analysis 216–218
  sensory nerve continuity, documentation 212
  thoracic-outlet syndrome 304
sensory ganglia
  short-term, long-term changes after injury 14–21
sensory system
  electrophysiological examination 42
shoulder joint
  CT, schwannoma 387
  Saha's transfer of trapezius muscle, paralysis of deltoid muscles 434
shoulder luxation
  axillary nerve injury, dorsal, ventral surgical view 381, 382, 384
skeletal muscles
  abductor pollicis brevis, motor units, after median nerve suture 221
  abductor pollicis brevis, thenar, atrophy, carpal tunnel syndrome 273, 274, 275
  acute posttraumatic changes 189
  after vein graft, electromyography 99
  anconaeus epitrochlear muscle, recurrent compression of median nerve 297
  atrophy, brachial plexus lesions 372
    loss of innervation, regeneration 7, 8, 10
    nerve-muscle continuity, interruption 38
  deltoid muscle function before and after surgery 383, 384
  denervation, delayed suture, motor recovery 70–72
    loss of activity, metabolism 8, 10
  electrical stimulation, metabolic changes 11
  electromyography, conduction velocity after neural anastomosis 91
    thoracic outlet syndrome 303, 304
  electrotherapy, indication 428
  evoked compound muscle response (ECMR), conduction block 32, 33, 34
    after neuronal anastomosis 93
    increasing denervation potentials 70
    nerve conduction block 32, 34
  extensor pollicis longus and brevis muscles, traumatic lesions, reconstruction by nerve graft 248–250

Subject Index

facial muscles, Bell's palsy, conduction velocity 33, 35
fibers, electrophysiological changes, following denervation 38
first dorsal interosseus, motor units, after ulnar nerve suture 222
functional restitution after nerve injury 7
lateral gastrocnemius muscle, calcified tendon, MRI 210
loss of innervation, changes of muscle membrane properties, changes after loss of innervation 8, 9
metabolism aerobic, anaerobic 10
motor endplates, degeneration, late nerve repair 71
neck-, anatomy 373, 374
nerve injury, reactions 38
nerve interaction, disturbances 7–13
physiotherapy, indications 428
reinnervation, after spinal nerve lesion, nerve suture 113
reinnervation of single fibers 189
Saha's transfer of trapezius muscle, paralysis of deltoid muscles 434
scalene muscle, broadened insertion, narrowing of axillary artery 311
structural integrity, innervation 27
supra-, infraspinatus, atrophy, paresis, entrapment neuropathy 261
thenar atrophy, carpal tunnel syndrome, differential diagnosis 275, 289, 292
transfer, incomplete brachial plexus injury, secondary reconstruction 435
transplants, histology, 1 year after implantation 67, 68
   regeneration of peripheral nerves, ultrastructural architecture 66, 67, 68
twitch force, recruitment threshold, relationship 221
somatosensory evoked potentials (SEP) thoracic-outlet syndrome 304
sonogram
   neurofibroma, tibialis anterior muscles 208
space occupying lesions
   differential diagnosis, computed tomography 207
spinal cord
   afferent neurones, electrical activity 53
   brachial plexus, root avulsion, medullary symptoms 376
   cervical, laminectomy, brachial plexus avulsion 418
   dorsal horn cells, functional alterations after peripheral nerve section 54
      reduction in opiate binding, axotomized neuron 15
   injury, molecularbiological responses 14–21
   meningioma 255
   microglial cells, reaction of sensory neurons to peripheral axotomy 16
   nerve growth factor, sympathetic and sensory neurons 29
   rhizotomy, tractotomy, relief of pain 420
spinal motoneurons
   crush lesions, posttraumatic metabolic responses 175–188
spinal nerves
   anatomy 373
   injuries, results of surgery 391
   lesions, regeneration with and without nerve suture 113–123
substance P
   sensory neurons, physiology 29, 30
supinator channel syndrome
   ganglion, elbow joint, CT 208
supraclavicular nerve
   Recklinghausen's disease 252
   entrapment neuropathy 260
sural nerve
   biopsy, nerve fiber regeneration, morphometric data 23, 24, 25
   donor, free vascularized graft, transplantation 328
   grafts, axillary nerve reconstruction, surgical view 383
   graft, neurofibromatosis, microsurgical reconstruction 251
   grafting, after removal of neurofibroma 255
   neuroma, traumatic, prognosis after microsurgical procedure 240
sympathectomy
   traumatic peripheral neuroma, outcome 239
sympathetic trunk
   C_1–C_7 roots, avulsion, brachial plexus lesions 376
synapses
   capacity not to degenerate after lesions with alteration of function 52, 55
   central nervous system, transsynaptic plasticity after peripheral lesions 48
   central synaptic transmission, changes, peripheral axonal injury 17
   efficacy, changes after nerve transection 55
   peripheral axonal injury, changes 17

synaptic transmission
  changes after injury of sensory ganglion cells 14
  reduction in opiate binding, spinal cord dorsal horn 15

tactile perception threshold
  carpal tunnel syndrome, findings before and after surgery 271
tarsal tunnel syndrome
  entrapment neuropathy 259, 265, 266
thoracic nerves
  caudal, entrapment neuropathy 264
thoracic outlet syndrome
  axillary artery, narrowing by a cervical rib 310
  brachial plexus entrapment 260
  costoclavicular space, narrowing, topography 311
  diagnosis, limitations 302–306
  diagnosis, surgical treatment 302–306, 307–314
  narrowing by a broadened insertion of medial scalene muscle 311
  plexus brachialis injury 408
  tumors, operative experience 359–366
thoracic spinal nerves
  entrapment neuropathy 259, 263
thymoma
  malignant, brachial plexus compression 360, 364
tibial nerve
  entrapment neuropathies 265
tibialis cranialis muscle
  fiber diameters, reinnervation with and without spinal nerve suture 120
transplant
  autologous nerve-, brachial plexus injury, technique of Samii 382
transplantation
  brachial plexus, C 5, C 6 reconstruction surgical view 379
  free vascularized nerve graft 326–334
  graft, autologous, centrocentral anastomosis, technique of Samii 75
  graft, autologous, revascularization conditions 143
  histocompatibility complex, immunological response 104
  laser-assisted, ultrastructural aspects 169–174
  muscle, nerve, regeneration 66–69
  rejection, MHC-, non-MHC systems 104–112
  venous interpositional, brachial plexus injury 377

trigeminal nerve
  rhizotomy, relief of pain 416
tumors
  brachial plexus, operative experience 359–366
  breast cancer, metastases, brachial plexus compression 360, 364
  meningioma, spinal cord 254
  neural sheath origin 359, 360
  neurilemmoma 251
  neurogenic, brachial plexus, classification, World Health Organization 386
  Pancoast-, brachial plexus 360, 364
  peripheral nerves, computed tomography 202
    diagnosis, MRI 205
  schwannoma, Recklinghausen's disease 251, 252
tunnel syndrome
  focal conduction block, slowed impulse conduction 36
tyrosine hydroxylase
  neurotransmitter, physiology 29

ulnar nerve
  anatomy 298
  compression, pathogenesis 296
  conduction velocity 302, 303
    after suture 219
  donor, free vascularized graft 326–334
  entrapment, computed tomography 201
  entrapment neuropathy, autoptic findings 279
  entrapment neuropathy, neurolysis 298–301
  entrapment syndromes, pathophysiology 262
  F-wave measurement, thoracic-outlet syndrome 304
  Guyon's tunnel syndrome 299
  indurated, operative situs 300
  irritation syndrome 295–297
  microsurgical repair, results 343–356
  microstimulation of single afferent fibers, interpretation 47, 48
  neurinoma, diagnosis, MRI 205
  neuroma, traumatic, prognosis after microsurgical procedure 240
  paralysis, compression, olecranon groove 299
  resuture, conduction velocity 219
  sensory disturbances, patterns 43, 44, 45
  sensory motor fascicle differentiation, intraoperative 217
  suture, clinical and electrophysiological

Subject Index

results, correlations 44, 45, 224–226
  motor units in first dorsal interosseous muscle 221, 222
ultrasound examination
  neurofibroma 208
ultrastructures
  dorsal column nuclei, substantia gelatinosa 16
  laser assisted nerve transplantation 169–174
  myelinated axons 283
  Renaut's body 282, 285
uremia
  neuropathy, sensory evoked potentials 212

Vater-Paccini bodies
  carpal tunnel ligament 279
vibration threshold
  carpal tunnel syndrome, before and after operation 271

Wallerian degeneration
  autologous nerve grafts 105, 108
  axon transection, electrophysiology 33, 34
  blood-nerve barrier alterations 138
wristdrop syndrome
  ganglion, CT diagnosis 207

X-ray damage
  brachial plexus, operative treatment, results 408, 411–415
X-ray examination
  brachial plexus, root avulsion 376, 377, 378, 379
  cervical rib, thoracic outlet syndrome 308, 309
X-ray lesions
  brachial plexus, free greater omentum transfer 411–415
X-ray therapy
  scar formation 427

M. Samii, Medizinische Hochschule Hannover;
W. Draf, Fulda

Surgery of the Skull Base

An Interdisciplinary Approach

With a Chapter on Anatomy by J. Lang

1989. XIV, 525 pp. 289 figs. in 841 sep. illus.
Geb. DM 490,– ISBN 3-540-18448-1

This is the first text to consider the skull base as a whole and from an interdisciplinary point of view. It analyzes the wide spectrum of pathological entitles which can affect this crossroad region, including anomalies, trauma, tumors and infectious processes.

The book considers general as well as specific surgical aspects and offers a wealth of excellent drawings and pictures to complement the text. All this is based on a detailed anatomical overview.

The reader will find himself equipped with a complete textbook on skull base surgery that emphasizes clinical applications and reflects valuable relevant experience from the fields of both ENT and neurosurgery.

Distribution rights for Japan:
EBS, Tokyo

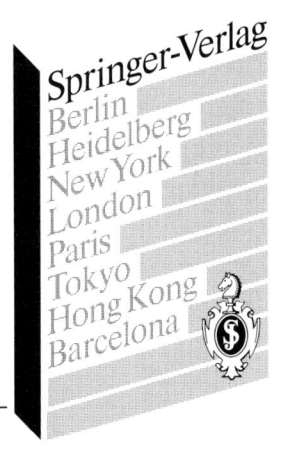

Springer-Verlag
Berlin
Heidelberg
New York
London
Paris
Tokyo
Hong Kong
Barcelona

M. Samii, Hannover (Ed.)

Surgery in and around the Brain Stem and the Third Ventricle

Anatomy. Pathology. Neurophysiology. Diagnosis. Treatment.

1986. XXIII, 599 S. 370 figs. Hardcover DM 346,–
ISBN 3-540-16581-9

This book covers the present state of possibilities and limitations for surgery in and around the brain stem and third ventricle, which was declared as an untouchable region for a long time. The complicated and interwoven anatomic structures with hundreds of nuclei and millions of pathways as well as the intrinsic vascular relationships are demonstrated from the surgical point of view. Furthermore, the study of metabolic disturbances and CBF-measurements are analyzed. The major breakthroughs in diagnostic means for pre-, intra- and postoperative control are considered in two different chapters on neurophysiology and neuroradiology.
Experienced authorities and trained scientists share and discuss their views and try to give answers to the different questions that face neuroscientists when dealing with lesions in this very difficult, dangerous and life-sustaining part of the brain.

Prices are subject to change without notice.

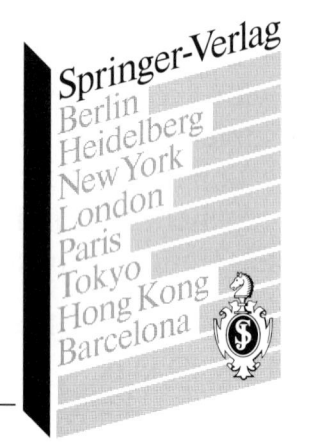

Springer-Verlag
Berlin
Heidelberg
New York
London
Paris
Tokyo
Hong Kong
Barcelona